Atlas of
Transesophageal Echocardiography

A Beginner's Perspective

With CD Containing Video Files of Important Clinical Conditions

Atlas of
Transesophageal Echocardiography

A Beginner's Perspective

Deepak K. Tempe MBBS, MD, FRCA (London), FAMS, FICA, FTEE, FIACTA
Dean, Maulana Azad Medical College and
Director-Professor of Anaesthesiology and Intensive Care
GB Pant Institute of Postgraduate Medical Education and Research
New Delhi

Suruchi Hasija MBBS, MD, DNB, DM (Cardiac Anaesthesia)
Associate Professor of Cardiac Anaesthesia
All India Institute of Medical Sciences
New Delhi

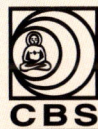

CBS

CBS Publishers & Distributors Pvt Ltd

New Delhi • Bengaluru • Chennai • Kochi • Kolkata • Mumbai
Hyderabad • Nagpur • Patna • Pune • Vijayawada

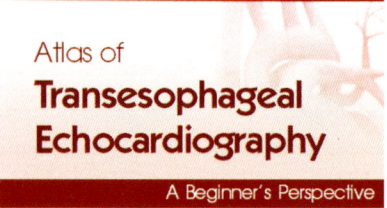

Atlas of
Transesophageal Echocardiography
A Beginner's Perspective

First Edition 2017

Published by Satish Kumar Jain and Produced by Varun Jain for
CBS Publishers & Distributors Pvt Ltd
4819/XI Prahlad Street, 24 Ansari Road, Daryaganj, New Delhi 110 002, India.
Ph: 23289259, 23266861, 23266867   Fax: 011-23243014   Website: www.cbspd.com
e-mail: delhi@cbspd.com; cbspubs@airtelmail.in.
Corporate Office: 204 FIE, Industrial Area, Patparganj, Delhi 110 092, India
Ph: 4934 4934   Fax: 4934 4935   e-mail: publishing@cbspd.com; publicity@cbspd.com

Branches

- **Bengaluru:** Seema House 2975, 17th Cross, K.R. Road,
  Banasankari 2nd Stage, Bengaluru 560 070, Karnataka, India
  Ph: +91-80-26771678/79   Fax: +91-80-26771680   e-mail: bangalore@cbspd.com
- **Chennai:** 7, Subbaraya Street, Shenoy Nagar, Chennai 600 030, Tamil Nadu, India
  Ph: +91-44-26260666, 26208620   Fax: +91-44-42032115   e-mail: chennai@cbspd.com
- **Kochi:** Ashana House, No. 39/1904, AM Thomas Road, Valanjambalam, Ernakulam 682 016, Kochi, Kerala, India
  Ph: +91-484-4059061-65   Fax: +91-484-4059065   e-mail: kochi@cbspd.com
- **Kolkata:** No. 6/B, Ground Floor, Rameswar Shaw Road, Kolkata-700014 (West Bengal), India
  Ph: +91-33-2289-1126, 2289-1127, 2289-1128   e-mail: kolkata@cbspd.com
- **Mumbai:** 83-C, Dr E Moses Road, Worli, Mumbai-400018, Maharashtra, India
  Ph: +91-22-24902340/41   Fax: +91-22-24902342   e-mail: mumbai@cbspd.com

Representatives

- **Hyderabad** 0-9885175004   • **Nagpur** 0-9021734563   • **Patna** 0-9334159340
- **Pune**   0-9623451994   • **Vijayawada** 0-9000660880

Printed at Nutech Print Services, Faridabad, India

to

My parents

Who have made me capable of what I am today and

Anjali (my wife), Anuradha (my daughter), and Tejas my son (in law)

For making my life so much more enjoyable

Deepak K. Tempe

My patients, who are also my teachers

Suruchi Hasija

Preface

The advances in ultrasound technology and its application for examining the heart and great vessels have revolutionized the field of diagnostic cardiology. The introduction of transesophageal echocardiography (TEE) in clinical practice, especially in the cardiac operating room has given a further boost to improving the patient care. The use of TEE during intraoperative as well as the postoperative period has become a standard practice nowadays. TEE allows continuous observation of the heart during operations without interfering with the surgical field. The cardiac anesthesiologists have acquired the skills of echocardiography over the years and the present day cardiac anesthesiologist has taken over this responsibility. The cardiac surgeon is appreciative of this fact and looks forward to knowing the TEE findings that will assist him in taking crucial surgical decisions. The anesthesiologist has also utilized TEE to obtain hemodynamic data to optimize the pharmacological intervention for his patient. Consequently, learning the TEE and acquiring the skills of echocardiographer have become a part of any cardiac anesthesia training programme.

TEE is an imaging technique and unlike some other imaging techniques, it is operator dependent. The basic step in learning echocardiography, therefore, is to understand the various normal images. During our discussions with the residents, it has often emerged that they struggle to get optimal images and hence have difficulty in interpreting them. This atlas has been published with the objective of helping the beginners in the field of TEE to understand the various normal images and the commonly encountered abnormal images. A CD showing most of the important clinical conditions in a chapterwise manner is also included for the benefit of the readers. It is advised that the readers simultaneously refer to the videos in the CD for better understanding of the subject. It is hoped that the Atlas along with the CD will strengthen the basic understanding of the beginners regarding the TEE images. This will reinforce the further training in the subject.

We wish to acknowledge our colleagues in our respective departments who have been very supportive in our endeavors and completion of this Atlas. In addition, we gratefully acknowledge the cooperation extended by the department of cardiothoracic surgery and its staff members in carrying out this work.

We are thankful to Mr YN Arujua, Mr SK Jain, Ritu Chawla and the artist Neeraj Prasad from CBS Publishers & Distributors (P) Ltd., New Delhi for their efforts in publishing this book.

Deepak K. Tempe
Suruchi Hasija

Contents

Preface   vii

1. PRINCIPLES OF ECHOCARDIOGRAPHY   1

2. IMAGE OPTIMIZATION   7

3. COMPREHENSIVE TRANSESOPHAGEAL ECHOCARDIOGRAPHY EXAMINATION   22

4. EVALUATION OF THE MITRAL VALVE   47

5. EVALUATION OF THE AORTIC VALVE   74

6. EVALUATION OF THE RIGHT SIDE OF THE HEART   96

7. EVALUATION OF LEFT VENTRICULAR FUNCTION   122

8. ARTIFACTS AND DIAGNOSTIC DILEMMA   147

9. EVALUATION OF INFECTIVE ENDOCARDITIS   166

10. EVALUATION OF INTRACARDIAC MASSES   175

11. EXAMINATION OF THE AORTA   197

12. EVALUATION OF PROSTHETIC VALVE FUNCTION   205

13. CONGENITAL HEART DISEASE   230

14. THREE-DIMENSIONAL TRANSESOPHAGEAL ECHOCARDIOGRAPHY   271

Index   289

Principles of Echocardiography

• **Deepak K. Tempe** • **Suruchi Hasija**

Echocardiography in the operating room was introduced in the 1970s and the use of transesophageal echocardiography (TEE) during surgery was first described in 1980. Its application grew subsequently with technical developments in high-frequency multi-plane, phased array transducers and color Doppler imaging. Its scope has further widened with the advent of three-dimensional echocardiography and strain echocardiography. The physical principles and instrumentation of TEE involve concepts similar to those of surface echocardiography and are briefly outlined in this chapter.

PHYSICAL PROPERTIES OF ULTRASOUND

Frequency of ultrasonic waves is above the audible range of human ear and exceeds 20 kilohertz (kHz). They can be directed in a beam and obey laws of reflection (Fig. 1.1). At the interface of two media with differing acoustic impedance, ultrasonic waves undergo reflection. Acoustic impedance (z) is the density of media (r) times the velocity (v) of sound in the media ($z = r \times v$). *Specular* or maximum reflection occurs when the angle of incidence is 90°. Incomplete reflection occurs when the angle of incidence is less than 90° (Fig. 1.1A). When an ultrasound beam encounters an irregular surface, the waves are reflected in all directions and that reaching the transducer are proportionately less (Fig. 1.1B, C). Ultrasonic waves are almost completely reflected when the absolute difference in the acoustic impedance of the two interfacing media is large such as soft tissue and metal, calcium, bone or air. The degree of penetration thus varies depending on the acoustic impedance of different media, being relatively poorer for gases and solids. Penetration also depends on the frequency of incidental wave; higher the frequency poorer is the penetration although, the near-resolution is superior. A reduction

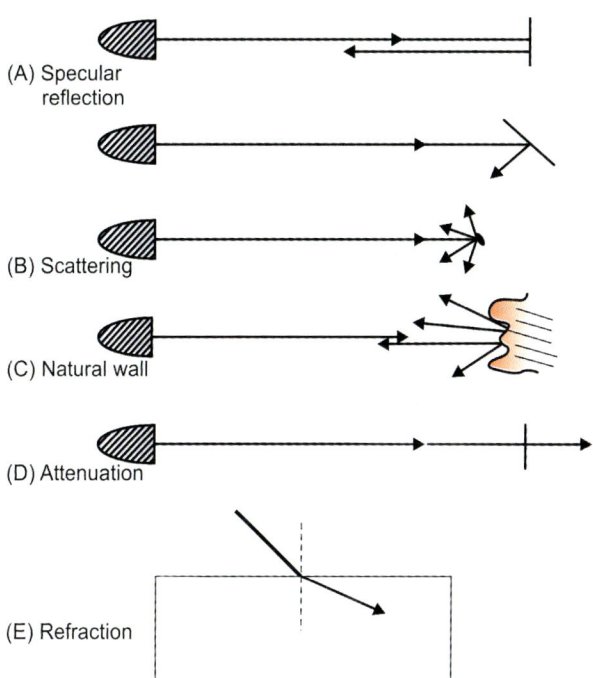

Fig. 1.1: Patterns of interference between an ultrasound wave and a target. Natural structures are inhomogenous and ultrasound waves undergo varying degrees of specular reflection (A), scattering (B and C), attenuation (D), and refraction (E).

in resolution occurs with increasing depth and is called attenuation (Fig. 1.1D). Bone and air produce higher attenuation than liquids such as blood and body fluids. Ultrasound waves change direction when they travel from one medium to another. The degree of refraction varies according to the angle of incidence and the difference in the acoustic impedance of the media (Fig. 1.1E). The total thickness that can be traversed by ultrasonic waves is about one-fourth of the wavelength of ultrasound. Since in transesophageal examination, heart is close to the transducer with little intervening

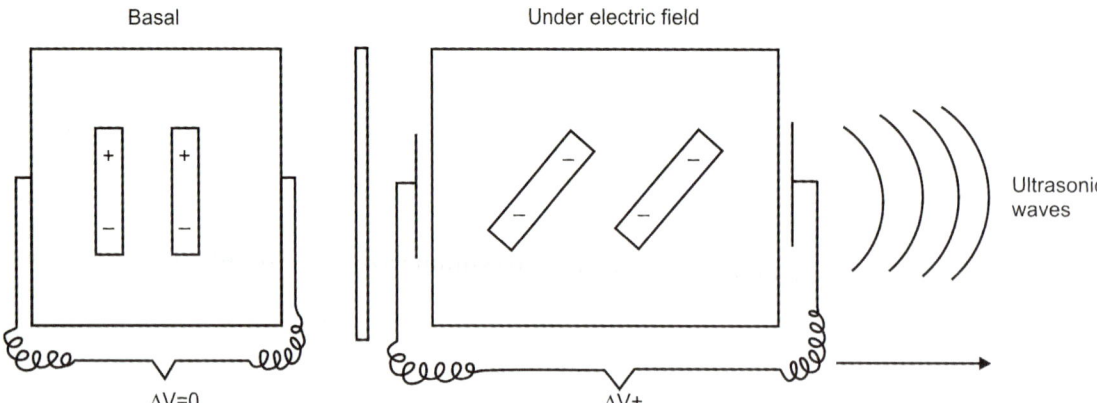

Fig. 1.2: Principles of piezoelectric crystals:The crystal generates and receives sound waves using a principle called the piezoelectric (pressure electricity) effect, which was discovered by Pierre and Jacques Curie in 1880. In the probe, there are one or more quartz crystals called piezoelectric crystals. When an electric current is applied to these crystals, they change shape rapidly. The rapid shape changes, or vibrations, of the crystals produce sound waves that travel outward. Conversely, when sound or pressure waves hit the crystals, they emit electrical currents. Therefore, the same crystals can be used to send and receive sound waves.

tissues, the frequency used is relatively higher (3.5–5 million hertz, mHz) than that used in transthoracic examination.

PRODUCTION OF ULTRASOUND AND TRANSDUCERS

In clinical practice, ultrasonic waves are produced from piezoelectric crystals. These crystals change their shape in electric field and produce alternate contraction and rarefaction of sound waves and conversely they also produce electrical impulses when struck by a sound wave (Fig. 1.2). If a single source (single crystal) were used, sound waves originating from it would resemble ripples in a pond. When multiple ripples from multiple elements originate, these coalesce to form a unidirectional wave front (Fig. 1.3). Such a wave-front can be advanced in a sector by rotating the elements. This can be done either mechanically or by electric motors. The most popular transducers are electronic real time scanners that use phased array principle. These transducers use multiple elements that are placed linearly and generate a linear wave front. The direction of the wave-front can be altered by delaying sequential activation of the elements. The crystals can be placed

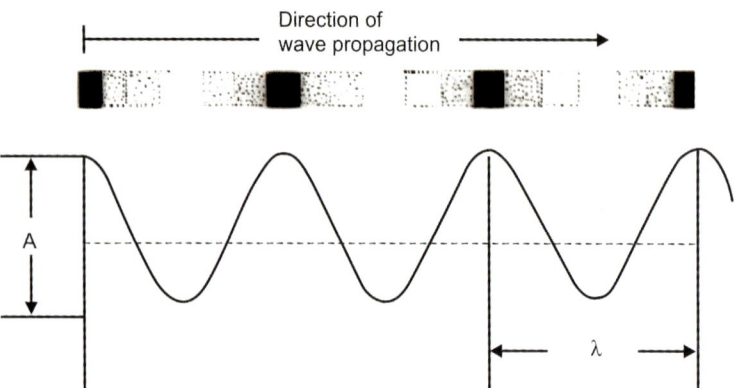

Fig. 1.3: Ultrasound propagates through the medium in the shape of a sinuous curve. The permanent transmission of kinetic energy from one molecule to the next is performed in the form of a continuous wave which is referred to as sound wave. During this process, alternating phases of compression (pressure phase) and decompression (suction phase) can be observed in the matter. The maximal height of a wave is the amplitude (A). The intensity of an ultrasound beam is proportional to the square of the amplitude. The ultrasound waves clinically used are low-intensity and do not cause injury. The wavelength (λ) of a wave is the minimum distance in which a wave repeats itself. The frequency (f) of a wave is the number of waves per second. The wavelength and frequency of a sound wave are related as: $c = f\lambda$, where c is the speed of propagation in the medium. As a wave travels from one medium to another, its frequency remains constant. However, the wavelength changes depending upon the speed of propagation.

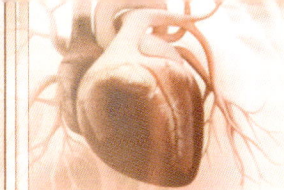

in sets, one horizontal and other vertical to produce a biplane transducer or a single set can be rotated through 180 degrees as in a multi-plane transducer.

Resolution

Resolution is the property of an ultrasound beam to discern echoes from sources related in close proximity with respect to space (spatial resolution), time (temporal resolution) or returned signal strength (contrast resolution). The resolution is better with shorter wavelength (depth) and higher frequency of the ultrasound wave.

Spatial resolution is axial, lateral or elevational depending on the ability of the ultrasound machine to identify objects along the axis of the ultrasound beam, horizontal to the beam's orientation or vertical to the beam's orientation, respectively (Fig. 1.4).

Variables for Real Time Imaging (Temporal Resolution)

A moving echo image on television screen is made of frames. Usually projection of at least 30 frames/sec is required for eliminating feeling of a stationary image. Each frame is made up of two fields separated by a black line, not appreciated on the screen due to persistence of vision. Each field originates from one ultrasonic sweep. The time required for one sweep is determined by the pulse repetition frequency and sector angle. The rate of emission of ultrasonic waves, which occurs in brief intervals of time (1–2 microseconds), determines the pulse repetition frequency. Similarly the sweep time is also dependent on the sector angle, smaller the sector angle more is the time available for sweeping a given area. The sweep time in turn determines the number of lines in

each sector. An image in ultrasound is made from multiple lines and its resolution depends upon the line density. More the number of lines in one sector, clearer would be the image. Since velocity of ultrasound is 1540 m/sec, each line takes about 0.28 sec to come and fly back. Thus smaller the sector angle, higher would be the number of lines per degree, more would be the line density and higher would be the image resolution. To summarize, the variables that determine an image resolution on screen include line density, pulse repetition frequency, angle of the sweep and the frame rate.

M-mode and Two-dimensional Imaging

Following emission of ultrasonic waves, the transducer becomes a receiver for the remaining (99%) period and receives the reflected wave. The reflected wave in turn hits the Piezo-electric crystal to produce an electric current. If one knows the time delay then the distance of object can be computed and shown on oscilloscope at a finite representative distance. The amplitude of the returning signal could be represented as a spike (A or amplitude mode) or in the form of varying brightness (B-mode). Subsequent frames over a period of time could be represented on one of the axis to produce motion and called M-mode or motion mode. The use of B-mode image to create exact image of an object in a field-sector and bringing in of subsequent frames with persistence of vision create real time B-mode imaging or the two-dimensional echocardiography. Since the returning signal strength is attenuated due to internal frictional heating, reflection and scattering, ultrasound machines are equipped with time-gain compensation to increase the gain progressively as signals return from deeper tissues. Similarly, the image dropout that occurs when ultrasound beam intersects a surface tangentially is compensated by lateral gain compensation (*refer* to Chapter 2).

Doppler Echocardiography

Doppler is a technique to detect the manner in which blood moves in the cardiovascular system. If the target is stationary, the frequency of transmitted wave and reflected wave is identical. If the target is moving towards the transducer, the received frequency is increased. If it moves away, then the frequency is decreased. The Doppler shift represents the difference between received and transmitted frequencies (Fig. 1.5). The mathematical relation between the velocity (v) of the target and Doppler frequency can be given by the following equation

Doppler equation: $v = fd.c / 2.ft \, (\cos \theta)$

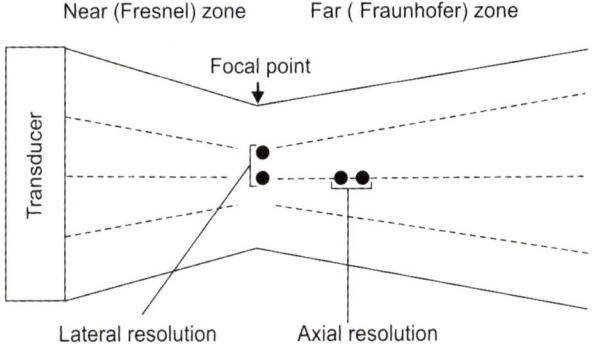

Fig. 1.4: The ultrasound wave is transmitted as a beam till the focal point beyond which it diverges like a cone. The lateral resolution is maximal at the focal depth and decreases in the near (Fresnel) zone and the far (Fraunhofer) zone.

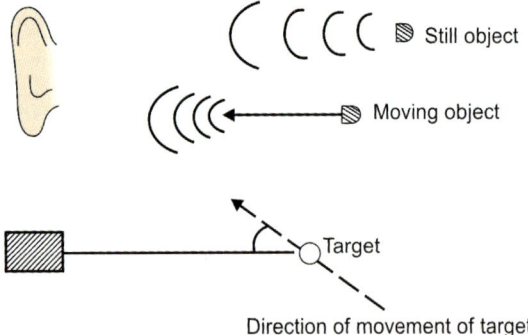

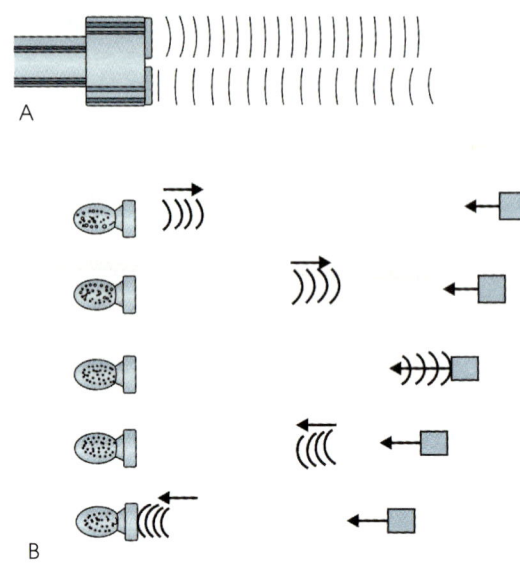

Fig. 1.5: Doppler effect. Sound waves that are emitted from an object moving towards a receiver are compressed causing an increase in the frequency.

where *fd* is the Doppler frequency, *ft* is the transmitted frequency, *c* is the speed of propagation in the medium and θ is the angle between path of travel and ultrasonic beam.

The best Doppler information is derived if the beam is parallel to moving target with an angle between the beam and direction of moving target not exceeding 20 degrees. This is paradoxical to 2-D echocardiography wherein the best information is derived if the beam is perpendicular to the region of interest. Two types of Doppler application are used in clinical practice: continuous wave and pulsed wave Doppler (Fig. 1.6). In continuous wave Doppler, a transducer is used with separate transmitting and receiving elements. This works continuously and hence there is no way to register the delay in receiving an incoming impulse, and thus the depth of an individual target or the location of a moving target cannot be estimated. On the contrary, in the pulsed wave Doppler, the same transducer initially sends a burst of waves and then works as a receiver. By knowing the delay, it is possible to compute the distance of a moving target or to obtain information from a given depth. However, the major limitation of pulsed wave Doppler is that it cannot measure velocities above a specific threshold. Since a finite time is required for transmitting a returning wave, frequency higher than a specific threshold cannot be registered. This is called an aliasing velocity and the limit is called Nyquist limit (Fig. 1.7). Usually the Nyquist limit equals one-half pulse repetition frequency.

The Doppler information is usually displayed graphically against time and is called the spectral Doppler. Use of spectral Doppler is useful for

Fig. 1.6: Principles of continuous wave (CW) and pulsed wave (PW) Doppler. The CW transducer (A) emits and receives simultaneously through two different crystals. The PW Doppler transducer (B) emits short pulses of ultrasound waves, the distance of interrogation is determined by the reception delay; the speed of the target is calculated by the difference between emitted and received frequencies.

computing velocity and pressure gradients, valve orifice areas and blood flow (Figs 1.8 and 1.9). Pulsed wave Doppler information from a given field sector can be represented at multiple points at multiple depths with different colors, each color denoting a particular frequency. This is called color Doppler and forms the basis of color-flow imaging. The Doppler flow is usually superimposed on the two-dimensional cardiac image. The physiologic motion of moving flow determines the direction; traditionally red color is assigned to motion towards the transducer and blue for motion away from the transducer with multiple shades of green and yellow for intermediate velocities in a turbulent flow. Since color Doppler uses the concept of pulsed wave Doppler, higher velocities are not properly represented and result in aliasing (Fig. 1.10). As image aliases, color changes from blue to red and vice-versa. Another limitation is the higher time required for color flow imaging that reduces the frame rate. Therefore for optimizing the image resolution, the sector angle and region of interrogation for color Doppler need to be much smaller than the actual 2-D image.

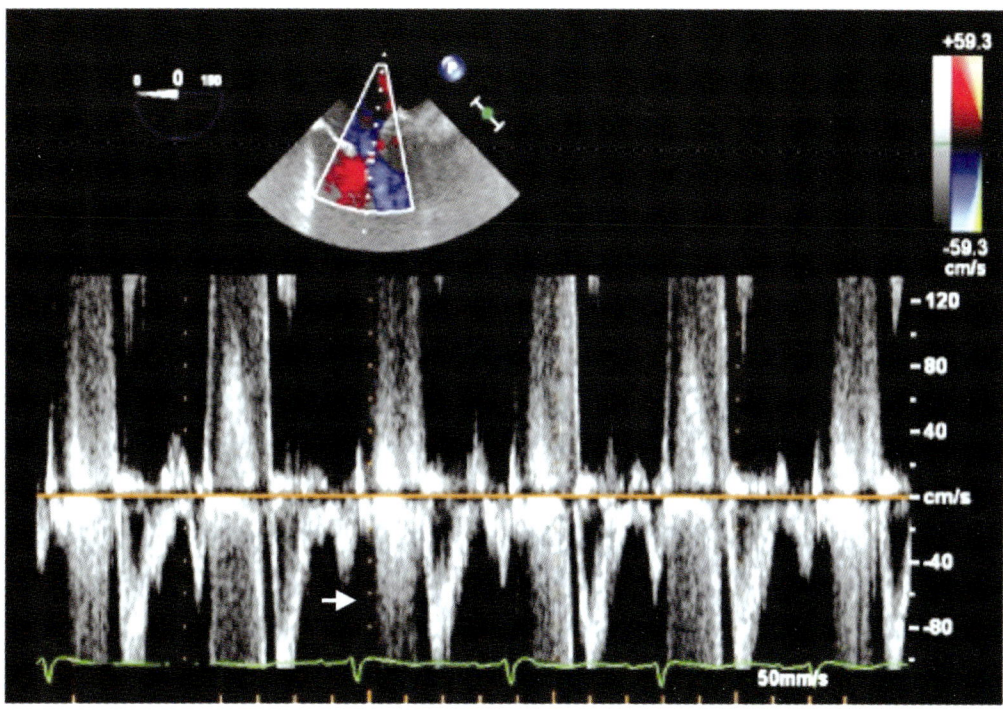

Fig. 1.7: A pulsed wave Doppler profile showing aliasing of the mitral regurgitation jet (arrow).

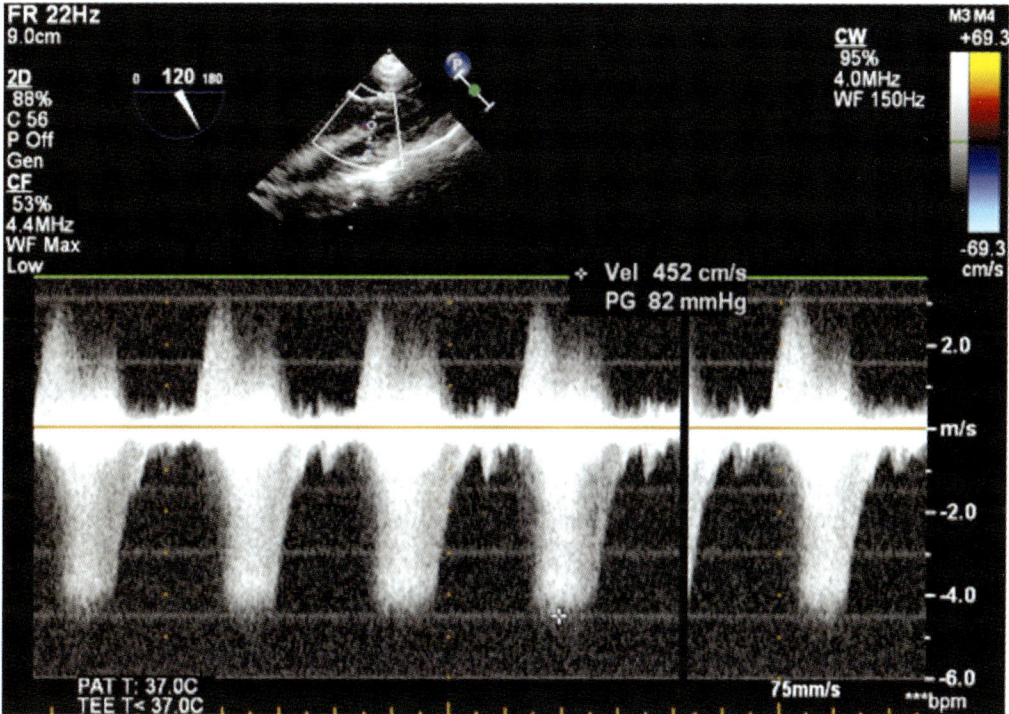

Fig. 1.8: A continuous wave Doppler profile depicting high velocity flow across a subaortic ventricular septal defect.

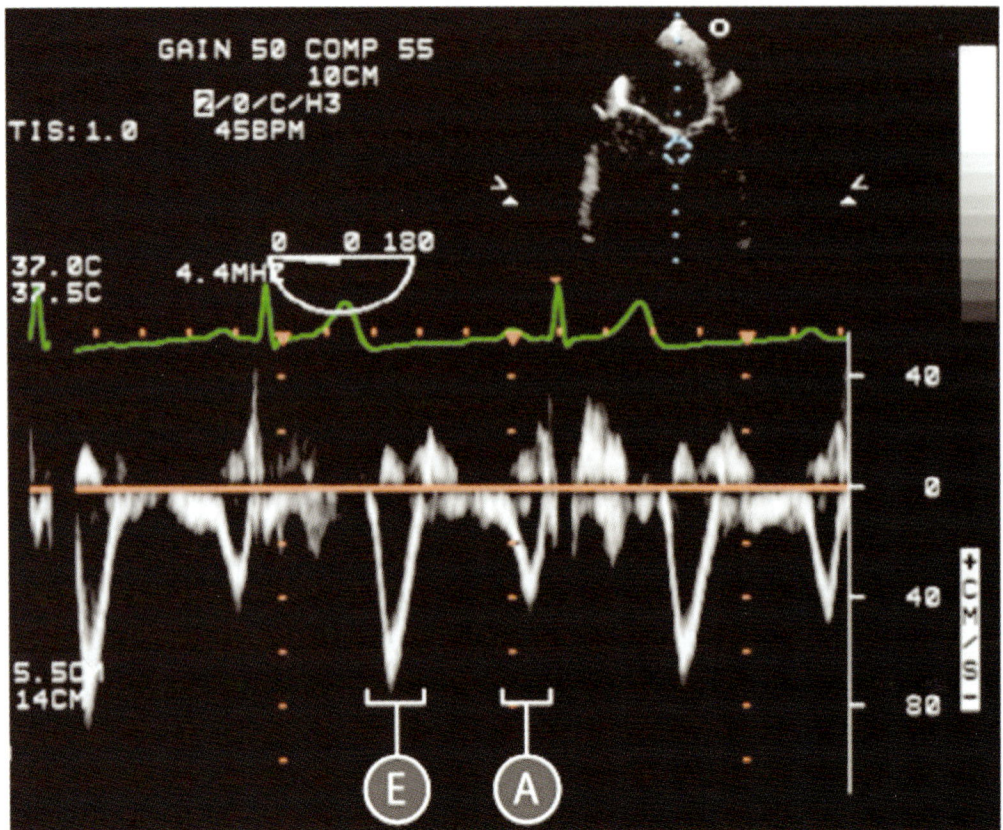

Fig. 1.9: A pulsed wave Doppler profile depicting the low velocity mitral inflow pattern during diastole. (E: early filling phase, A: atrial contraction).

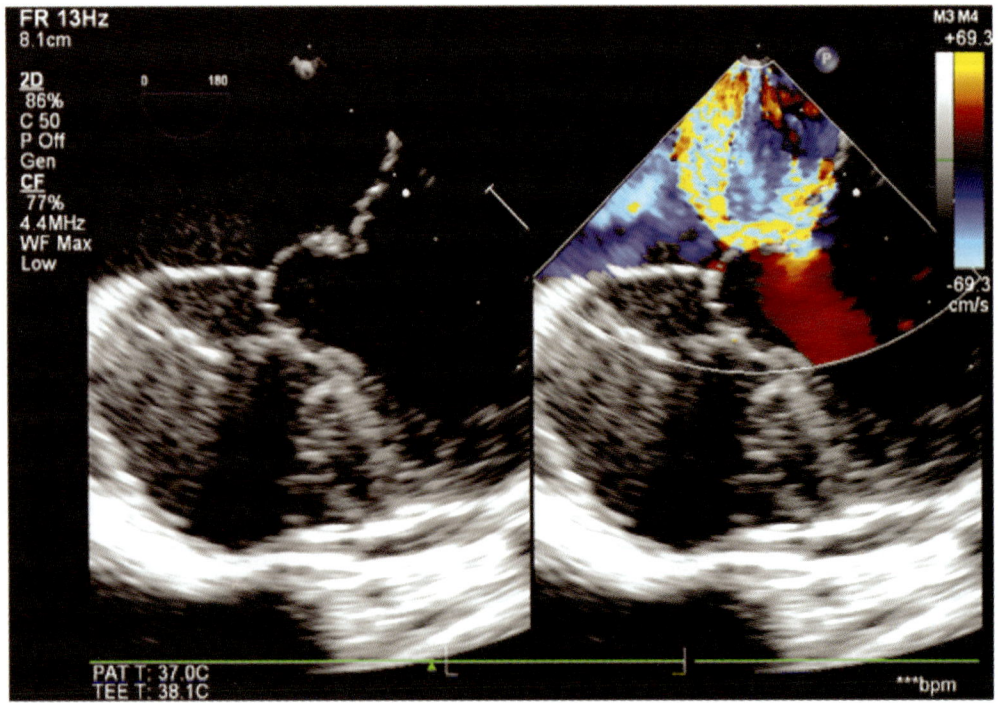

Fig. 1.10: A color flow Doppler image showing aliasing of the mitral regurgitation jet. The hue changes from red towards blue across the shades of 'Vibgyor'.

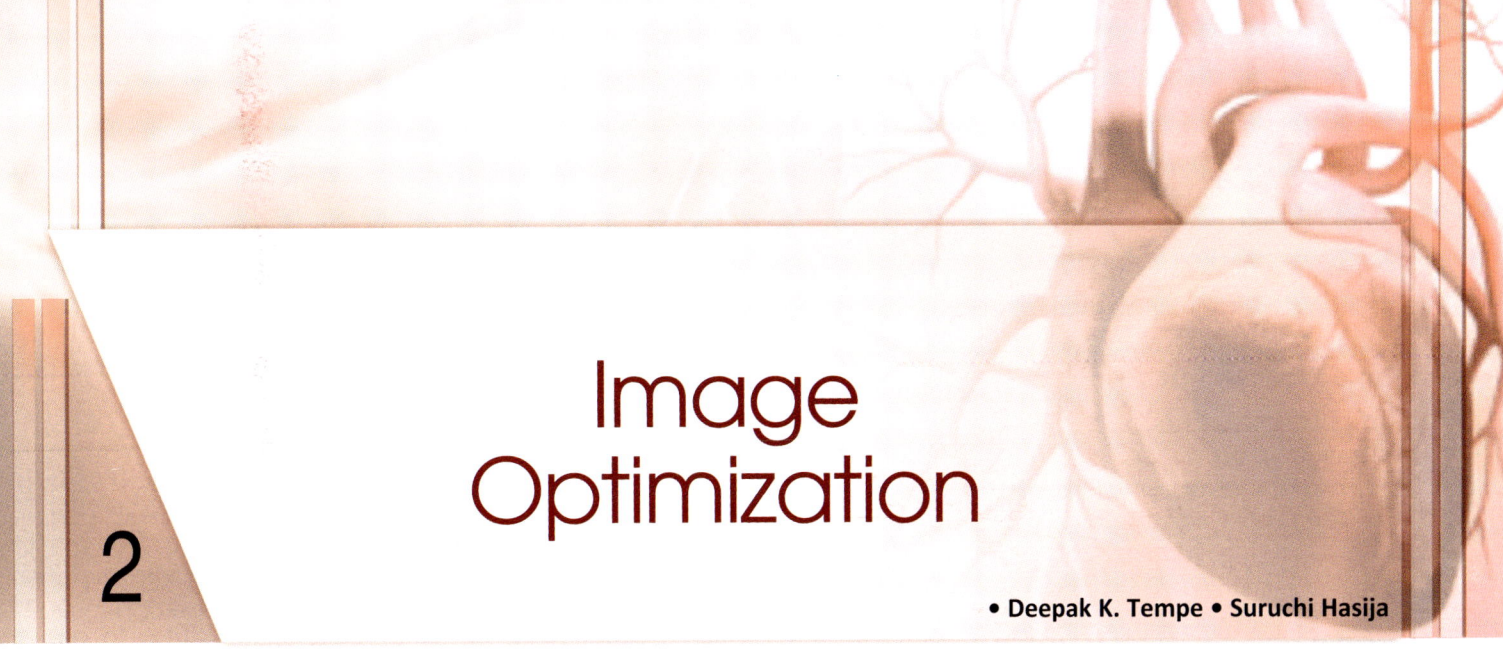

Image Optimization

2

• Deepak K. Tempe • Suruchi Hasija

A beginner in the field of transesophageal echocardiography (TEE) often struggles to obtain a good quality image. It is important to note that unlike other imaging techniques (computerised tomography, magnetic resonance imaging), getting a good image on TEE is operator dependent. Nevertheless, some equipment (defective probe) or patient related factors (fluid/air in the stomach, emphysematous lung, calcified intracardiac structures, presence of mechanical heart valves) can influence the quality of image. The operator can learn to optimise the image by understanding the function of various knobs and buttons available on the console of the TEE machine (Fig. 2.1). In addition, the operator should also understand the physics related to ultrasound.

The typical controls of every echocardiography machine that enable the operator to obtain a good image include the following (also *refer* to Chapter 1).

TRANSDUCER FREQUENCY

Higher transmitted ultrasound frequency is chosen for interrogating shallow structures and lower frequency for deeper structures. Higher frequency ultrasound permits increased frame rate and improved temporal resolution.

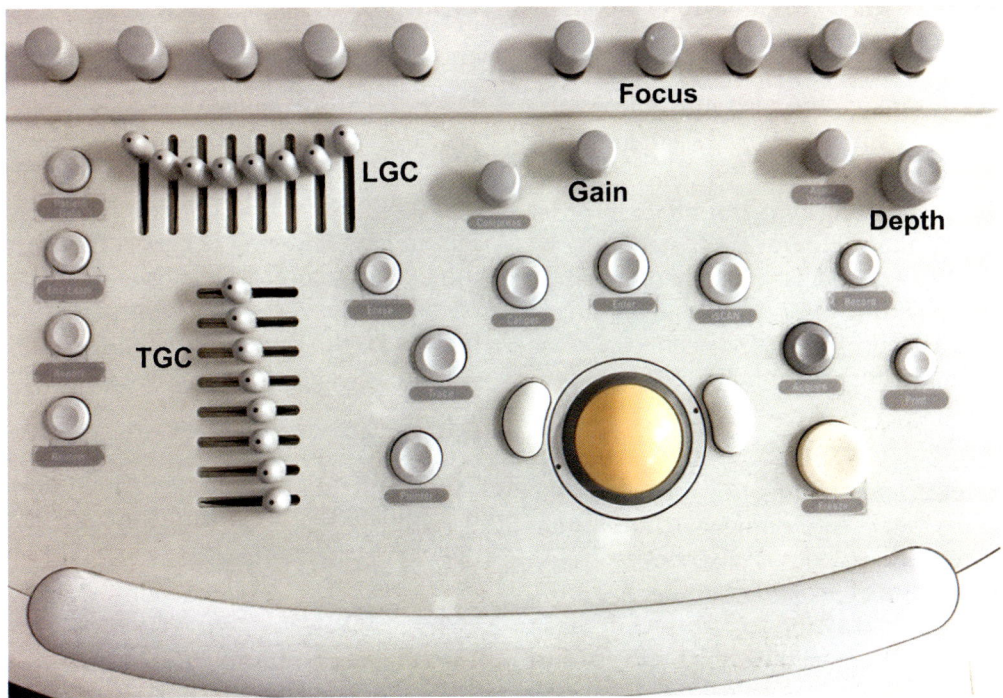

Fig. 2.1: The TEE machine console showing the various knobs and controls.

Wavelength

Longer wavelengths (lower frequency) enable greater tissue penetration, but at the cost of resolution.

Pulse Repetition Frequency

Pulse repetition frequency is the frequency at which ultrasound pulses are generated. The resolution is improved with frequent ultrasound pulses. The velocity scale enables adjustment of the pulse repetition frequency so as to match the velocities of interest and prevent aliasing.

Frame Rate

A lower frame rate decreases the temporal resolution, i.e., the ability to locate moving structures.

Sector Width/Scan Line Density

The angle of the sector displayed on the monitor can vary from 15 to 90°. The temporal resolution and frame rate can be improved by reducing the sector width (increasing the line density and pulse repetition frequency) (Figs 2.2 and 2.3).

Most of the images can be considerably improved by adjustment of 3 controls, i.e. gain, depth, and time gain compensation (TGC).

Gain

The receiver gain increases the amplitude of the returning ultrasound signals. It serves to compensate for signal loss due to attenuation. It is set at a level that permits rare noise signals into the image. A high gain setting brightens the image but also introduces false signals, whereas a low gain setting masks actual signals (Figs 2.4–2.6).

In general, the gain settings are around 75 in order to obtain a good image. However, it needs to be adjusted according to a particular image. For instance, in Fig. 2.8, the gain setting is only 14, but the image quality is quite good. Hence, there is no need to increase the gain setting here (compare with Fig. 2.7).

Depth

Increasing the depth of interrogation increases the wavelength but decreases the frequency (frame rate) and thereby, the resolution. Conversely, the resolution is improved by decreasing the depth (Figs 2.9 and 2.10). It is ideally set to just display the structure of interest. In general, the depth setting is 8–10 cm, 10–15 cm and 15–20 cm for upper-esophageal, midesophageal and transgastric views respectively.

There are no fixed depth settings and it should be adjusted according to the area of interest. For instance, visualization of interatrial septum can be considerably improved in midesophageal view by decreasing the depth (Figs 2.11 and 2.12).

Time Gain Compensation

Time gain compensation allows selective depth-dependent amplification. As the ultrasound reaches the far field, the returning signal becomes weak. This can be amplified by TGC. Figure 2.13A and B shows the TGC controls. It can be used to amplify weaker signals returning from far field more compared to those returning from near field (Figs 2.14 and 2.15).

Lateral Gain Control

When the directioin of ultrasound is parallel to the object, there is little reflection resulting in a weak signal. This can be augmented by lateral gain control (LGC). For instance, in transgastric midpapillary view, the lateral wall and the interventricular septum are parallel to the ultrasound waves hence, there can be a dropout of these structures. This can be improved by adjusting the LGC (Figs 2.16 and 2.17).

Lateral gain compensation allows for selective amplification along adjacent scan lines within a sector scan.

Focus

The optimal focal depth is kept at the point of interest as the lateral resolution is maximal at this point. Sound energy travels as a beam until the focal point (near field) beyond which it diverges (far field) (Figs 2.18 and 2.19).

COLOR CONTROLS

Color Box Size and Position

Figure 2.20 shows the TEE machine console highlighting the Doppler controls. Color is displayed in the region of interest. As the sector width or depth of color box is increased, the frame rate, and therefore, the temporal resolution, is decreased (Figs 2.21 and 2.22).

Color Gain

Color gain amplifies the returning ultrasound signals. It is adjusted by decreasing the color gain until speckles of color disappear outside the blood pool.

Color Scale

The color scale must be adjusted according to the blood velocity being evaluated as aliasing occurs when velocities outside the range are sampled.

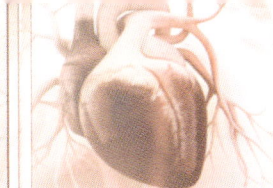

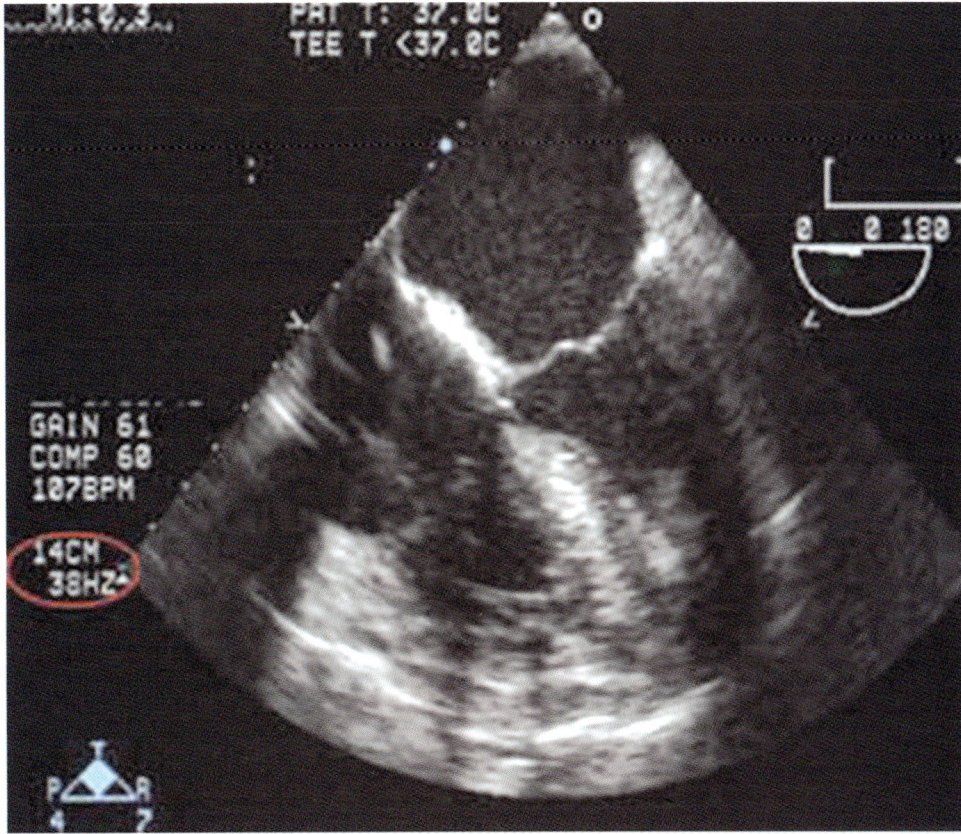

Fig. 2.2: Midesophageal 4-chamber view with maximum width of the sector scan.

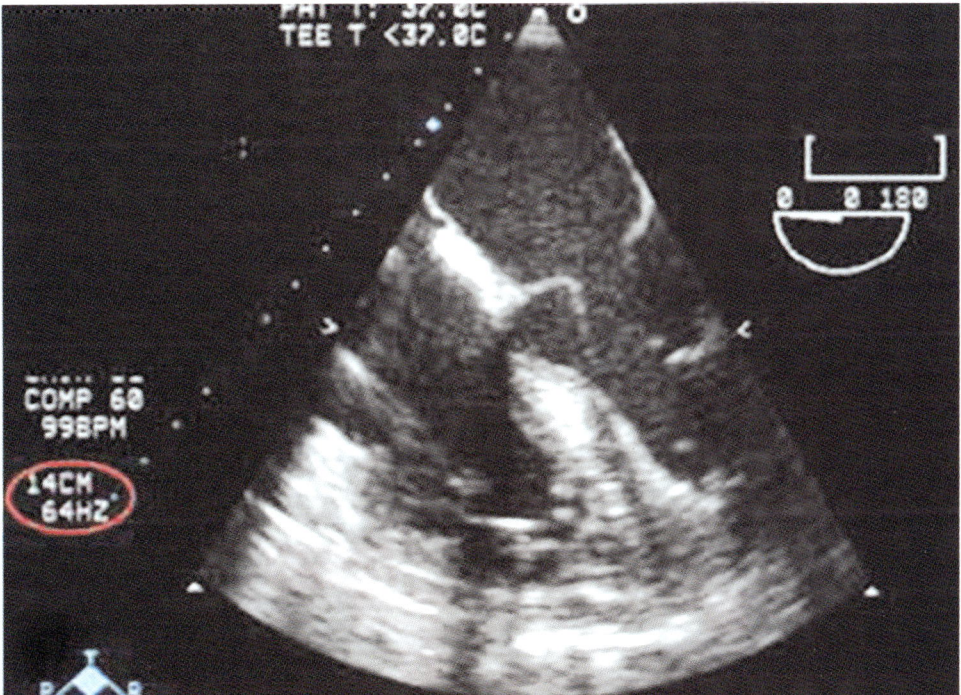

Fig. 2.3: Midesophageal 4-chamber view depicting how a reduction in sector scan leads to an increase in frame rate (64 Hz) for the same depth (compare with Fig. 2.2).

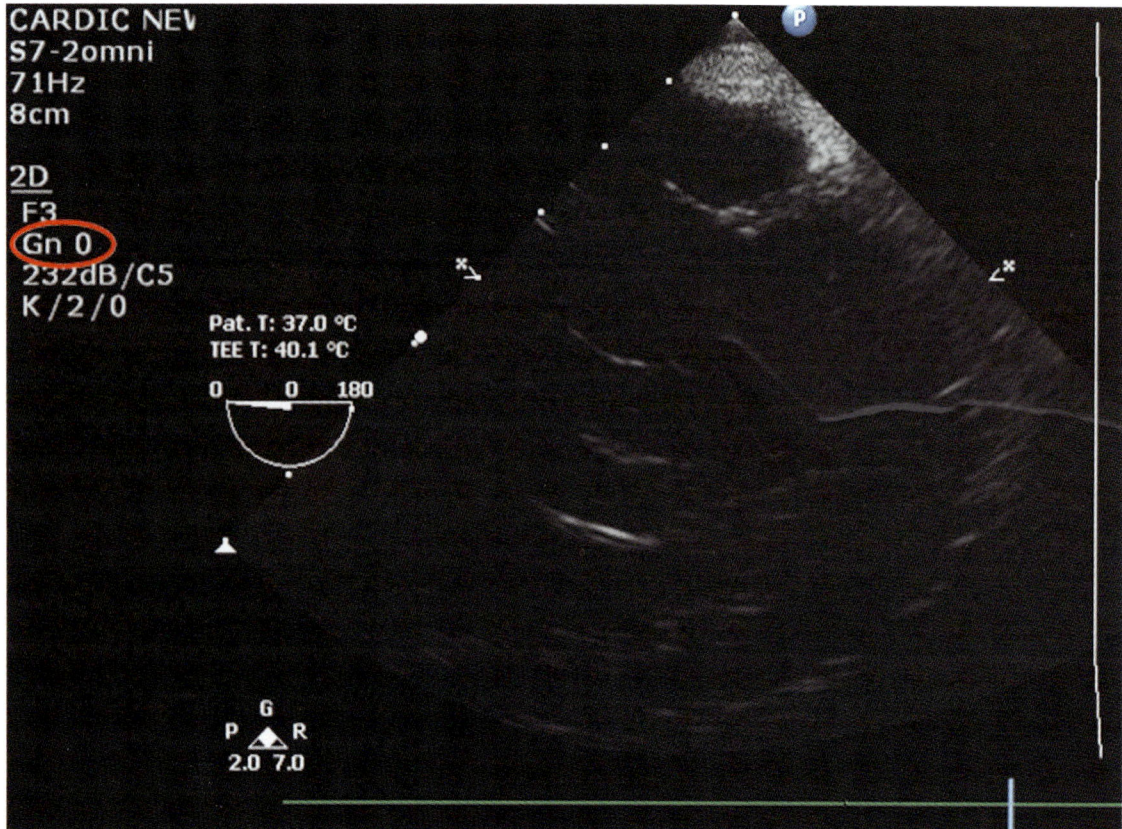

Fig. 2.4: The image is not visible when the gain is set at minimum.

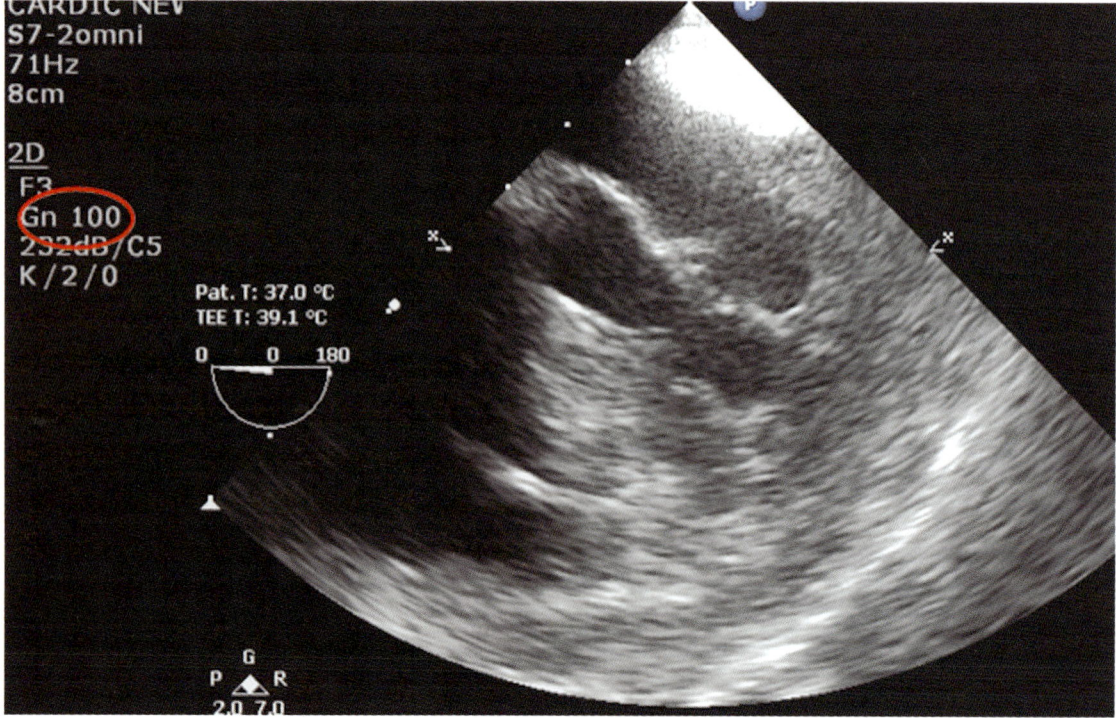

Fig. 2.5: The image appears unduly bright when the gain is set at maximum.

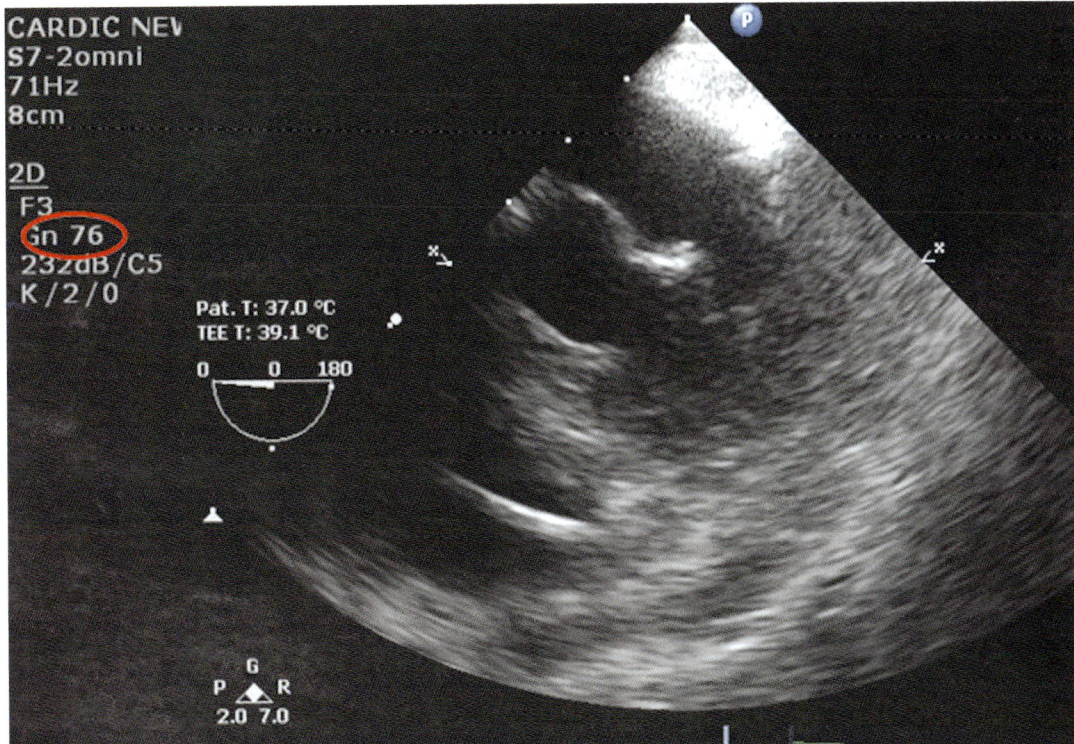

Fig. 2.6: The gain is set to permit image detailing.

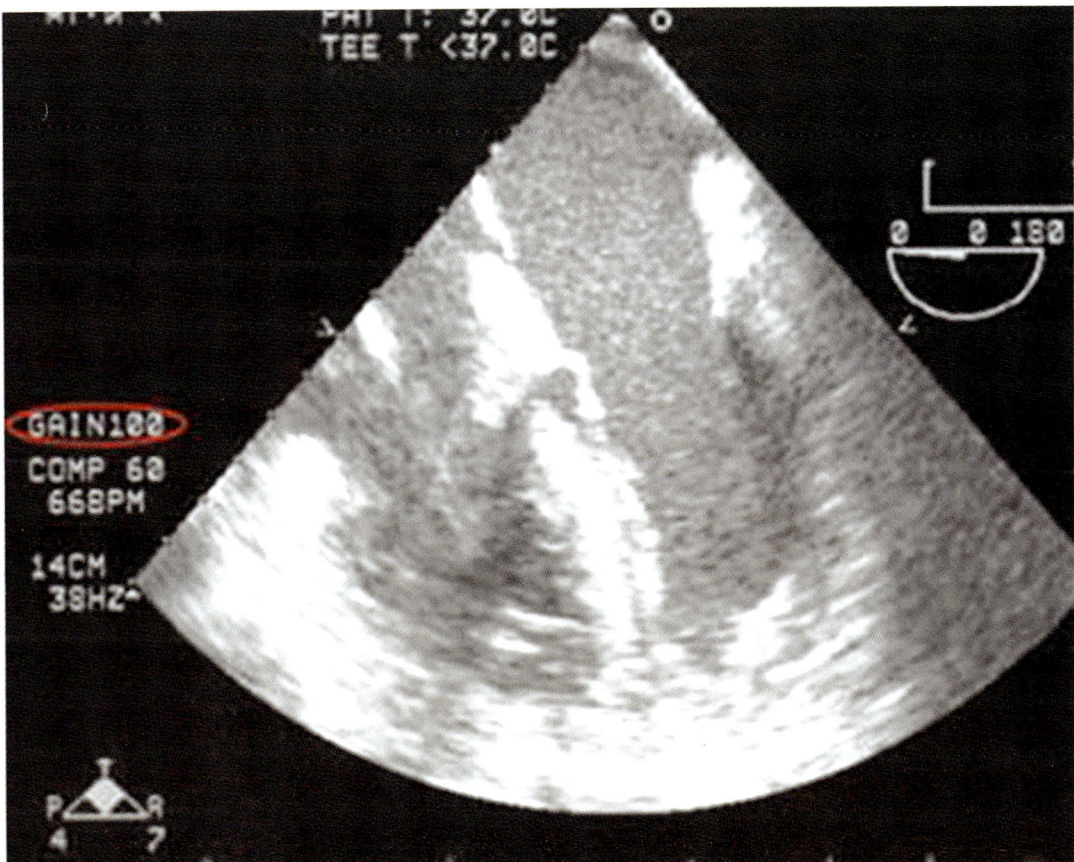

Fig. 2.7: Midesophageal 4-chamber view with increased overall gain in 2-D ultrasound.

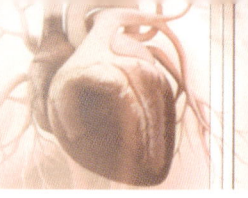

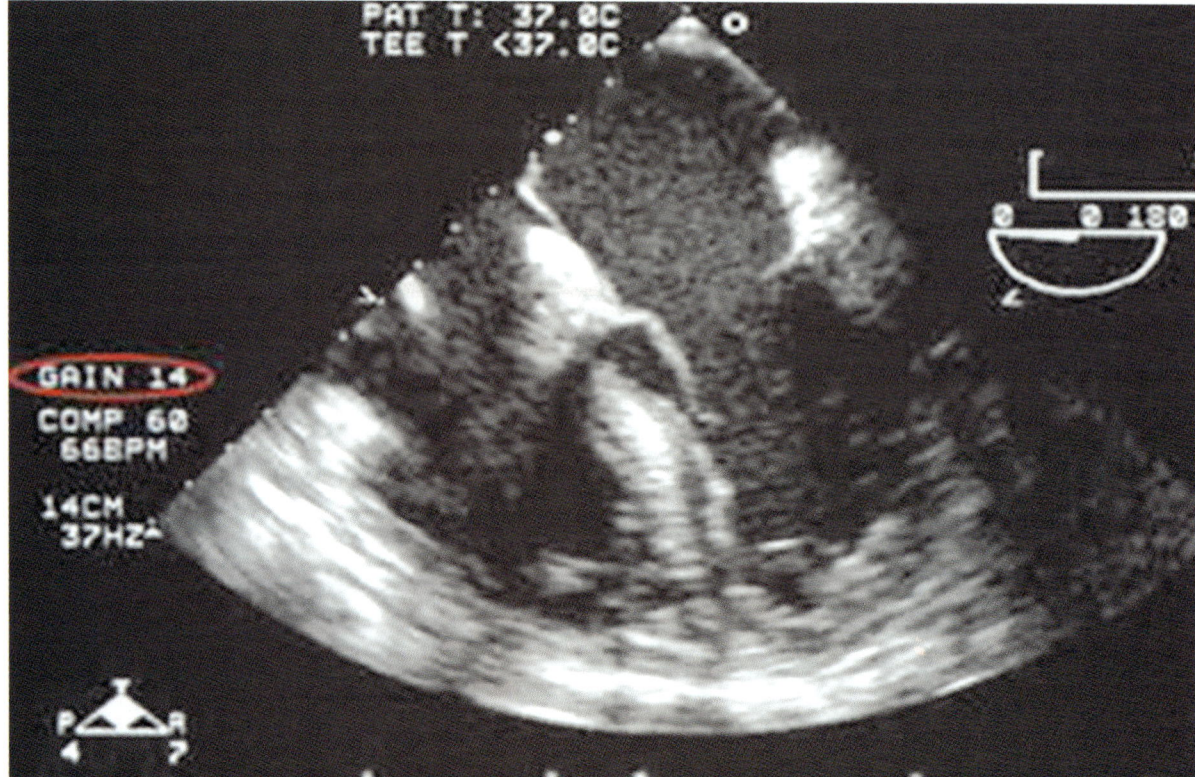

Fig. 2.8: Midesophageal 4-chamber view wherein gain has been reduced to optimize the 2-D ultrasound image.

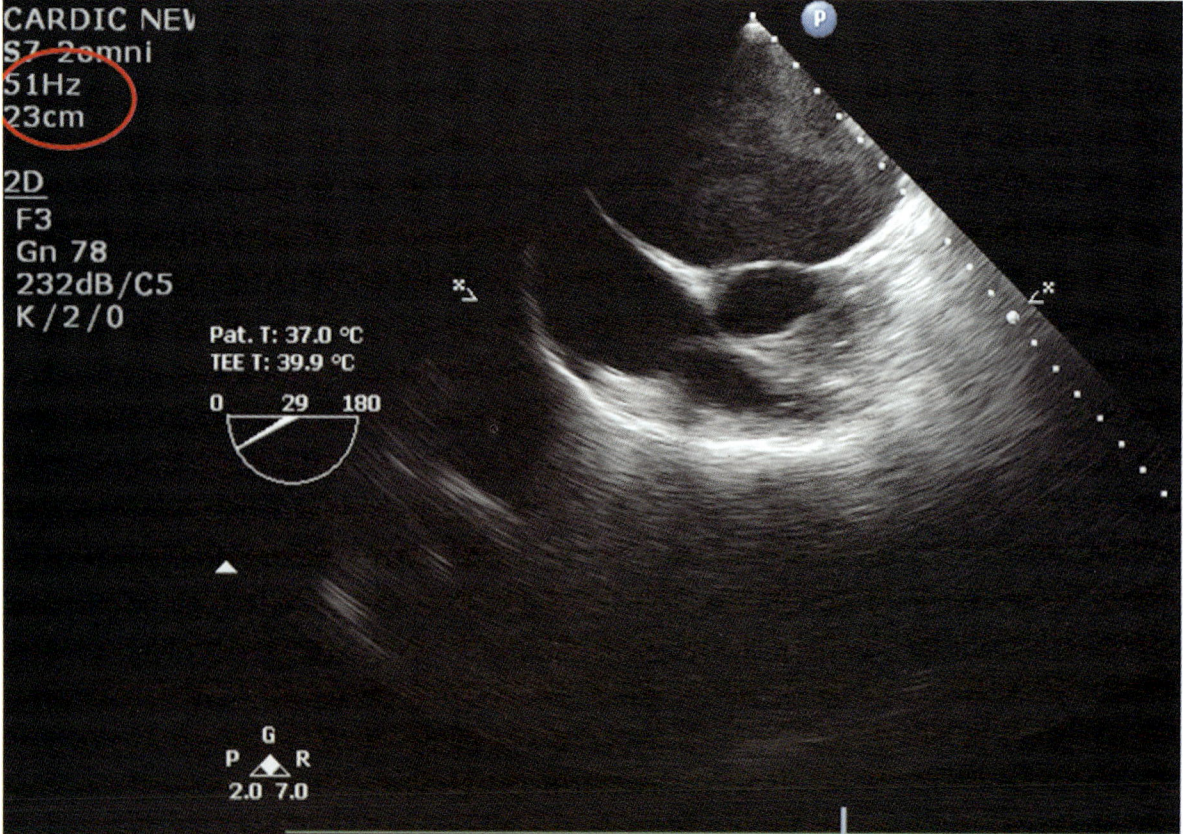

Fig. 2.9: Midesophageal aortic valve short-axis view showing a greater depth setting (23 cm) resulting in lower frequency and resolution. Note the frequency is 51 Hz.

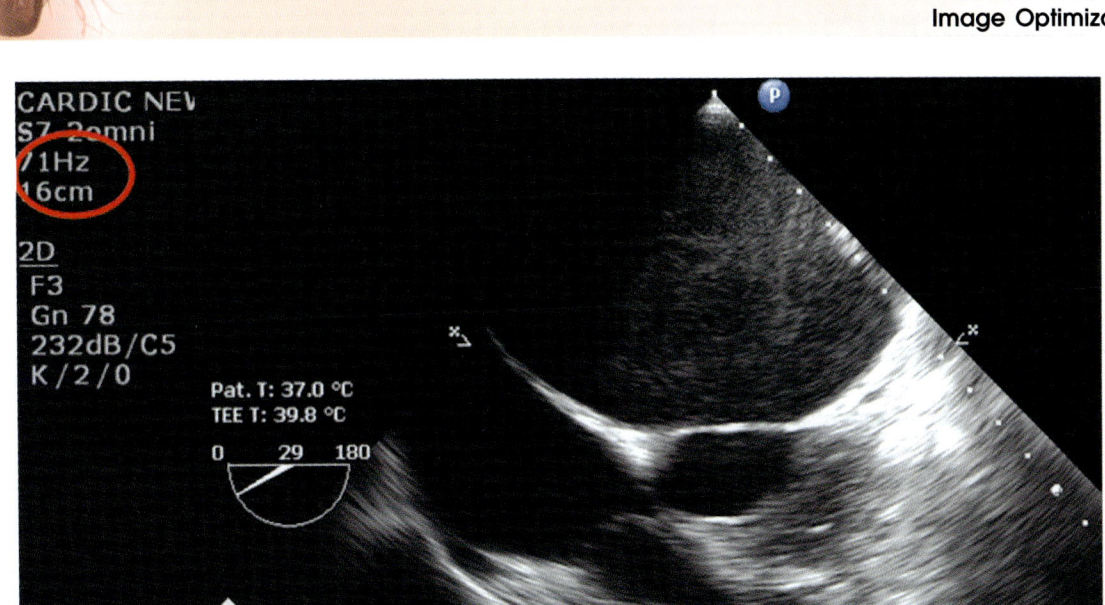

Fig. 2.10: Midesophageal aortic valve short-axis view showing a lower depth setting (16 cm) resulting in higher frequency and resolution. Note that the frequency has improved to 71 Hz (compare with Fig. 2.9).

Variance

A variance in flow, i.e., turbulent flow may be color-coded (e.g.: shades of green) to distinguish it from laminar flow which is coded on the red-blue color flow map.

Baseline

Adjustment of the baseline of the spectral display is performed to accommodate the entire velocity range in the direction of interest and prevent aliasing (Figs 2.23 and 2.24). For higher velocities, aliasing can be prevented by utilising continuous wave Doppler and increasing the scale to accommodate the velocity (Fig. 2.25).

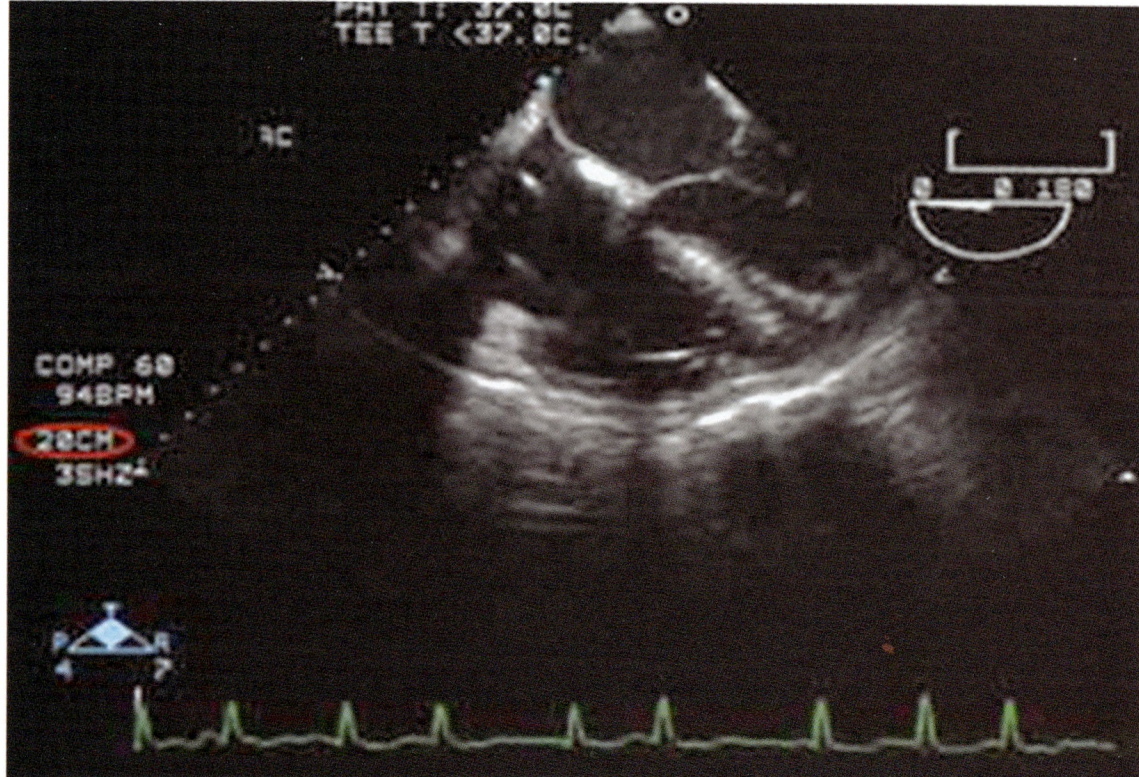

Fig. 2.11: Midesophageal 4-chamber view showing the depth set at 20 cm and the resultant frequency 35 Hz resulting in compromised resolution.

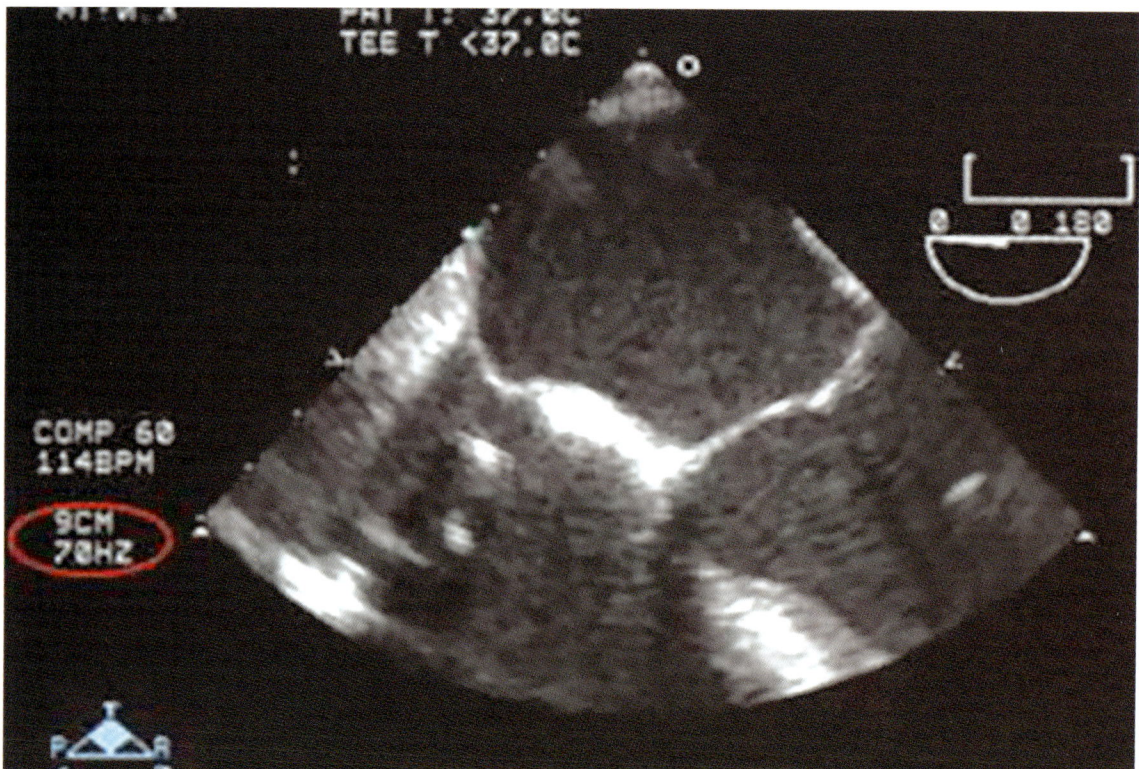

Fig. 2.12: Midesophageal 4-chamber view wherein the depth of imaging has been decreased to 9 cm resulting in increased frequency and improved resolution. In this case, it is useful for examination of inter-atrial septum.

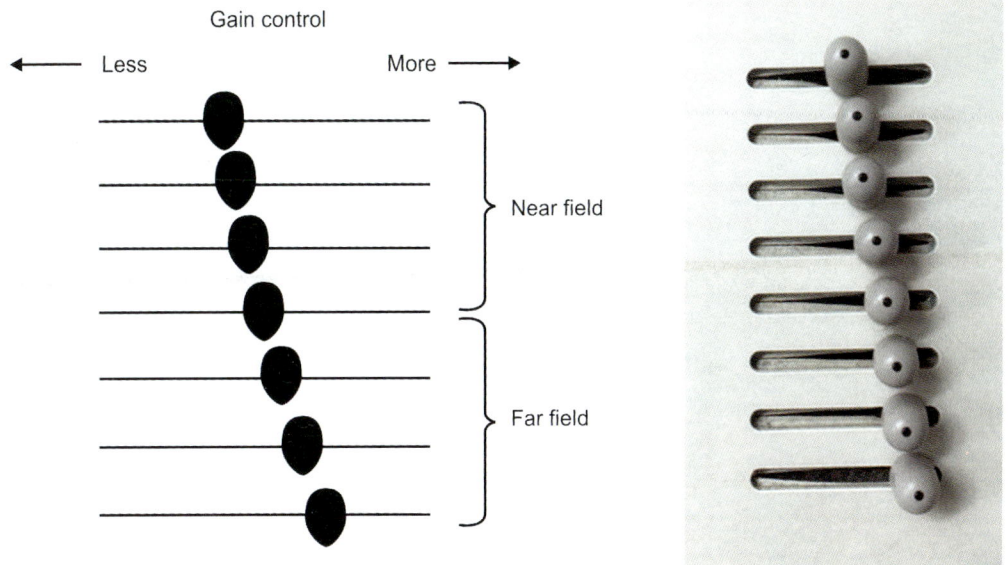

Fig. 2.13: The time gain compensation controls on the TEE machine console.

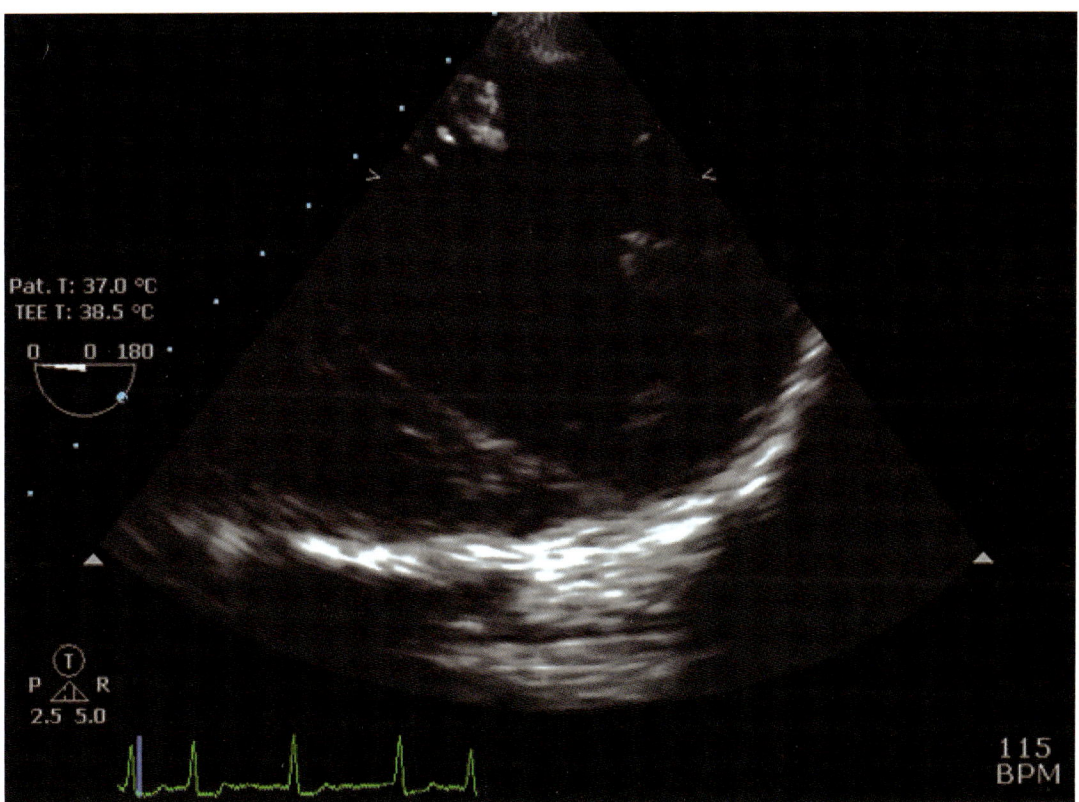

Fig. 2.14: The time gain compensation setting is low in this figure, the image appears less bright.

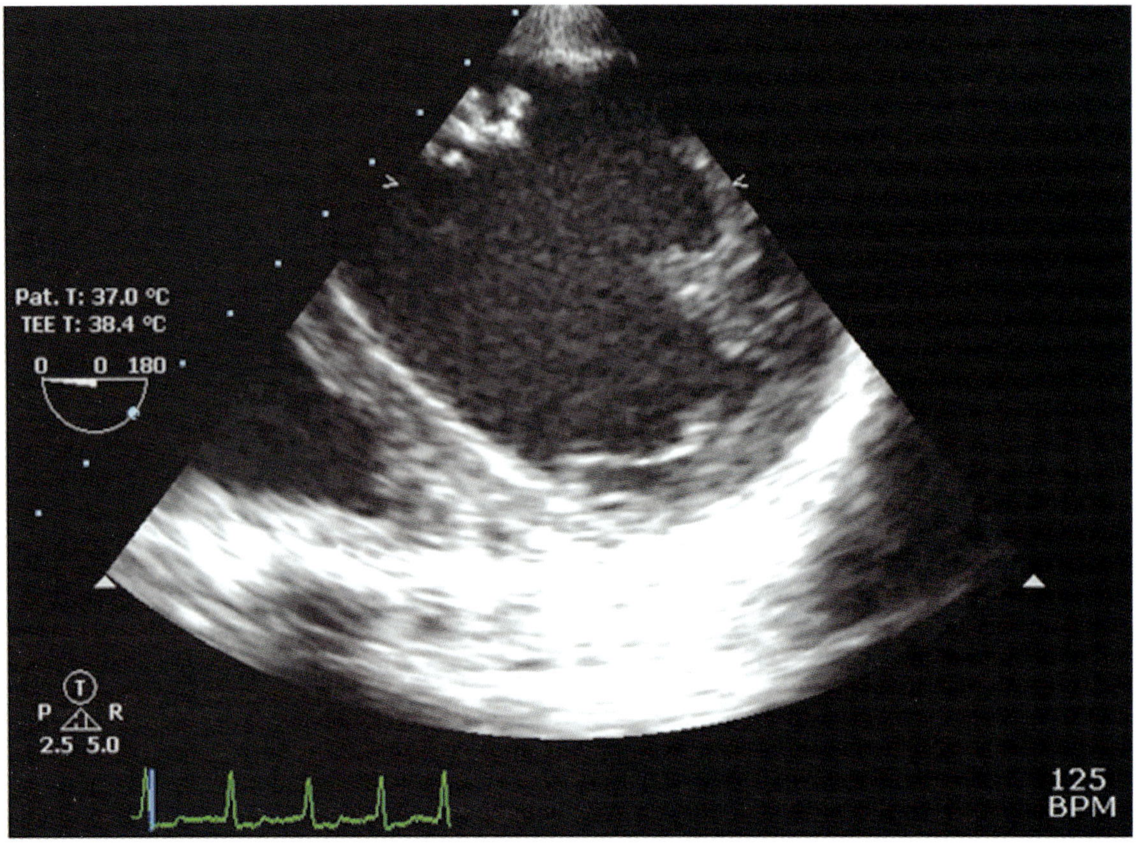

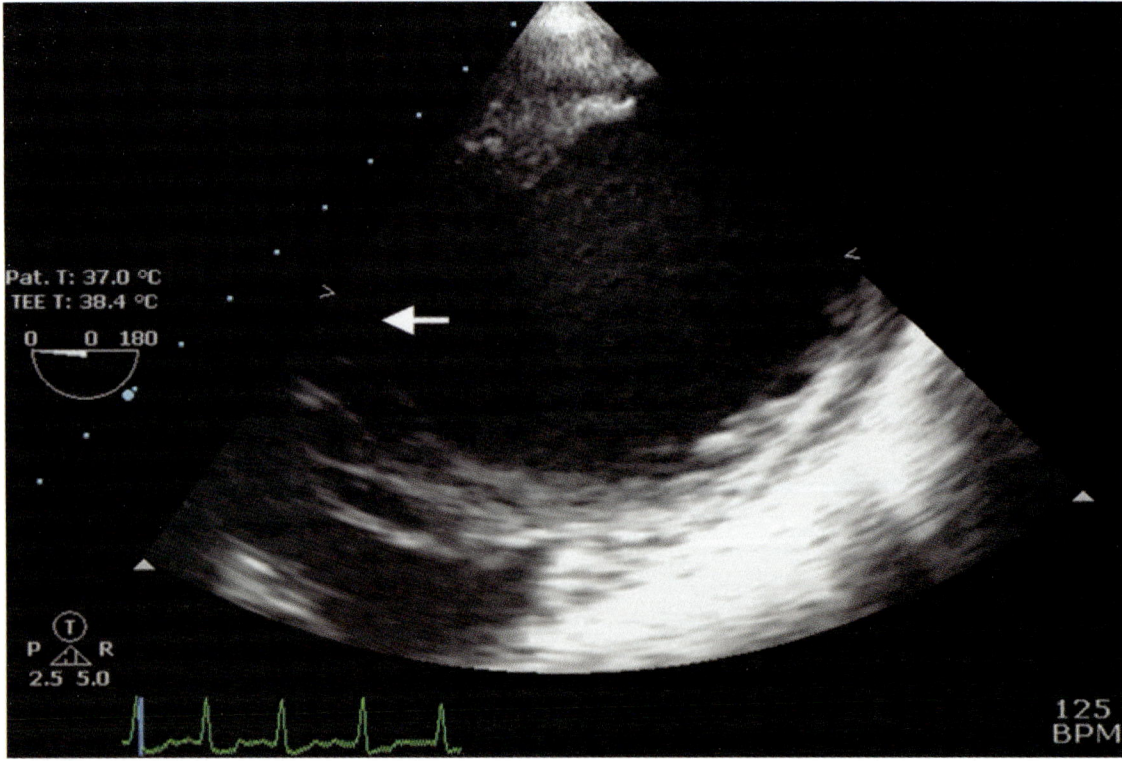

Fig. 2.15: The image is brighter at the bottom as the time gain compensation has been increased in the far field.

Fig. 2.16: Transgastric mid-papillary short-axis view. Note the image drop out of the interventricular septum as the ultrasound wave strikes parallel to the septum (arrow).

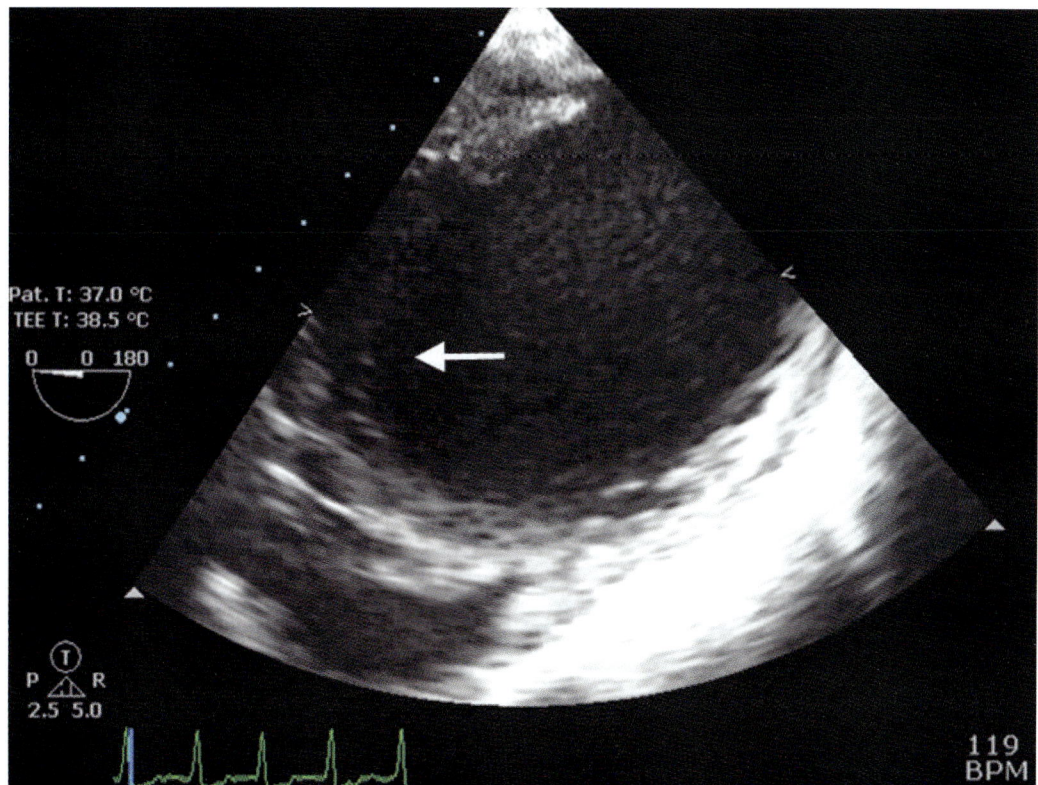

Fig. 2.17: The same image as in Fig 2.16. Note the improved visualization of the interventricular septum by adjusting the lateral gain control.

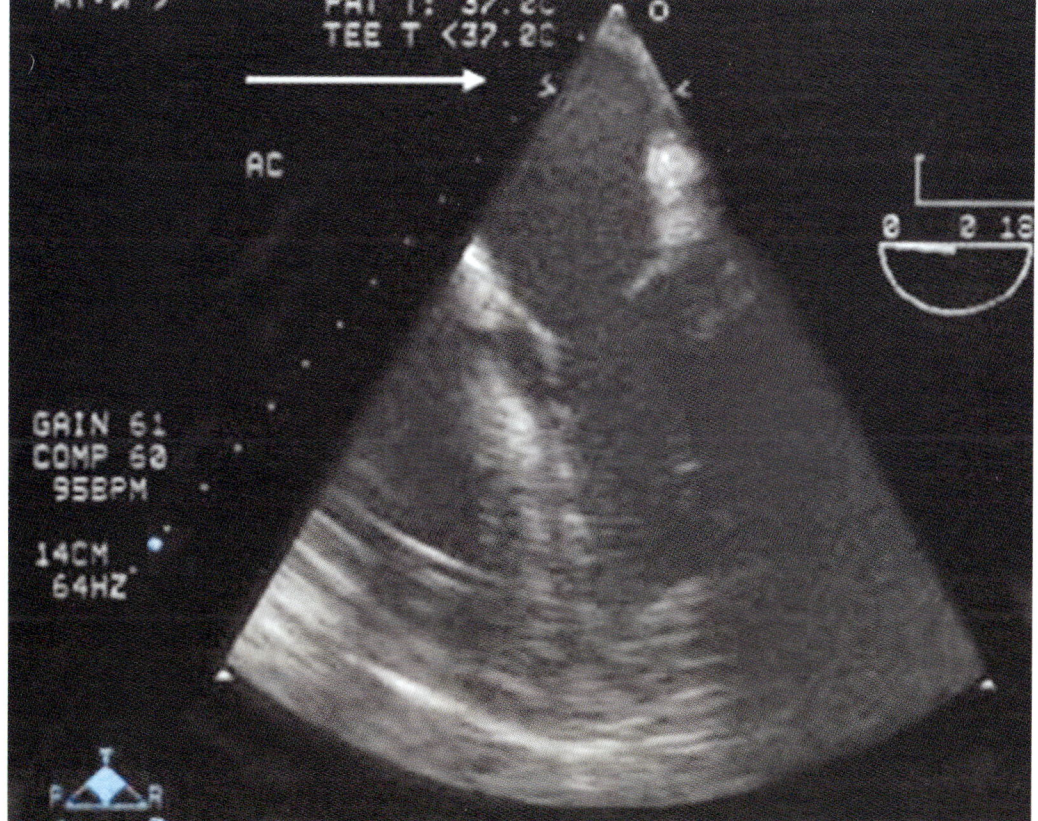

Fig. 2.18: With the focus set close to the probe (arrow), the far zone increases and resolution is poor beyond the focal point.

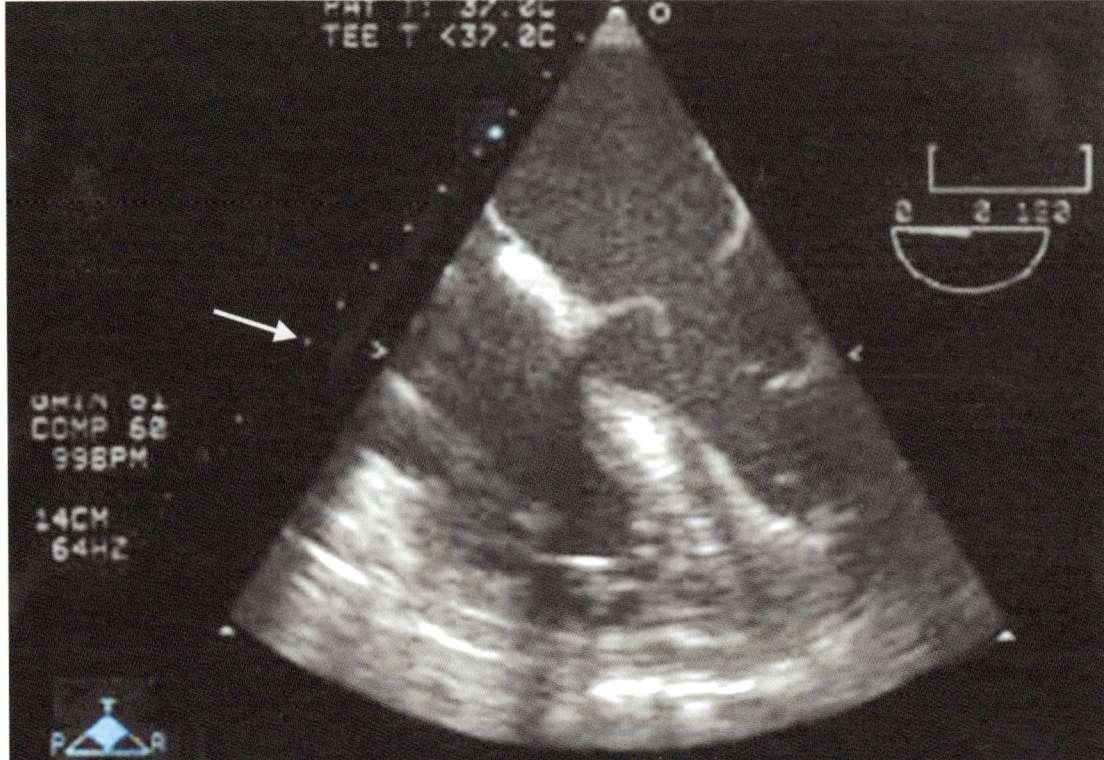

Fig. 2.19: The focus is now set at the point of interest (valvular level) resulting in improvement of image quality.

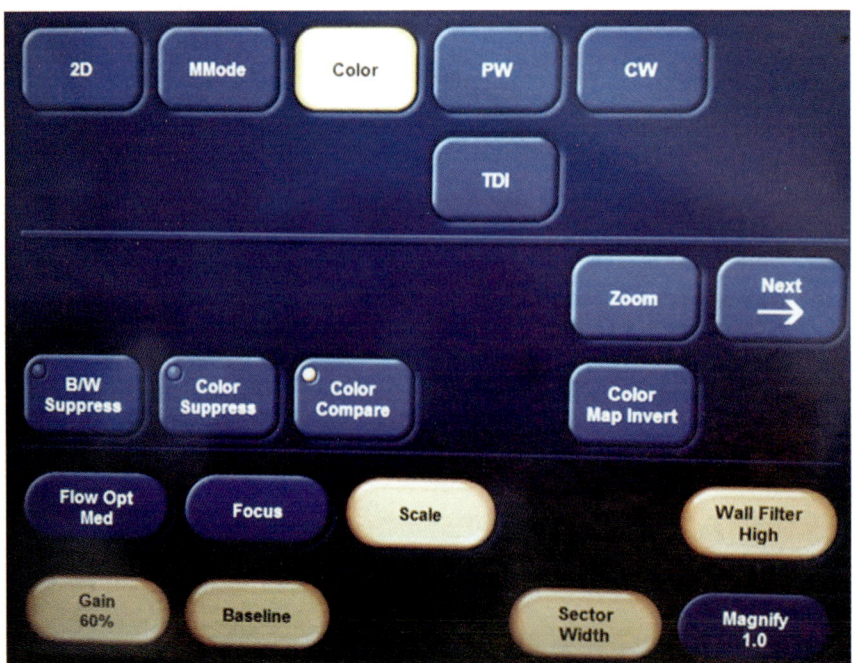

Fig. 2.20: The TEE machine console highlighting the color Doppler controls.

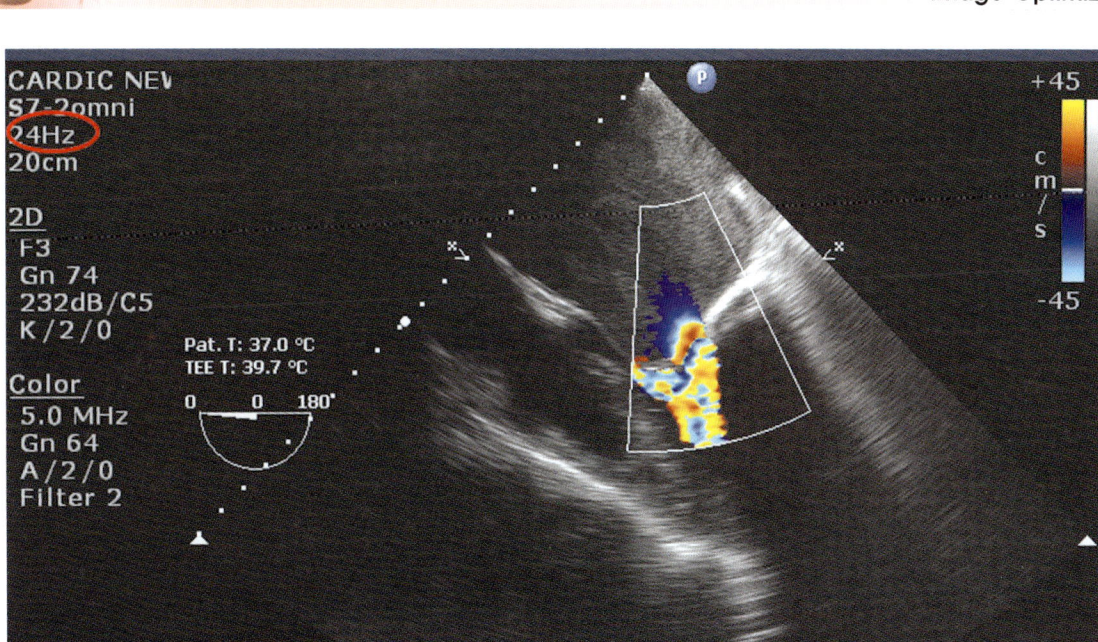

Fig. 2.21: Midesophageal 4-chamber view showing that a narrow color box increases the frequency (24 Hz) and thereby, the resolution.

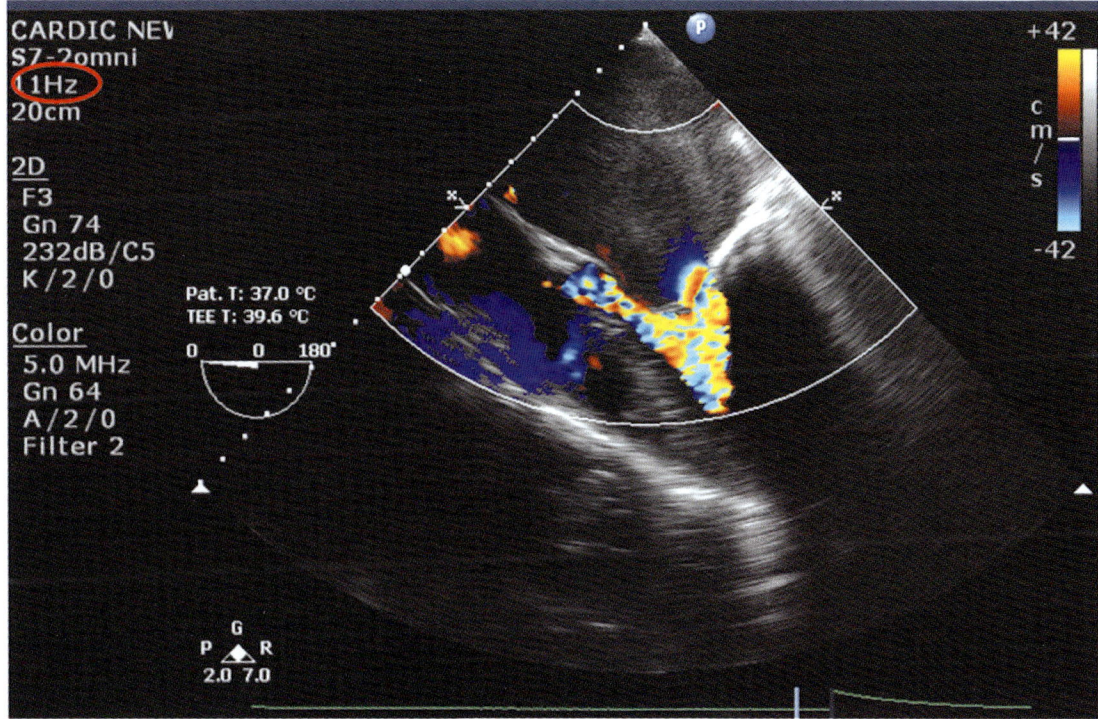

Fig. 2.22: Midesophageal 4-chamber view showing that a wider color box decreases the frequency (11 Hz) and thereby, the resolution (compare with Fig. 2.21).

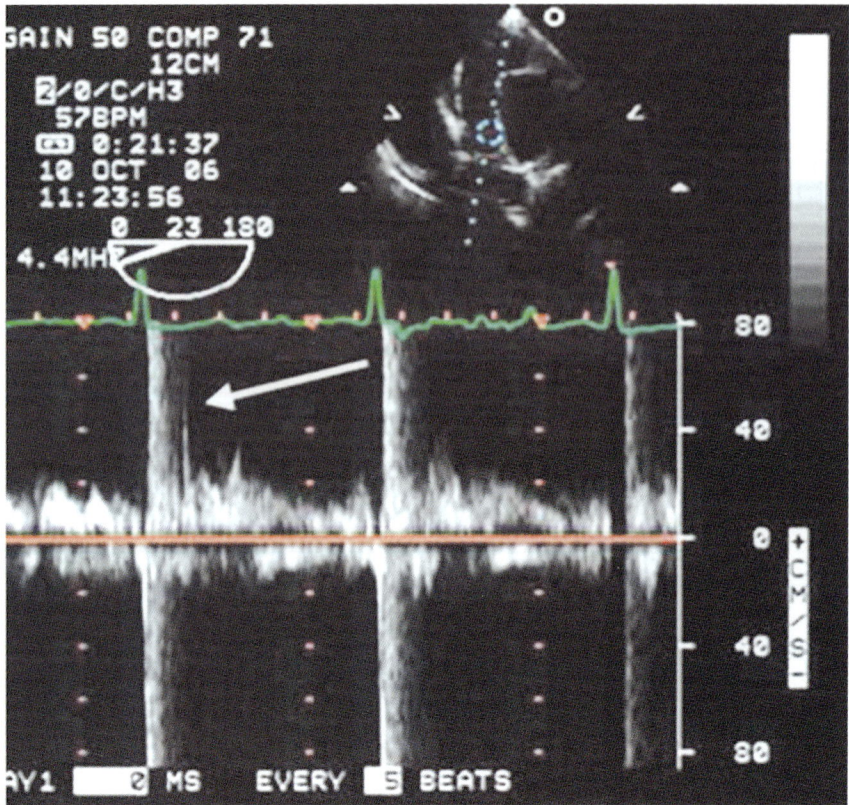

Fig. 2.23: Deep transgastric view showing cut-off of the aortic flow profile and its appearance above the baseline (arrow), implying aliasing.

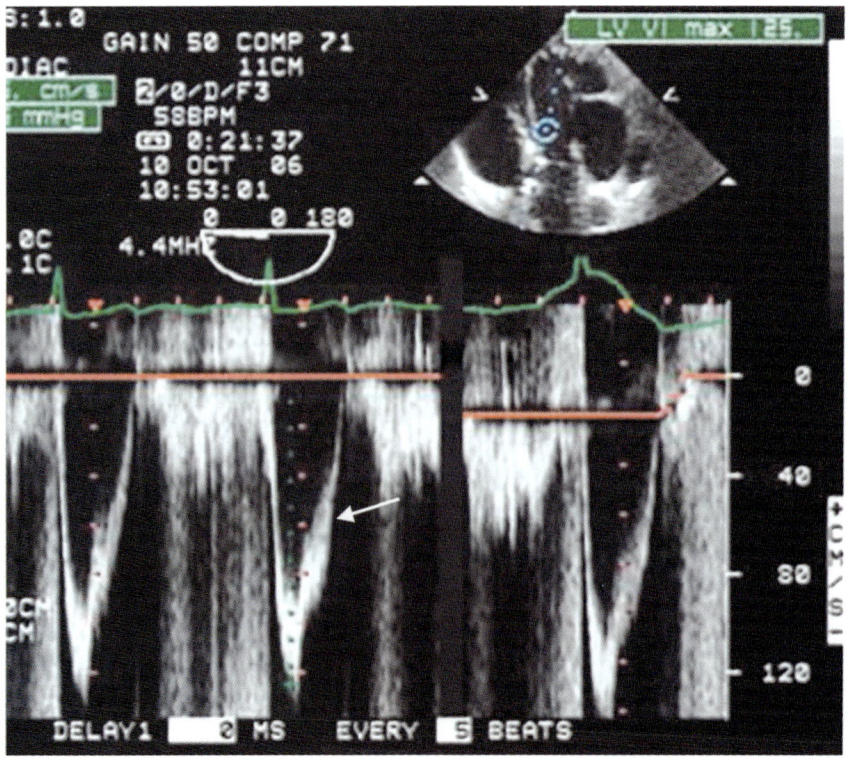

Fig. 2.24: Shifting the baseline upwards accommodates the entire pulse wave Doppler envelope (arrow).

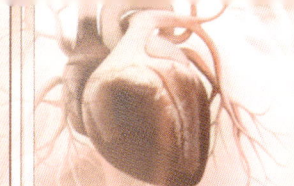

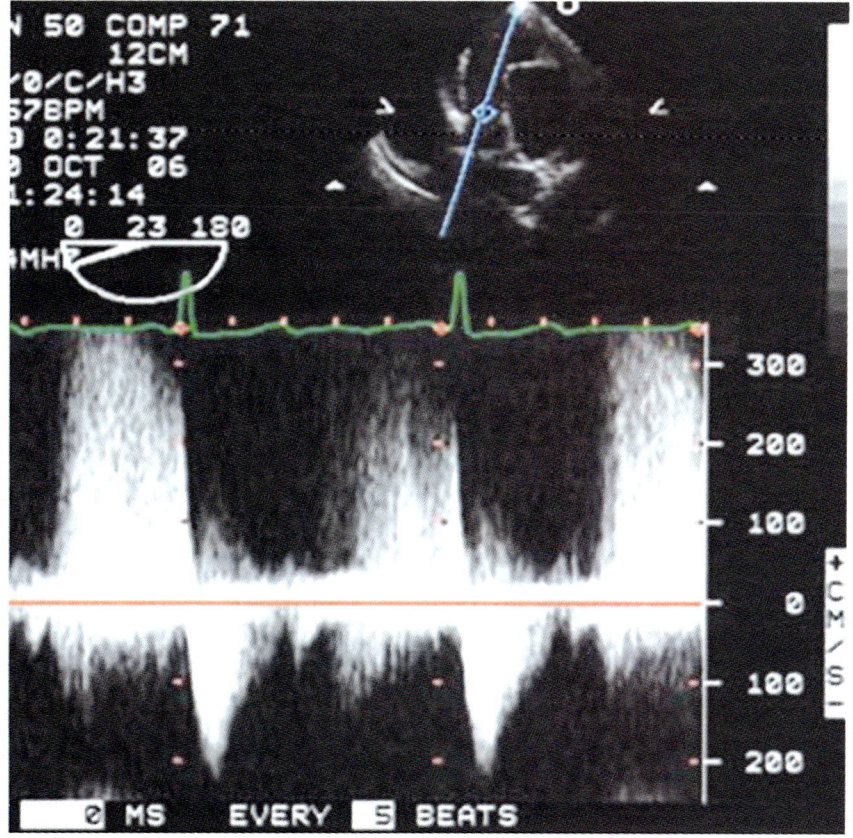

Fig. 2.25: Aliasing can also be prevented by resorting to the use of continuous wave Doppler and increasing the scale to accommodate the velocity.

3

Comprehensive Transesophageal Echocardiography Examination

• Deepak K. Tempe • Suruchi Hasija

INTRODUCTION

Transesophageal echocardiography (TEE) is an accepted monitoring tool inside the cardiac operation theater. Although, its use was first described in 1980, it did not become commonplace until high-frequency transducers and color Doppler imaging became available in the mid-1980s. In India, it became available only in the late 1990s. The improvement in the quality of the acoustic image has enabled the anesthesiologists and surgeons to use TEE intraoperatively to diagnose myocardial ischemia, confirm the adequacy of valve and other surgical repairs, determine the cause of hemodynamic disorders and other intraoperative complications, and provide diagnostic information that could not be obtained preoperatively. Indeed, the use of TEE has facilitated the prevention and early treatment of perioperative complications. The advantages of TEE over the conventional transthoracic echocardiography include better acoustic images and continuation of monitoring even when the chest is open during the surgery.

Anesthesiologists using the TEE must have adequate knowledge of the cardiac anatomy, physiology and ultrasound technology. In addition, he must acquire the essential technical skills for the use of TEE.

TECHNIQUE OF TEE EXAMINATION

Initially, a monoplane probe was used for TEE. With the advances in the ultrasound technology, a biplane probe was introduced in the early 1990s and was soon replaced by the omniplane (multiplane) probe. Perioperatively, TEE is performed in the supine position in an anesthetized and intubated patient or sedated or unconscious patient in the operation theater or intensive care unit.

It should be ensured before the insertion of the probe that it has been disinfected and that the control wheels are working and unlocked. Basically, the probe is a gastroscope equipped with ultrasound instead of fiberoptic technology. The phased-array transducer is integrated into the flexible tip of the probe that has a diameter of 10–15 mm and length of 20–45 mm. The shaft of the probe has a diameter of 9–10 mm and is about 100 cm long. The position of the flexible tip can be varied by rotation of the two steering wheels at the handle of the probe. The bigger wheel helps anteflexion or retroflexion, whereas the smaller wheel provides left and right lateral flexion. The wheels and, therefore, the tip of the probe can be locked in an optimum position for monitoring purposes (Fig. 3.1).

Probe Insertion

The ultrasound machine is positioned behind the patient's head at the left side. The insertion of the probe must be smooth and no force should be applied. The stomach should be aspirated and gastric tube removed before insertion of the probe. This helps to remove the

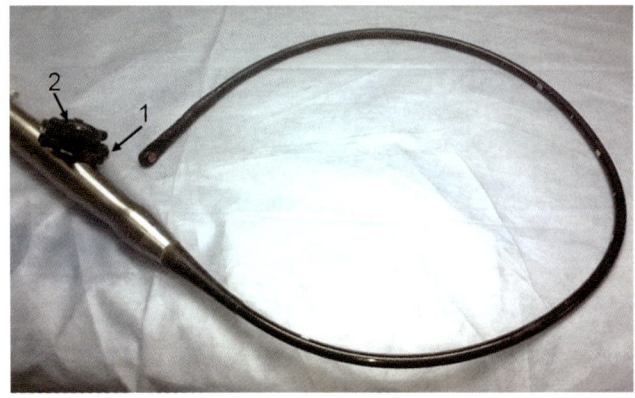

Fig. 3.1: Adult TEE Probe. The probe is a 100 cm modified gastroscope. There are two control knobs present on the handle of the probe. The larger inner knob (arrow 1) controls anterior and posterior flexion and the smaller outer knob (arrow 2) controls leftward and rightward angulation.

gastric secretions as well as air that might degrade the quality of the image. The assistant holds the handle of the probe and the operator opens the mouth and lifts the jaw of the patient with the left hand and with the right hand he gently introduces the tip (that is lubricated with lignocaine jelly) into the oropharynx and esophagus. A slight degree of anteflexion of the tip may be required for the entry into the esophagus. The biting block should be used in all patients (except those who are edentulous) so that the injury to the probe by teeth is prevented during movement of the probe. Some operators use index and middle finger of the left hand to guide the probe through the pharynx. This blind technique of probe insertion is almost always successful but increased jaw and chin lift or slight rotation of the head may be required. Very rarely, laryngoscope may be necessary to facilitate the insertion. The probe is advanced approximately 30 cm from the teeth and is connected to the console. A hyperinflated tracheal cuff of the endotracheal tube may offer resistance high in the esophagus, while stenosis or stricture of the hiatus may do so lower down in the esophagus. It must be remembered that force should not be applied to overcome resistance at any stage during the probe insertion.

Manipulation of the Probe

With the omniplane probe, the steering of the ultrasound beam is automated, usually by pressing a knob on the handle. However, some manually controlled movement of the probe will be necessary to obtain the optimum image in a given patient. Transverse plane imaging (usually 0° angle on the multiplane probe) usually provides transverse or horizontal sections of the heart, whereas longitudinal plane imaging gives longitudinal or vertical sections. During longitudinal plane examination, right (clockwise) or left (anticlockwise) rotation of the probe can shift the vertical plane to the right or left. With the right rotation, the vertical plane shifts to the right so that right sided structures such as superior vena cava

and right pulmonary veins are visualized, whereas left rotation helps to visualize left sided structures such as left atrial appendage and the left pulmonary veins. Thus, the probe requires up (withdrawing the probe) and down (advancing the probe) movements in order to obtain transverse sections of the heart at various levels (Fig. 3.2) and rotation of the probe to obtain vertical sections. With the help of the knobs on the handle and the manual movement of the probe, a comprehensive examination of various cardiac structures can be performed using the multiplane probe (Fig. 3.3).

A small semicircular icon on the screen displays the position of the imaging plane between 0° and 180°. The transducer scanning sector is fan-shaped, and appears as such on the monitor screen. The narrowest portion of the fan lies closest to the transducer (posterior aspect). The wide portion of the fan represents anterior aspect of the image.

The practice guidelines of the American Society of Echocardiography (ASE), Council for Intraoperative Echocardiography, and the Society of Cardiovascular Anesthesiologists Task Force for Certification in Perioperative Transesophageal Echocardiography recommend 20 standard views for comprehensive TEE examination (Table 3.1).

The order in which the examination proceeds may vary from examiner to examiner. In general, the midesophageal (ME) views are obtained first. The author recommends a simplified following method for obtaining all the views, which is especially useful for the beginners. The method involves minimal probe movement and allows four views at each step of examination by merely changing the angle of the ultrasound imaging plane.

Step 1: The ME 4-chamber view is obtained first at 0 degree (Figs 3.4 and 3.5). Keeping the probe at the same position, by increasing the angle to 60–75°, 80–100° and 110–135°, ME commissural (Fig. 3.6), ME 2-chamber (Figs 3.7 and 3.8), and ME long-axis (Fig. 3.9) views are obtained respectively.

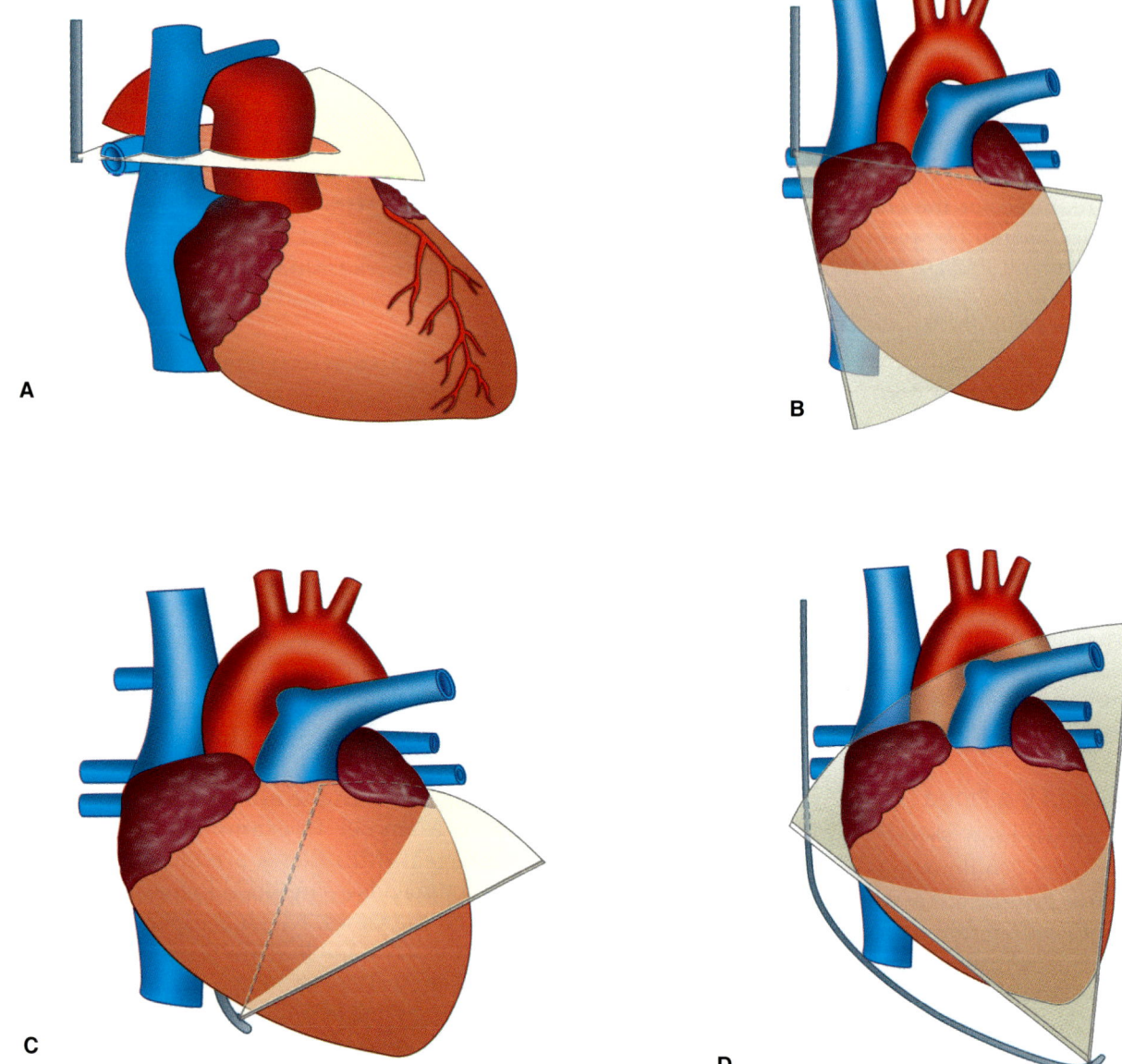

Fig. 3.2: Diagrammatic representation of ultrasound beam: (A) Upper esophageal view, (B) Mid esophageal view, (C) Transgastric view; (D) Deep transgastric view.

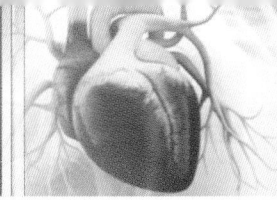

Table 3.1: Standard TEE views and additional views

	View	Angle (°)	Sector depth (cm)	Probe adjustments	Structures visualized
	STANDARD VIEWS				
1.	ME 4-chamber	0–10	12–14	Retroflexed	LA, LV, RA, RV, MV, TV
2.	ME mitral commissural	60–75	12	Neutral	LA, LV, MV, papillary muscles
3.	ME 2-chamber	80–100	12–14	Neutral	LAA, MV, LV
4.	ME LV LAX	110–130	12–14	Neutral	LA, MV, LV, LVOT, AV, proximal ascending aorta
5.	ME AV SAX	25–45	10–12	Neutral	AV leaflets, commissures, coaptation point
6.	ME RV inflow-outflow	50–70	10–12	Neutral	TV, RV, PV, proximal main PA
7.	ME AV LAX	115–130	8–10	Neutral	LVOT, AV, ascending aorta
8.	ME bicaval	100–110	8–10	Rightward	RA, SVC, IAS, IVC, LA
9.	TG basal SAX	0	12	Neutral, Anteflexed	Mitral leaflets, LV (basal segment)
10.	TG midpapillary SAX	0	12	Anteflexed	LV cavity, LV walls, papillary muscles
11.	TG 2-chamber	90	12	Neutral	Mitral leaflets, mitral subvalvular apparatus, LV
12.	TG LAX	110–130	12	Neutral to leftward	Mitral leaflets, mitral subvalvular apparatus, LV, LVOT, AV, proximal ascending aorta
13.	TG RV inflow	110–130	12	Neutral to rightward	RA, TV, tricuspid subvalvular apparatus, RV
14.	Deep TG LAX	0	16	Anteflexed	LV, AV, ascending aorta
15.	Descending aorta SAX	0	6	Leftward	Descending aorta
16.	Descending aorta LAX	90	6	Neutral	Descending aorta
17.	ME ascending aorta SAX	10–30	12	Withdraw 1–2 cm from AV SAX view	Aorta, main and proximal right PA
18.	ME ascending aorta LAX	100	10–12	Neutral	Ascending aorta, right PA
19.	UE aortic arch LAX	0	10	Withdraw from descending aorta SAX view, rightward, downward	Distal ascending aorta, aortic arch
20.	UE aortic arch SAX	90	10	Neutral	Aortic arch, main PA
	ADDITIONAL VIEWS				
1.	ME 5-chamber	0–10	12–14	Neutral, retroflexed	LA, LV, RA, RV, MV, TV, IVS, AV, LVOT
2.	ME modified bicaval	110	8–10	Rightward	RA, LA, IAS, coronary sinus, TV, SVC, IVC
3.	ME left atrial appendage	90–110		Neutral	LAA, left upper pulmonary vein
4.	ME right pulmonary vein	0–30		Neutral	Mid-ascending aorta, SVC, right pulmonary veins
5.	UE right and left pulmonary veins	90–110		Rightward or leftward for right or left pulmonary veins, respectively	Pulmonary veins, pulmonary artery
6.	TG RV basal	0–20		Anteflex	LV (mid), RV (mid), RVOT, TV, PV
7.	TG RV inflow-outflow	0–20	16	Rightward	RA, RV, RVOT, PV, TV
8.	TG apical SAX	0–20		Anteflex	LV (apex), RV (apex)
	MORE VIEWS				
1.	LE hepatic	20		Rightward	RA, hepatic vein, IVC
2.	LE coronary sinus	0–10	12–14	Retroflexed	Coronary sinus, TV

TEE: transesophageal echocardiography, ME: midesophageal, LA: left atrium, LV: left ventricle, RA: right atrium, RV: right ventricle, MV: mitral valve, TV: tricuspid valve, IAS: interatrial septum, IVS: interventricular septum, LAA: left atrial appendage, LAX: long-axis, LVOT: left ventricular outflow tract, RVOT: right ventricular outflow tract, AV: aortic valve, SAX: short-axis, PV: pulmonary valve. PA: pulmonary artery, SVC: superior vena cava, IVC: inferior vena cava, TG: transgastric, UE: upper esophageal, LE: lower esophageal

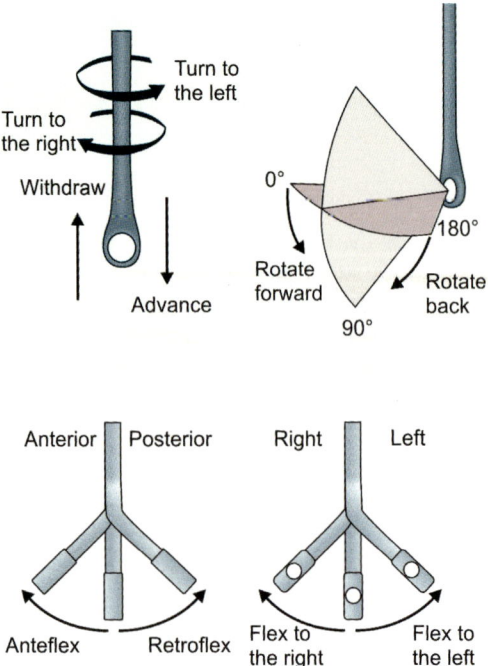

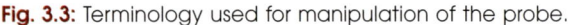

Fig. 3.3: Terminology used for manipulation of the probe.

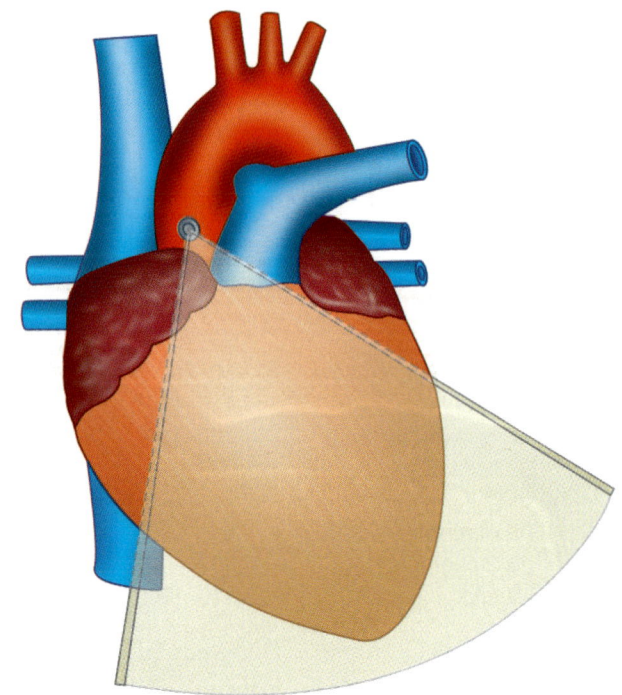

Fig. 3.4: Diagrammatic representation of ultrasound beam in midesophageal 4-chamber view.

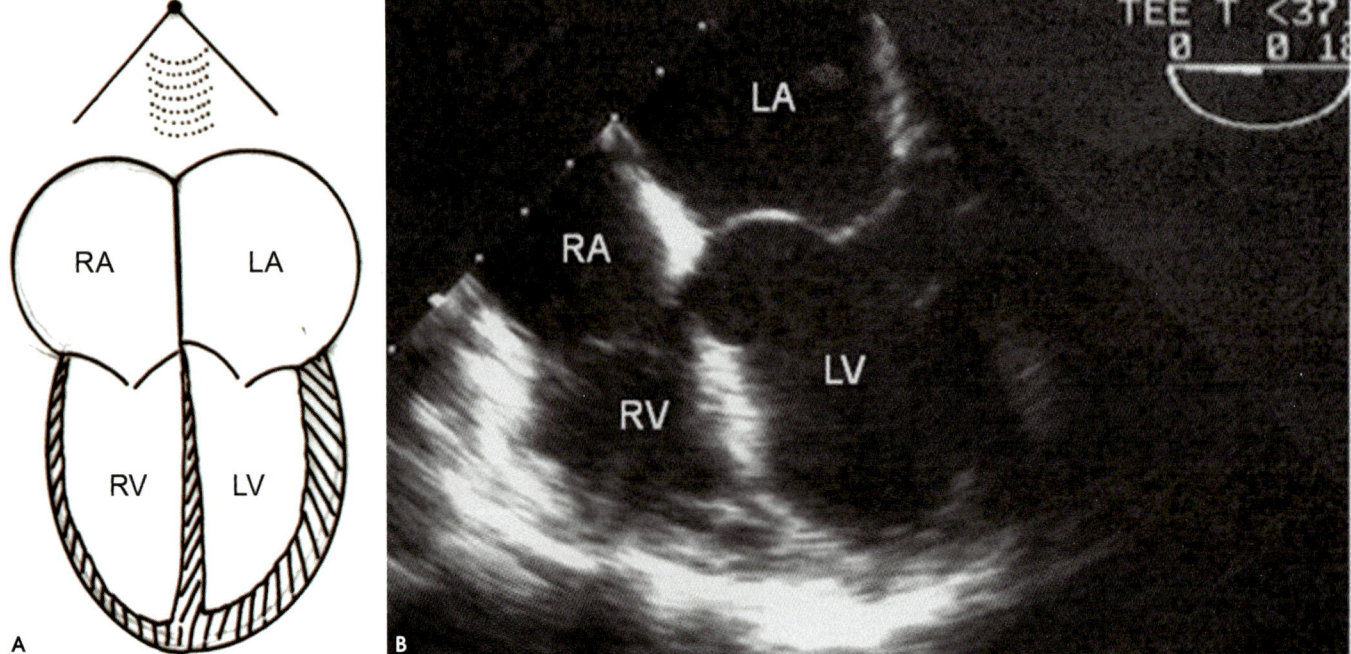

Fig. 3.5: Midesophageal 4-chamber view (0–10°). (A) Diagrammatic representation of the 4-chamber view; (B) This is the standard four-chamber view showing both atria and both ventricles. The lateral free walls of both ventricles and the posterior portion of the interventricular septum are seen. The mitral valve is close to the transducer and can be examined in detail. (LA: Left atrium, RA: right atrium, LV: Left ventricle, RV: right ventricle).

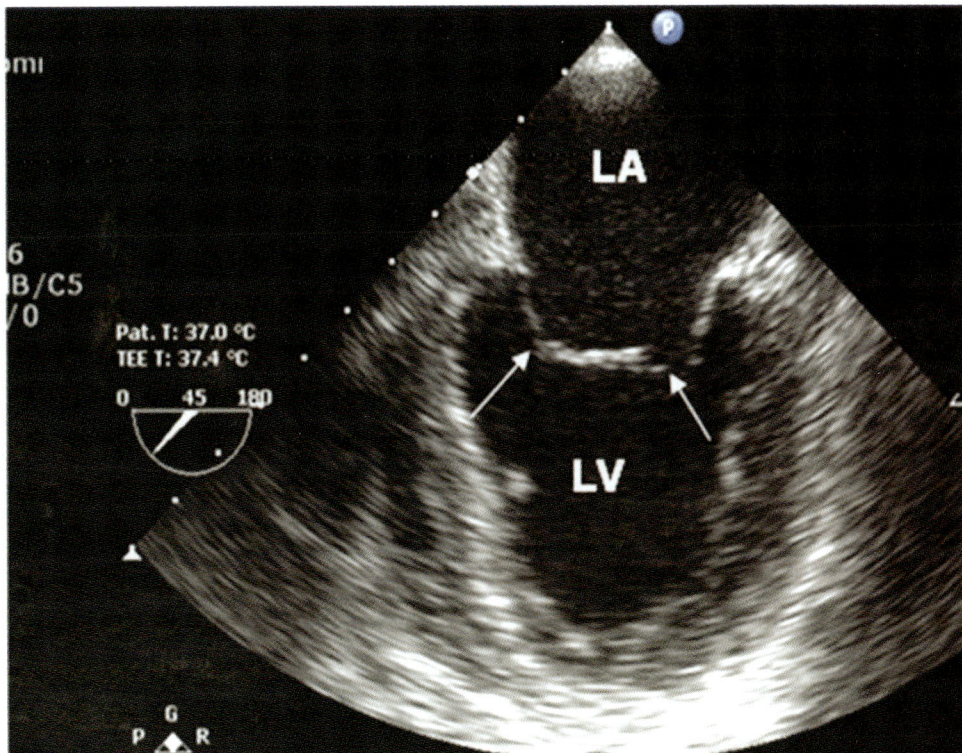

Fig. 3.6: Midesophageal mitral commissural view. By rotating the plane to 60–75°, the two chamber view with the left atrium at the top and the left ventricle below is obtained. The arrows indicate the coaptation points between A2–P3 (left arrow) and A2–P1 (right arrow) segments of the mitral valve leaflets (LA: left atrium, LV: left ventricle).

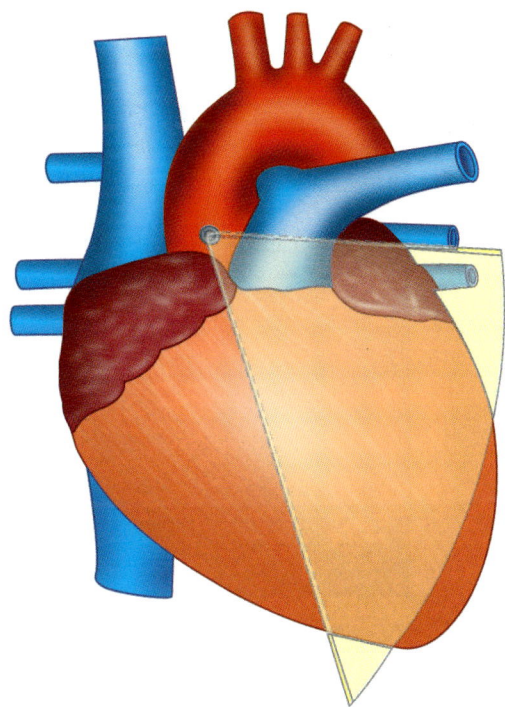

Fig. 3.7: Diagrammatic representation of the ultrasound beam in midesophageal 2-chamber view.

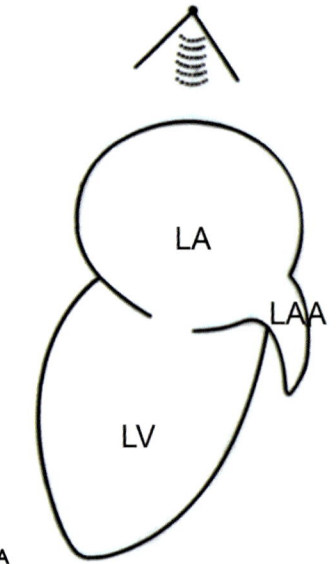

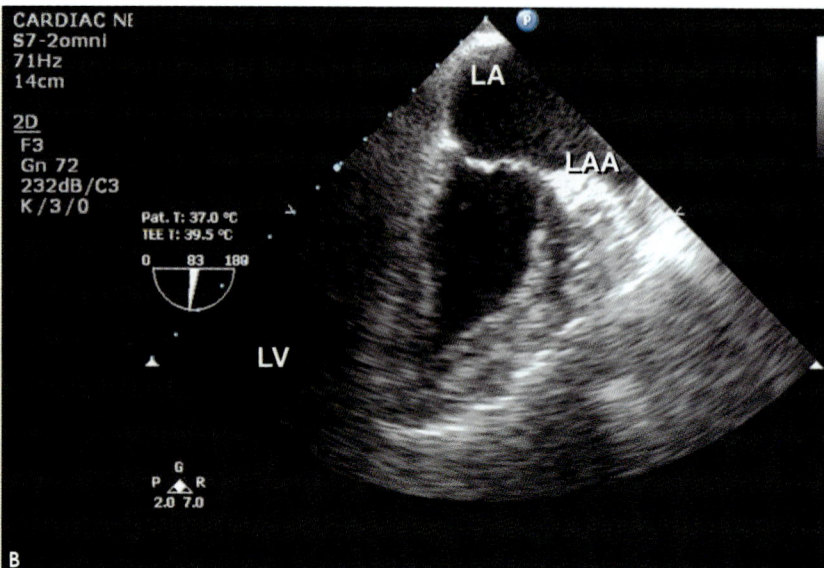

Fig. 3.8: Midesophageal two-chamber view (90°). (A) Diagrammatic representation; (B) By rotating the plane to 90°, the two-chamber view with the left atrium at the top and the left ventricle below is obtained. The view helps to examine the mitral valve and the left ventricular wall motion abnormality of the inferior wall (left of the sector) and anterior wall (right of the sector). The left atrial appendage can also be seen. (LA: left atrium, LV: left ventricle, LAA: left atrial appendage).

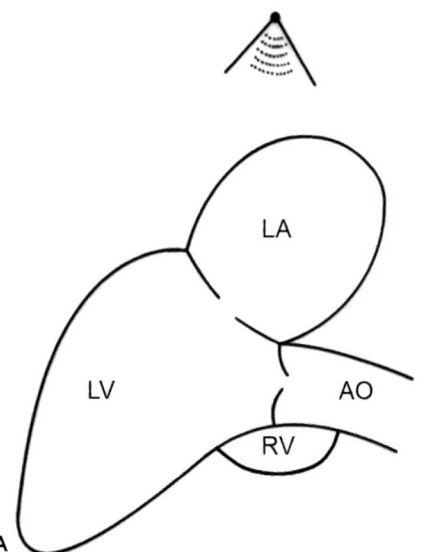

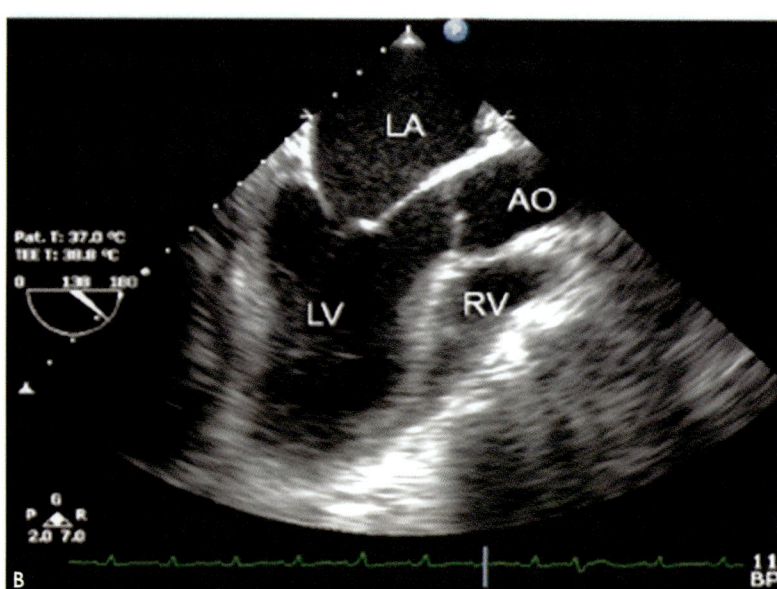

Fig. 3.9: Midesophageal long-axis view (110–130°). (A) Diagrammatic representation; (B) Rotation of the plane to 110–130° shows the midesophageal long-axis view. The long-axis view of the left atrium, left ventricular outflow, aortic valve and a part of the ascending aorta is obtained. The noncoronary (top) and right coronary cusps of the aortic valve are visible. This view helps to examine aortic and mitral valves, subaortic ventricular septal defect and regional wall motion abnormality of the anteroseptal and inferolateral walls of the left ventricle. (LA: left atrium, LV: left ventricle, RV: right ventricle, Ao: aorta).

Step 2: Next, the ME aortic valve (AV) short-axis view (Figs 3.10 and 3.11) is obtained by withdrawing the probe by 3–5 cm and adjusting the multiplane angle to 20–30°. The probe may have to be rotated rightward in order to display the AV. The image depth is adjusted to 10–12 cm as required to position the AV in the centre of the display screen. Keeping the probe at same position, by increasing the angle to 60–80°, and 115–130°, ME right ventricular (RV) inflow-outflow view (Figs 3.12 and 3.13) and ME AV long-axis views (Figs 3.14 and 3.15) respectively are obtained. By rotating the probe to right from the ME AV long-axis view, bicaval view (Figs 3.16 and 3.17) is obtained.

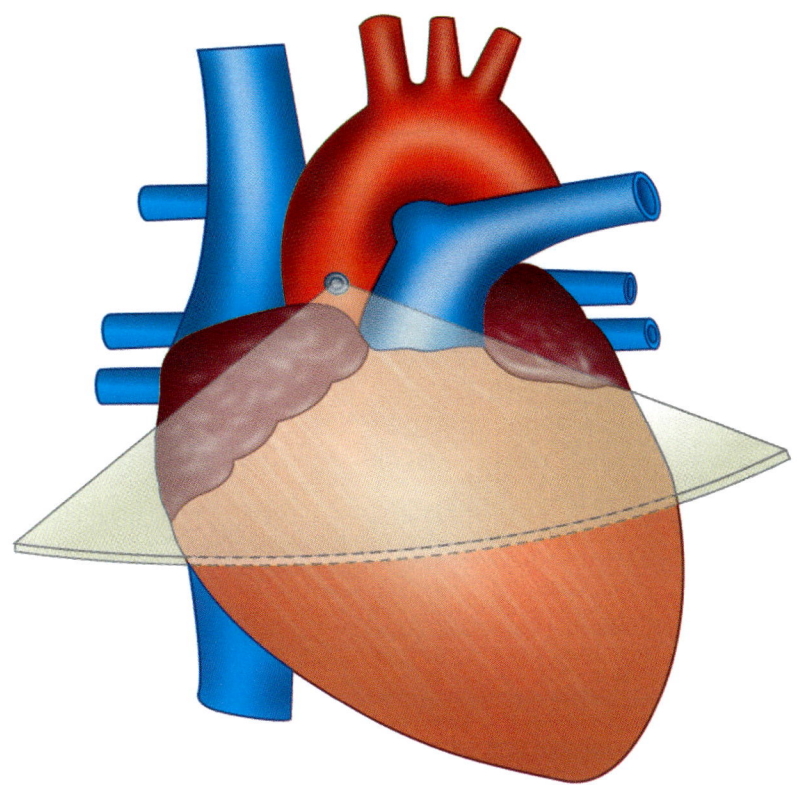

Fig. 3.10: Diagrammatic representation of ultrasound beam in midesophageal aortic valve short-axis view.

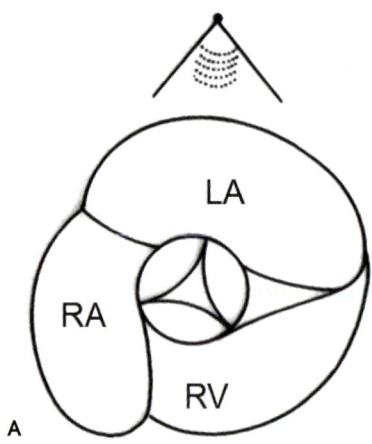

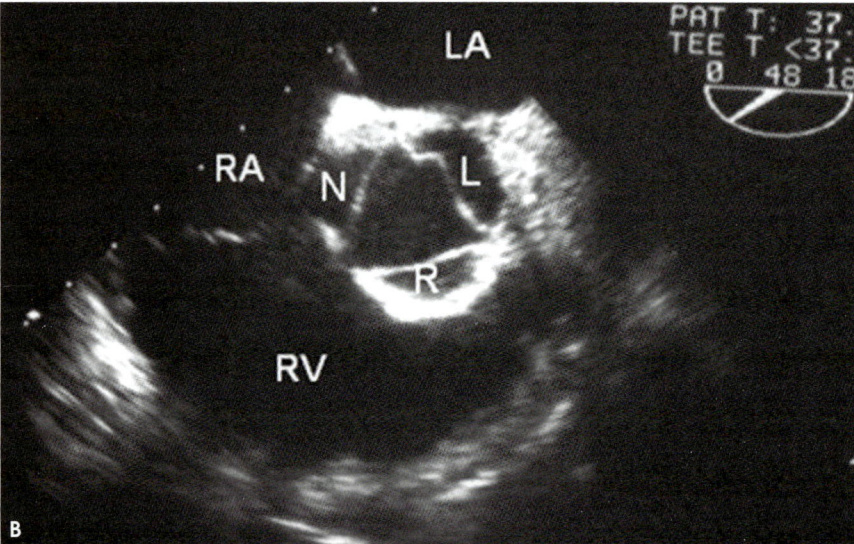

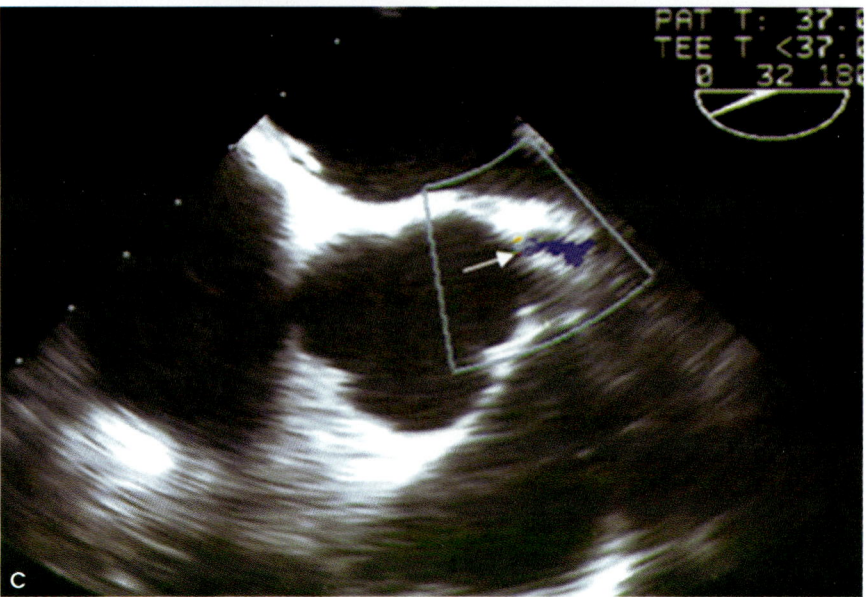

Fig. 3.11: Midesophageal aortic valve short-axis view (25–45°). (A) Diagrammatic representation; (B) This is an important view that images the aortic valve in short axis. The left coronary cusp (L) is on the right side of the image, the right coronary cusp (R) is at the bottom and the noncoronary cusp (N) lies on the left side of the image. (C) By withdrawing the probe, the left main coronary artery can be seen originating at this level (arrow) and can be followed further till its bifurcation.

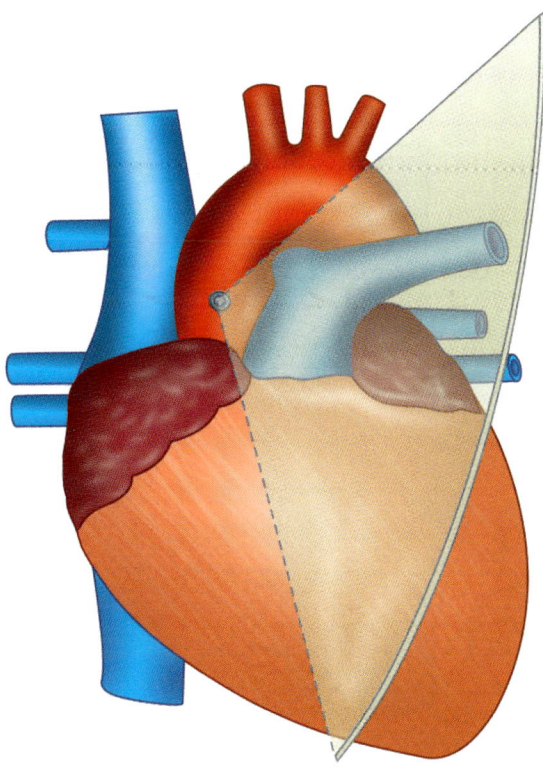

Fig. 3.12: Diagrammatic representation of the ultrasound beam in midesophageal right ventricular inflow-outflow view.

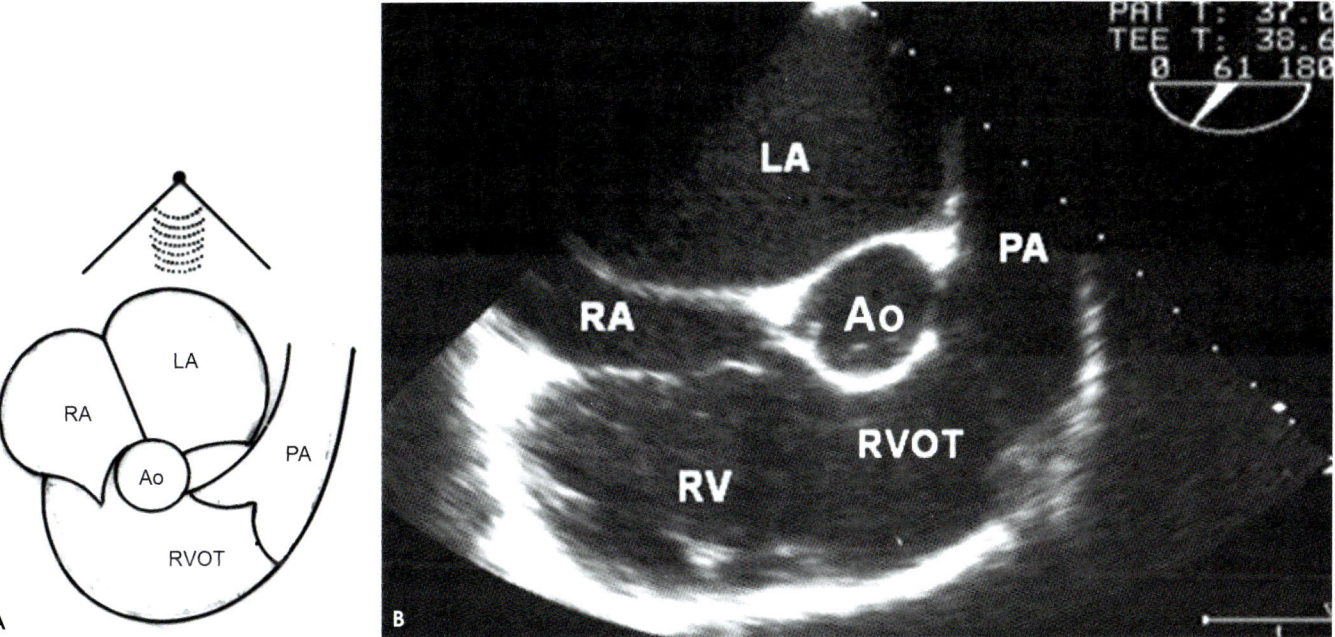

Fig. 3.13: Midesophageal right ventricular inflow-outflow view (50–70°). (A) Diagrammatic representation; (B) The transverse section of the aorta remains in the middle and left atrium lies at the top of the screen, while from left to right of the image, the right atrium, tricuspid valve, right ventricle, pulmonary valve, and the main pulmonary artery are visualized as they circle around the aorta. The view is useful for the evaluation of the right ventricular outflow tract, especially in the congenital lesions involving the right ventricle and pulmonary artery (LA: left atrium, RA: right atrium, RV: right ventricle, Ao: aorta, RVOT: right ventricular outflow tract, PA: pulmonary artery).

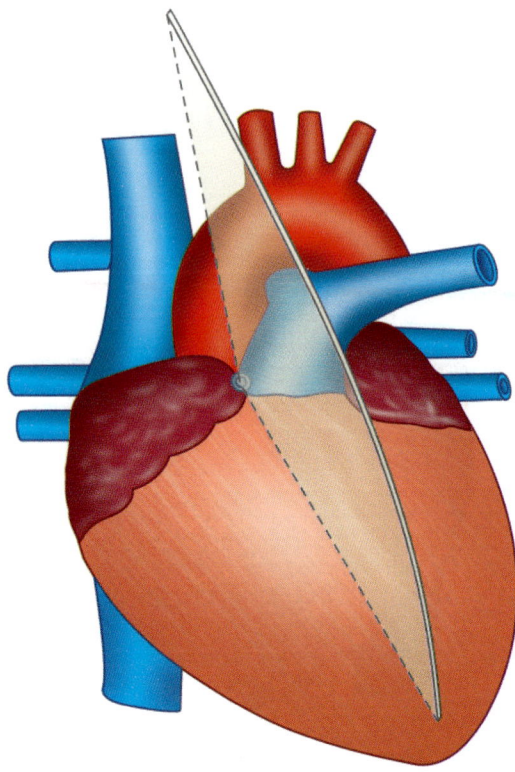

Fig. 3.14: Diagrammatic representation of the ultrasound beam in midesophageal aortic valve long-axis view.

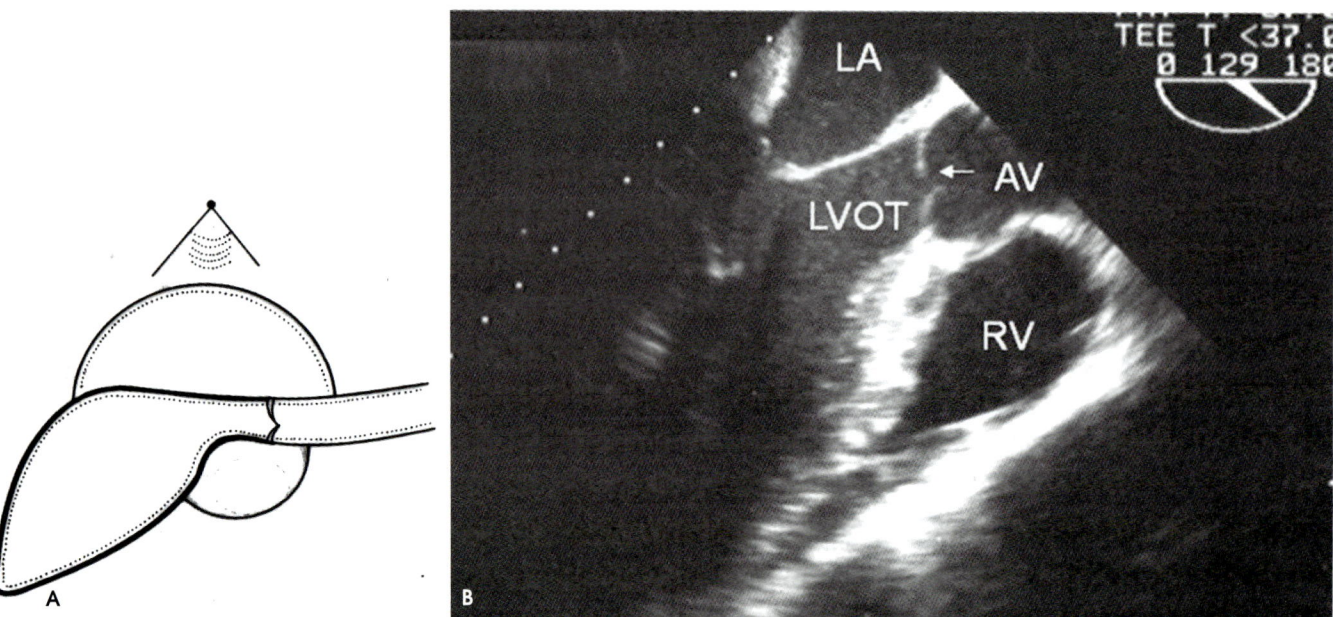

Fig. 3.15: Midesophageal aortic valve long-axis view (115–130°). (A) Diagrammatic representation; (B) The imaging plane beyond 110° displays the distal part of the left ventricular outflow tract, the aortic valve and ascending aorta in the longitudinal axis. (LA: left atrium, LVOT: left ventricular outflow tract, AV: aortic valve, RV: right ventricle).

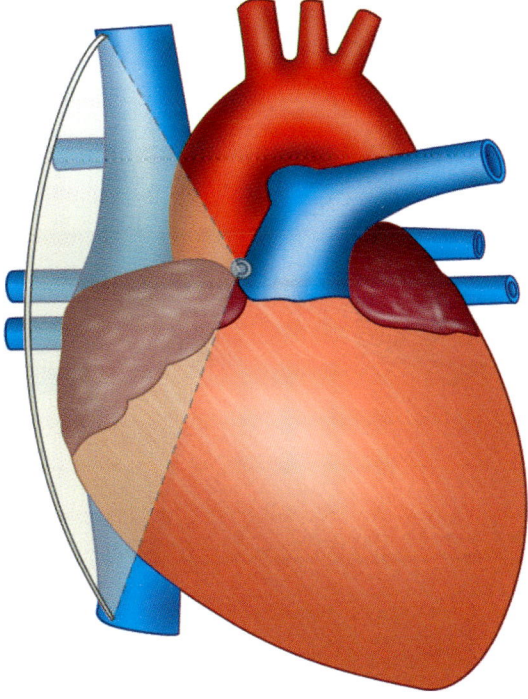

Fig. 3.16: Longitudinal beam through superior vena cava, inferior vena cava and atria (bicaval view).

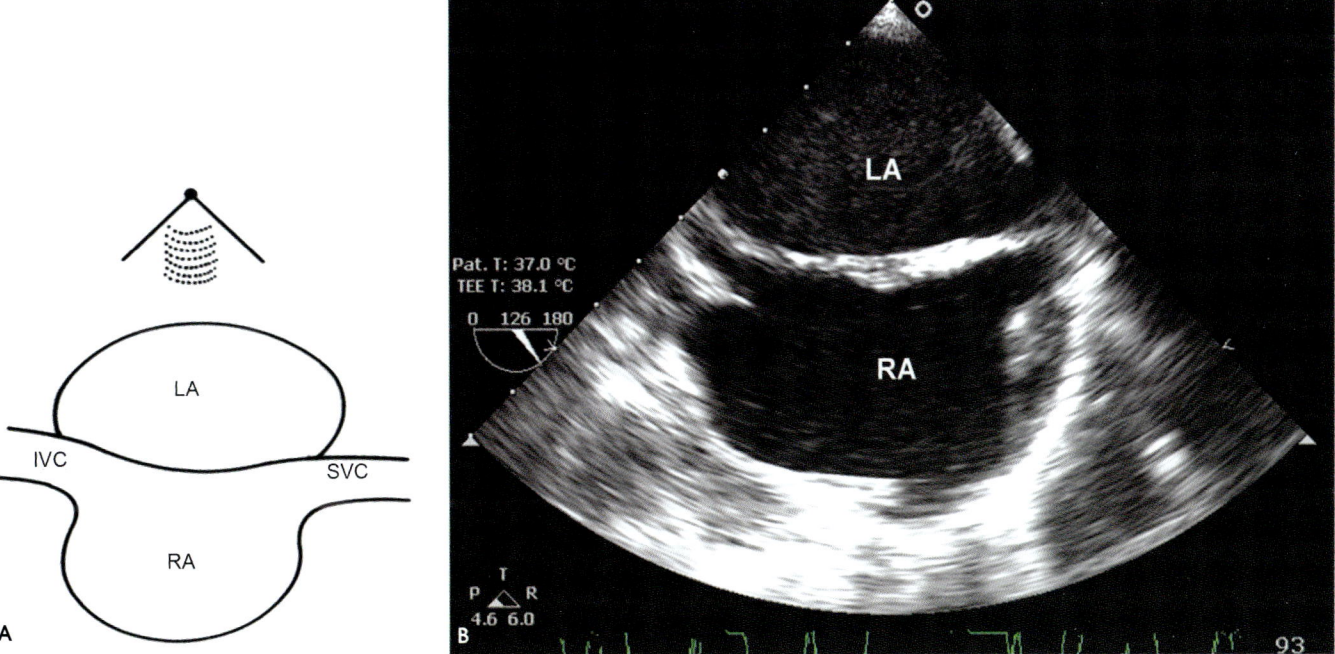

Fig. 3.17: Bicaval view (100–110°). (A) Diagrammatic representation; (B) This is an extremely important view for evaluating the anatomy of the interatrial septum. Left atrium lies at the top. (LA: left atrium, RA: right atrium).

Step 3: Next, the multiplane angle is set at zero and the probe is advanced into the stomach to obtain the transgastric (TG) views. By anteflexing the tip and right rotation of the probe, the transverse section, mid-papillary short-axis view is visualized (Figs 3.18 and 3.19). By withdrawing the probe upwards by 2–5 cm, the basal transgastric view of the LV is seen (Fig. 3.20). Keeping the probe at the same position, by increasing the angle to 90° and 110–135°, TG 2-chamber view (Fig. 3.21) and TG long-axis view (Fig. 3.22) are produced respectively.

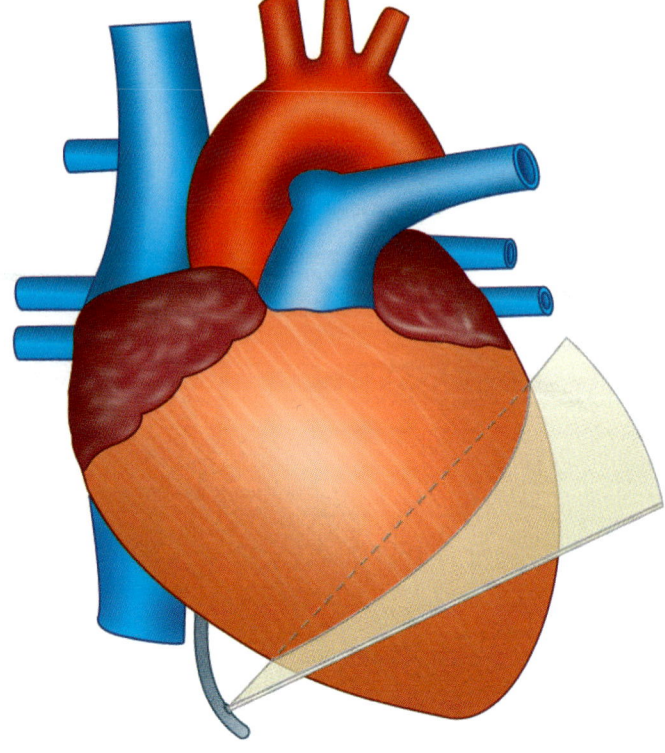

Fig. 3.18: Transverse beam through short-axis of the left ventricle at the level of papillary muscle (transgastric midpapillary view).

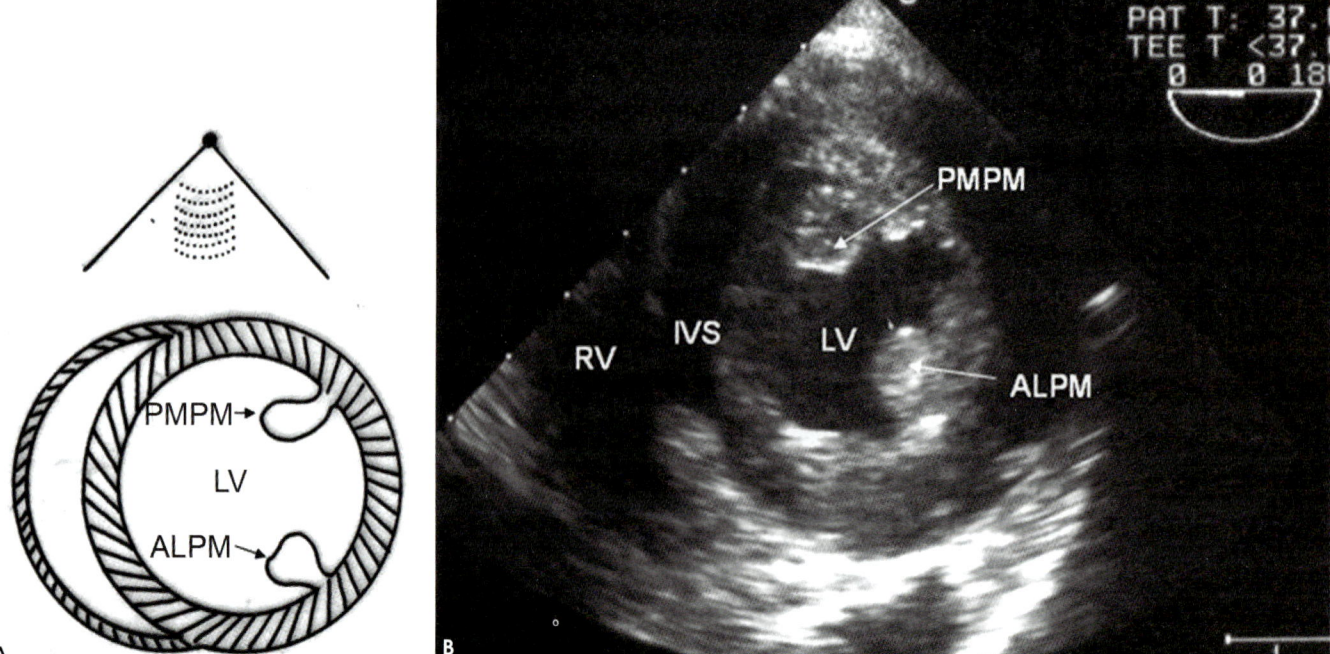

Fig. 3.19: Transgastric midpapillary short-axis view (0°). (A) Diagrammatic representation; (B) The standard short-axis view of the left ventricle at mid-papillary muscle level is the most commonly employed view. The inferior left ventricular wall lies at the top of the section, close to the transducer, and the anterior wall at the bottom. The interventricular septum is located on the left of the image and the lateral wall is seen on the right side. (PMPM: posteromedial papillary muscle, ALPM: anterolateral papillary muscle, IVS: interventricular septum, LV: left ventricle, RV: right ventricle).

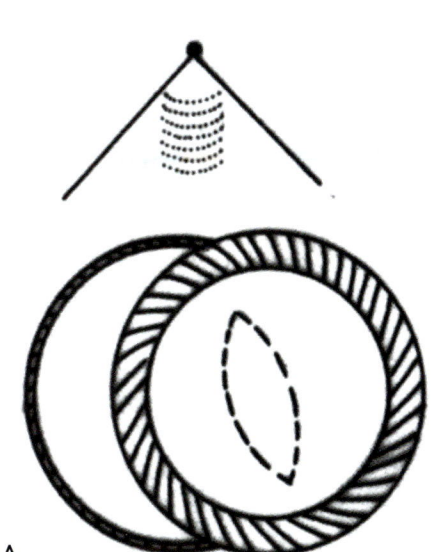

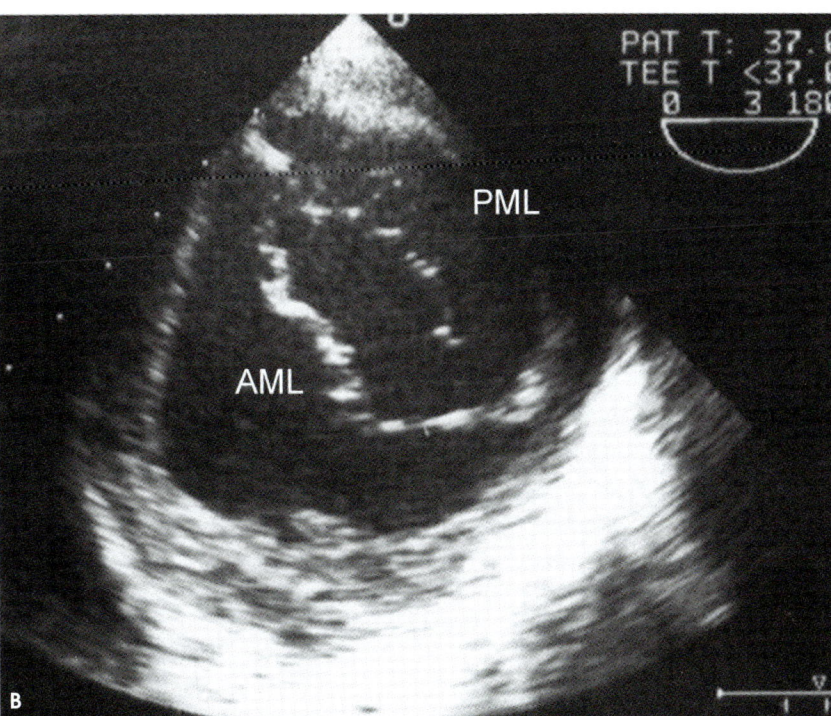

Fig. 3.20: Transgastric basal short-axis view (0°). (A) Diagrammatic representation; (B) This view displays the anterior mitral leaflet (AML), posterior mitral leaflet (PML), anterior and posterior commissures.

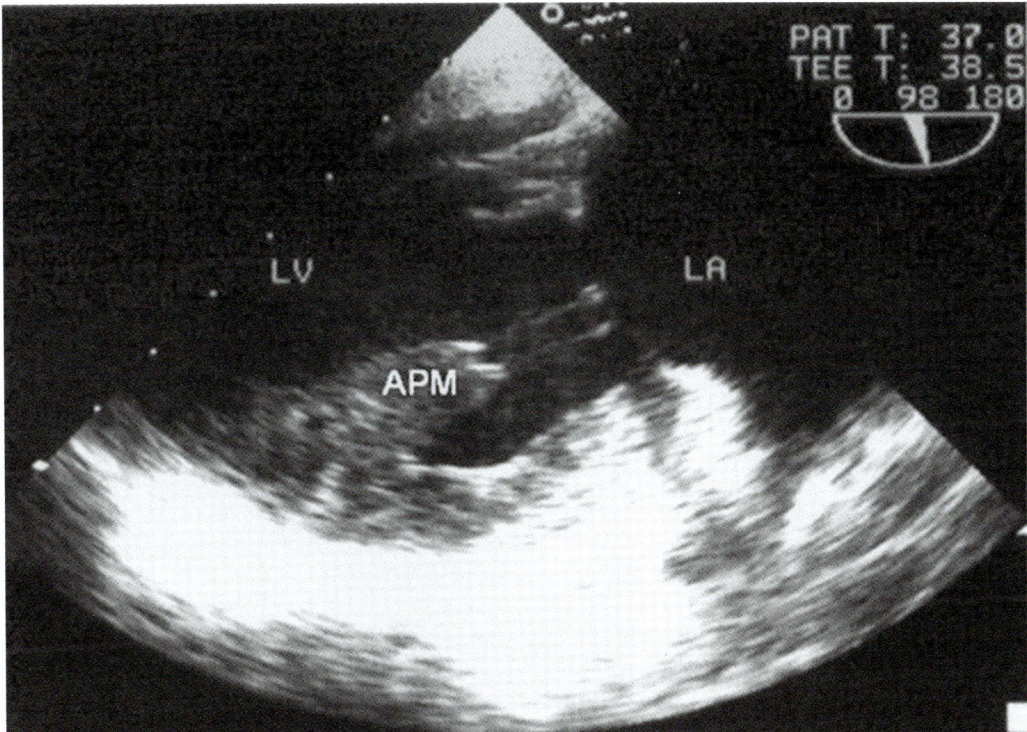

Fig. 3.21: Transgastric two-chamber view (90°). This view is derived from the short axis view of the left ventricle by rotating the imaging plane from 0–90° and beyond. At 90°, the long-axis view of the left atrium, mitral valve, two papillary muscles and the left ventricle is obtained. The anterior wall of the left ventricle is at the bottom, while the inferior wall is at the top (LA: left atrium, LV: Left ventricle, APM: anterior papillary muscle).

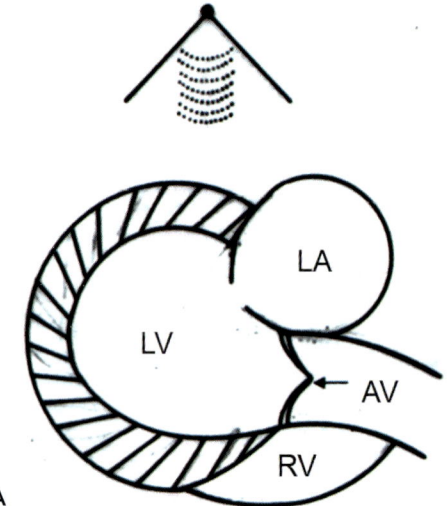
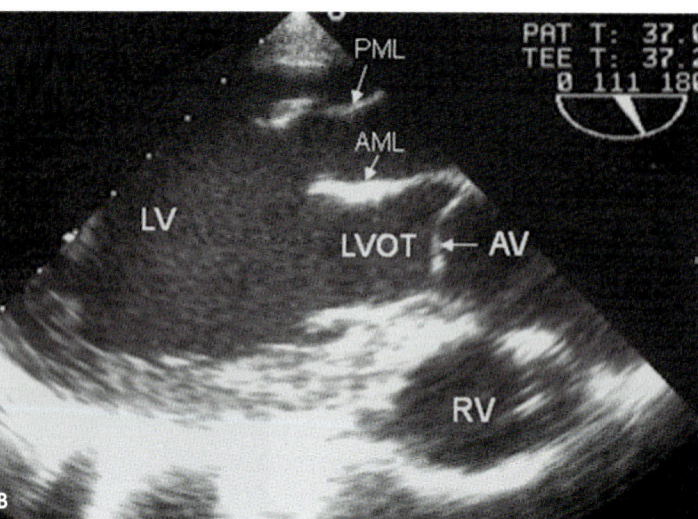

Fig. 3.22: Transgastric long-axis view (110–130°). (A) Diagrammatic representation. (B) At 110 to 130° the left ventricular outflow tract is seen to open into the aorta in its longitudinal course. This view can be used to perform Doppler interrogation of the aortic valve since the ultrasound beam is parallel to the direction of blood flow across the aortic valve in this view. (LA: left atrium, LV: left ventricle, AML: anterior mitral leaflet, PML: posterior mitral leaflet, LVOT: left ventricular outflow tract, AV: aortic valve, RV: right ventricle).

The deep TG view is obtained by advancing the probe deep into the stomach and positioning it adjacent to the LV apex. The probe is anteflexed to direct the imaging plane towards the base of the heart. The probe is then withdrawn gradually until the longitudinal section of the heart appears (Fig. 3.23). The image depth should be increased as required to position the image at the center of the display screen.

The tip of the probe may have to be moved sideways (by the knob on the handle or by rotating the probe) to center the image. This is a difficult view to obtain, but with a little practice, it can be obtained in most patients.

The TG RV inflow view is obtained by turning the probe to right after getting the TG mid-papillary view and increasing the angle to 100–110° (Fig. 3.24).

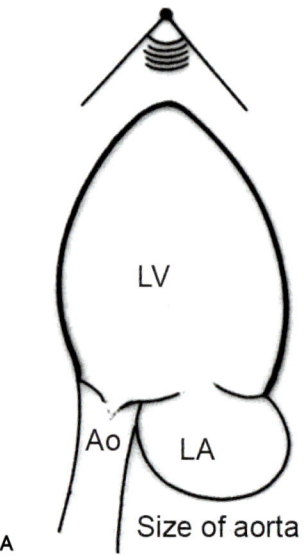
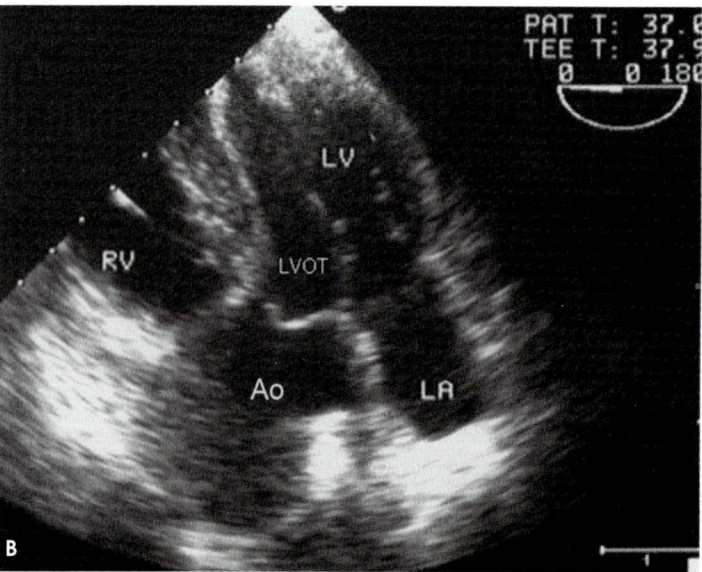

Fig. 3.23: Deep transgastric long-axis view (0°). (A) Diagrammatic representation; (B) With the imaging plane at 0°, a three chamber view with the left ventricular outflow tract, aortic valve and a proximal portion of ascending aorta in the center (left of the left atrium) is obtained. As this view allows an excellent alignment of the ultrasound beam and the blood flow out of the left ventricle, it remains the best view for Doppler measurement of cardiac output and the Doppler quantification of aortic stenosis. (LV: left ventricle, LVOT: left ventricular ourflow tract, Ao: aorta, LA: left atrium, RV: right ventricle).

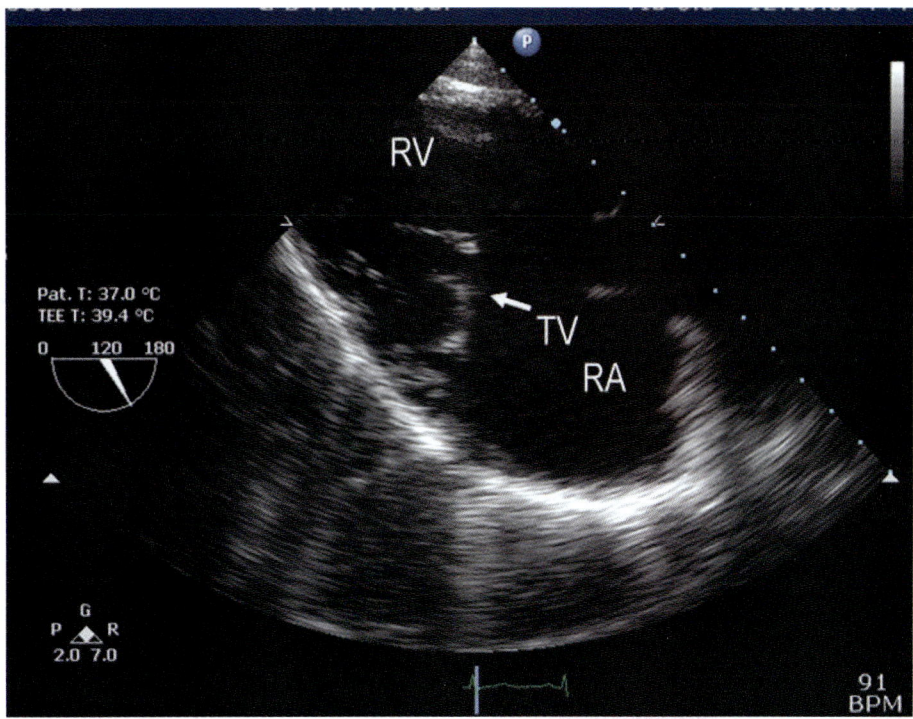

Fig. 3.24: Transgastric right ventricular inflow view (RA: right atrium, RV: right ventricle, TV: tricuspid valve).

Step 4: Aorta: The aorta can be examined almost completely barring the part of the ascending aorta where the trachea is interposed between the esophagus and the aorta. The AV short-axis view is achieved (step 2 above) and the probe is slowly withdrawn 1–3 cm while keeping the aorta in the center of the screen (Fig. 3.25). As the probe is withdrawn further, the sections of ascending aorta are seen until the image is lost due to interposed trachea.

The probe is reinserted and the multiplane angle is increased to 90–100° to view the ascending aorta in long-axis (Fig. 3.26). Next, the transducer angle is returned to 0° and the probe turned to left to reveal the descending thoracic aorta in short-axis (Fig. 3.27). By increasing the angle to 90°, descending thoracic aorta in long-axis (Fig. 3.28) is seen. The probe can be advanced to examine the entire length of the descending thoracic aorta.

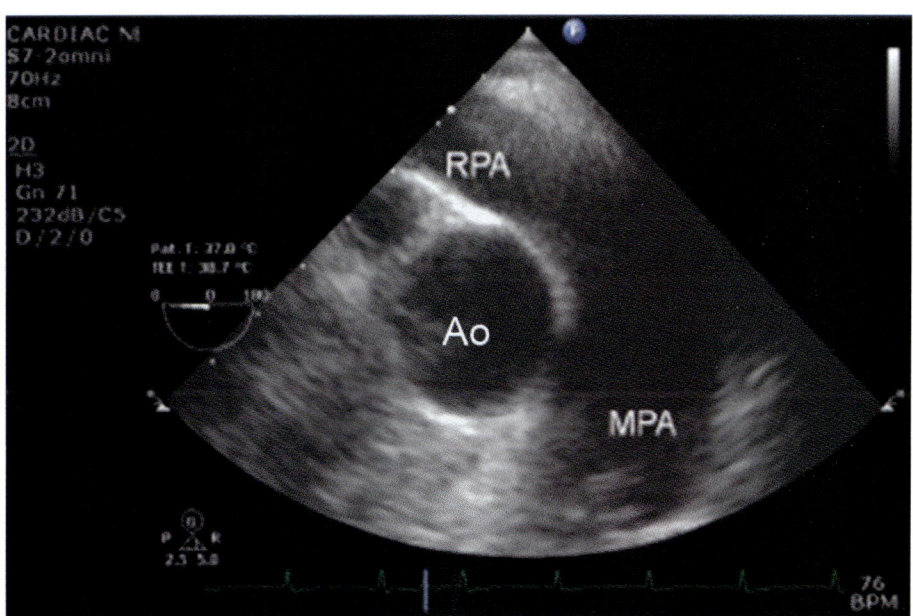

Fig. 3.25: Midesophageal ascending aortic short-axis view (RPA: right pulmonary artery, MPA: main pulmonary artery, Ao: aorta).

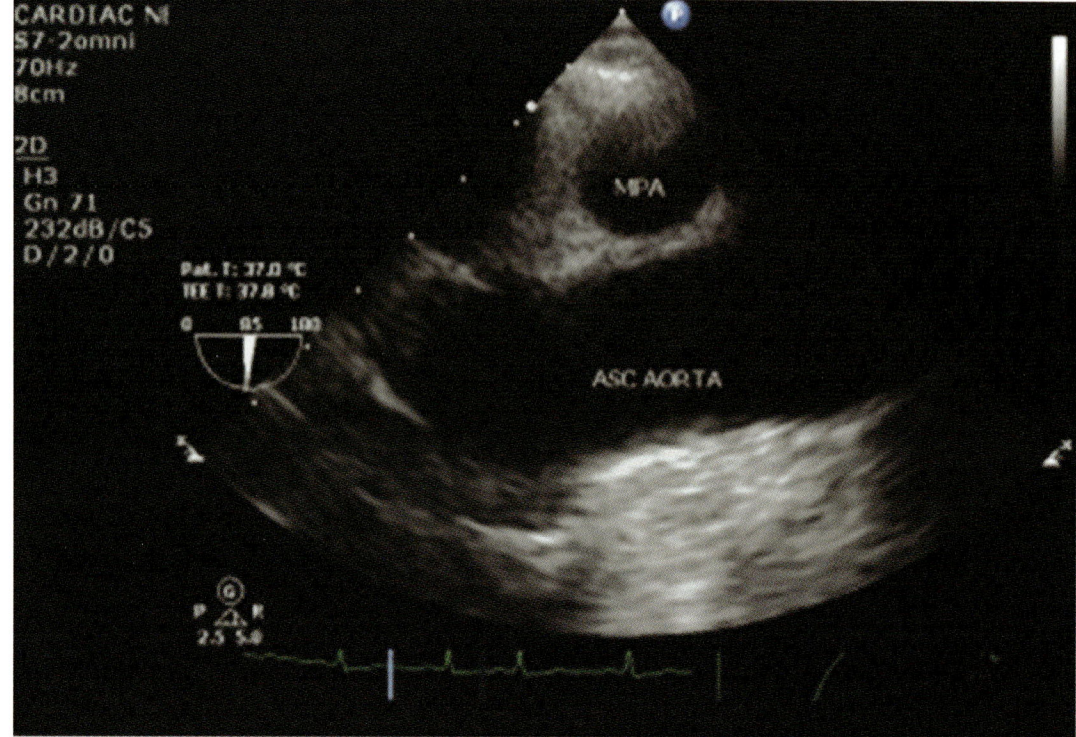

Fig. 3.26: Midesophageal ascending aortic long-axis view (MPA: main pulmonary artery).

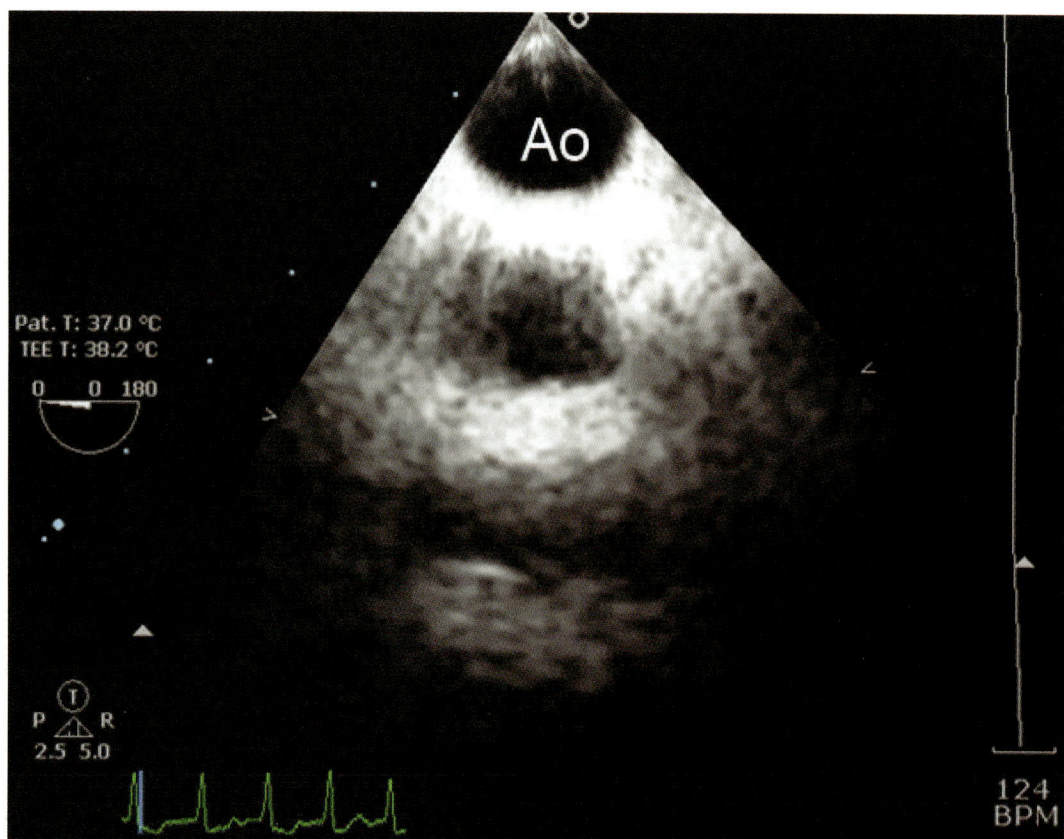

Fig. 3.27: Midesophageal descending aortic short-axis view (Ao: aorta).

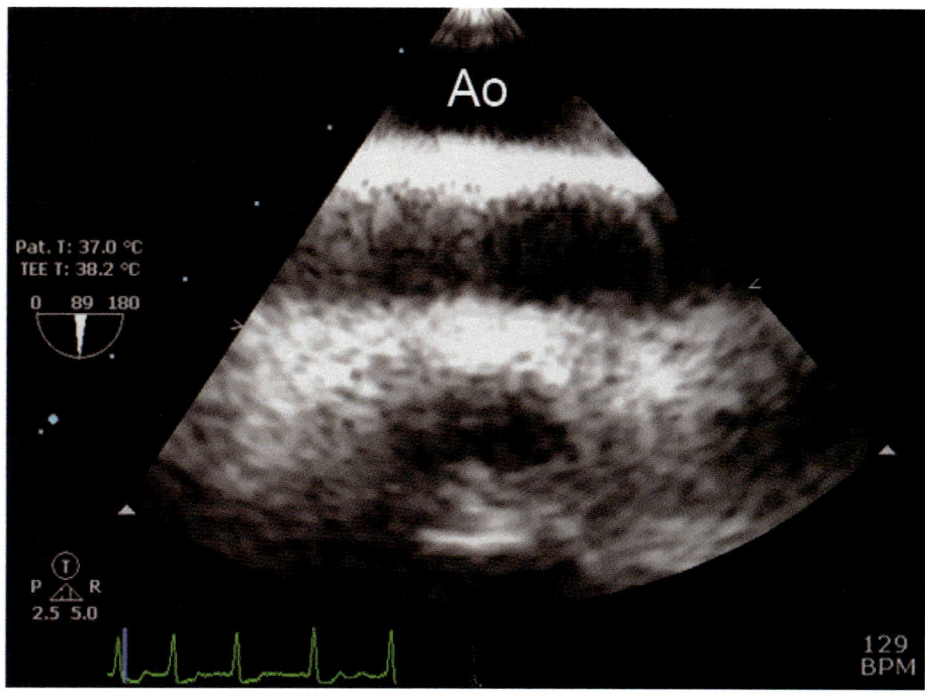

Fig. 3.28: Midesophageal descending aortic long-axis view (Ao: aorta).

Next, the transducer is returned to 0° and the probe is withdrawn until the distal aortic arch is reached when the circular aortic image changes to oval (upper esophageal aortic arch long-axis view, Fig. 3.29).

Increasing the angle to 90° reveals the distal aortic arch in short-axis with pulmonary artery in long-axis (Fig. 3.30).

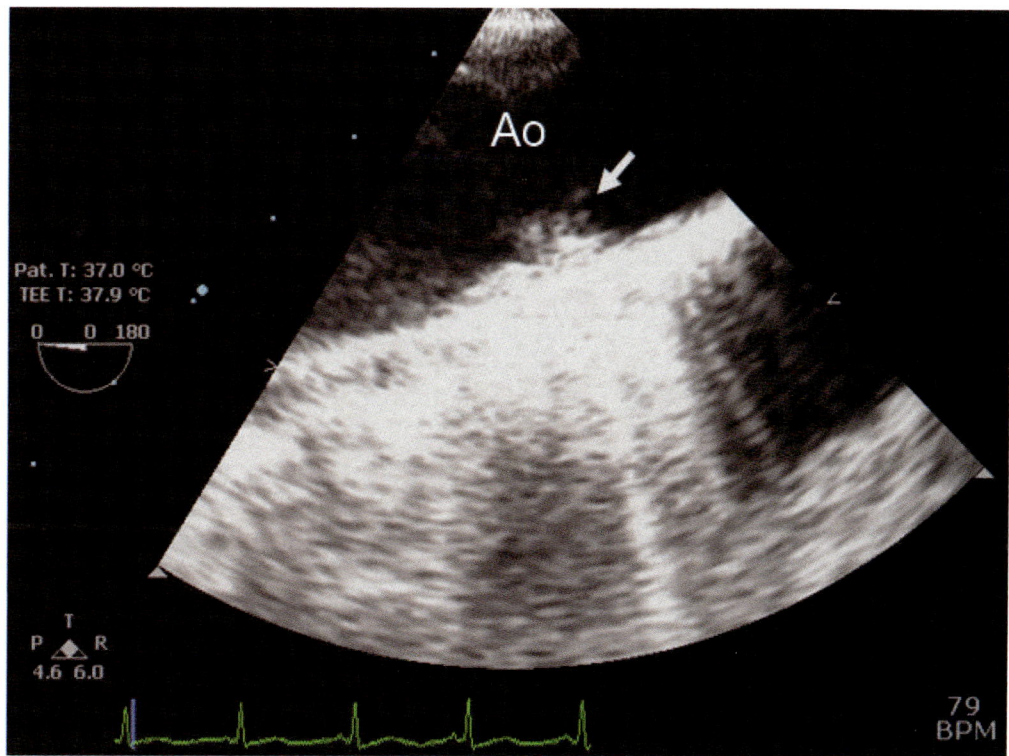

Fig. 3.29: Upper esophageal aortic arch long-axis view. An atheromatous plaque is also seen (arrow) (Ao: aorta).

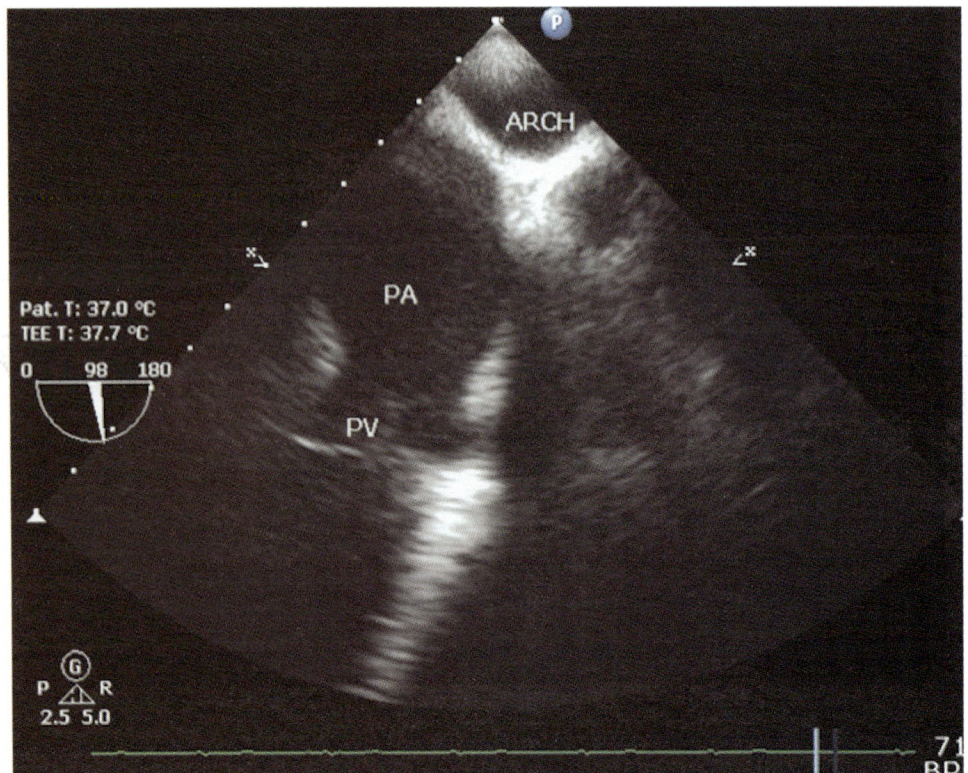

Fig. 3.30: Upper esophageal aortic arch short-axis view (PA: pulmonary artery, PV: pulmonary valve).

This completes the visualization of 20 standard views. Recently, 8 more additional views have been described as a part of comprehensive examination.

These include:
- ME 5-chamber view (Fig. 3.31)
- ME modified bicaval view (Fig. 3.32)

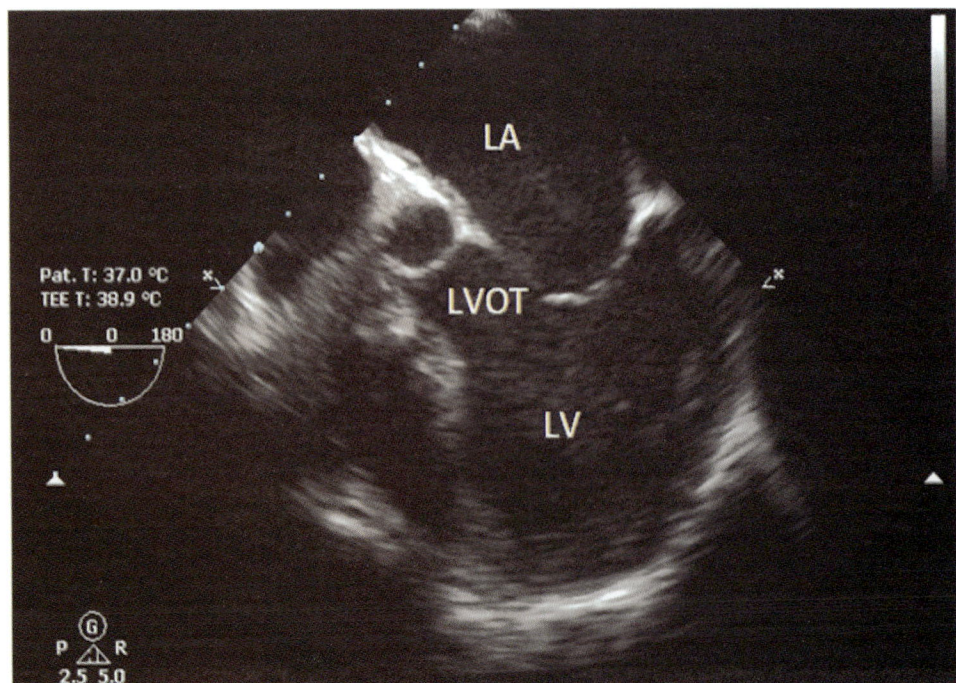

Fig. 3.31: Midesophageal 5-chamber view (LA: left atrium, LV: left ventricle, LVOT: left ventricular outflow tract).

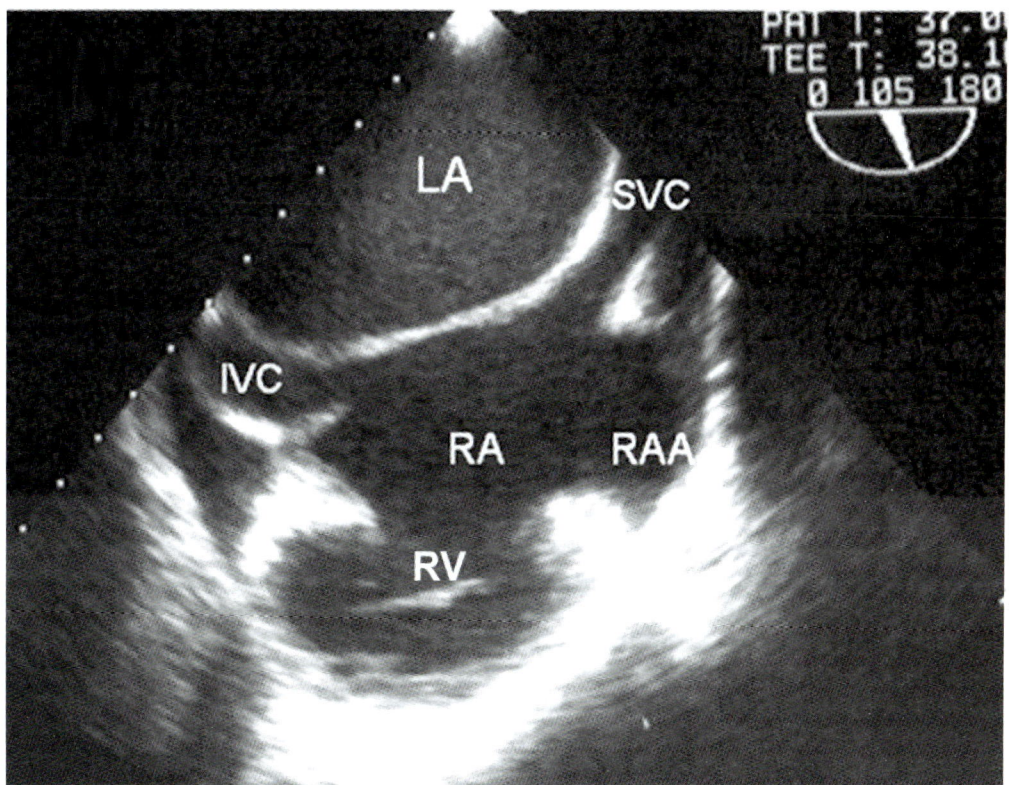

Fig. 3.32: Midesophageal modified bicaval view (LA: left atrium, RA: right atrium, SVC: superior vena cava, IVC: inferior vena cava, RAA: right atrial appendage, RV: right ventricle).

- ME left atrial appendage view (Fig. 3.33)
- ME right pulmonary vein view (Fig. 3.34)
- UE right and left pulmonary vein views (Fig. 3.35)
- TG RV inflow-outflow view (Fig. 3.36)

- TG RV basal view (Fig. 3.37)
- TG apical short-axis view (Fig. 3.38)

A few more views are also utilized in clinical practice. These are, hepatic vein view (Fig. 3.39), and coronary sinus view (Fig. 3.40).

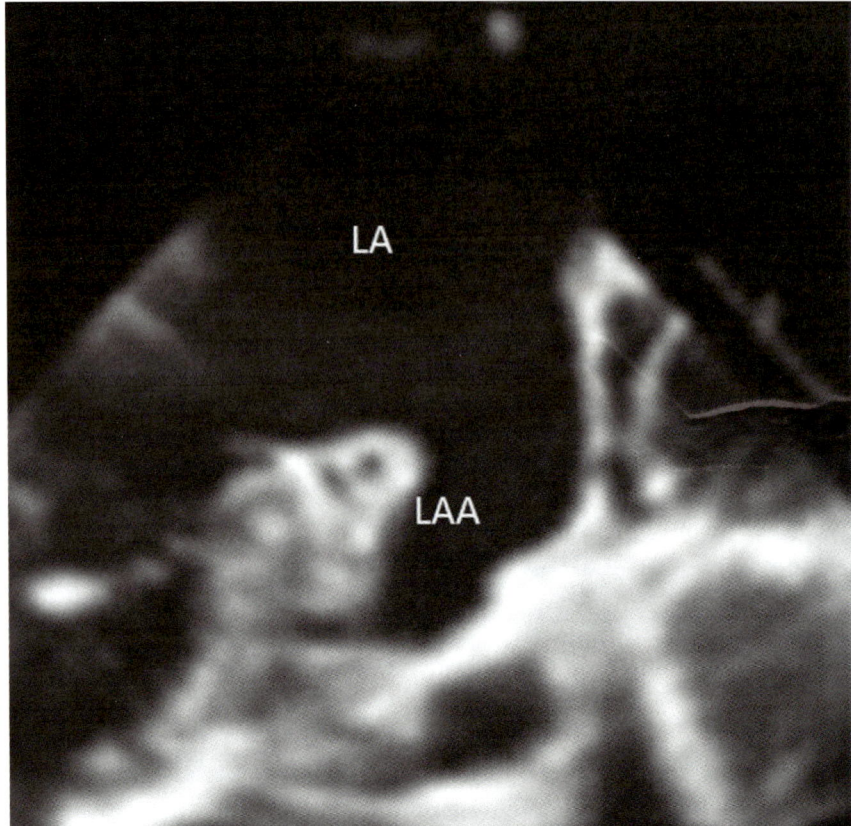

Fig. 3.33: Midesophageal left atrial appendage view (LA: left atrium, LAA: left atrial appendage).

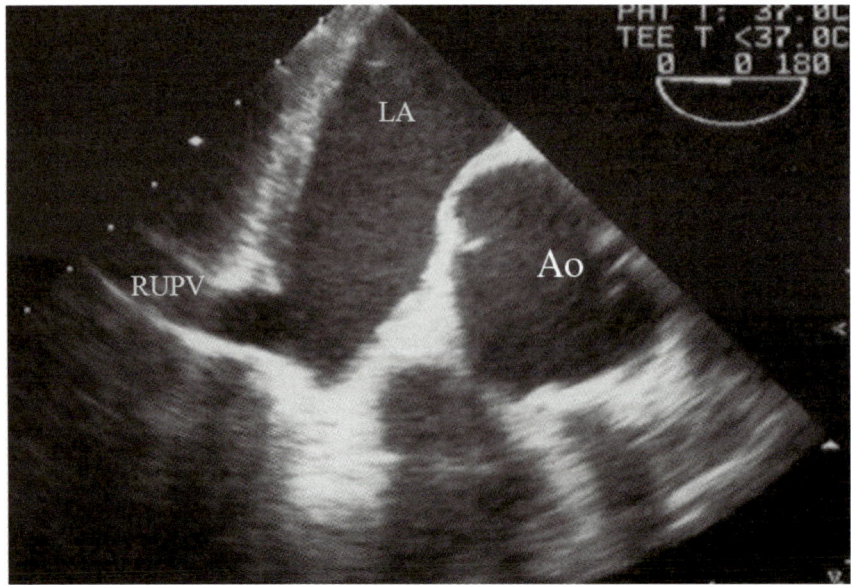

Fig. 3.34: Midesophageal right pulmonary vein view (0°). The right upper and lower pulmonary veins can be visualized on the left of the sector at 0° as they enter the left atrium from the right. Rotation of the imaging plane to facilitate the best view is required. (RUPV: right upper pulmonary vein, LA: left atrium, Ao: aorta).

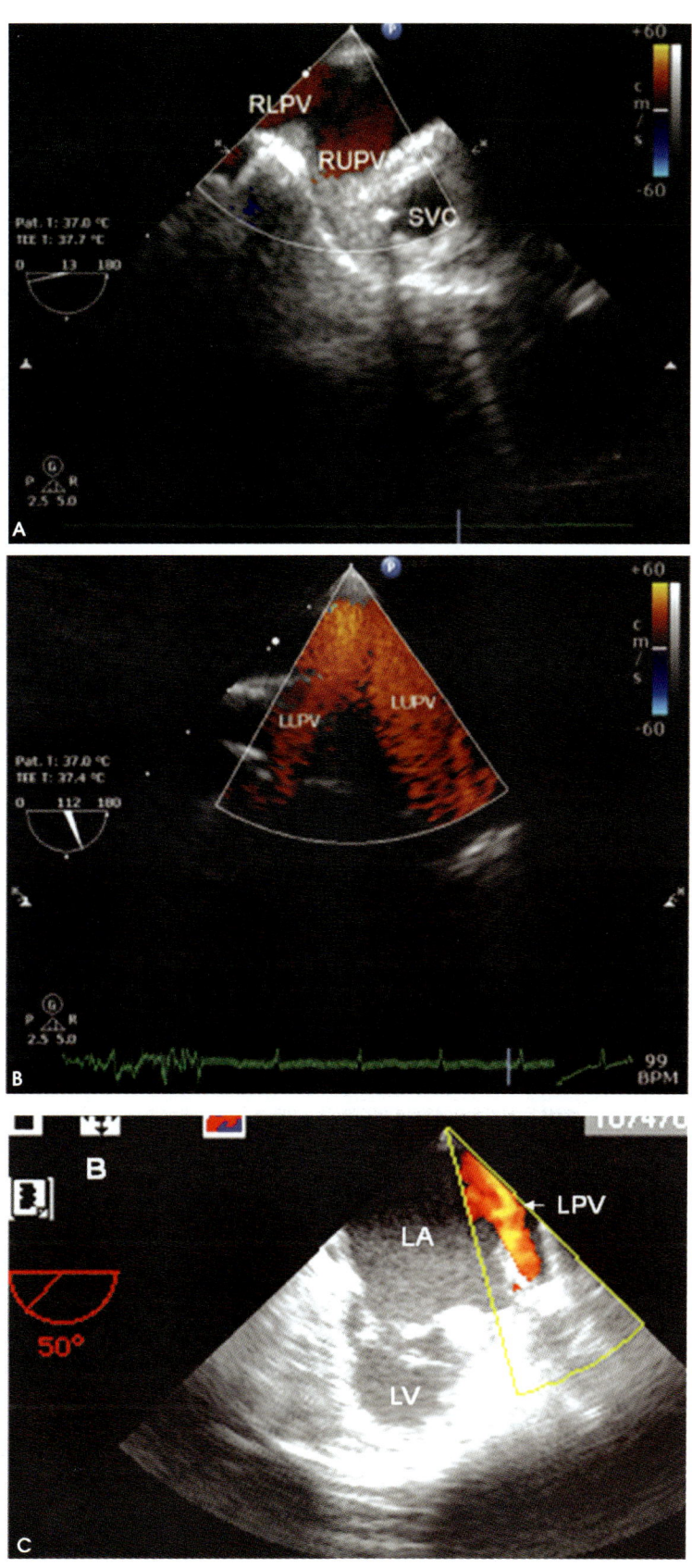

Fig. 3.35: Upper esophageal right (A) and left (B and C) pulmonary vein views. (RUPV: right upper pulmonary vein, RLPV: right lower pulmonary vein, LUPV: left upper pulmonary vein, LLPV: left lower pulmonary vein, SVC: superior vena cava, LA: left atrium, LV: left ventricle, LPV: left pulmonary vein).

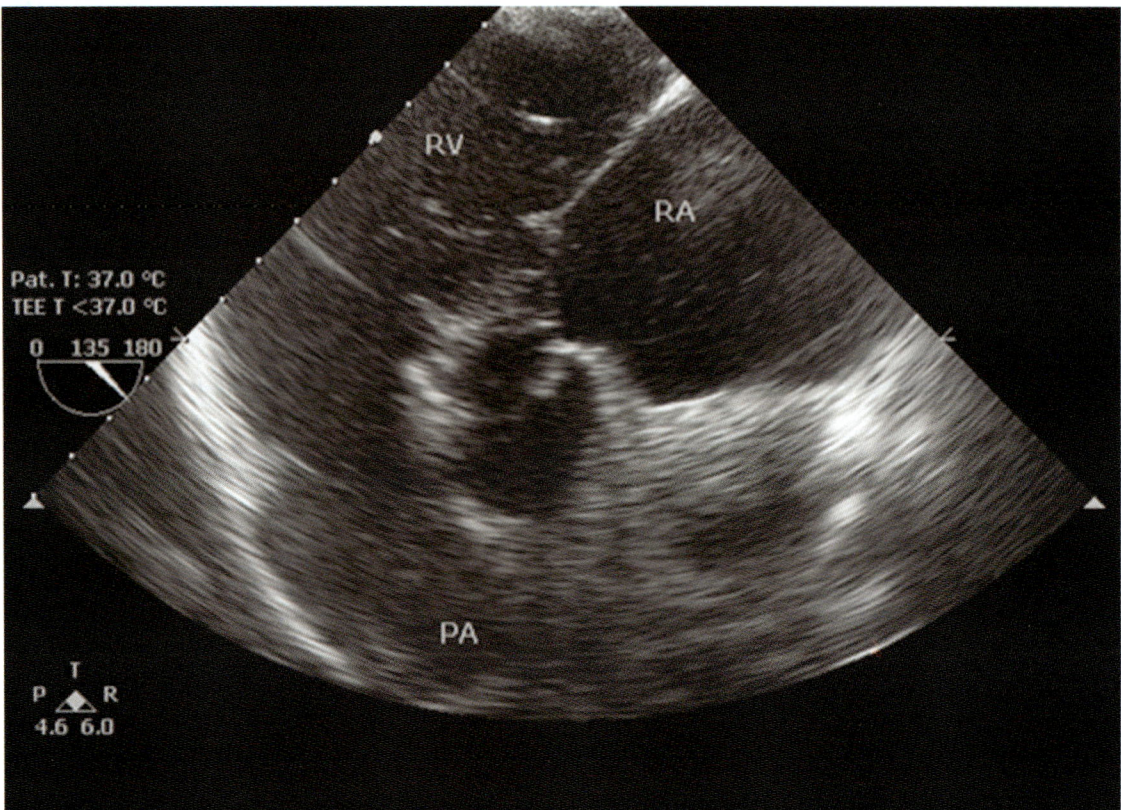

Fig. 3.36: Transgastric right ventricular inflow-outflow view. (RA: right atrium, RV: right ventricle, PA: pulmonary artery).

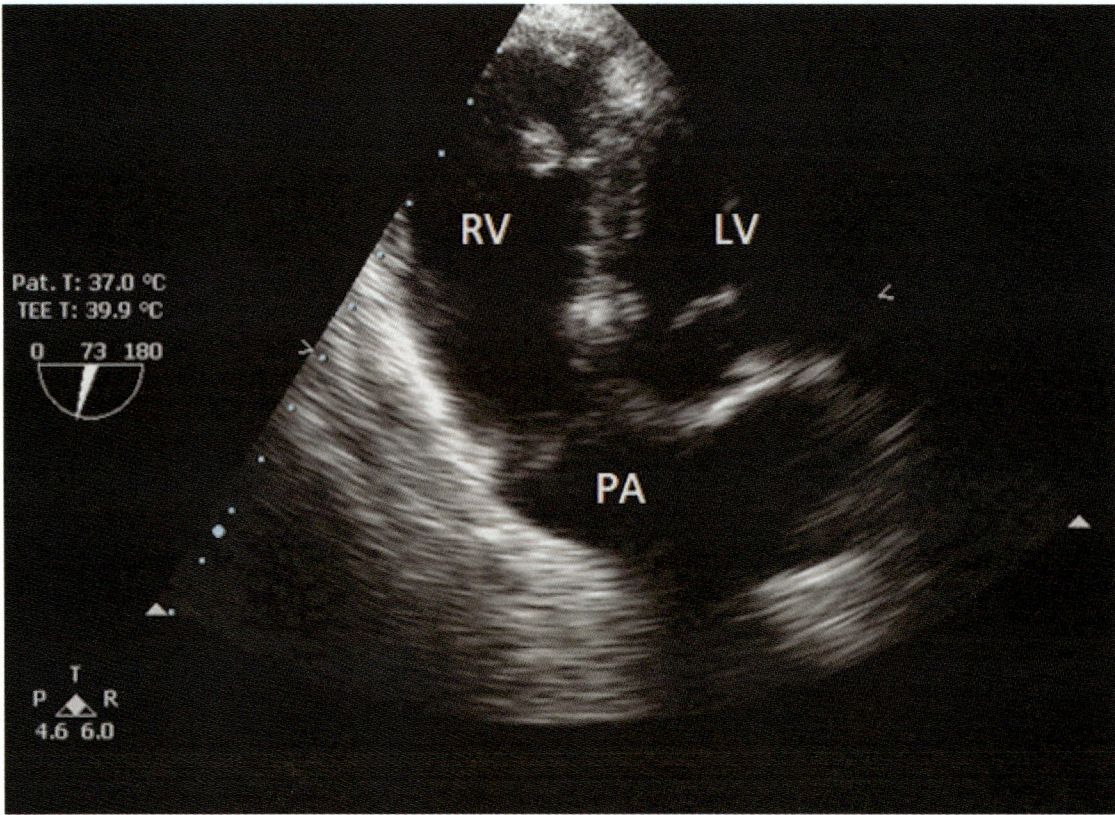

Fig. 3.37: Transgastric right ventricular basal view. (LV: left ventricle, RV: right ventricle, PA: pulmonary artery).

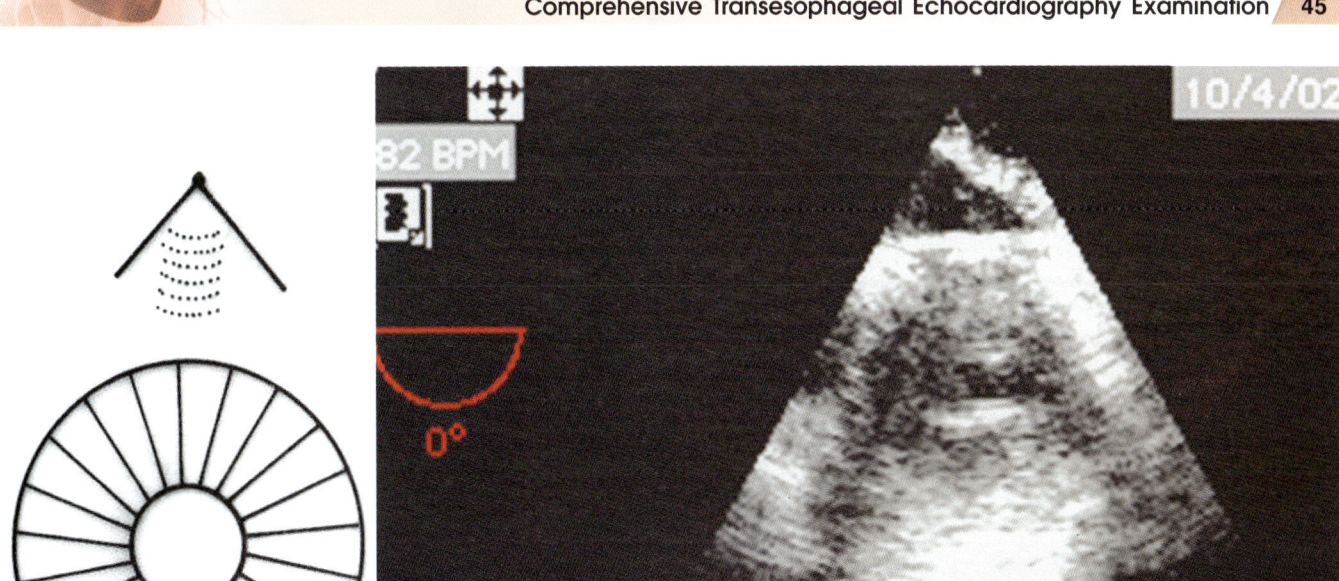

Fig. 3.38: Transgastric apical short-axis view (0°). (A) Diagrammatic representation; (B) Apical short-axis view of the left ventricle.

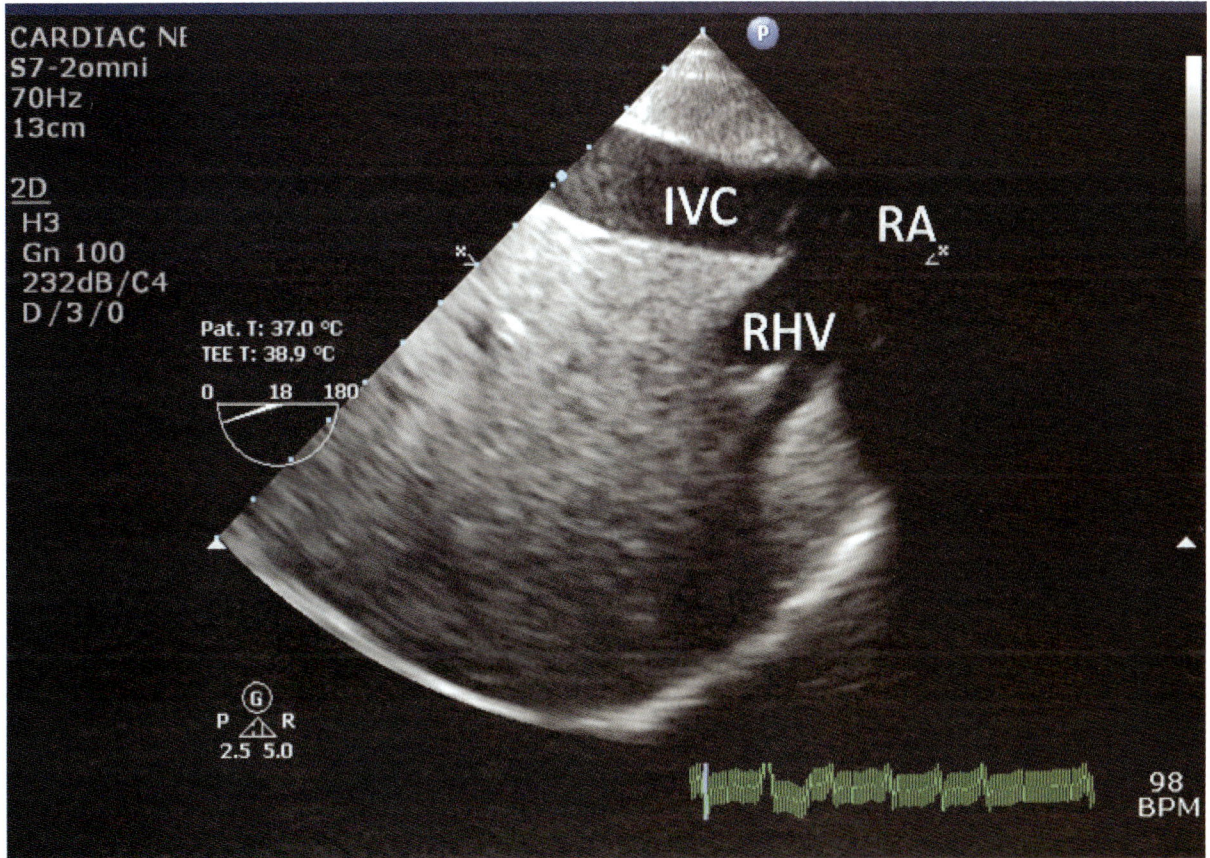

Fig. 3.39: Hepatic vein view. (IVC: inferior vena cava, RHV: right hepatic vein, RA: right atrium).

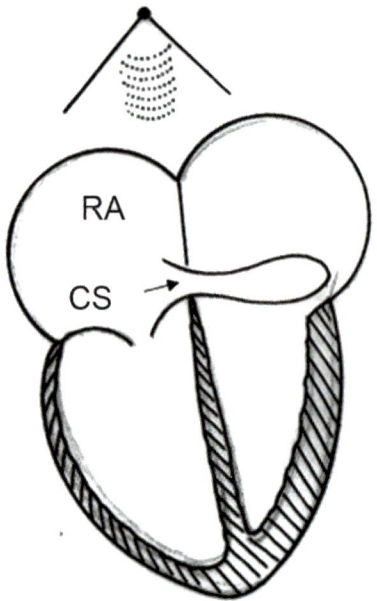

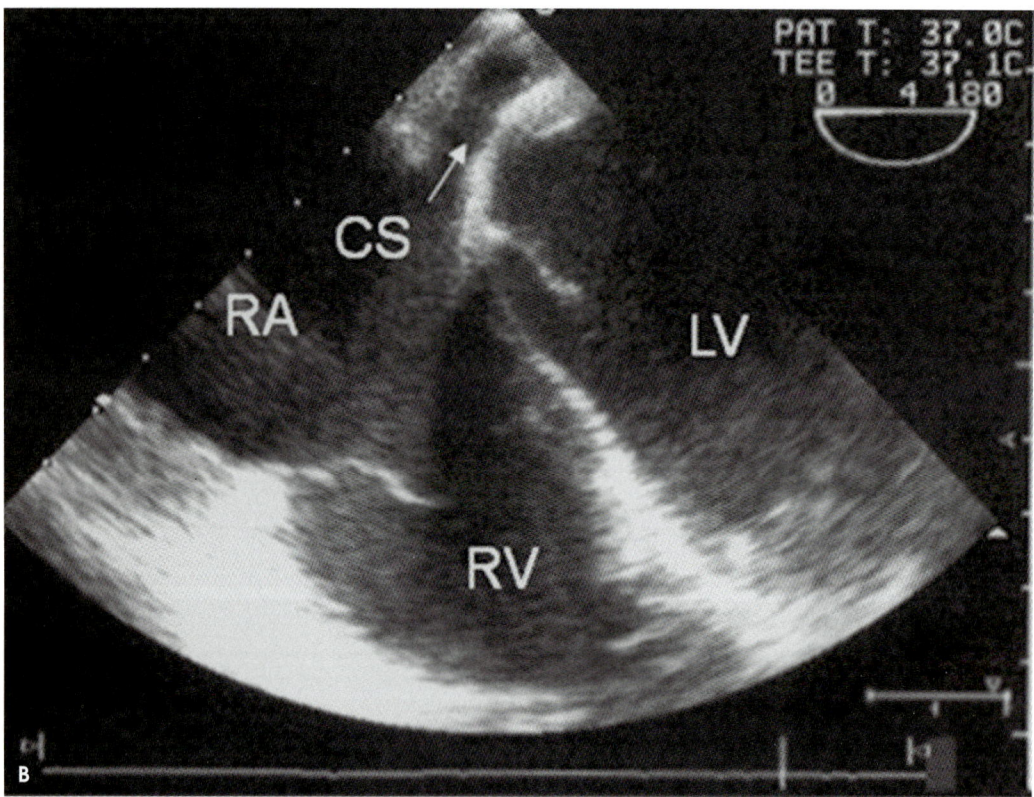

Fig. 3.40: Lower esophageal coronary sinus view (0–10°). (A) Diagrammatic representation; (B) By advancing the probe a little further from midesophageal 4-chamber view (1 cm), coronary sinus can be profiled opening into the right atrium (RA: right atrium, RV: right ventricle, LV: left ventricle, CS: coronary sinus).

Reference

1. Shanewise JS, Chenng AT, Aranson S, *et al.* Anesth Analg 89:870;1999.

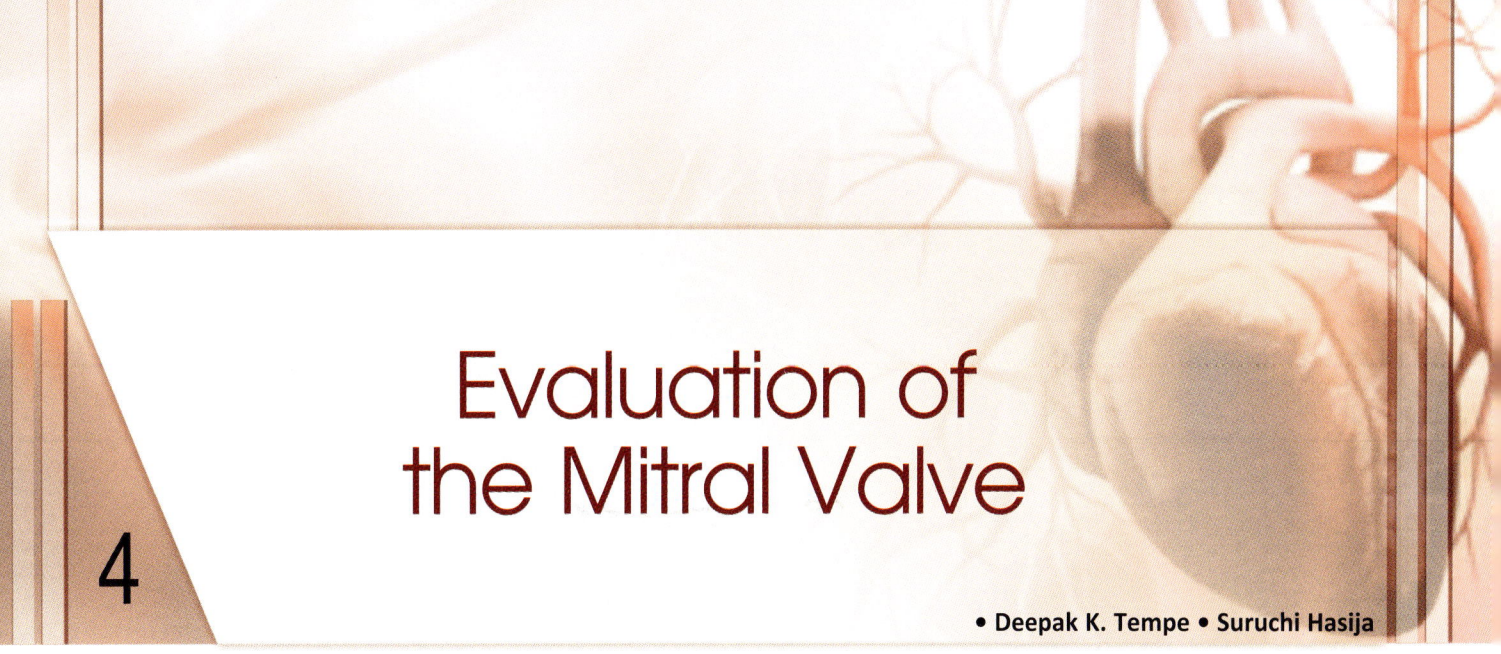

Evaluation of the Mitral Valve

4

• Deepak K. Tempe • Suruchi Hasija

The potential for suboptimal surgical outcome is always present in patients undergoing valvular surgery. It is important to recognise the need for additional corrections in the immediate postoperative period. Transesophageal echocardiography (TEE) during valvular surgery is therefore widely used in this setting.

TEE constitutes an important tool for assessing the mitral valve (MV) and provides an excellent anatomical visualization, clear delineation of transmitral flow, and is highly sensitive for detecting valve regurgitation. It plays an important role in the accurate assessment of the MV function, especially following valve replacement and repair. In addition, it reliably detects left atrial thrombi and vegetations. Before initiating cardiopulmonary bypass (CPB), TEE at times can detect thrombi and vegetations and this is important for modifying the surgical strategies. In post-CPB period, TEE can identify significant valve dysfunction (if present) for necessitating additional surgical correction. It should be remembered however, that the post-CPB detection of valvular regurgitation is confounded by mitral leakage that occurs in the presence of abnormal loading conditions or due to myocardial ischemia. These need to be kept in consideration before additional therapeutic strategies are initiated.

Percutaneous transluminal mitral commissurotomy is a commonly performed procedure for patients with mitral stenosis (MS). TEE can be used for guiding the procedure. In this chapter important images related to the MV abnormalities are shown.

Anatomy

The MV is named after its resemblance to 'mitre', a type of folding cap consisting of two similar parts that rise to a peak. A thorough understanding of the normal MV anatomy is extremely important in order to identify the exact pathophysiology. The mitral apparatus includes the annulus, leaflets, chordae tendinea, and papillary muscles with their supporting LV walls. The MV is located cephalad in comparison with the tricuspid valve. The annulus comprises fibroelastic tissue, which completely encircles the valve orifice in a cone-like shape. The annulus is elliptical in shape during systole and round in diastole. The two leaflets are different in shape. The anterior leaflet is triangular in shape and is in continuity with the aortic annulus. It encircles only one-third of the annulus, but covers two-thirds of the valve orifice area. The posterior leaflet is quandrangular in shape and occupies two-thirds of the annulus. It covers only one-third of the valve area. The Carpentier nomenclature is followed for understanding of the echocardiographic images as well as uniformity in communicating with the surgical team. The anterior leaflet is termed A and divided into 3 parts; lateral third (A1), middle third (A2) and medial third (A3). The posterior leaflet is termed P and divided into lateral (P1), middle (P2) and medial (P3) scallops. The leaflets are thick at the base and the tips with central thinning. The anterior leaflet is more mobile, while the posterior leaflet fulfills a supporting role.

The MV can be examined in considerable detail by TEE due to its proximity to the esophagus. The MV can be examined in the midesophageal (ME) four-chamber view (Fig. 4.1), ME commissural view (Fig. 4.2), ME two-chamber view (Fig. 4.3), ME long-axis view (Fig. 4.4), transgastric (TG) basal short-axis view (Fig. 4.5) and TG two-chamber view (Fig. 4.6). The TG two-chamber view best delineates the subvalvular anatomy of the MV.

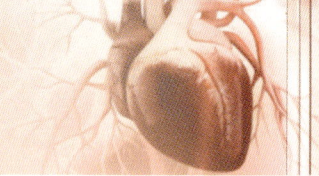

MIDESOPHAGEAL VIEWS

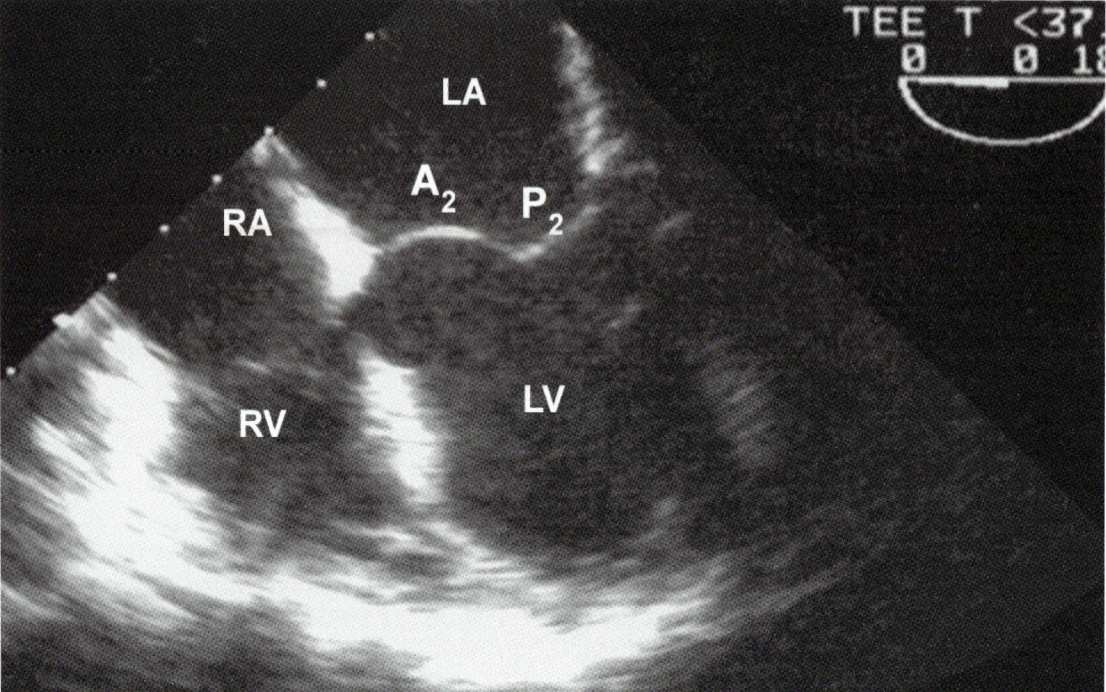

Fig. 4.1: Midesophageal 4-chamber view showing the A2,P2 segments of the mitral valve. (LA: left atrium, LV: left ventricle, RA: right atrium, RV: right ventricle).

MITRAL STENOSIS

Echocardiographic mitral valve assessment is performed under the following headings: 2-D imaging to demonstrate the valve morphology (Fig. 4.7), color flow imaging to delineate the blood flow profile (Fig. 4.8A), Doppler evaluation of velocities and gradients (Fig. 4.8B) and hemodynamic calculations of the extent of stenosis or regurgitation. The key features to be identified on 2-D echocardiographic examination include the extent of leaflet thickening, calcium deposition, subvalvular involvement, leaflet mobility, and chamber dimensions and function (Figs 4.9 and 4.10). The mitral valve leaflets get thickened due to variable degrees of tissue fibrosis and calcification. The chordal tendons also display thickening and contracture. Because of commissural fusion, the leaflets exhibit restricted motion at the annulus with relative mobility of the midsection during diastole (diastolic doming or 'hockey stick' deformity). In advanced stages, there is minimal movement of the valve throughout the cardiac cycle. The left atrial dimension may be increased with signs of blood stasis in the form of spontaneous echo contrast or a thrombus (Figs 4.11–4.15).

The severity of MS can be estimated by the following methods (Figs 4.16 to 4.20 and Table 4.1):

1. According to the simplified Bernoulli equation,
   $$P_1 - P_2 = 4V^2$$
   where, $P_1 - P_2$ is the pressure gradient across the valve (mm Hg) and V represents the instantaneous velocity of blood distal to the stenotic valve (m/s) (Fig. 4.18).

2. *Planimetry:* The MV area is directly measured in the transgastric basal short-axis view at the level of the leaflet tips in early diastole when the MV is maximally open.

3. *Pressure half-time (PHT)* (Fig. 4.17B)
   MV area (cm^2) = 220/PHT (msec)

Table 4.1: Assessment of severity of mitral stenosis				
Method	*Valve area (cm^2)*	*Mean gradient (mm Hg)*	*Pressure half-time (msec)*	*Peak velocity (m/s)*
Normal	4–6		40–70	< 1.0
Mild	1.5–2.5	<6	70–150	1.0–1.5
Moderate	1.0–1.5	6–12	150–220	1.5–3.0
Severe	<1.0	>12	>220	>3.0

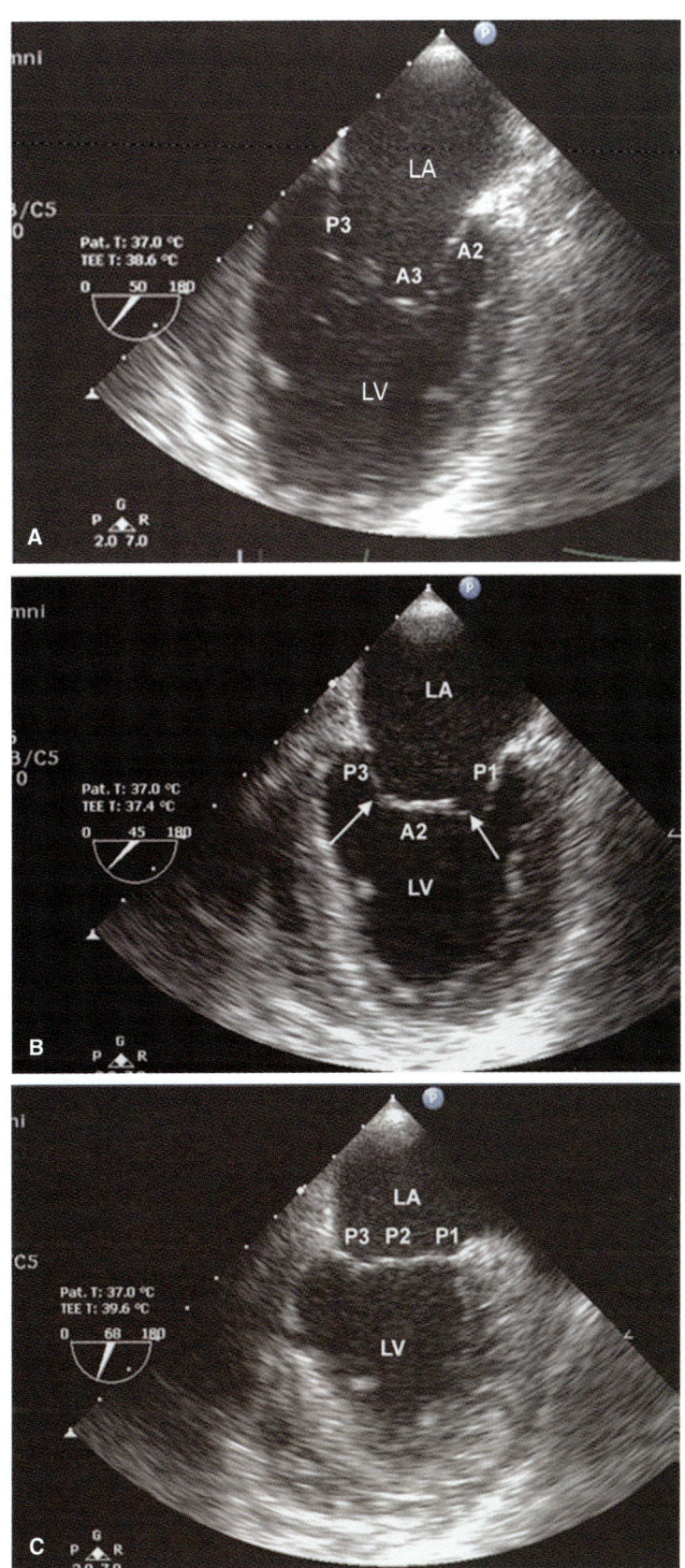

Fig. 4.2: Midesophageal commissural view showing the mitral valve. (A) Anterior cross-section showing anterior and posterior mitral leaflets (A2, A3, P3); (B) Mid cross-section showing 2 coaptation points (arrows, P1, A2, P3); (C) Posterior cross-section showing the P1, P2, P3 scallops. (LA: left atrium, LV: left ventricle).

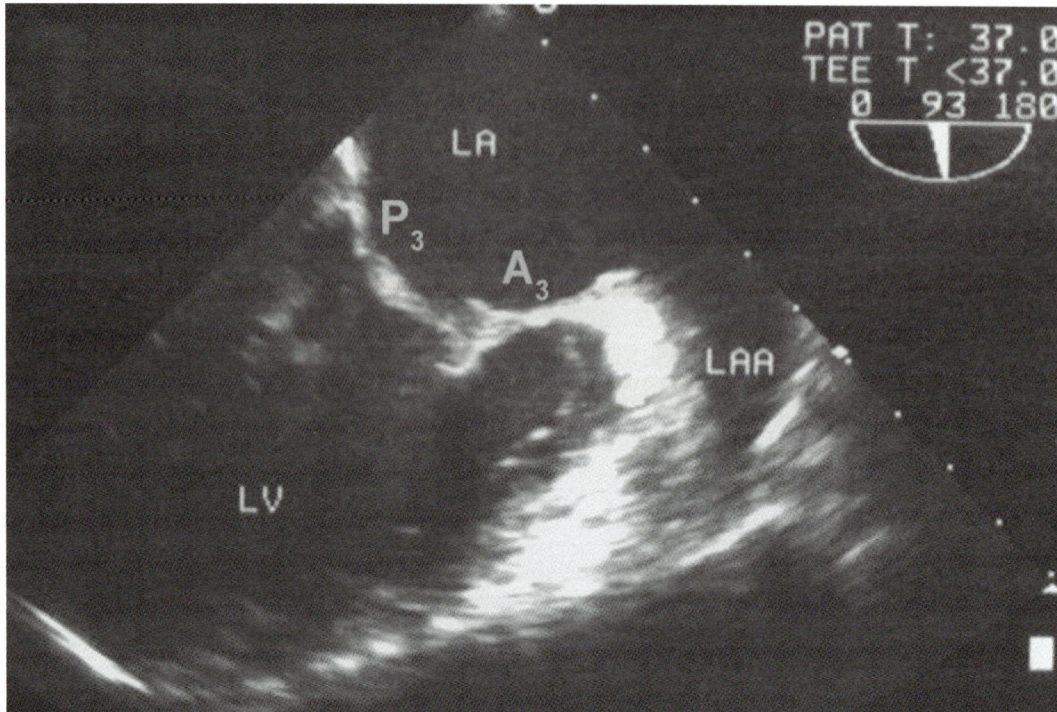

Fig. 4.3: Midesophageal two-chamber view showing the A3,P3 segments of the mitral valve (LA: left atrium, LV: left ventricle, LAA: left atrial appendage).

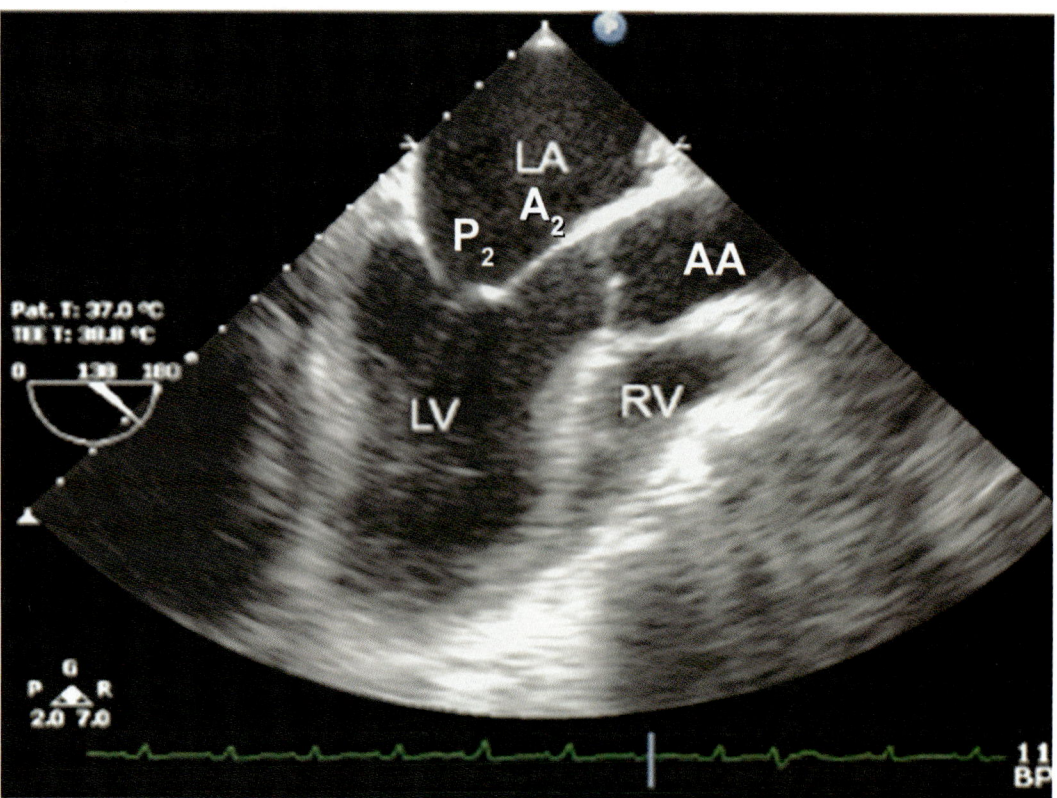

Fig. 4.4: Midesophageal long-axis view showing the A2,P2 segments of the mitral valve (LA: left atrium, LV: left ventricle, RV: right ventricle, AA: ascending aorta).

TRANSGASTRIC VIEWS

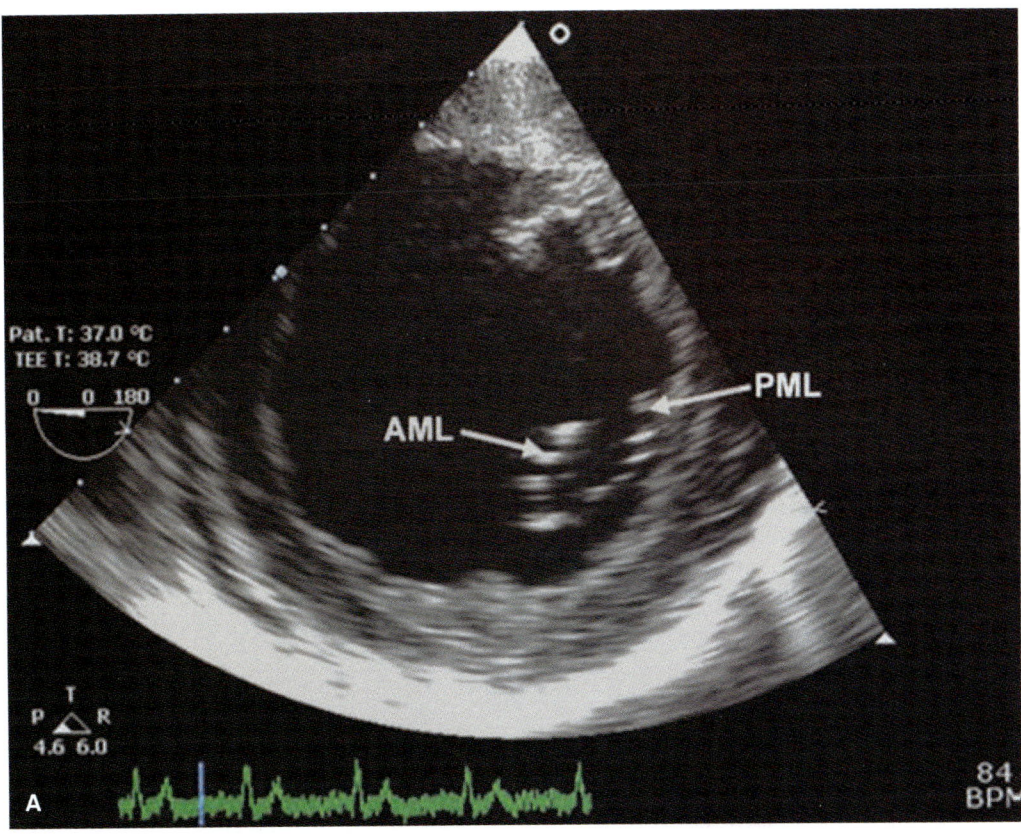

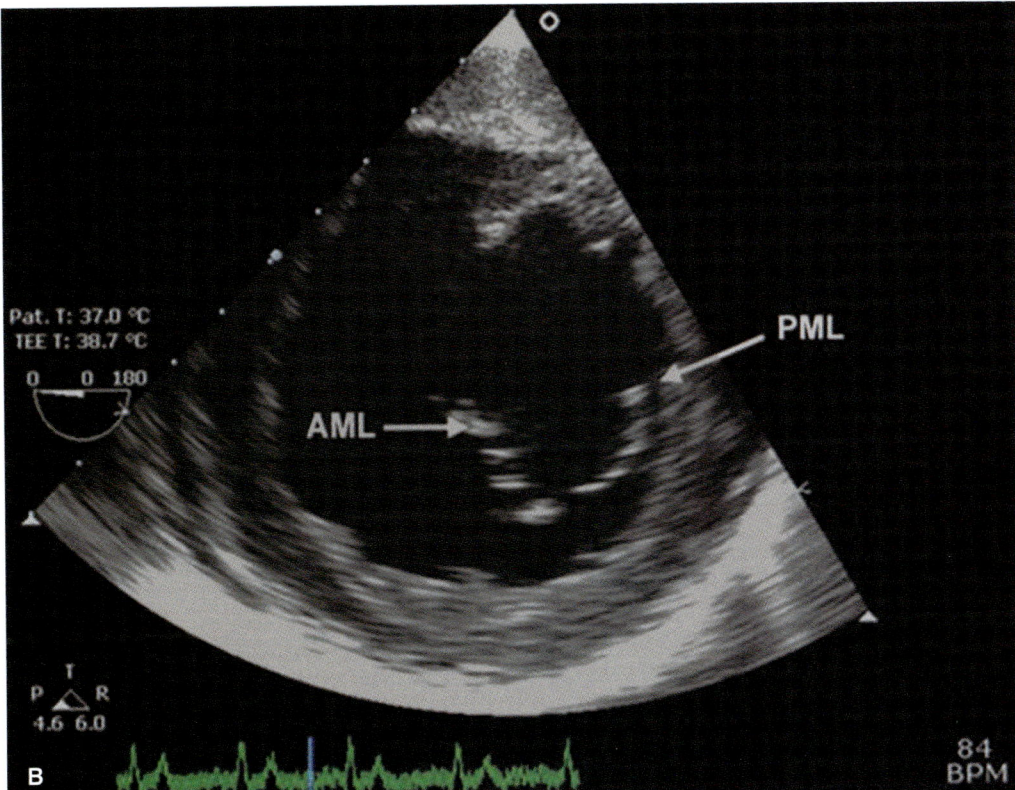

Fig. 4.5: Transgastric basal short-axis view of the left ventricle showing the mitral valve in systole (A) and diastole (B). (AML: anterior mitral leaflet, PML: posterior mitral leaflet).

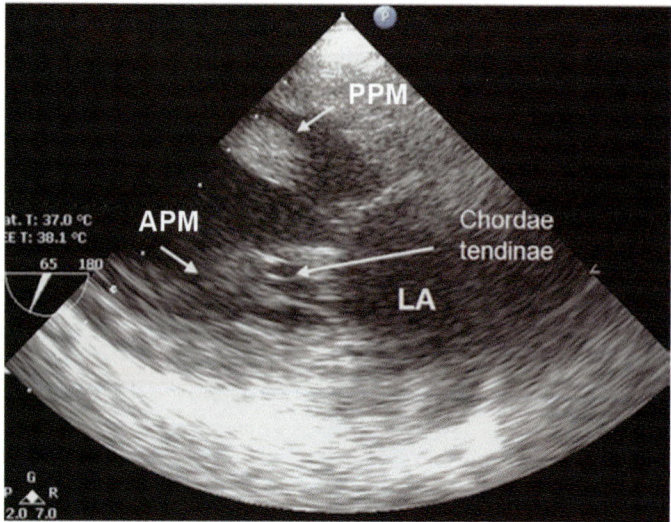

Fig. 4.6: Transgastric two-chamber view of the left ventricle showing the mitral subvalvular apparatus (APM: anterior papillary muscle, PPM: posterior papillary muscle, LA: left atrium).

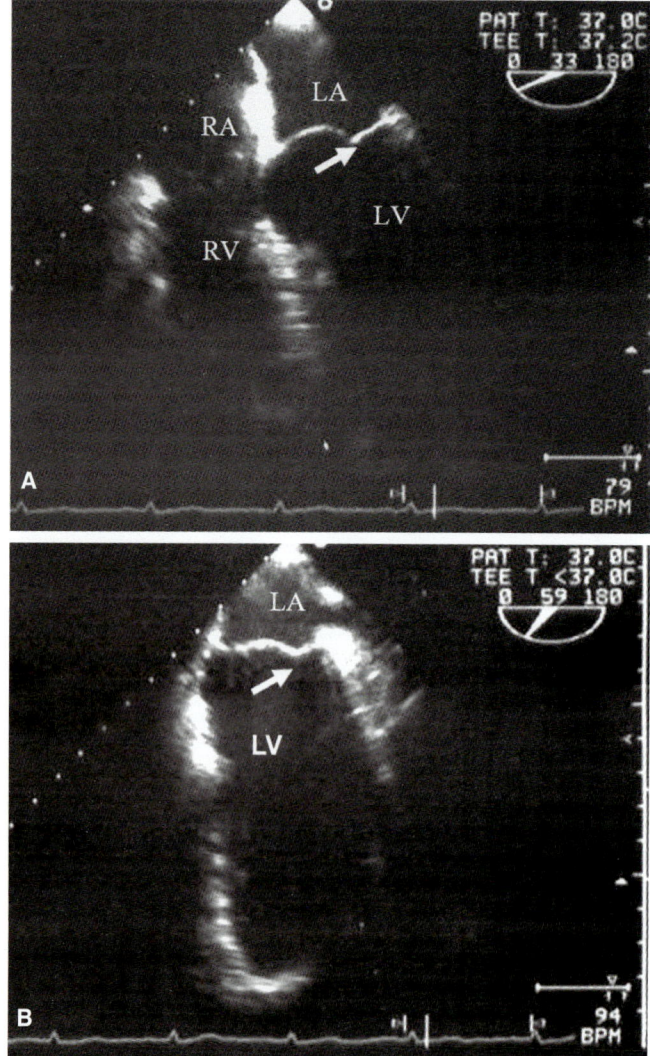

Fig. 4.7: Appearance of the mitral valve on two-dimensional echocardiography in midesophageal four (A) and two (B) chamber views. Note the proper coaptation of the leaflets (arrow) during systole (LA: left atrium, RA: right atrium, LV: left ventricle, RV: right ventricle).

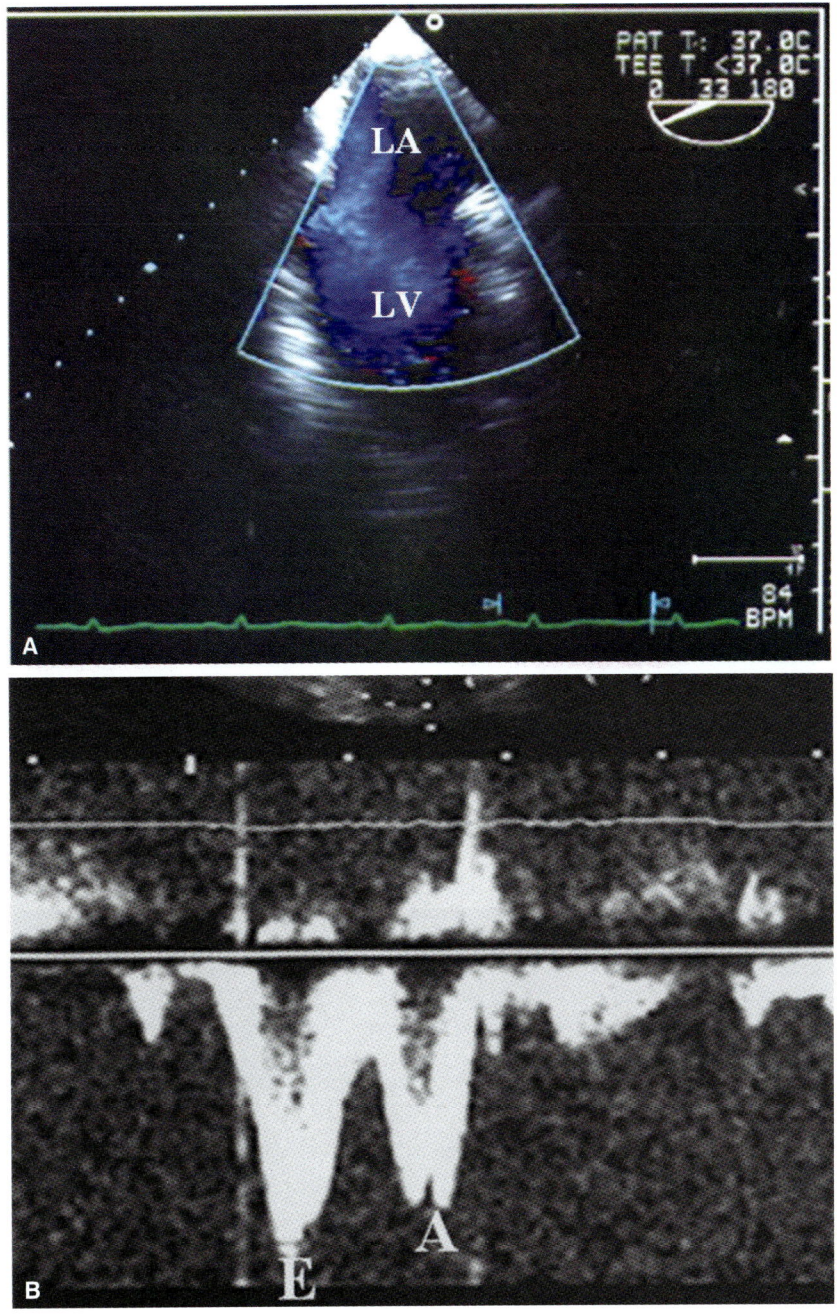

Fig. 4.8: Appearance of the normal transmitral flow on color Doppler imaging (A) and pulsed wave Doppler imaging (B). (E—early diastolic flow, A—late diastolic flow) (LA: left atrium, LV: left ventricle).

4. *Deceleration time (DT)*

   MV area (cm^2) = 759/DT (msec)

   PHT = 0.29 × DT

5. *Continuity equation*

   MV area = (LVOT$_{area}$ X LVOT$_{TVI}$) / MV$_{TVI}$

   where, LVOT$_{area}$ is the cross sectional area of the left ventricular outflow tract, LVOT$_{TVI}$ is the velocity time integral across the left ventricular outflow tract and MV$_{TVI}$ is the velocity time integral across the MV.

6. Proximal isovelocity surface area (PISA) (Figs 4.19 and 4.20)

   MV area (cm^2) = Q / Vp (cm/s) or $2\pi r^2 \times \alpha/180° \times$ Va/Vp

   where, Q is the instantaneous flow rate, r is the radius of the flow convergence shell , α is the angle subtended by the mitral leaflets, Va is the aliasing velocity and Vp is the peak transmitral inflow velocity.

   Figures 4.21 to 4.24 depict the sequence of steps involved in performing Balloon Mitral Valvotomy.

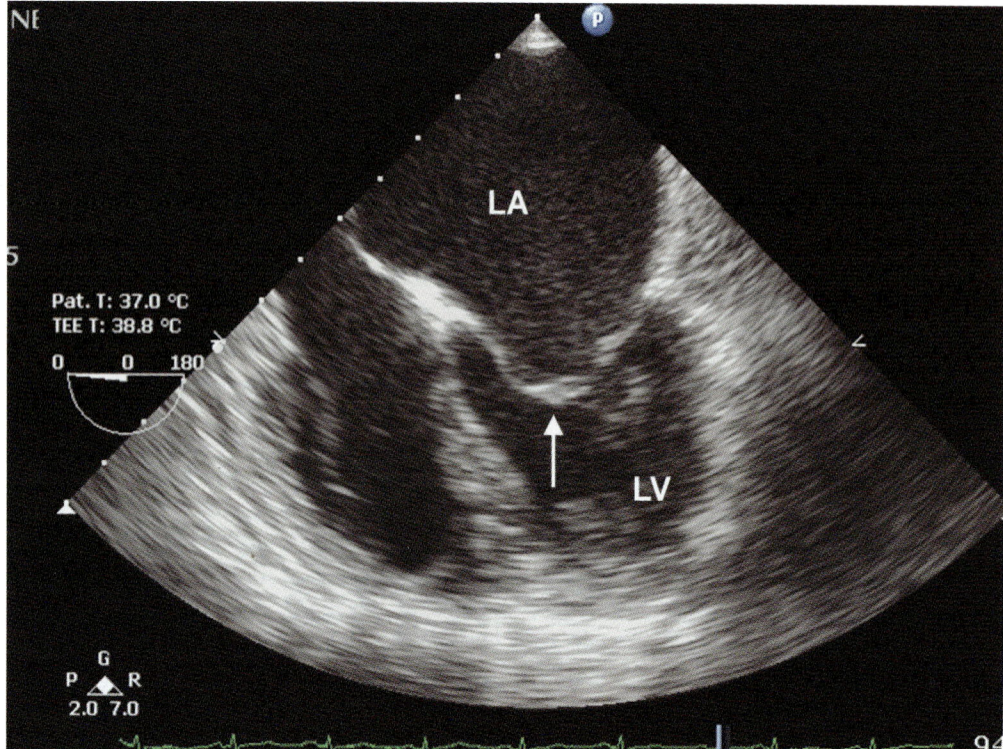

Fig. 4.9: Midesophageal 4-chamber view showing thickened mitral valve leaflets. Note the doming anterior leaflet giving it a hockey stick appearance (arrow) (LA: left atrium, LV: left ventricle).

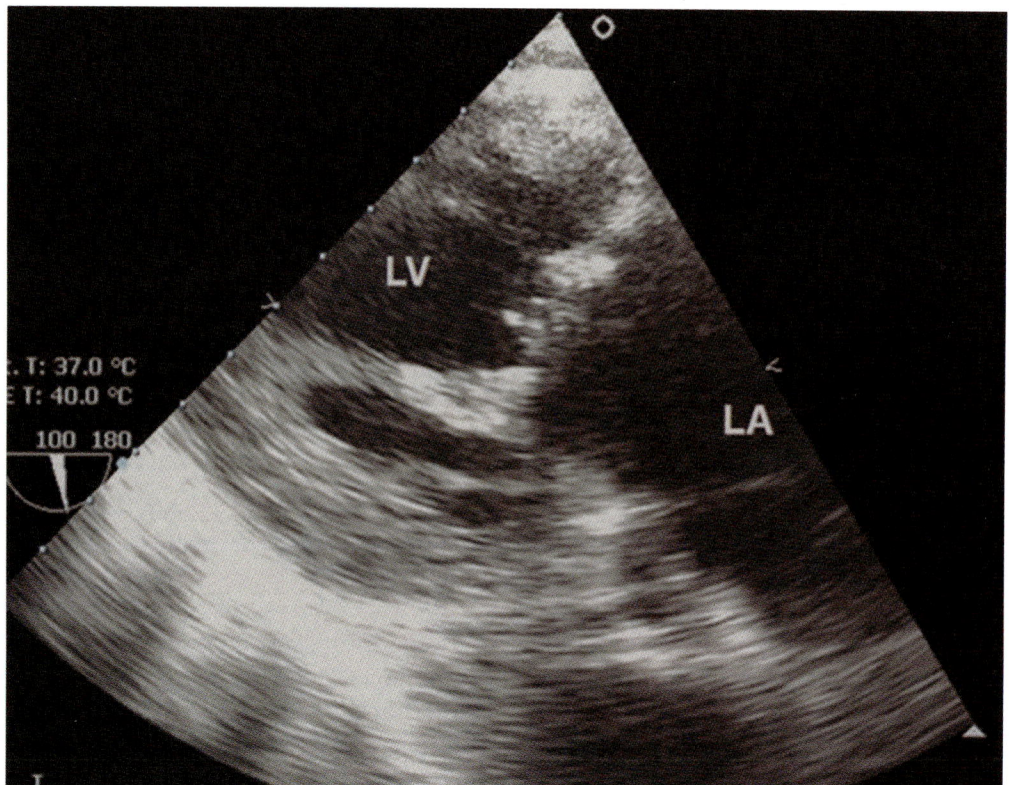

Fig. 4.10: Transgastric view of the left ventricle at 100° showing the mitral subvalvular apparatus. Note the thickened and fused chordae tendinea (LA: left atrium, LV: left ventricle).

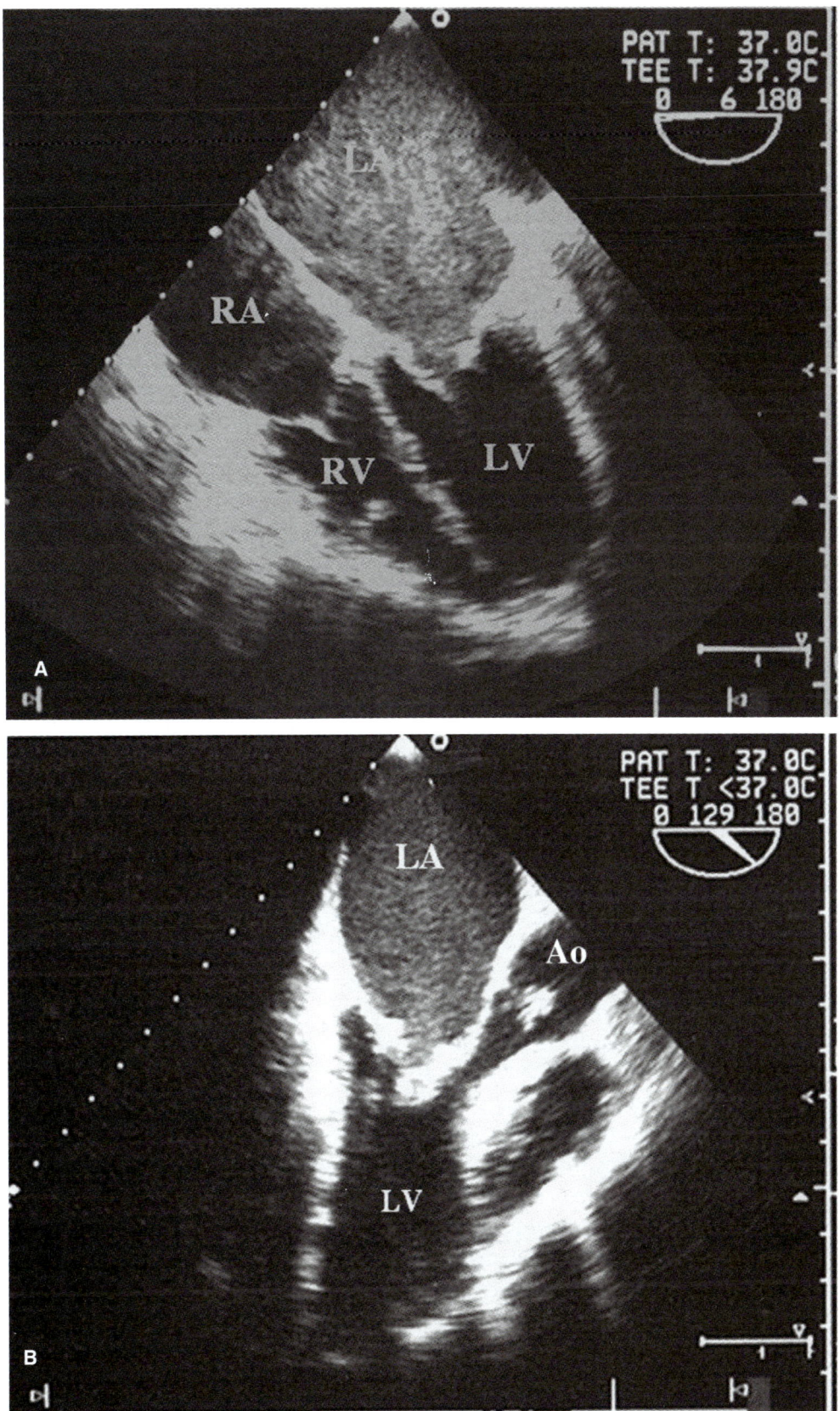

Fig. 4.11: Midesophageal 4-chamber view (A) and long-axis view (B) in a patient with severe mitral stenosis showing doming of mitral leaflets and dense left atrial spontaneous echo contrast (RA: right atrium, RV: right ventricle, LA: left atrium, LV: left ventricle, AA: ascending aorta).

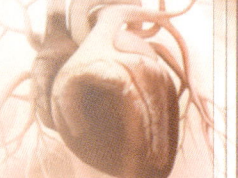

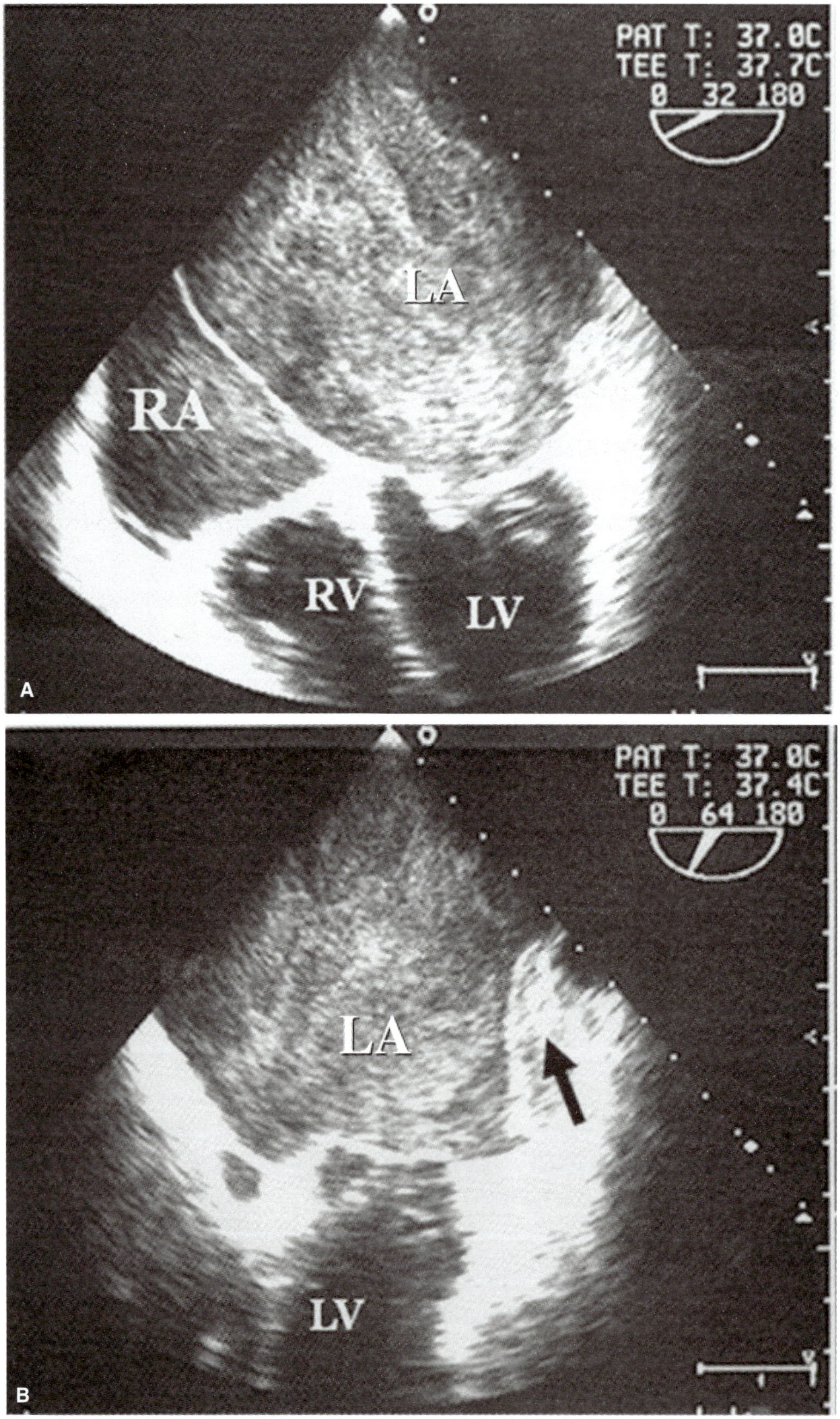

Fig. 4.12: Appearance of the left atrium in midesophageal 4-chamber view (A) and 2-chamber view (B) in a patient with mitral stenosis. Note the bulging inter-atrial septum and the dense spontaneous left atrial contrast in 4-chamber view and a well formed left atrial body thrombus (arrow) in the 2-chamber view (LA: left atrium, RA: right atrium, RV: right ventricle, LV: left ventricle).

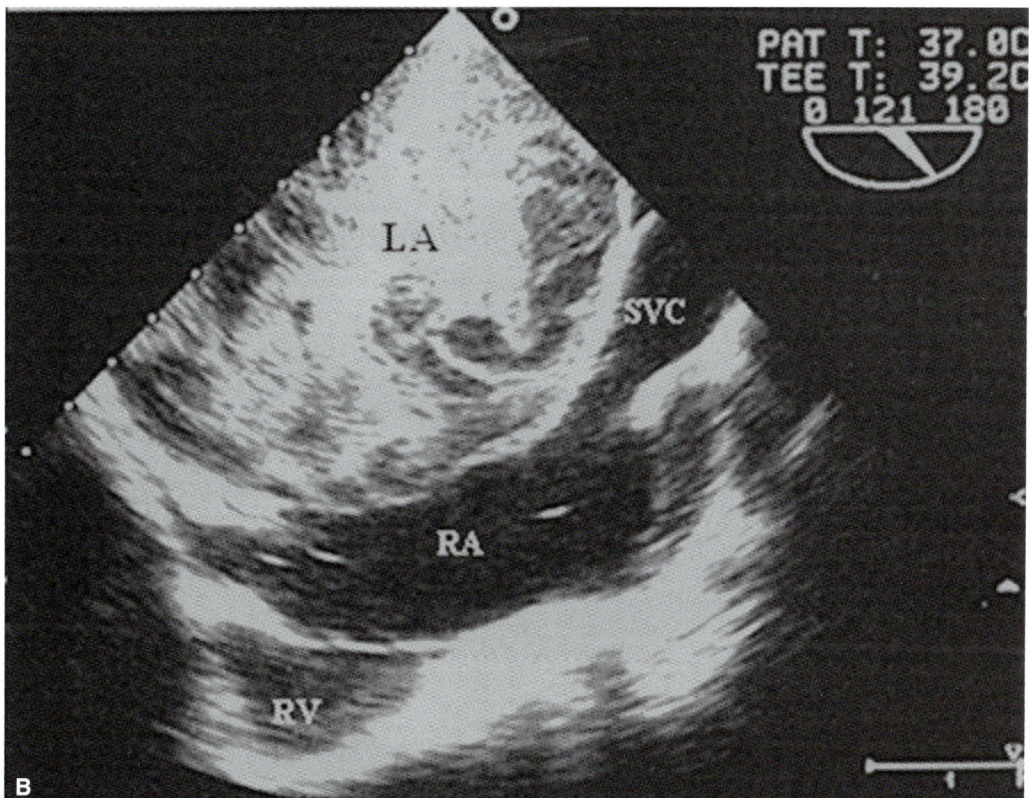

Fig. 4.13: Midesophageal bicaval view in mitral stenosis. Note the difference in the size of atrium in two patients. Left atrium of the patient in panel B is larger and shows denser spontaneous echo contrast (LA: left atrium, RA: right atrium, RV: right ventricle, SVC: superior vena cava).

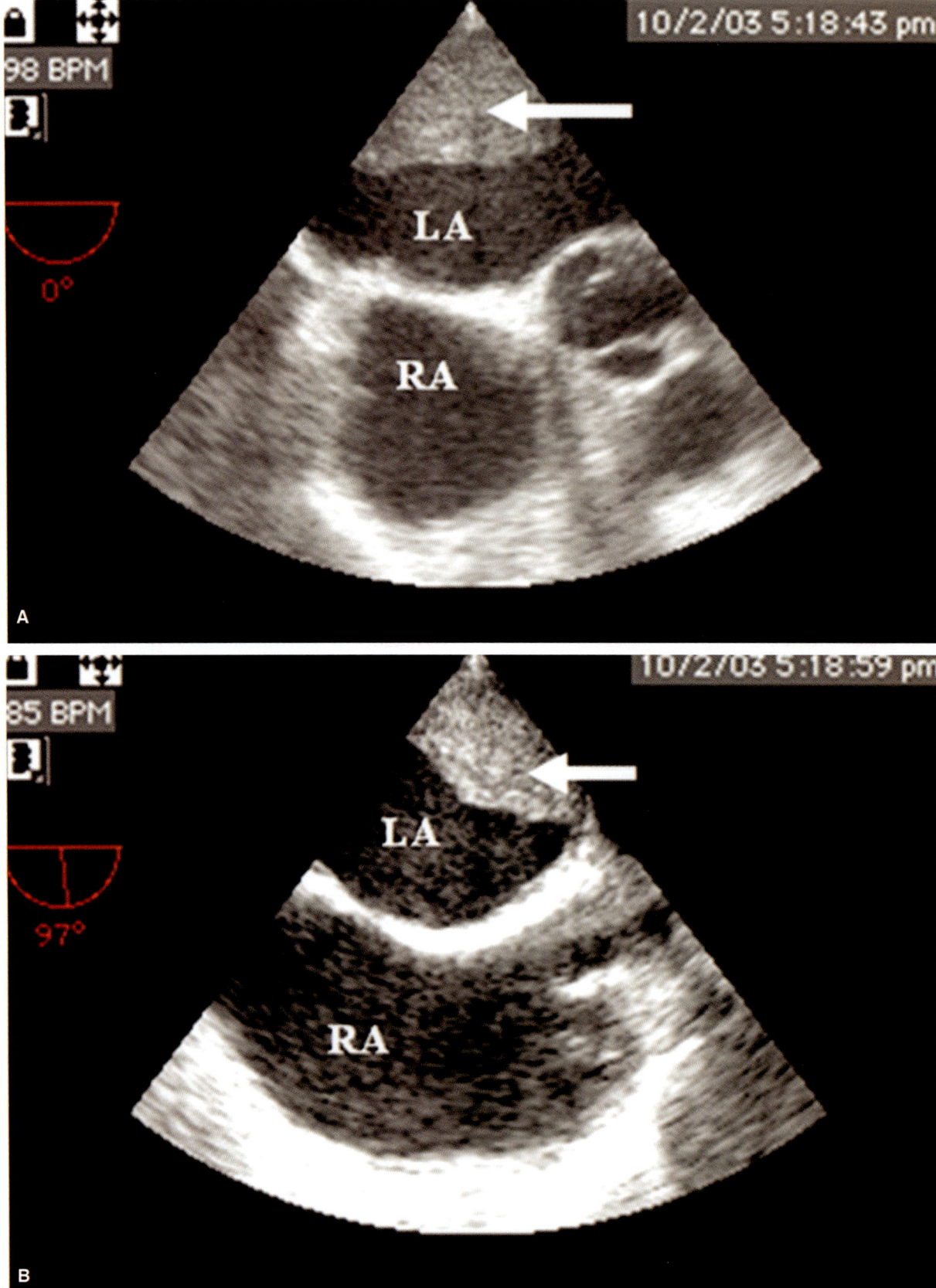

Fig. 4.14: Large left atrial body thrombus (arrow) in a patient with severe mitral stenosis seen in short-axis (A) and bicaval view (B) (LA: left atrium, RA: right atrium).

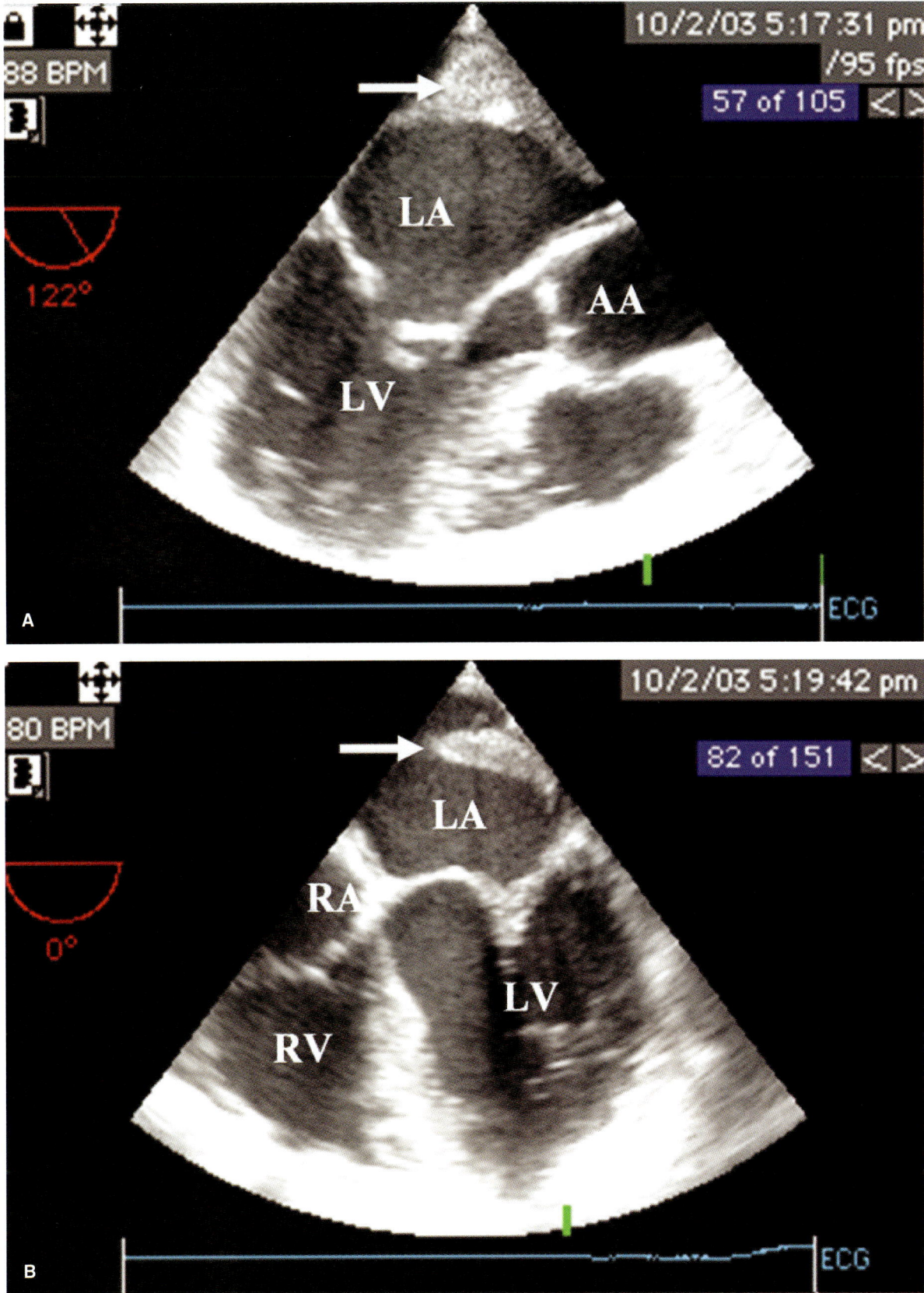

Fig. 4.15: Panel A: Large left atrial body thrombus (arrow) in a patient with severe mitral stenosis layered across the posterior wall of the left atrium. Panel B: A left atrial body thrombus (arrow) in another patient with mitral stenosis. (LA: left atrium, LV: left ventricle, RV: right ventricle, AA: ascending aorta, RA: right atrium).

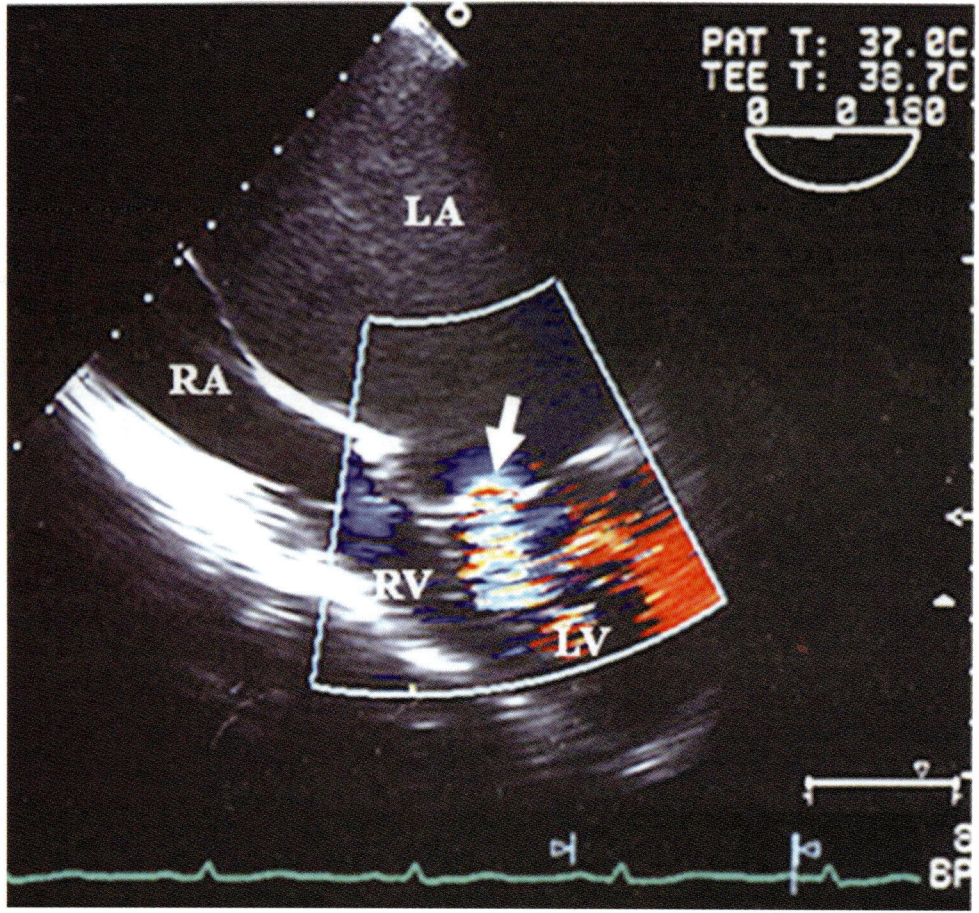

Fig. 4.16: Transmitral flow showing turbulent flow during diastole (arrow) in a patient with severe mitral stenosis. Compare with low velocity laminar nontubulent flow in a normal patient in Fig. 4.8A (LA: left atrium, LV: left ventricle, RA: right atrium, RV: right ventricle).

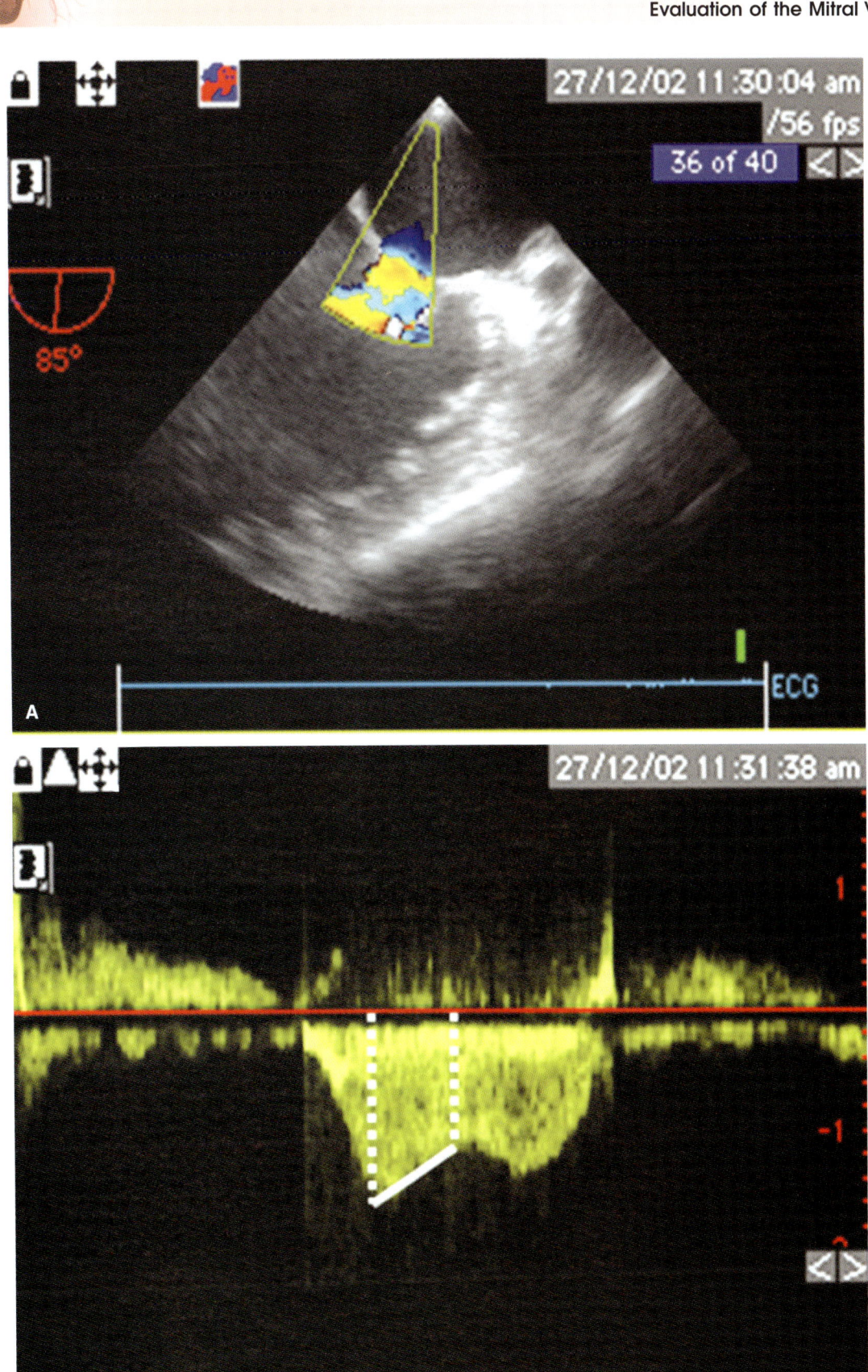

Fig. 4.17: Antegrade transmitral color flow (A) in a patient with severe mitral stenosis. Continuous wave Doppler across the mitral valve (B) is used for calculating severity of the mitral stenosis by knowing the deceleration slope (pressure half time-method).

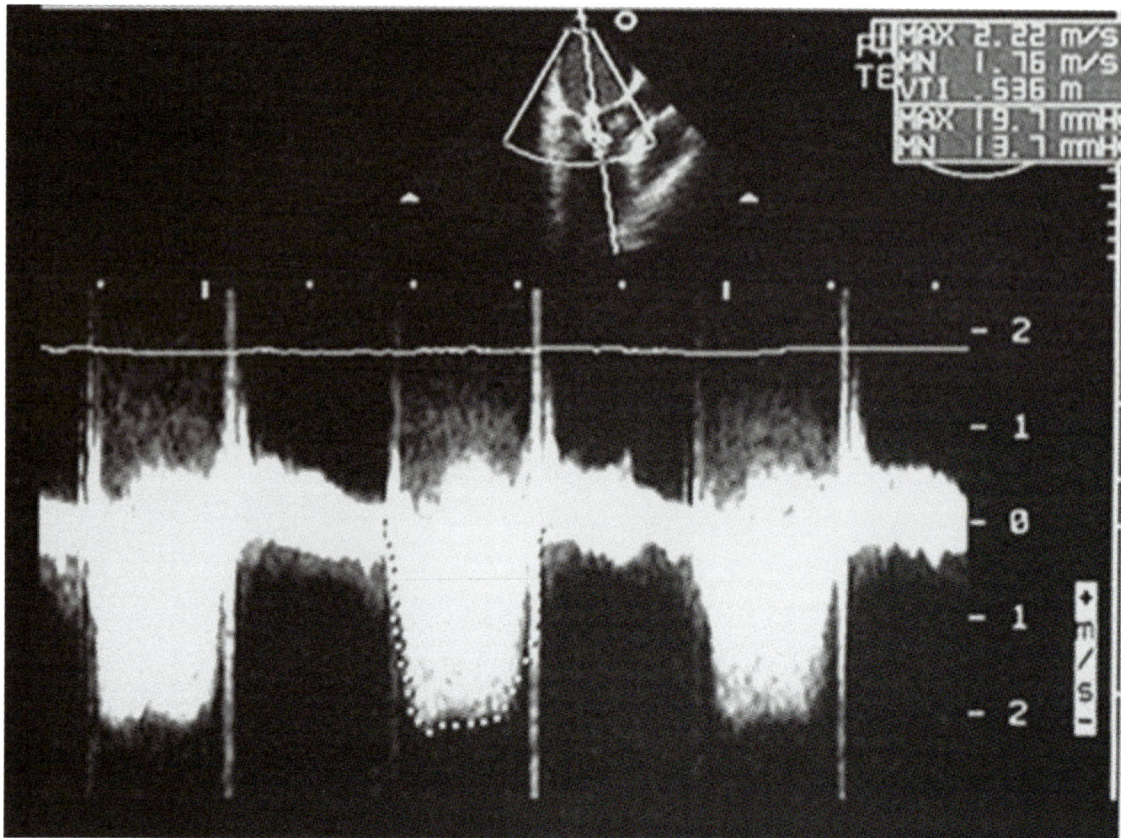

Fig. 4.18: Continuous wave Doppler across the mitral valve in a patient with severe mitral stenosis. The spectral envelope in this view can be traced for calculating peak and mean mitral gradients. Compare with the normal bimodal flow seen on pulsed wave Doppler in a normal valve (Fig. 4.8B) that shows early diastolic flow (E wave) and late diastolic flow (A wave) due to atrial contraction.

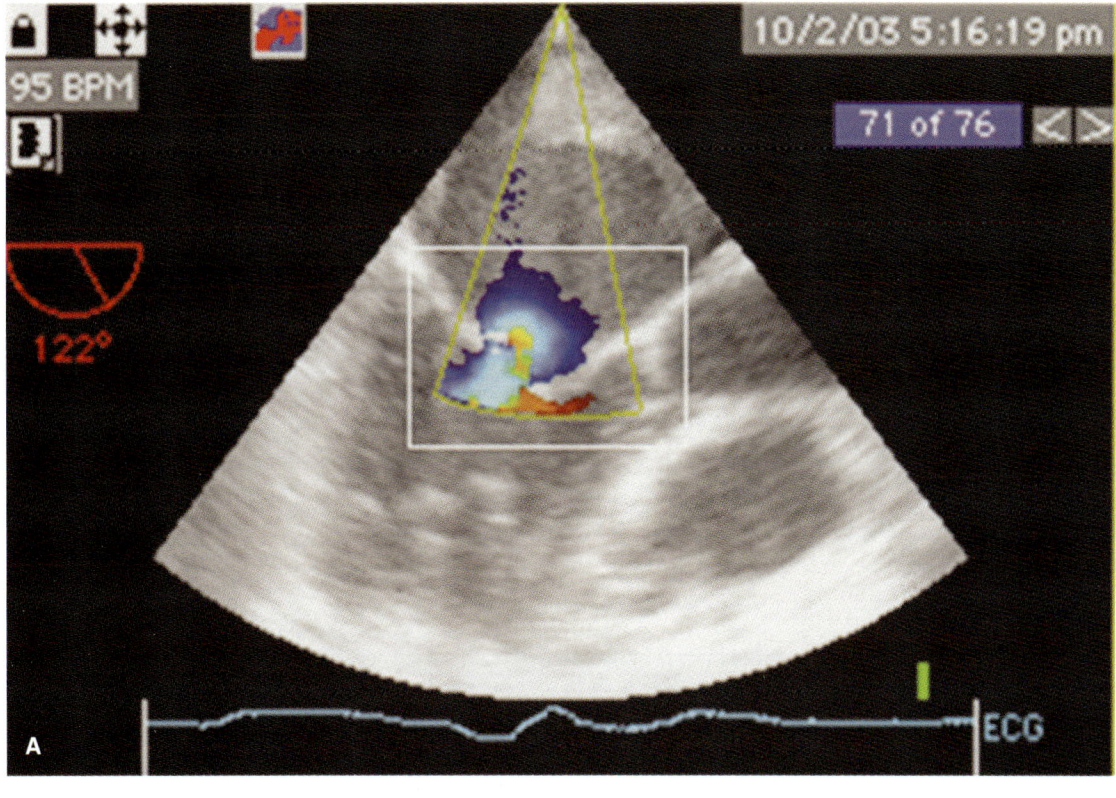

A

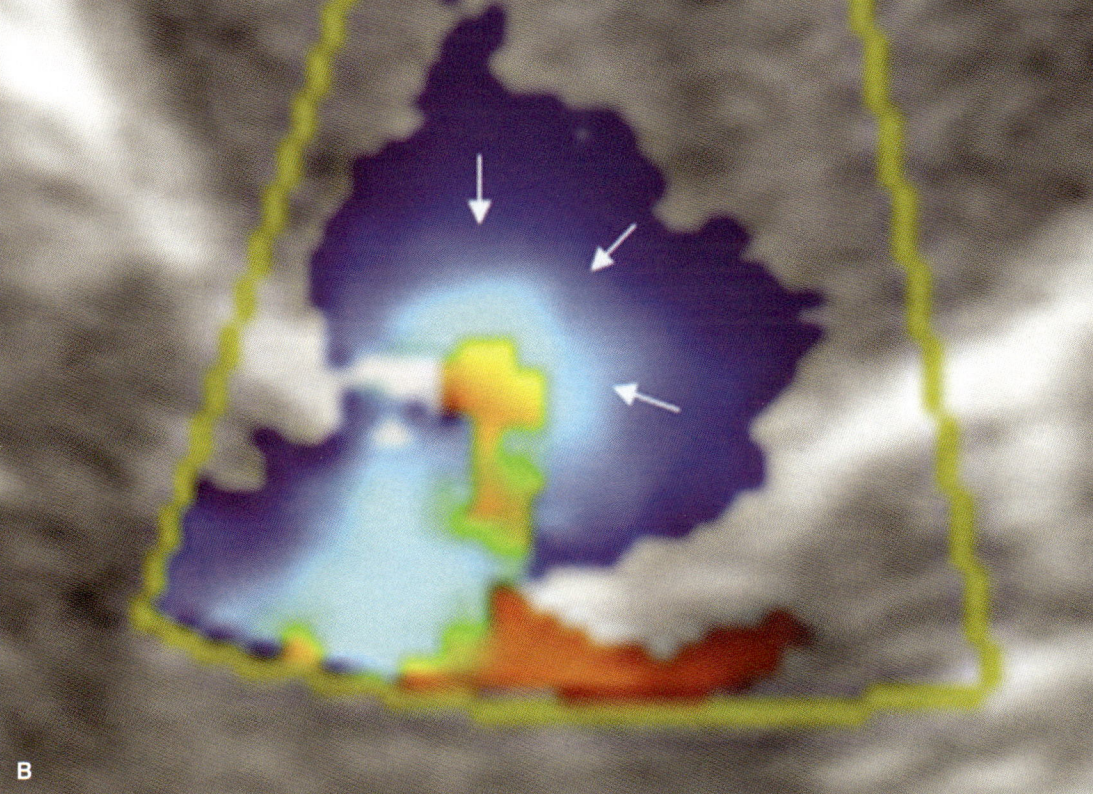

B

Fig. 4.19: Midesophageal long-axis view showing antegrade color flow across the mitral valve in severe mitral stenosis (A). Note the appearance of proximal iso-velocity area (PISA) shown by arrows in zoomed panel B image. As the flow converges towards the stenotic valve there is aliasing since the velocity of blood flow exceeds the Nyquist limit. The area of hemisphere formed by this color is calculated and multiplied by the velocity of blood to give the flow across the stenosed valve. This is used to quantify the severity of valve stenosis.

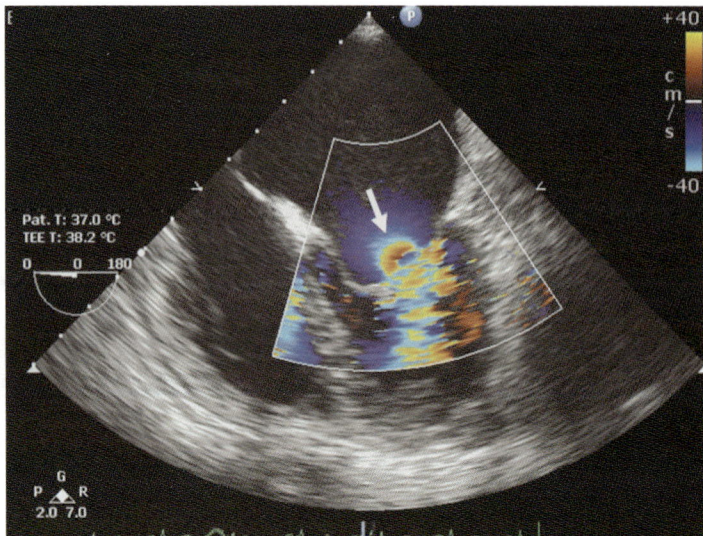

Fig. 4.20: Midesophageal 4-chamber view showing the appearance of proximal isovelocity area (PISA) (arrow) in the left atrium in another patient with severe mitral stenosis.

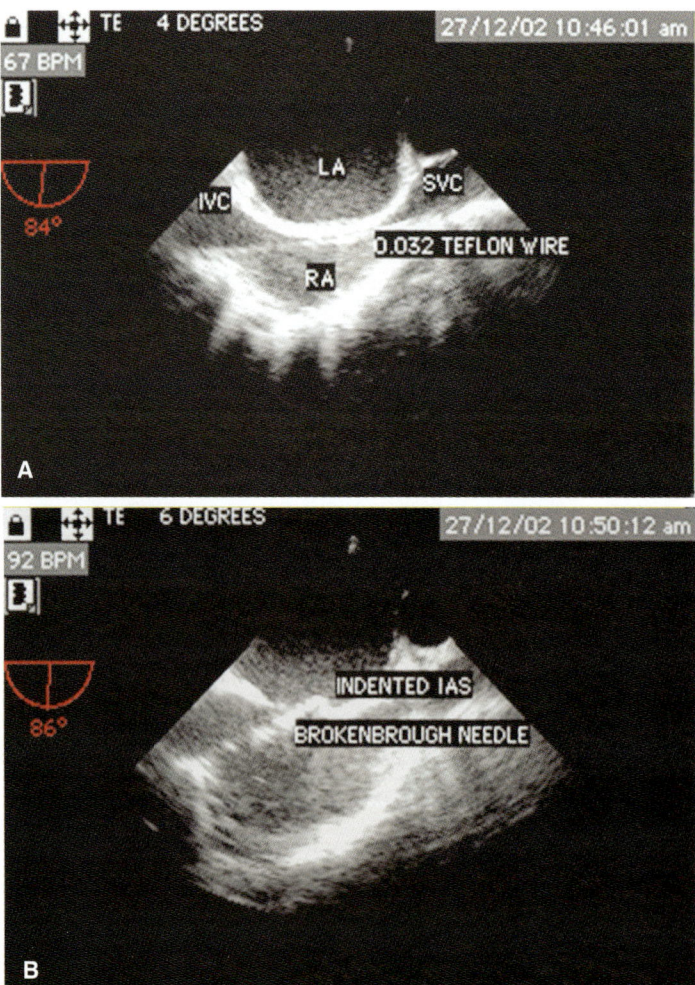

Fig. 4.21: Transesophageal echocardiography (bicaval view) for guiding percutaneous balloon mitral valvuloplasty. Panel A shows the placement of a 0.032 wire in superior vena cava used for placing Mullin's sheath. A trans-septal needle is introduced into this sheath and the entire assembly is moved down to a desirable point on the inter-atrial septum (panel B) (LA: left atrium, RA: right atrium, SVC: superior vena cava, IVC: inferior vena cava).

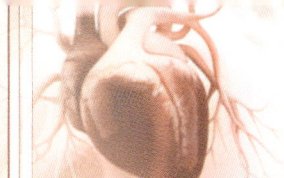

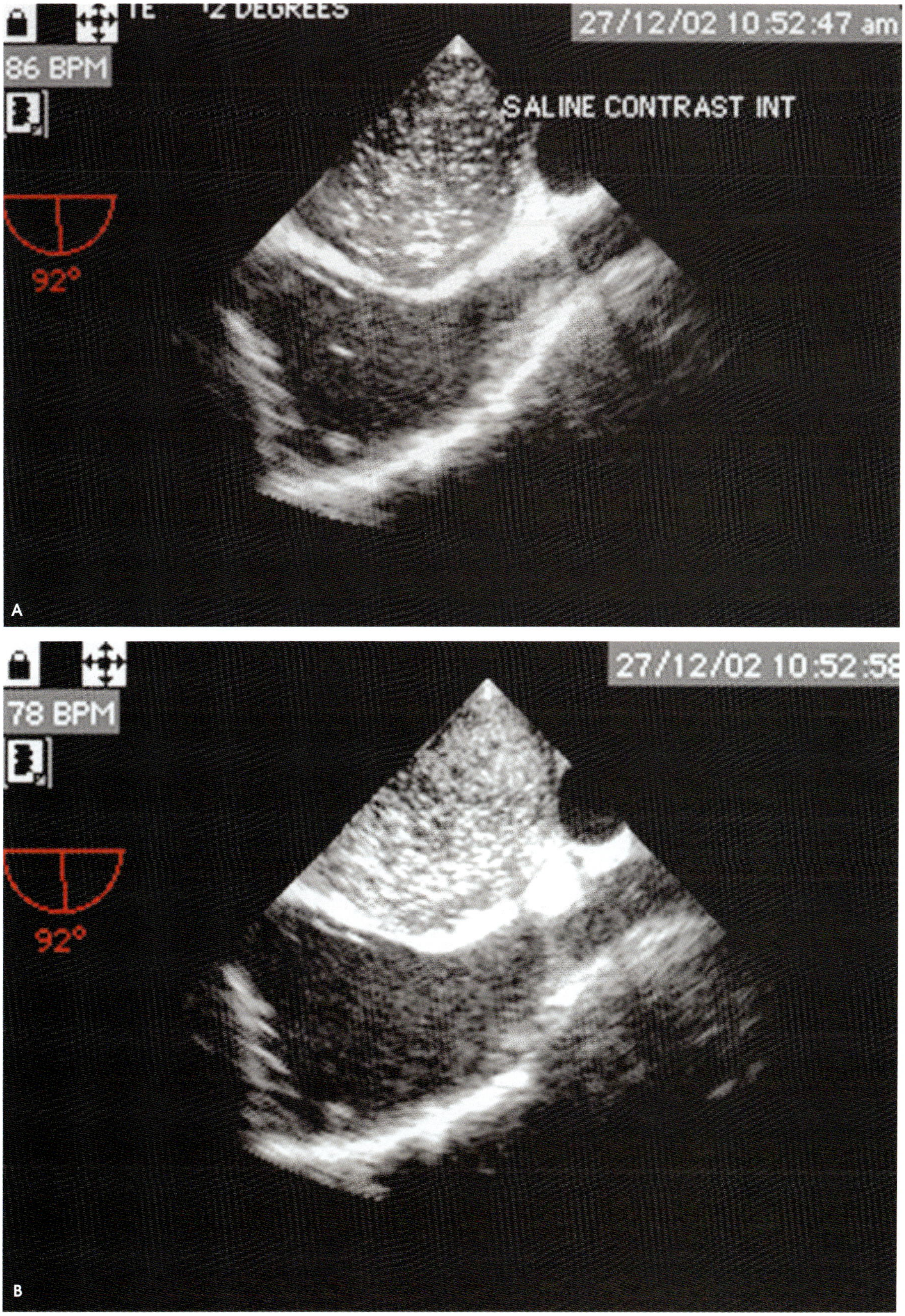

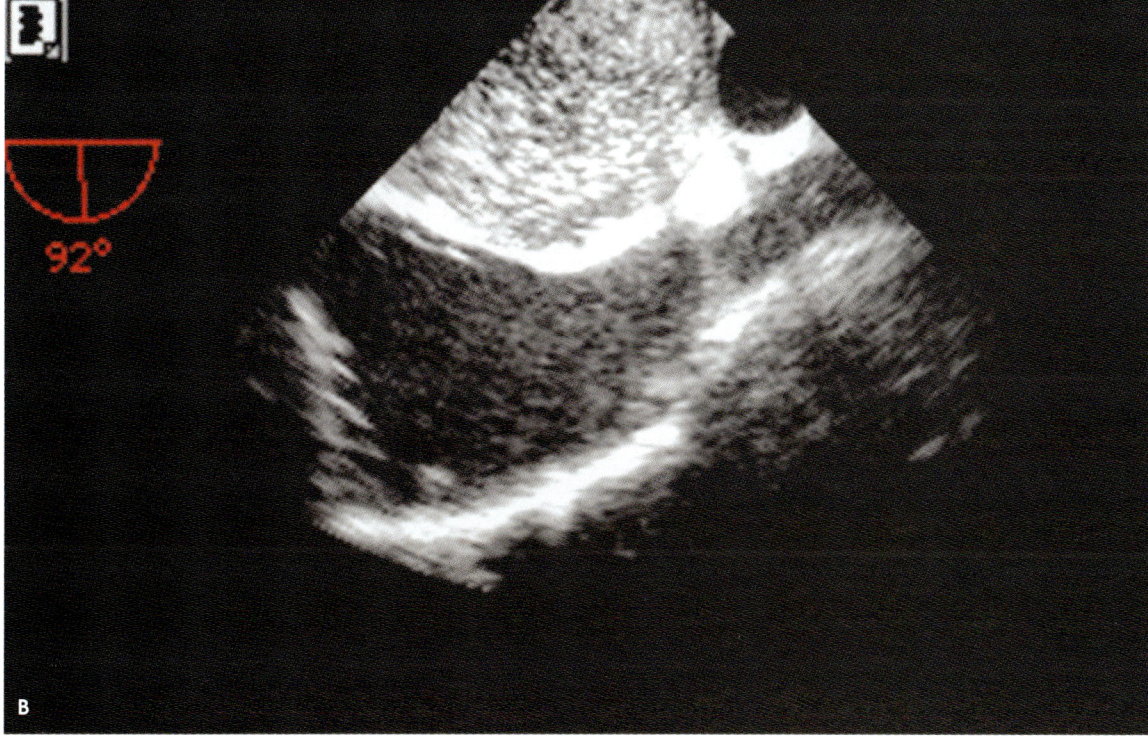

Fig. 4.22A and B: Inter-atrial septum is punctured and the position of the needle inside the left atrium is confirmed by injecting saline contrast which opacifies the left atrium.

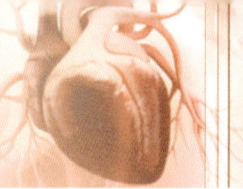

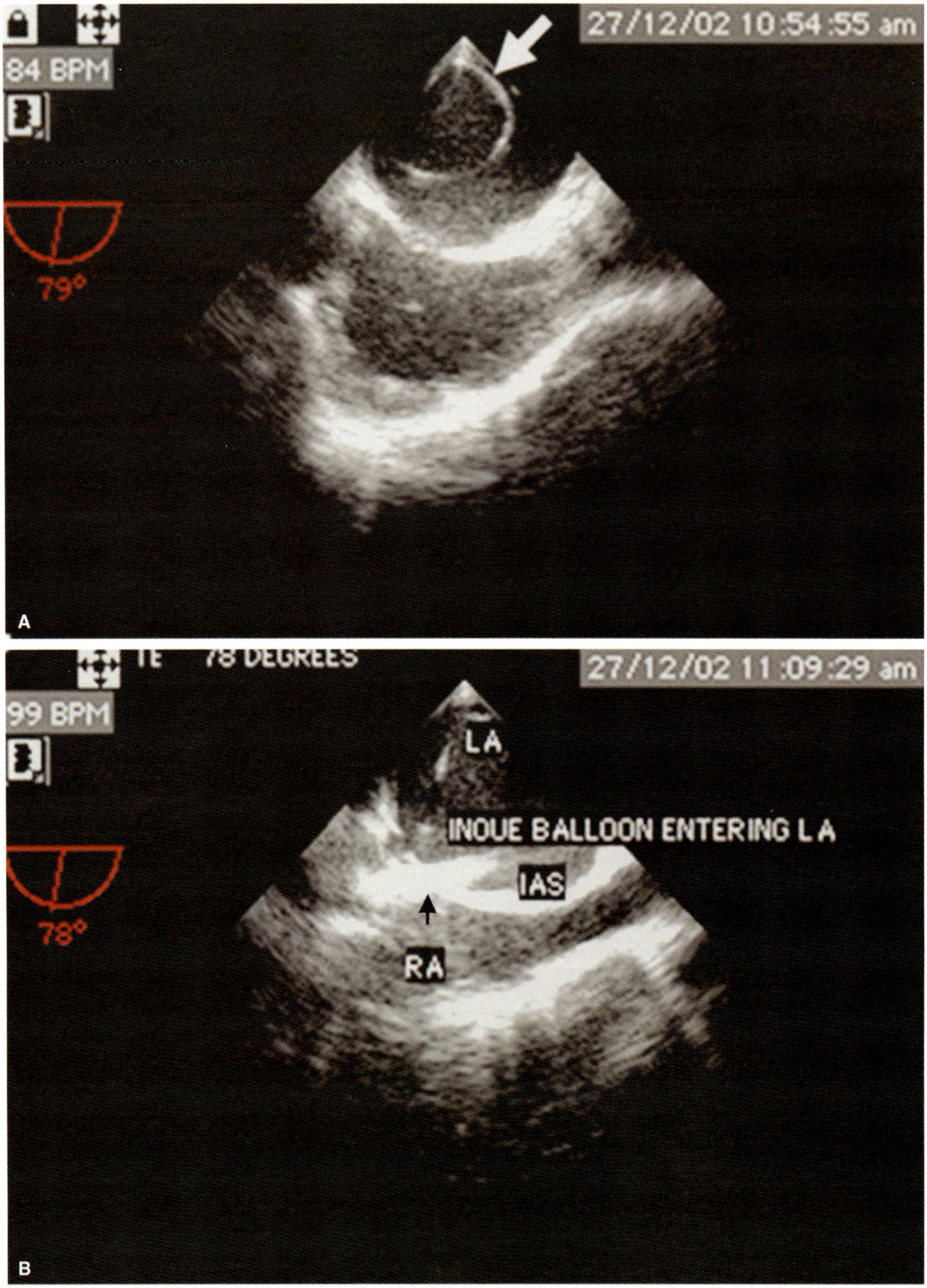

A

B

Fig. 4.23: The trans-septal needle is removed, keeping the Mullin's sheath in place and a coil wire is introduced in the left atrium (arrow in panel A). The Mullin's sheath is removed keeping the coil wire in the left atrium, inter-atrial septum puncture site is dilated with a dilator and a Inoue balloon is introduced (arrow in panel B) in its place over the coil wire. (LA: left atrium, RA: right atrium, IAS: inter-atrial septum).

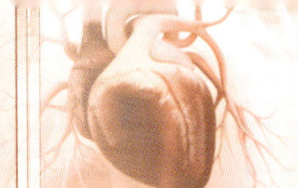

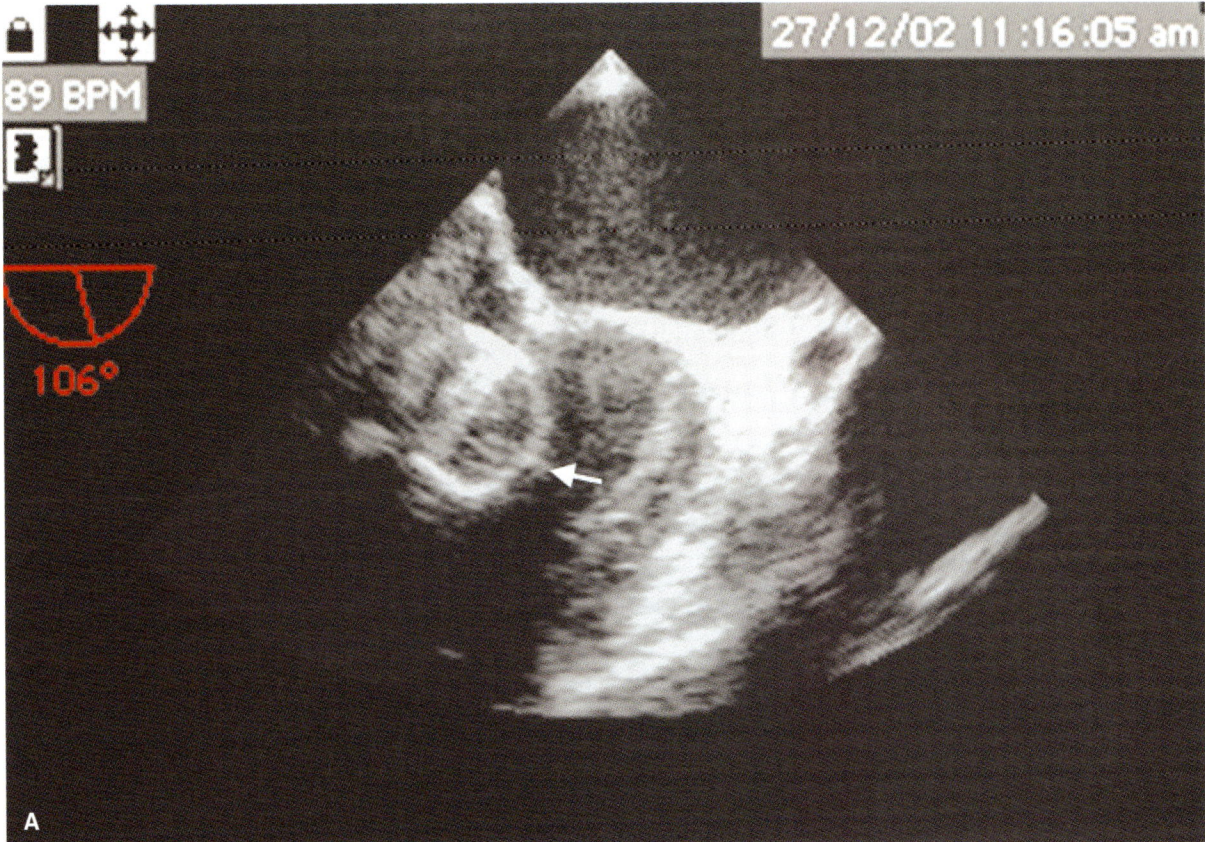

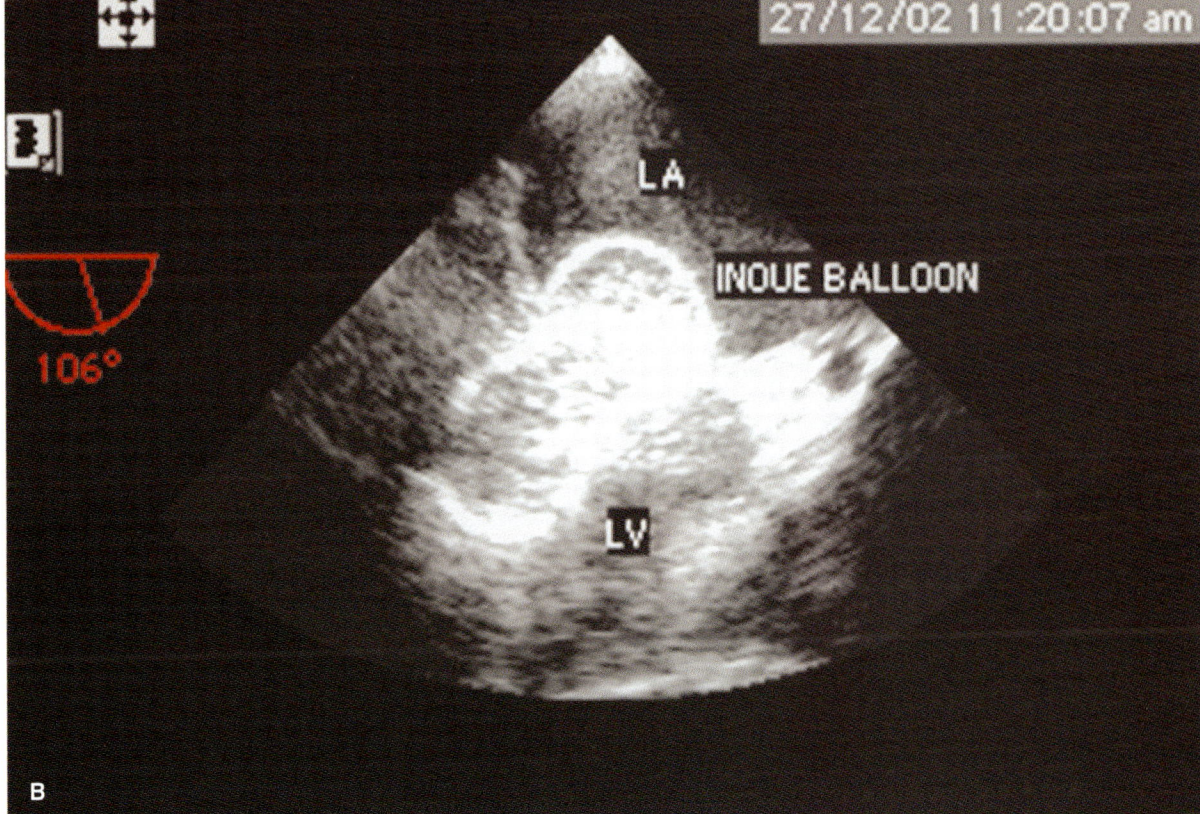

Fig. 4.24: Balloon is negotiated across the stenotic mitral valve (A). Partly inflated balloon (arrow) is then pulled back across the mitral valve and inflated completely for dilating the mitral valve (B). (two chamber views; LA: left atrium, LV: left ventricle).

MITRAL REGURGITATION

As in MS, the TEE assessment of mitral regurgitation (MR) is performed under the headings of 2-D imaging (to demonstrate valve morphology) (Fig. 4.25A), color-flow imaging (to examine blood flow profile) (Fig. 4.25B to 4.29), and Doppler evaluation (to measure velocities and calculations) (Figs 4.30–32). All the views described for examination of the mitral valve should be utilized. In addition, multiple probe manipulations are necessary to interrogate the entire mitral valve to localize the pathology.

The various methods used for assessment of the severity of MR are shown in Table 4.2.

Table 4.2: Assessment of severity of mitral regurgitation

Method	Mild	Moderate	Severe
CWD signal strength	Faint	Moderate	Dense
Jet area (cm^2)	<4	4–8	>8
Vena contracta (mm)	<3	4–6	>6
Pulm vein Doppler (S wave)	Normal	Blunt	Reverse
Regurgitant volume (cc)	<30	30–60	>60
Regurgitant fraction (%)	<30	30–50	>50
EROA (cm^2)	<0.2	0.2–0.4	>0.4
PISA radius (mm)	<4	4–10	>10

(CWD: continuous wave Doppler, EROA: effective regurgitant orifice area, PISA: proximal isovelocity surface area)

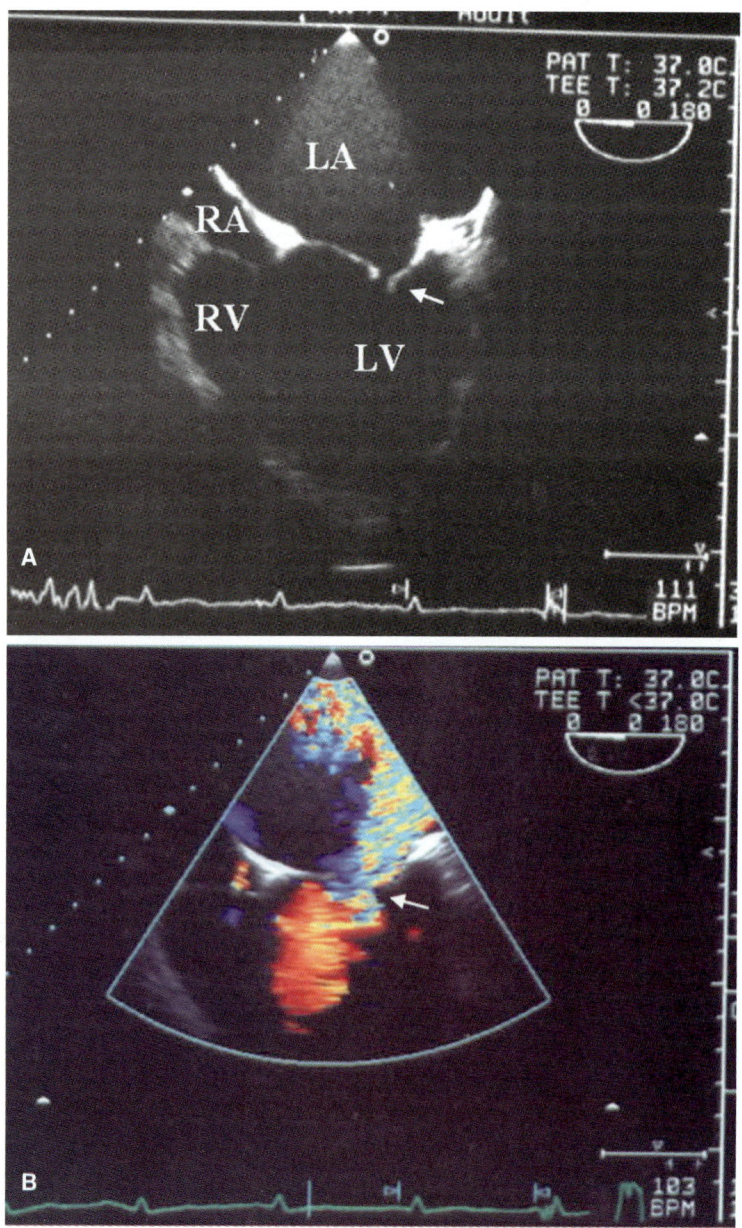

Fig. 4.25: Severe mitral regurgitation due to incomplete coaptation of the mitral leaflets (arrow) in 4-chamber views (A and B). (LA: left atrium, LV: left ventricle, RA: right atrium, RV: right ventricle).

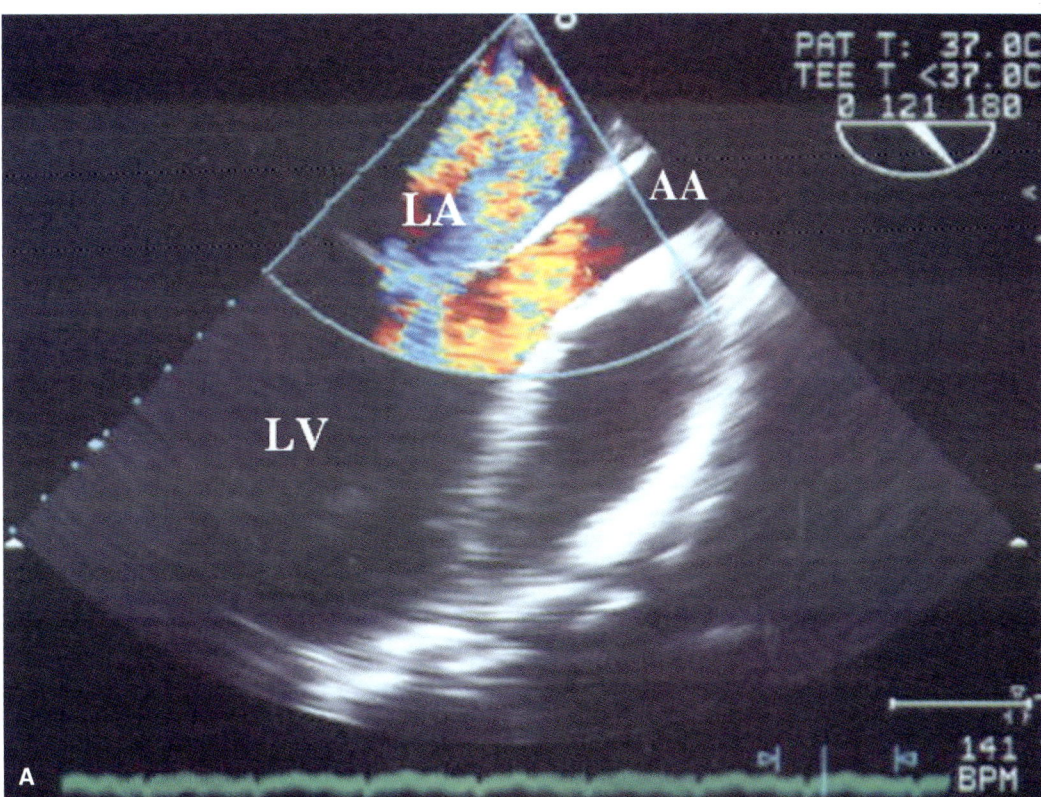

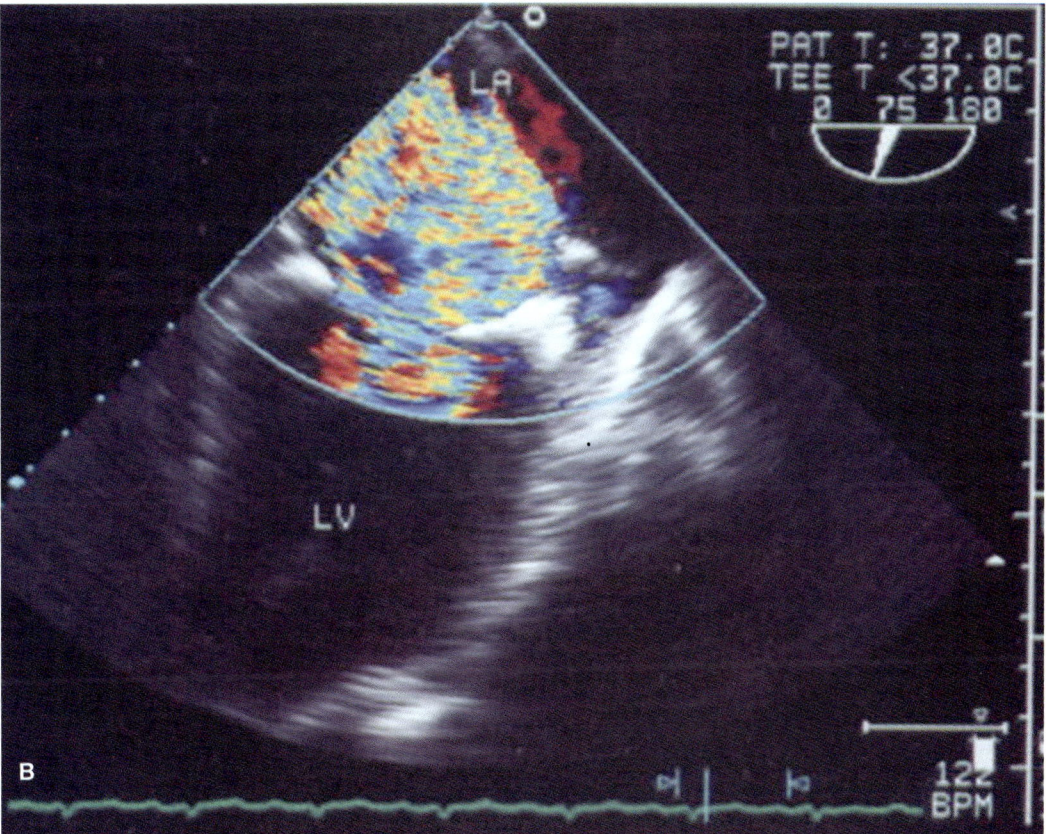

Fig. 4.26: Appearance of severe mitral regurgitation on color flow imaging in midesophageal aortic valve long-axis view (A) and two chamber view (B) (LA: left atrium, LV: left ventricle, AA: ascending aorta).

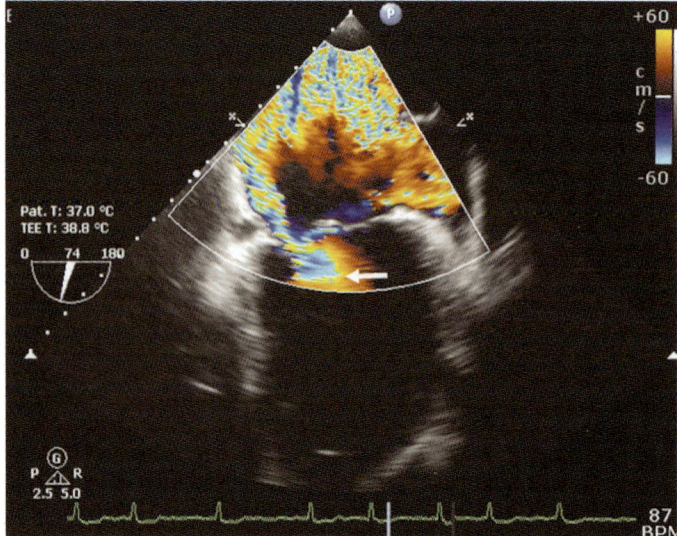

Fig. 4.27: Midesophageal two-chamber view showing the convergence of blood at the mitral valve and formation of a hemisphere of proximal isovelocity area (PISA) (arrow) in the left ventricle in a patient with severe mitral regurgitation.

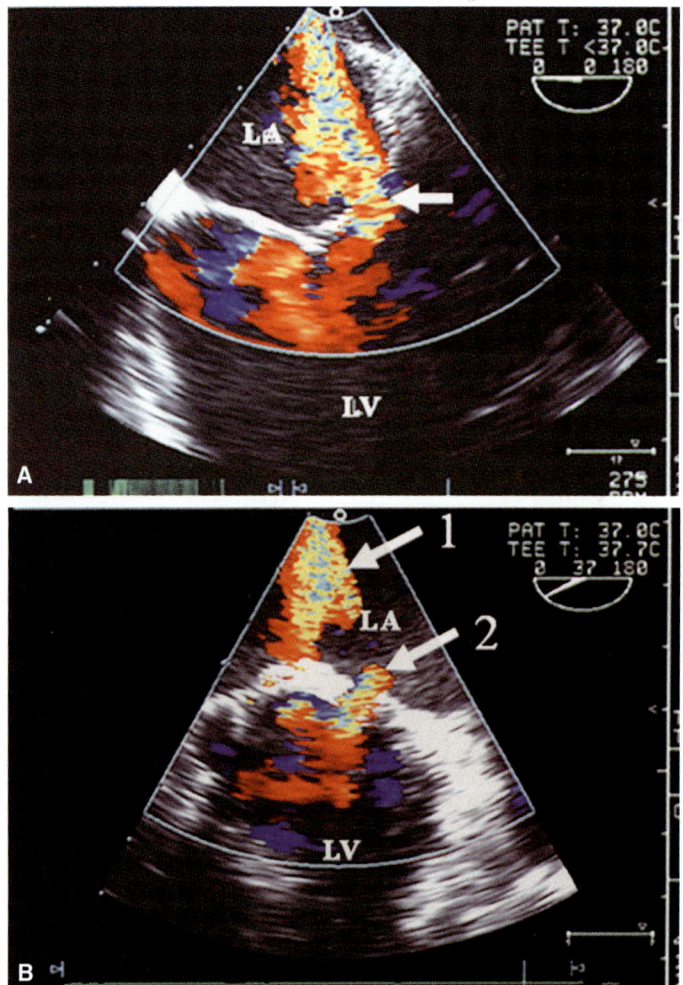

Fig. 4.28: Mitral regurgitation due to perforation of the mitral valve leaflet (A). Note the regurgitant orifice which is located at the base of the posterior mitral leaflet (arrow). Panel B shows the echo picture with two regurgitant orifices (arrows 1 and 2) in the mitral valve. (LA: left atrium, LV: left ventricle).

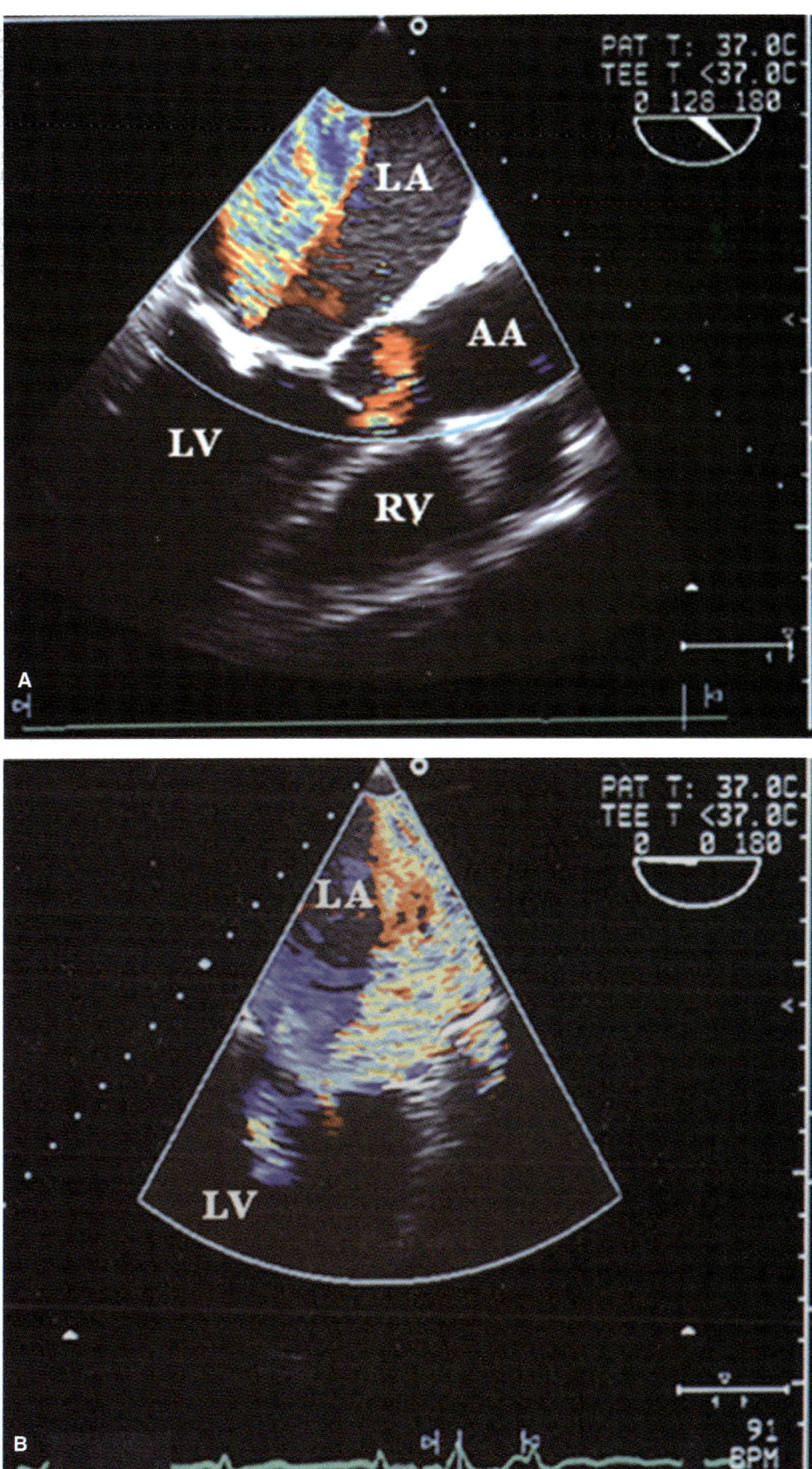

Fig. 4.29: Appearance of mitral regurgitation (MR) on TEE. Panel A shows a central jet in a patient with moderate MR, while panel B shows an eccentric jet that is directed posteriorly. (LA: left atrium, LV: left ventricle, RV: right ventricle, AA: ascending aorta).

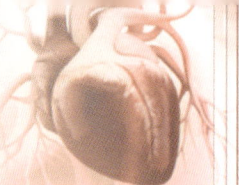

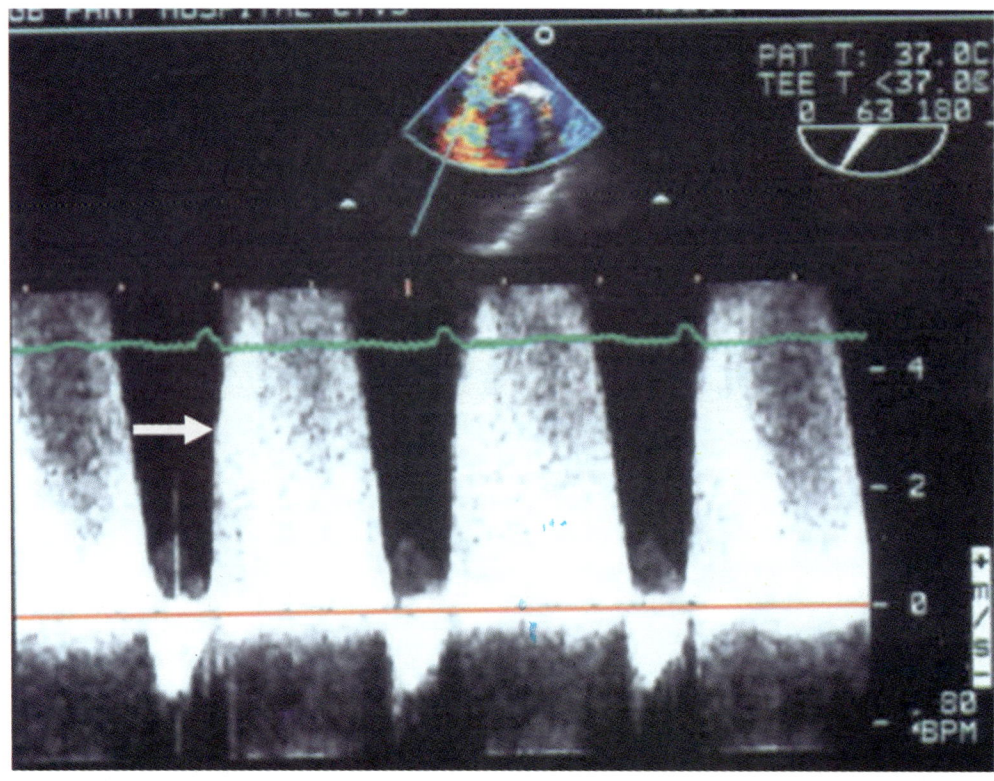

Fig. 4.30: Continuous wave Doppler across the mitral valve in a patient with mitral regurgitation (MR). Note the spectral trace of MR (arrow).

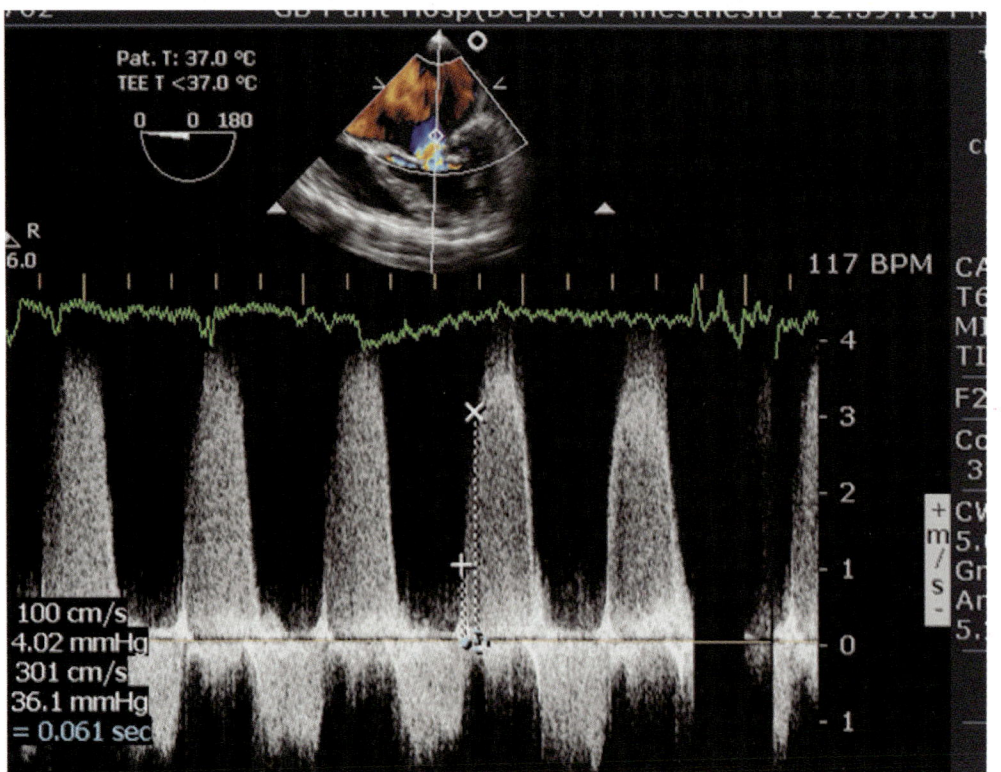

Fig. 4.31: Continuous wave Doppler profile in mitral regurgitation (MR). The MR velocity (V_{max}) greater than 400 cm/s indicates severe MR. The rate of ventricular pressure rise (dP/dt) is a measure of left ventricular function that can be measured in the presence of MR. Here, it equals (36-4)/0.06 = 533.3 mmHg/s.

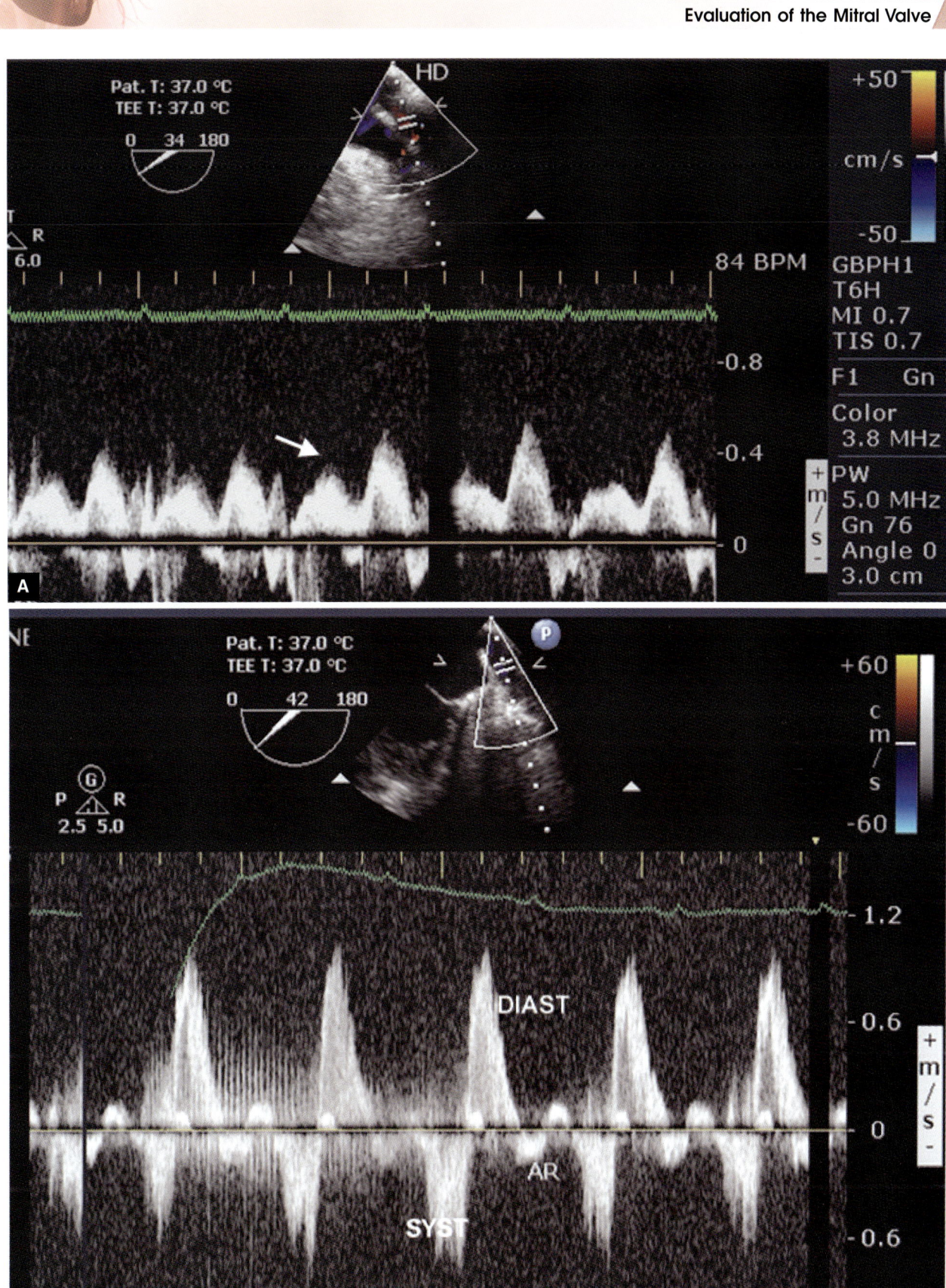

Fig. 4.32: Pulmonary venous flow velocity profile on pulsed wave Doppler showing obtundation of systolic wave (arrow, panel A) and reversal of systolic wave (panel B) in severe mitral regurgitation (SYST: systole, DIAST: diastole, AR: atrial reversal).

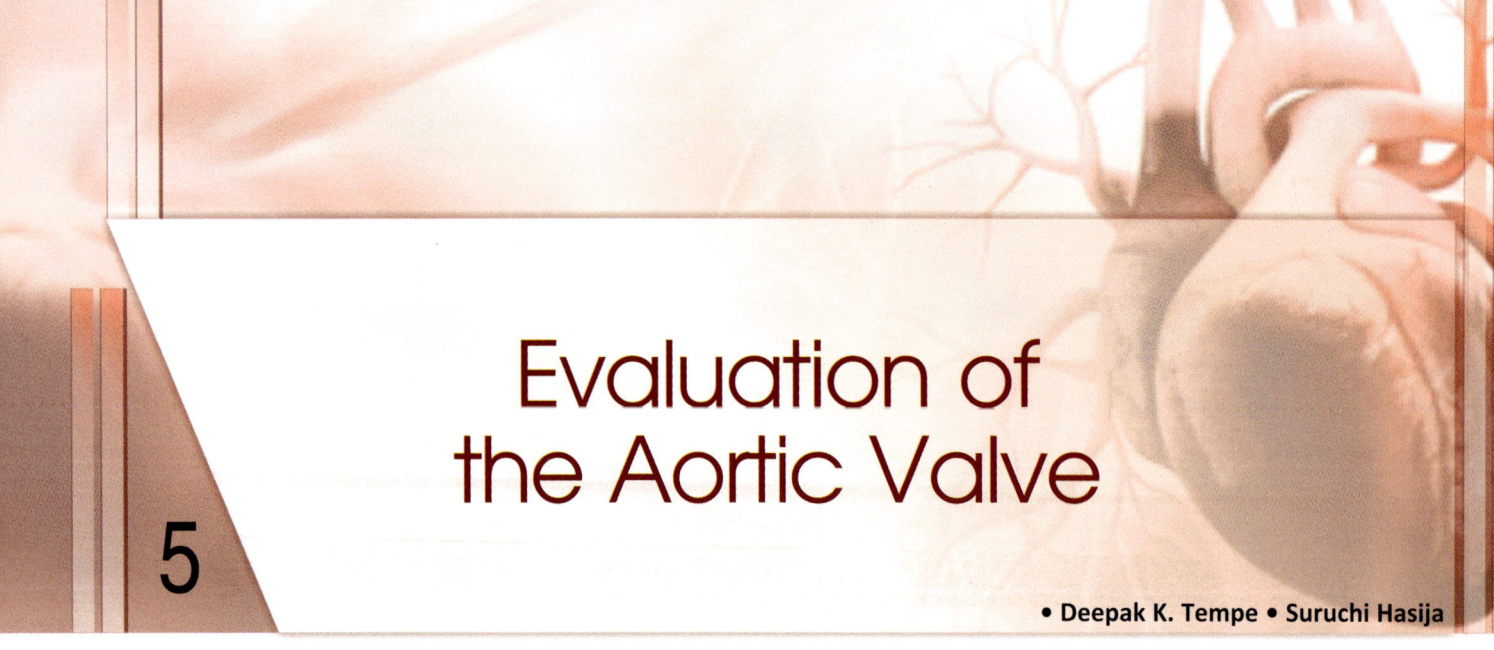

Evaluation of the Aortic Valve

5

• **Deepak K. Tempe** • **Suruchi Hasija**

A careful and complete assessment of the aortic valve is a part of every transesophageal echocardiographic (TEE) examination. The TEE examination of the aortic valve should include two-dimensional images from multiple transducer locations and angle as well as color flow and spectral Doppler interrogation. Three-dimensional imaging completes the examination of the aortic valve. This chapter illustrates the common pathological states affecting the aortic valve encountered during the perioperative period. The pre- and post-cardiopulmonary bypass assessment of the aortic valve in patients undergoing aortic valve replacement is useful to detect the adequacy of the valve function so that immediate surgical correction of the paravalvular leaks can be carried out. Information obtained from TEE also aids in assessing the feasibility of repair, sizing the valve from the annular diameter, adequacy of surgical repair, prosthetic valve function, and other possible complications.

ANATOMY

The aortic valve is a part of the aortic valve apparatus, which consists of the left ventricular outflow tract, aortic

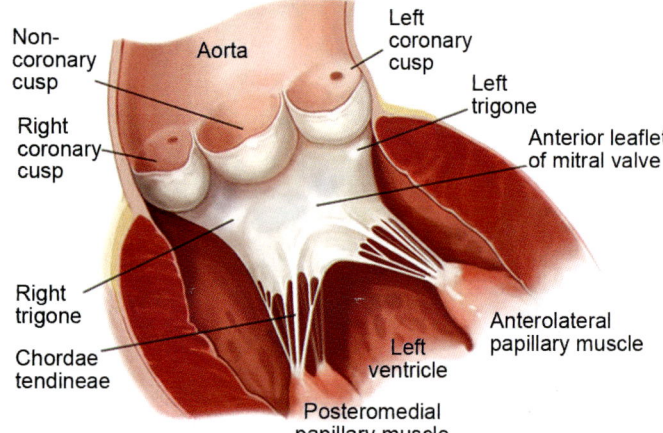

Fig. 5.1: The aortic valve apparatus.

valve cusps, sinuses of Valsalva and proximal ascending aorta (Fg. 5.1). The aortic root extends from the aortic valve annulus to the sinotubular junction and includes the sinuses of Valsalva. Aortic valve dysfunction can occur consequent to disruption of any component of this apparatus.

The following views are useful in examining the aortic valve:

1. Midesophageal 5-chamber View (0–10°) (Fig. 5.2)

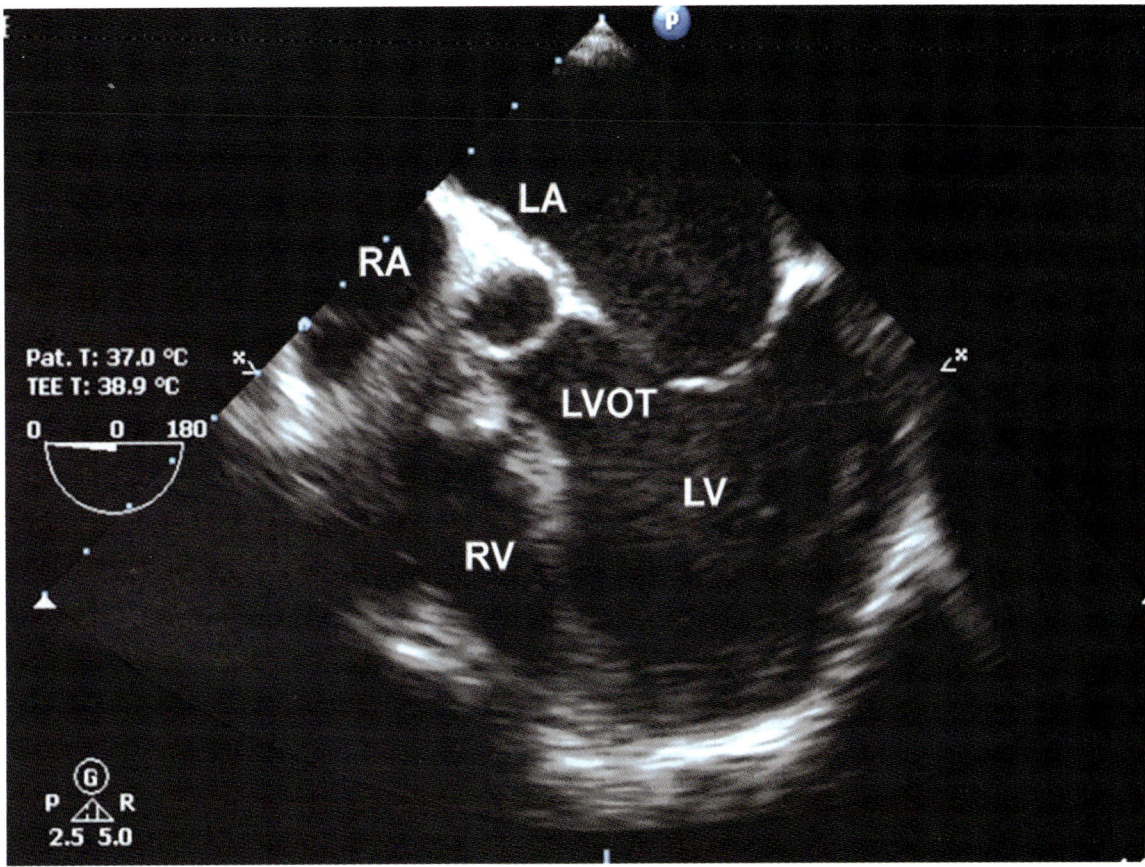

Fig. 5.2: Midesophageal 5-chamber view. (RA: right atrium, LA: left atrium, RV: right ventricle, LV: left ventricle, LVOT: left ventricular outflow tract).

2. Midesophageal Aortic Valve Short-axis View (25–45°) (Figs 5.3–5.5)

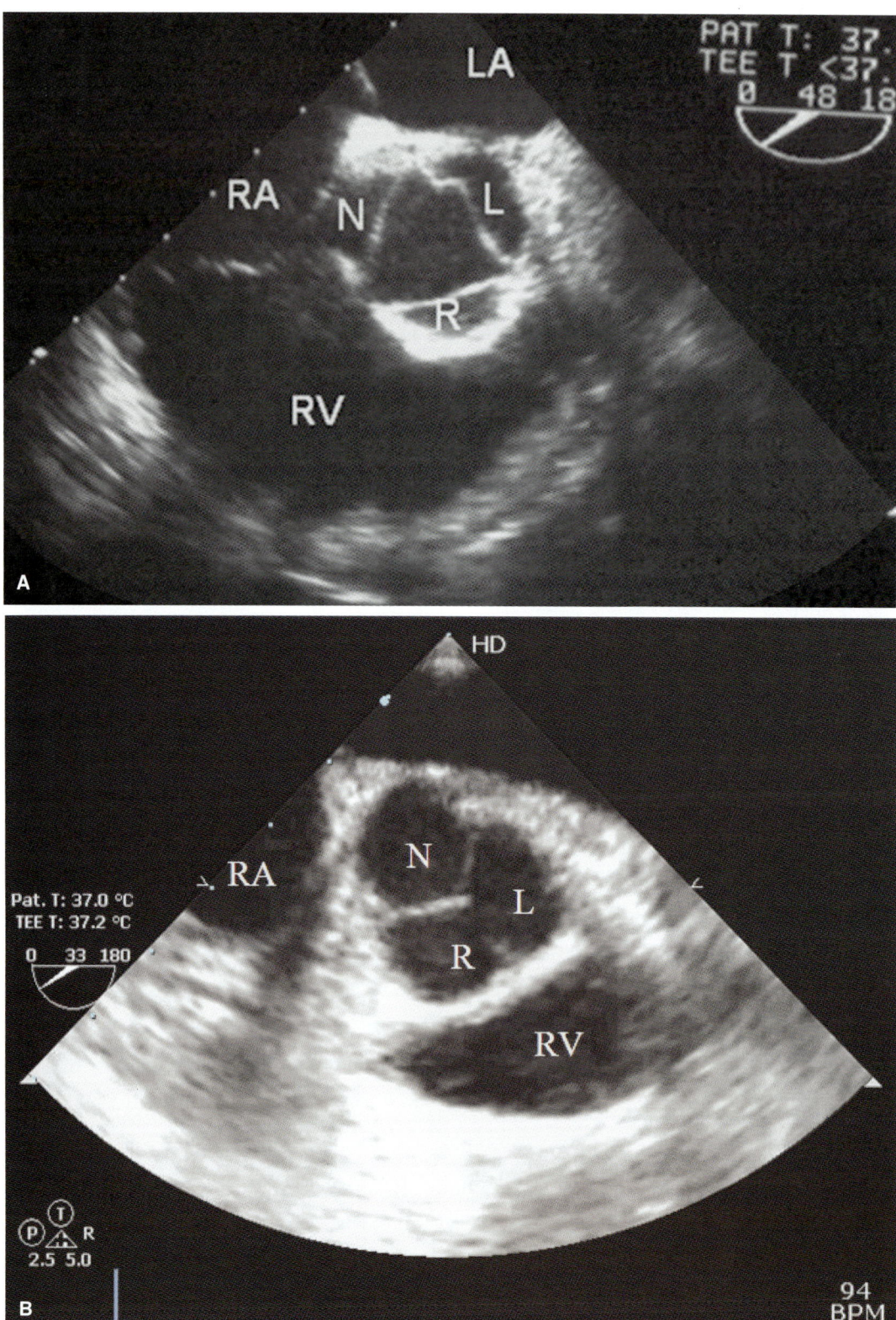

Fig. 5.3: Midesophageal aortic valve short-axis view of the normal aortic valve in systole (A) and diastole (B). (RA: right atrium, LA: left atrium, RV: right ventricle, N: non-coronary cusp, L: left coronary cusp, R: right coronary cusp).

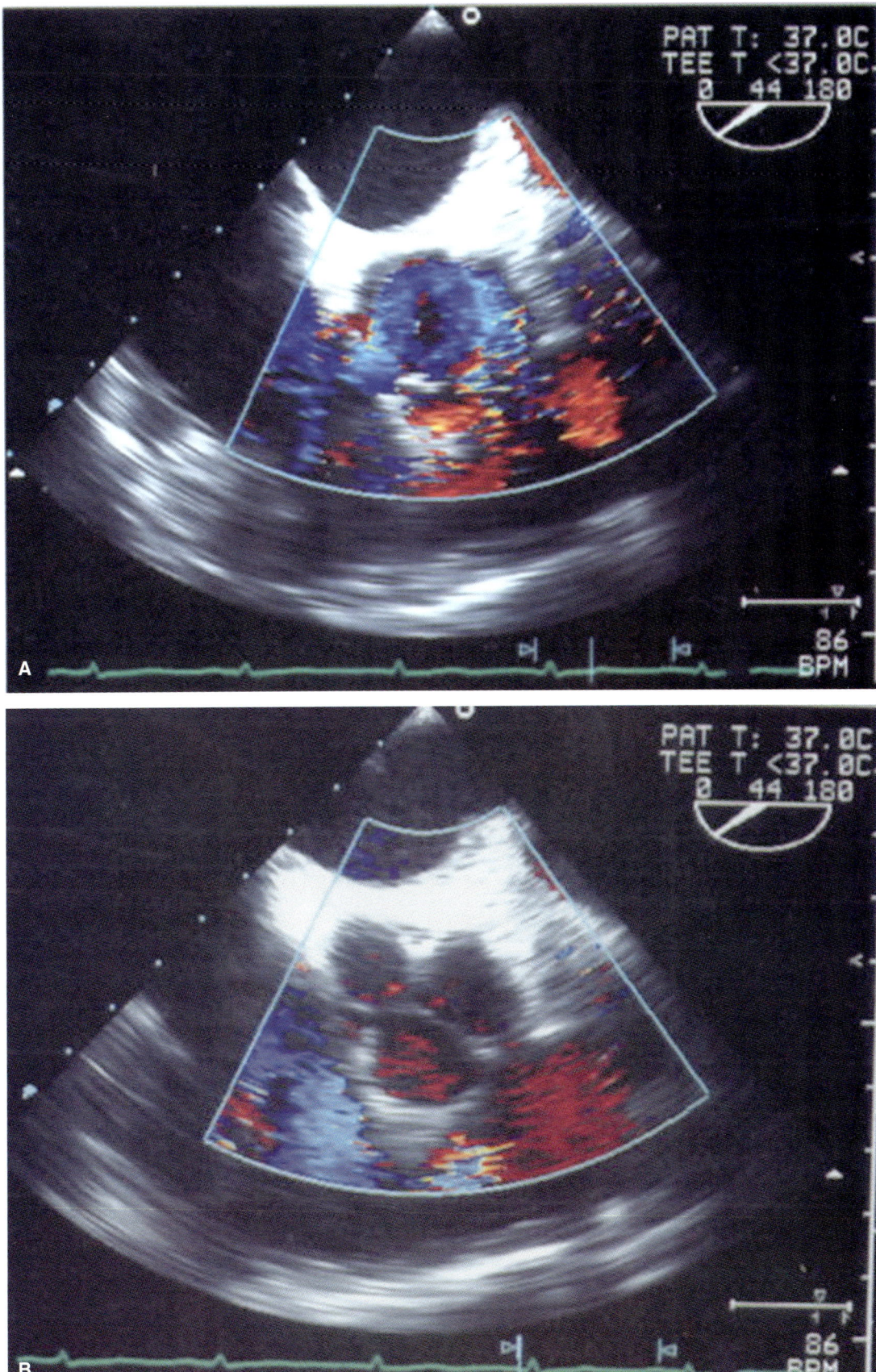

Fig. 5.4: Color flow across a normal aortic valve in systole (A) and diastole (B).

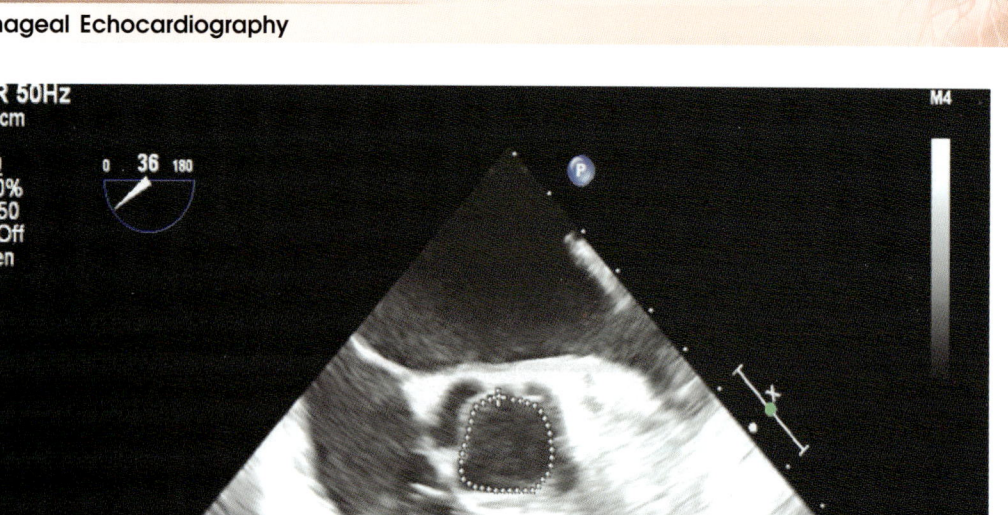

Fig. 5.5: Midesophageal aortic valve short-axis view showing the calculation of aortic valve area by planimetry in a non-stenotic aortic valve.

3. Midesophageal Aortic Valve Long-axis View (120–140°) (Fig. 5.6)

This view is used to measure the aortic valve annulus between the hinge points of the leaflets.

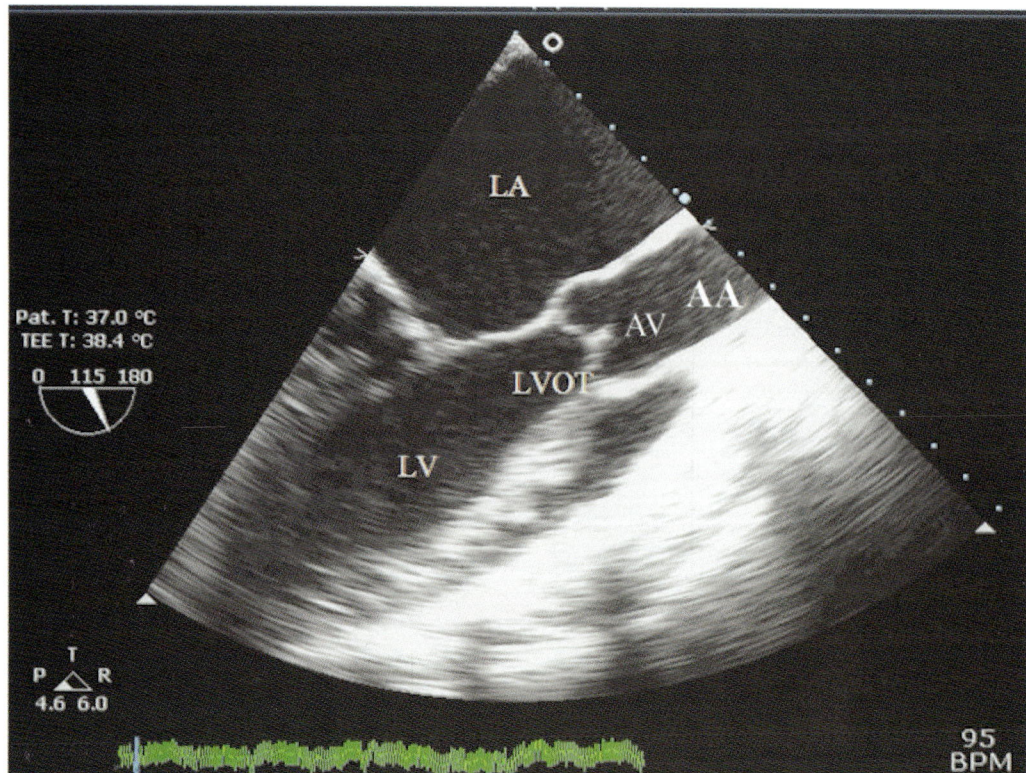

Fig. 5.6: Midesophageal aortic valve long-axis view showing the aortic valve in closed position. (LA: left atrium, LV: left ventricle, LVOT: left ventricular outflow tract, AV: aortic valve, AA: ascending aorta).

4. Deep Transgastric Long-axis View (0–20°) (Figs 5.7 and 5.8)

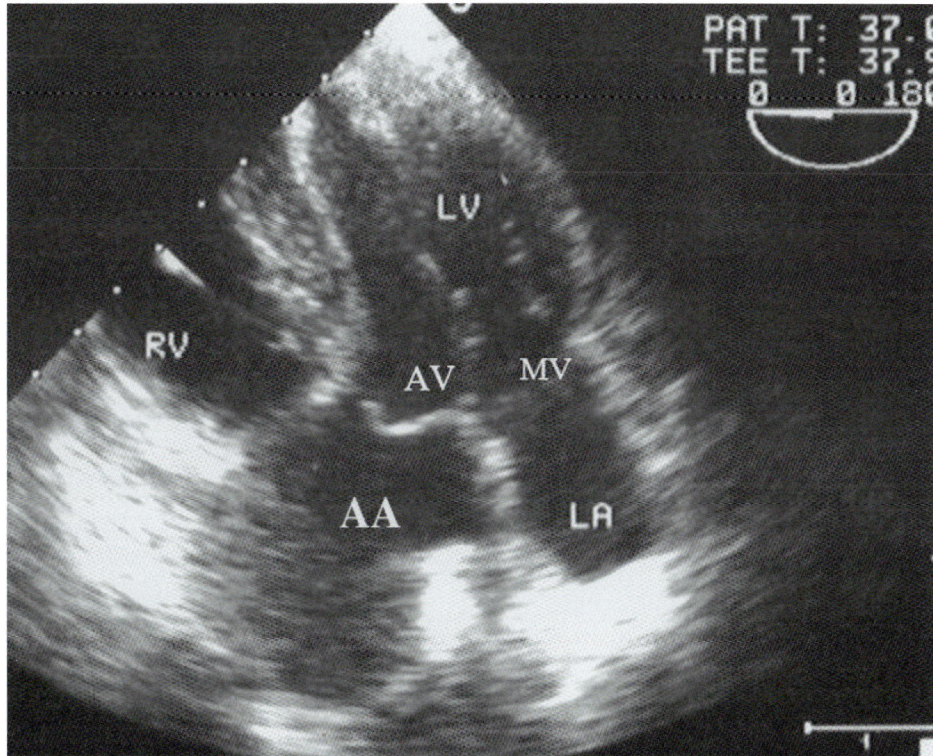

Fig. 5.7: Deep transgastric long-axis view. Blood flow velocity and pressure gradient across the aortic valve can be calculated in this view as the ultrasound beam is parallel to the direction of blood flow. (LA: left atrium, MV: mitral valve, LV: left ventricle, RV: right ventricle, AV: aortic valve, AA: ascending aorta).

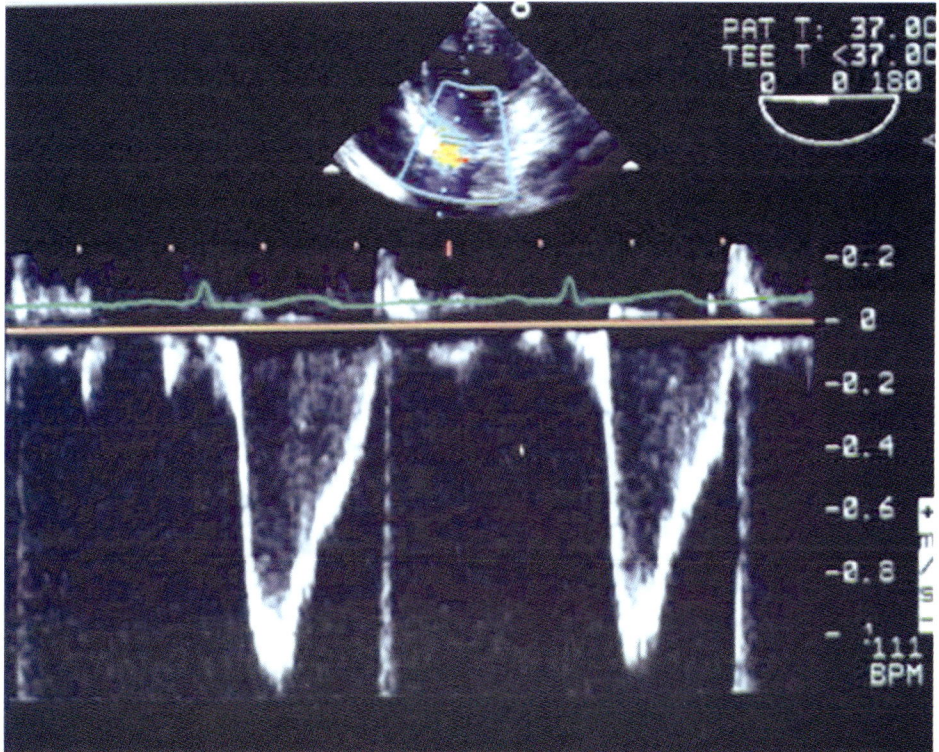

Fig. 5.8: Pulsed wave Doppler flow across the normal aortic valve in deep transgastric long-axis view.

5. Transgastric Long-axis View (120–140°) (Fig. 5.9)

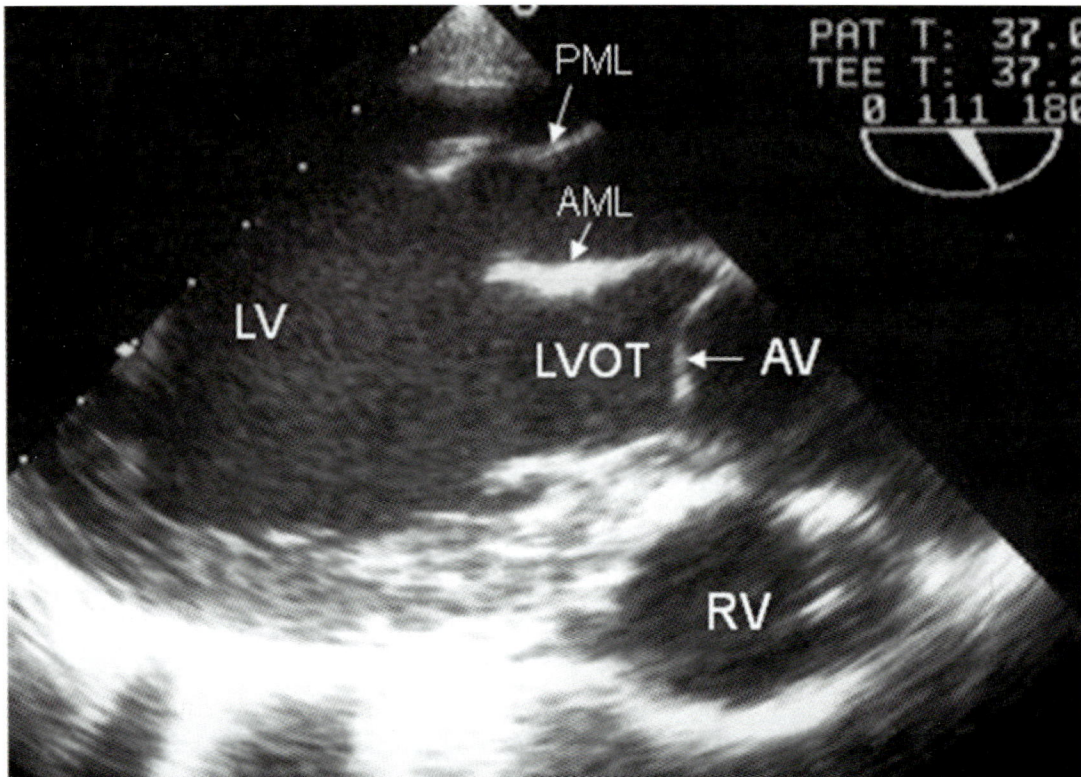

Fig. 5.9: Transgastric long-axis view. This view also allows spectral Doppler analysis of the aortic valve. (LV: left ventricle, RV: right ventricle, LVOT: left ventricular outflow tract, AV; aortic valve, AML: anterior mitral leaflet, PML: posterior mitral leaflet).

AORTIC STENOSIS

The etiology of aortic stenosis is rheumatic heart disease, degenerative or congenital (bicuspid, unicuspid, quadricuspid valve). Rheumatic heart disease causes valvular fibrosis resulting in stenosis/ insufficiency. The underlying mechanism of aortic stenosis in the elderly and congenitally malformed valves is progressive calcification of the leaflets.

The severity of aortic stenosis can be estimated by the following methods (Table 5.1) (Figs 5.10–5.18).

1. *Peak aortic stenosis jet velocity:* The ultrasound beam is oriented parallel to the direction of blood flow and the highest systolic velocity across the aortic valve is measured using continuous wave Doppler (Fig. 5.16).

2. *Pressure gradient:* The mean and peak transaortic pressure gradients are derived from the continuous wave Doppler profile of blood flow across the aortic valve (Fig. 5.16).

3. *Planimetry:* The aortic valve area is measured by manually tracing the inner edges of the aortic valve leaflets in the same plane (Fig. 5.17).

4. *Continuity equation:* The area of aortic valve can be derived using the following equation:

$$AV \ area \times VTI_{AV} = LVOT \ area \times VTI_{LVOT}$$
$$AV \ area = LVOT \ area \times VTI_{LVOT}/VTI_{AV}$$
$$AV \ area = 0.785 \ d^2 \times VTI_{LVOT}/VTI_{AV}$$

Where; AV is aortic valve, VTI is velocity time integral, LVOT is left ventricular outflow tract, and d is diameter of LVOT (Fig. 5.18).

5. *Proximal isovelocity surface area (PISA) method:* The ultrasound beam is oriented parallel to the direction of blood flow and color flow Doppler view of the aortic valve is obtained.

$$AVA = \frac{2\pi r^2 \times V_A \times (\alpha/180)}{V_{max}}$$

Where, AVA is aortic valve area, r is the radius from the center of the PISA formation to its first aliasing

Table 5.1: Assessment of severity of aortic stenosis				
	Valve area (cm²)	Indexed valve area (cm²/m²)	Peak jet velocity (m/s)	Pressure gradients (mm Hg)
				Peak	Mean
Mild	>1.5	>0.85	< 3.0	20–40	<25
Moderate	1.0–1.5	0.6–0.85	3.0–4.0	40–70	25–40
Severe	<1.0	<0.6	>4.0	>70	>40

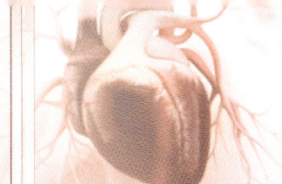

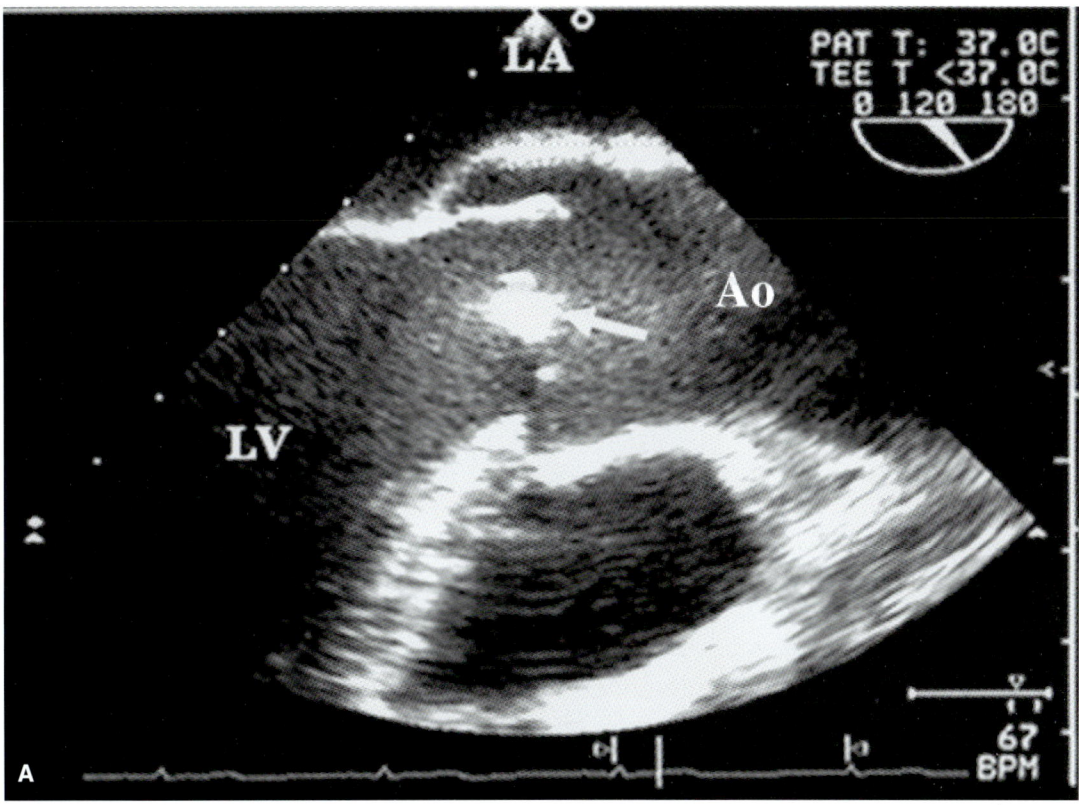

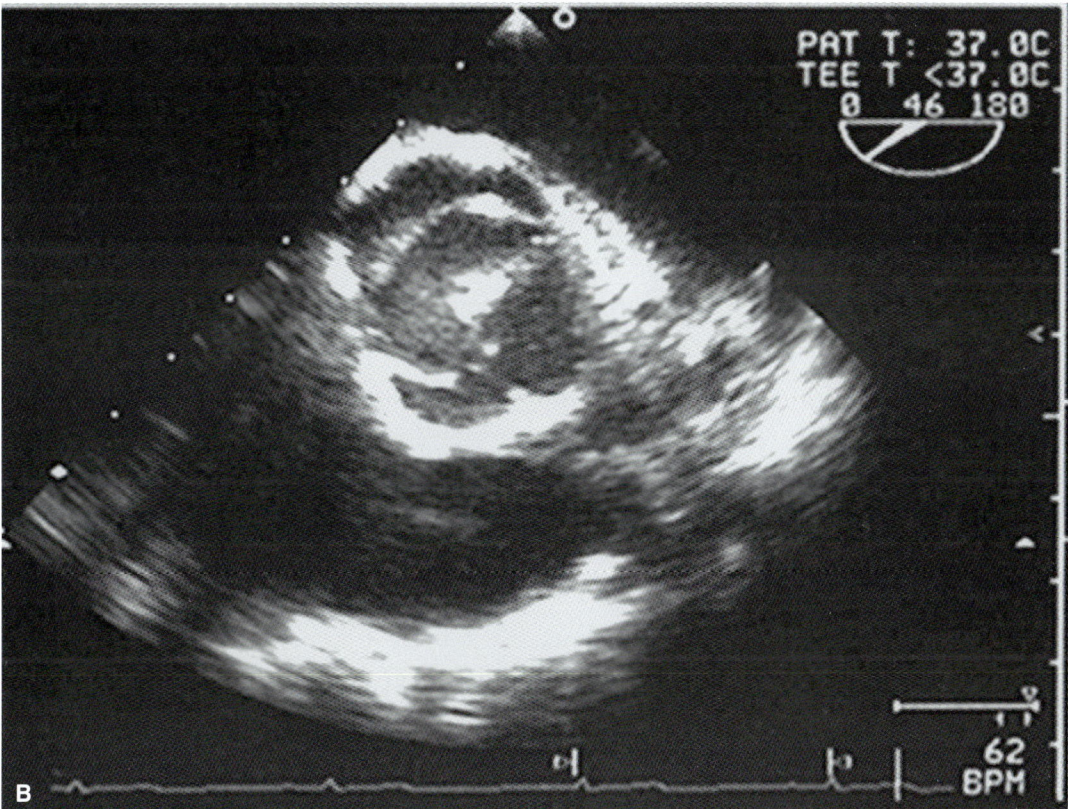

Fig. 5.10: A patient with rheumatic aortic valve disease. Note the doming aortic valve in long axis (A). Also note the calcific nodule on the aortic valve leaflet (arrow). Appearance of the stenosed aortic valve in short axis (B). This view can be used for performing aortic valve planimetry. (LA: left atrium, LV: left ventricle, Ao: aorta).

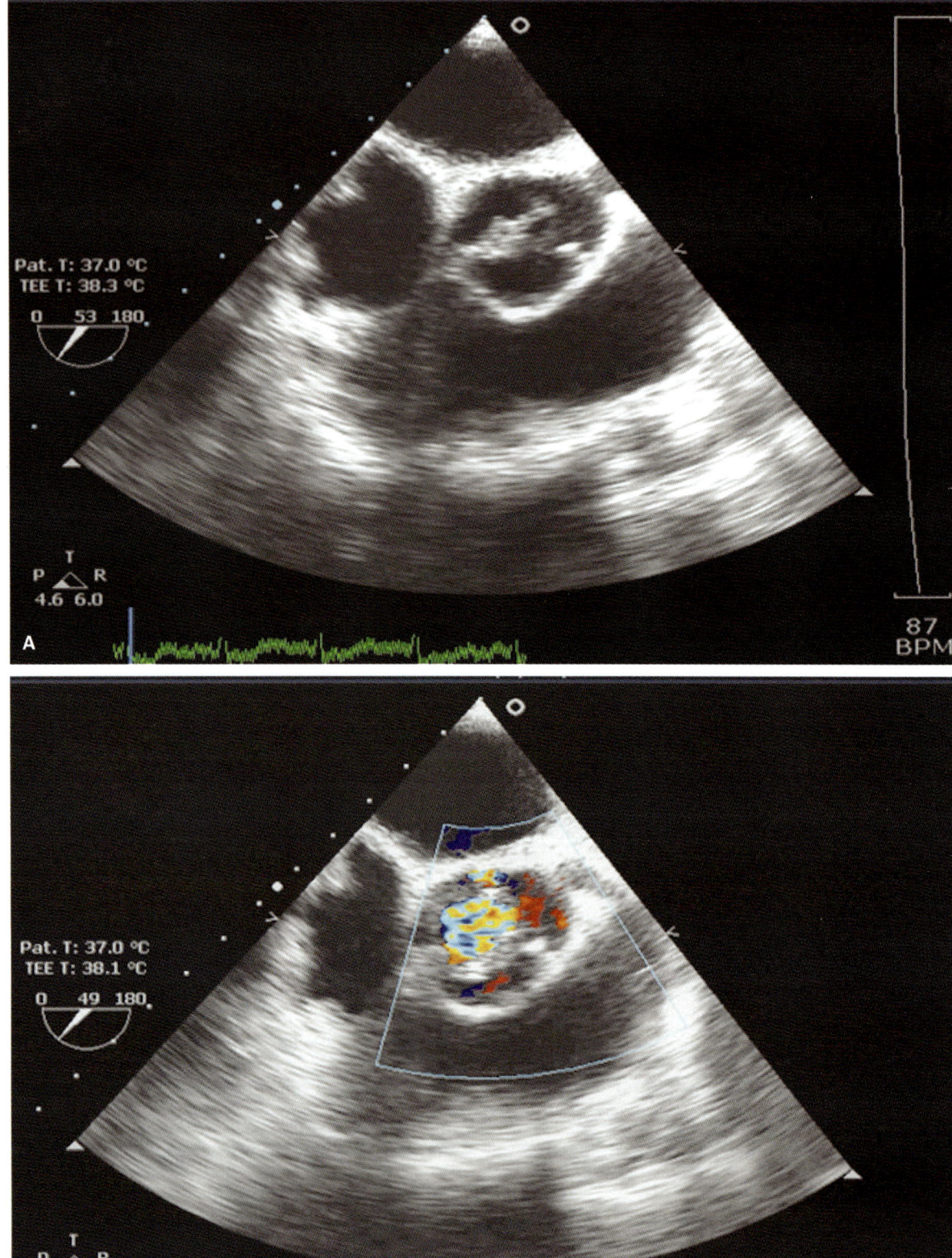

Fig. 5.11: Midesophageal aortic valve short-axis view in a patient with severe aortic stenosis showing thickened aortic leaflets with a narrowed orifice (A) and turbulent flow across it (B).

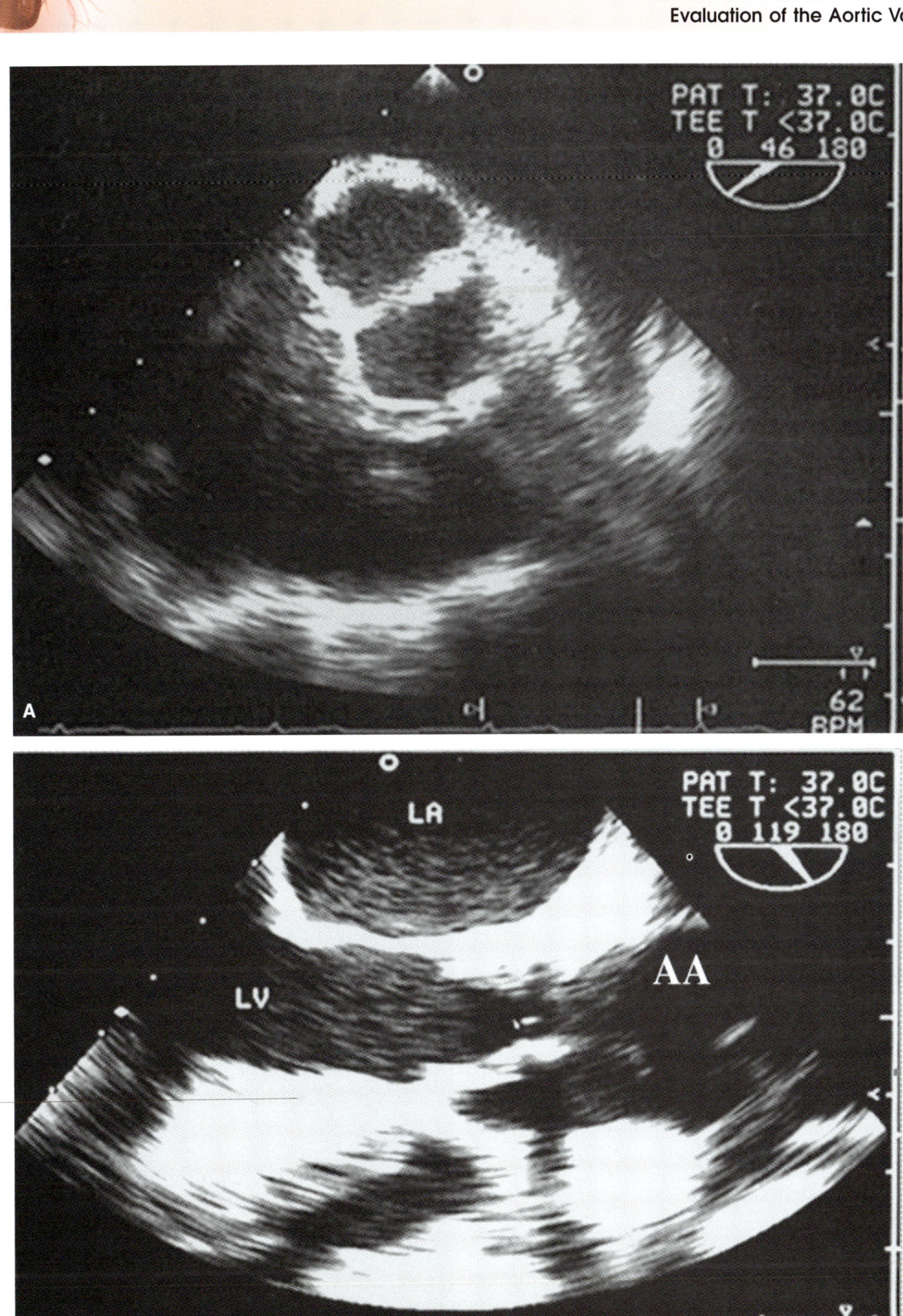

Fig. 5.12 : A patient with bicuspid aortic valve (A). Note the doming of stenosed aortic valve in long axis (B). (LA: left atrium, LV: left ventricle, AA: ascending aorta).

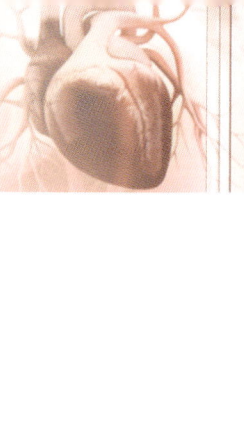

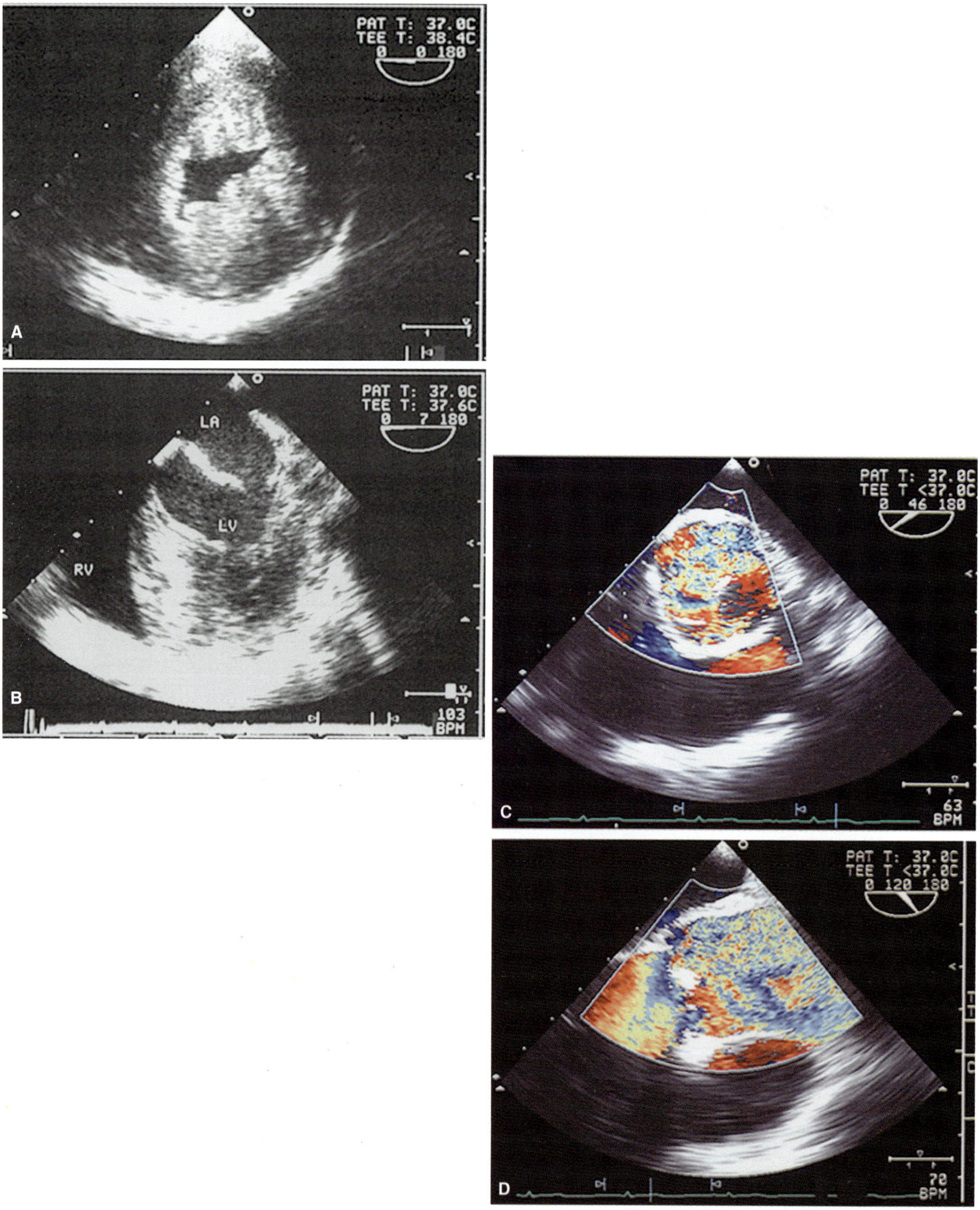

Fig. 5.13: Left ventricular function assessment in a patient with aortic stenosis. Note the concentric left ventricular hypertrophy in transgastric mid-papillary short-axis view (A) and midesophageal four-chamber view (B). Systolic flow across the stenosed aortic valve in short-axis (C) and long-axis (D) revealing marked turbulence on color flow (LA: left atrium, LV: left ventricle, RV: right ventricle).

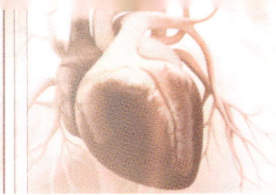

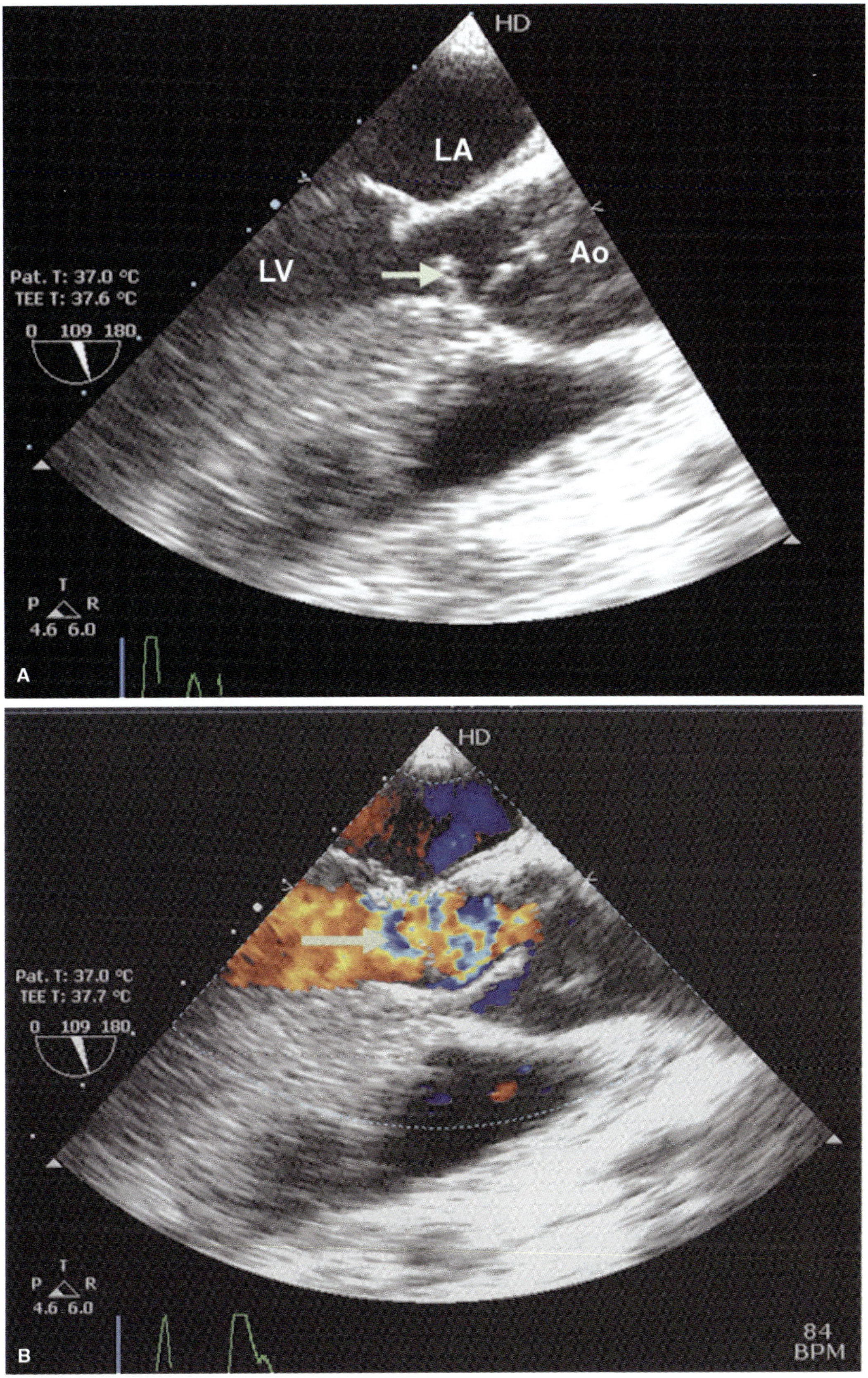

Fig. 5.14: Midesophageal aortic valve long-axis view showing a circumferential sub-aortic membrane (A, arrow) causing obstruction to blood flow. Note the proximal isovelocity area (PISA) formation in the left ventricular outflow tract (B, arrow) (LA: left atrium, LV: left ventricle, Ao: aorta).

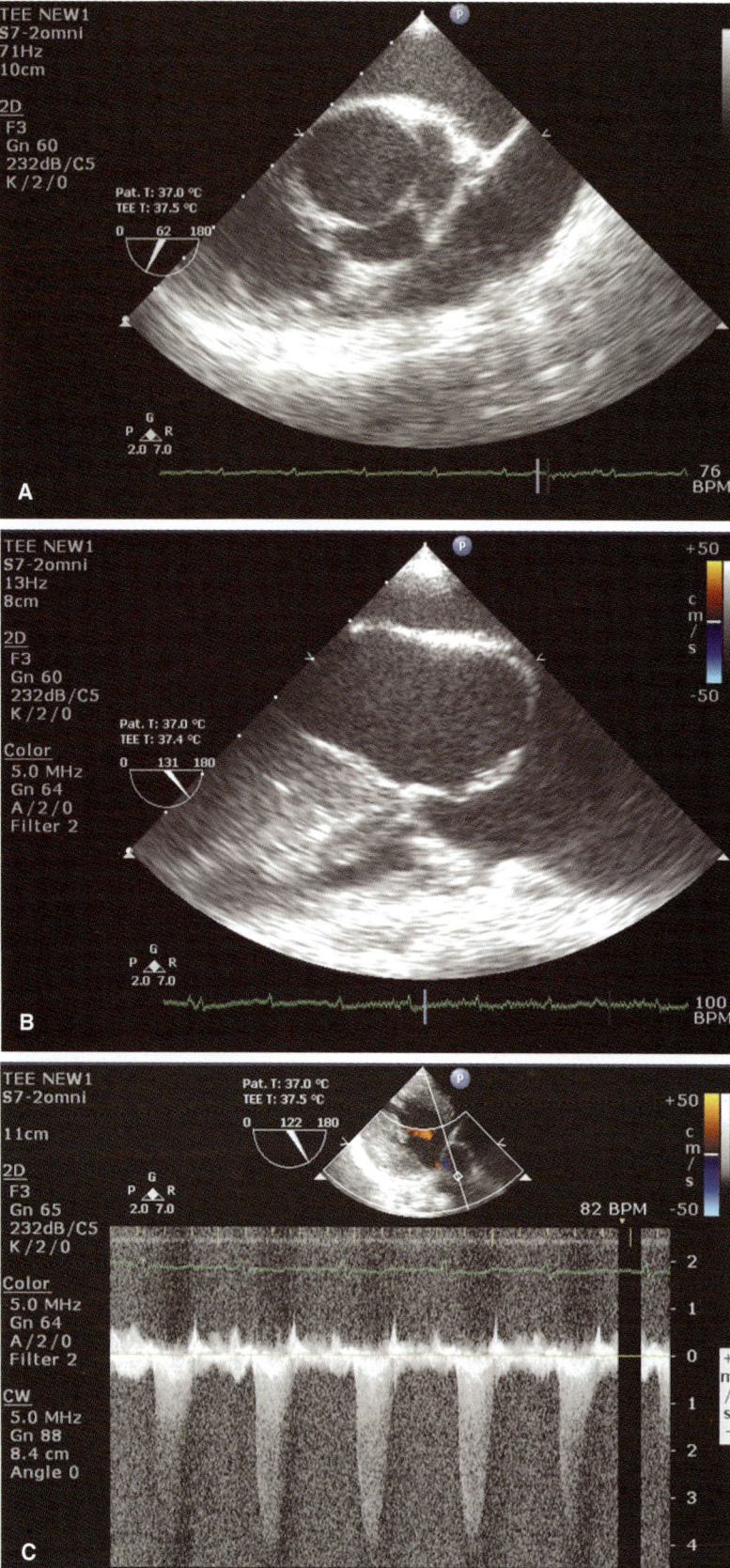

Fig. 5.15: Unicuspid aortic valve in short-axis (A), long axis (B) showing doming and continuous wave Doppler (C) showing high velocity (around 4 m/s) flow across it.

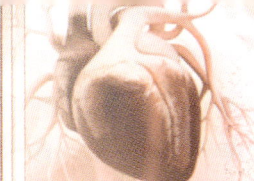

PRESSURE GRADIENT

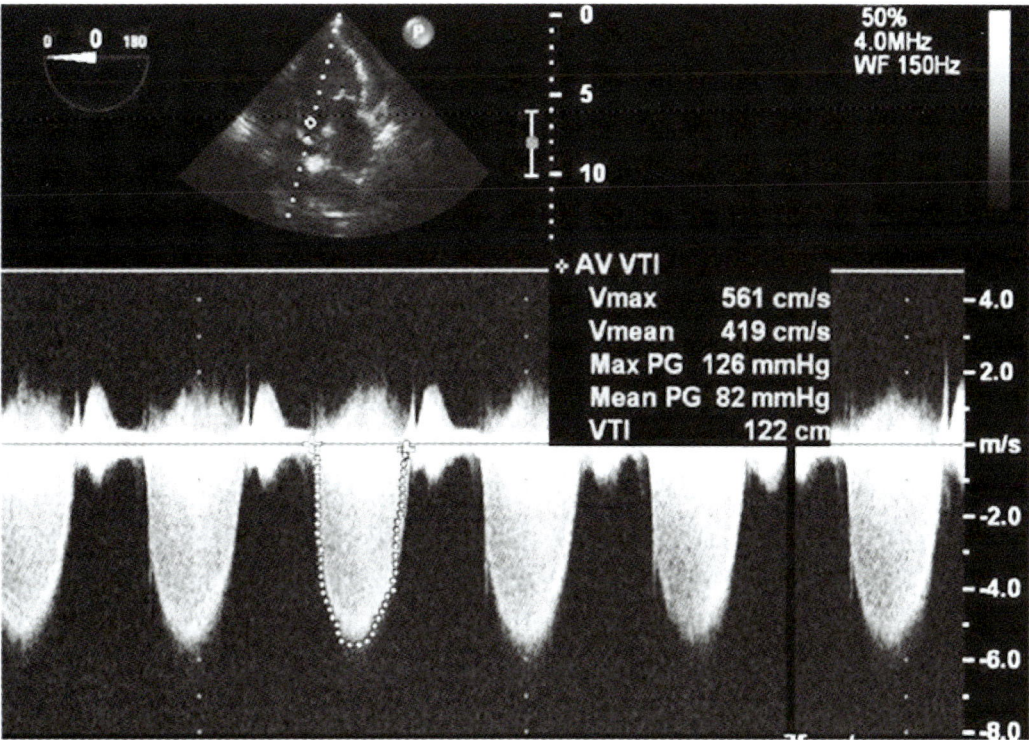

Fig. 5.16: Continuous wave Doppler across the aortic valve in deep transgastric view showing the calculation of peak and mean gradients (by enveloping the spectral Doppler) in the setting of aortic stenosis.

PLANIMETRY

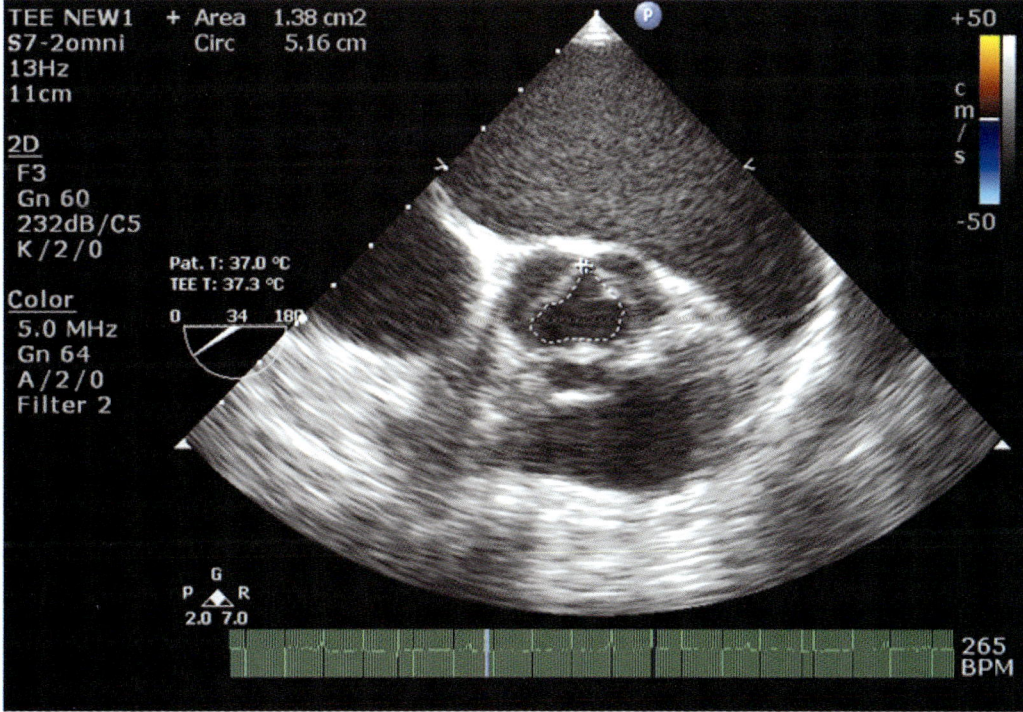

Fig. 5.17: Midesophageal aortic valve short-axis view showing the calculation of aortic valve area by planimetry in a patient with moderate aortic stenosis.

CONTINUITY EQUATION

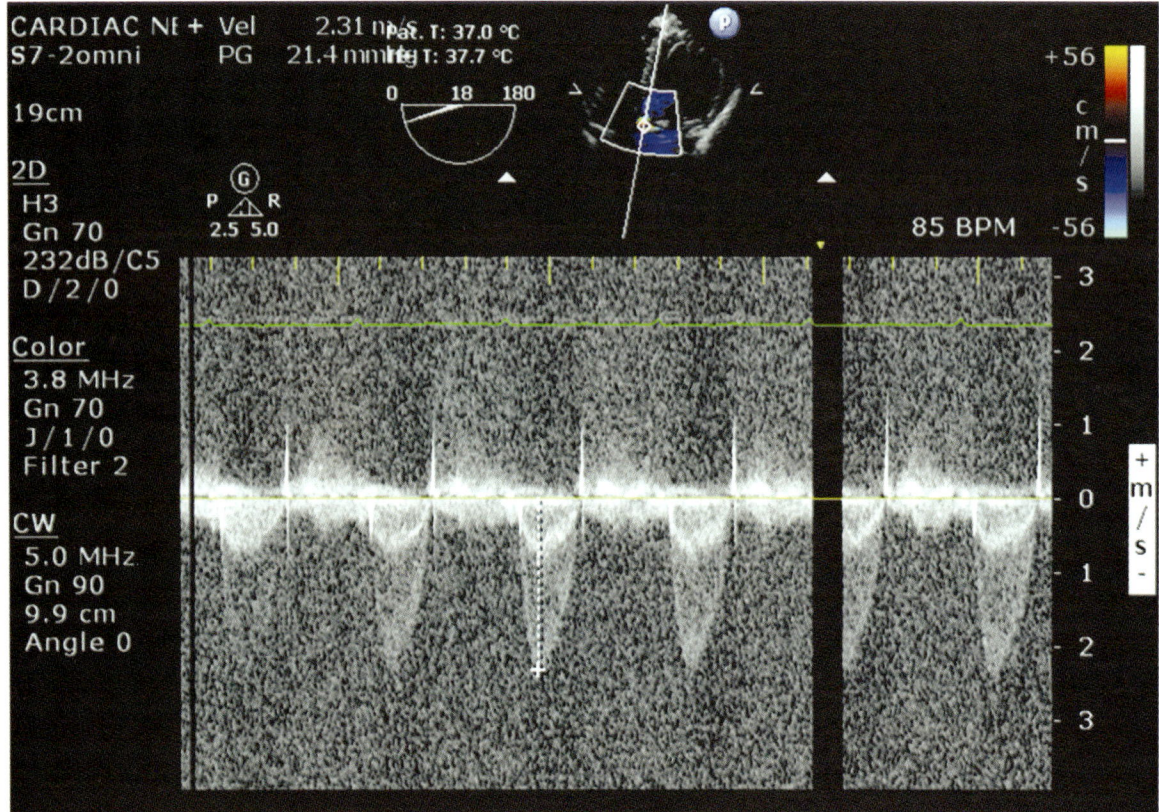

Fig. 5.18: Deep transgastric long-axis view showing the application of continuous wave Doppler for calculation of aortic valve area using the continuity equation. The velocity time integral is obtained from the spectral tracing across the aortic valve (larger light flow profile) and left ventricular outflow tract (LVOT-smaller dense flow profile). The diameter of the LVOT can also be obtained from the same view.

velocity edge, V_A is the aliasing velocity, α is the angle of PISA formation and V_{max} is the peak velocity across the aortic valve.

AORTIC REGURGITATION

The etiology of aortic regurgitation is rheumatic, calcific, myxomatous, endocarditis, traumatic and congenital (bicuspid aortic valve). Conditions involving the ascending aorta that lead to aneurysm formation / dissection such as connective tissue disorders, hypertension, trauma, cystic medial necrosis, mycotic aneurysm, etc. also cause aortic regurgitation. Table 5.2 summarizes the methods to quantify aortic regurgitation. Also refer to Figs 5.19 to 5.26.

Table 5.2: Assessment of severity of aortic regurgitation			
Method	*Mild*	*Moderate*	*Severe*
Jet width /LVOT width (%)	<25	25–65	>65
Jet CSA / LVOT CSA (%)	<5	5–60	>60
CWD density	Weak "flat top"	↑ angle on CWD	Dense steep slope
Decay slope (m/s²)	<2	2–3.5	>3
PHT (ms)	>500	200–500	<200
Descending aorta flow reversal	Early mild	Intermediate	Holodiastolic, in abdominal aorta
Vena contracta (mm)	<3	3–6	>6
ERO area (cm²)	< 0.1	0.1–0.3	>0.3
Regurgitant volume (ml)	<30	30–60	>60
Regurgitant fraction (%)	20–30	30–50	>50

(LVOT: left ventricular outflow tract, CSA: cross sectional area, PHT: pressure half time, ERO: effective regurgitant orifice, CWD: continous wave Doppler)

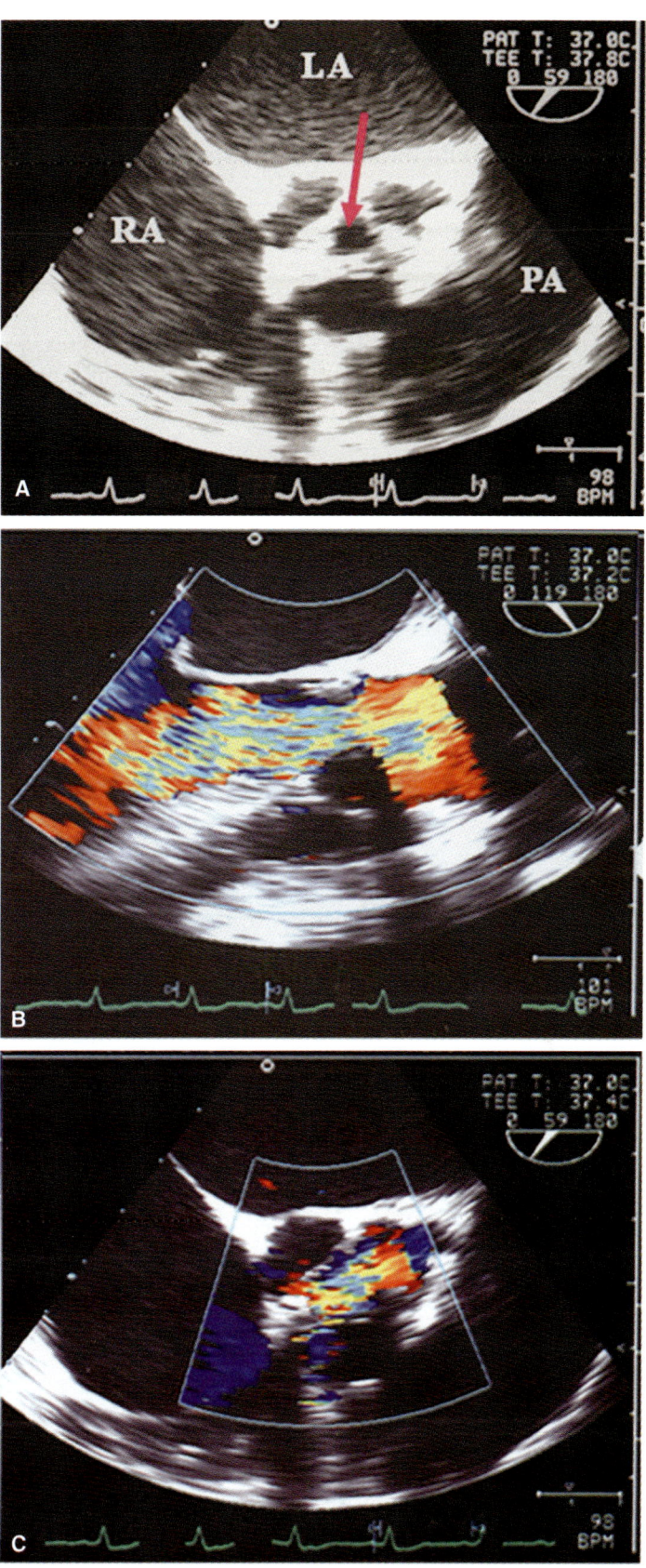

Fig. 5.19: Appearance of the regurgitant orifice of aortic valve in short-axis (arrow, A) in a patient with rheumatic aortic regurgitation. Note the color flow across the aortic valve showing severe aortic regurgitation in long-axis (B) and short-axis (C) (LA: left atrium, RA: right atrium, PA: pulmonary artery).

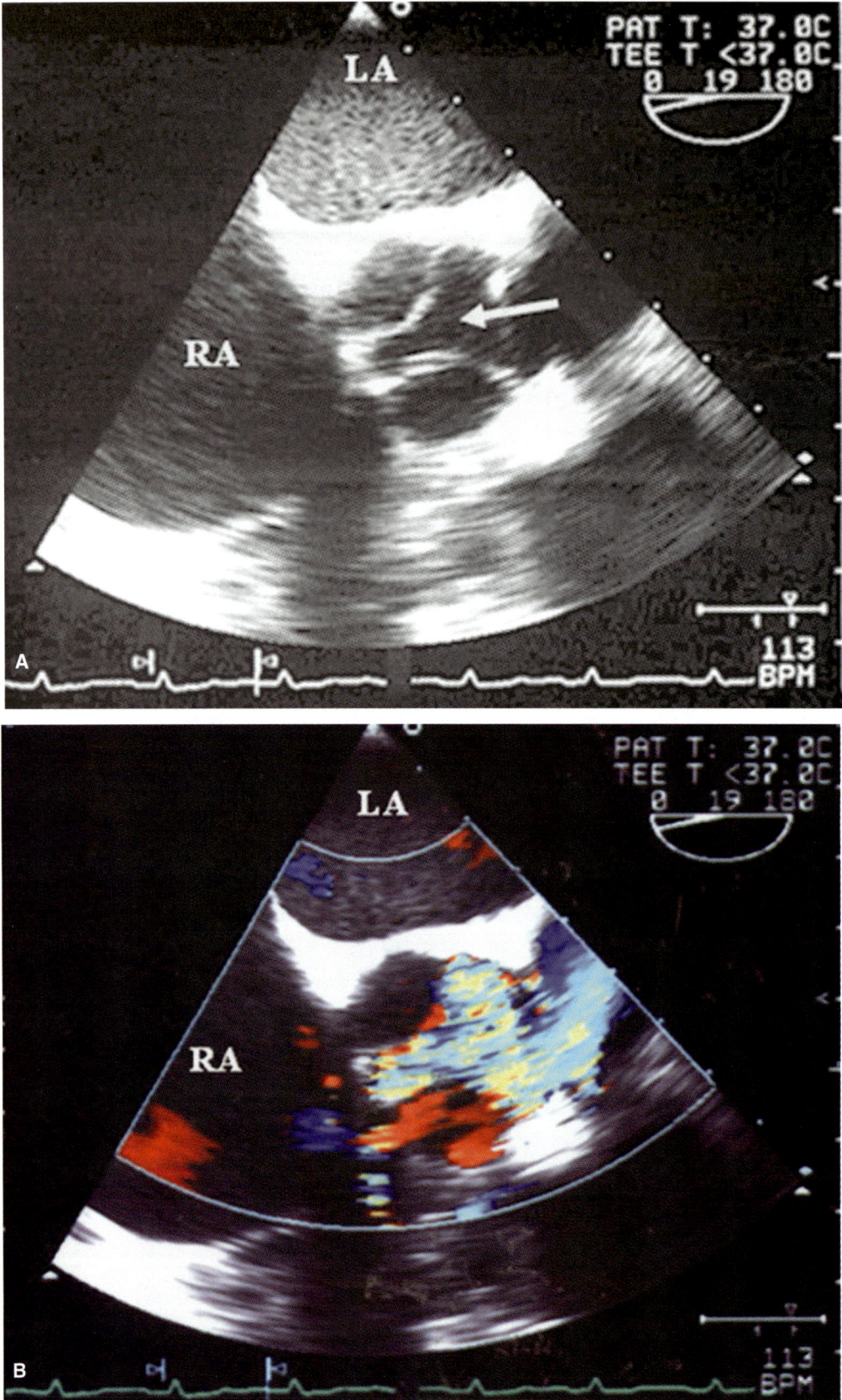

Fig. 5.20: Incomplete coaptation of the aortic valve in short-axis. Note the closed leaflets with a wide gap in between (arrow, A). Color flow across the aortic valve (B) in diastole showing aortic regurgitation. (LA: left atrium, RA: right atrium).

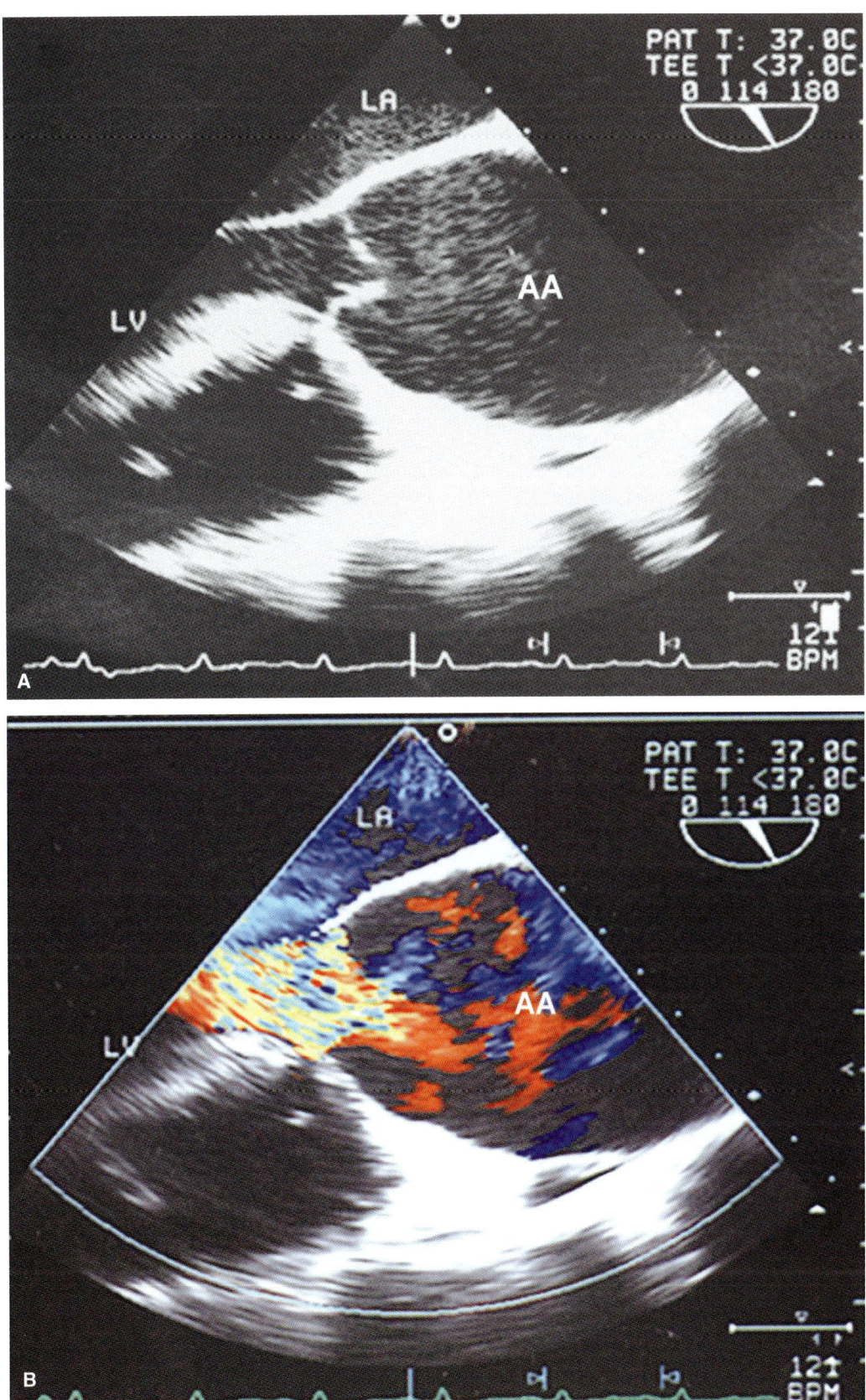

Fig. 5.21: Dilatated ascending aorta in a patient with Marfan's syndrome. Note the incomplete coaptation of the aortic leaflets (A). Color flow across the valve (B) in diastole showing severe aortic regurgitation. (LA: left atrium, LV: left ventricle, AA: ascending aorta).

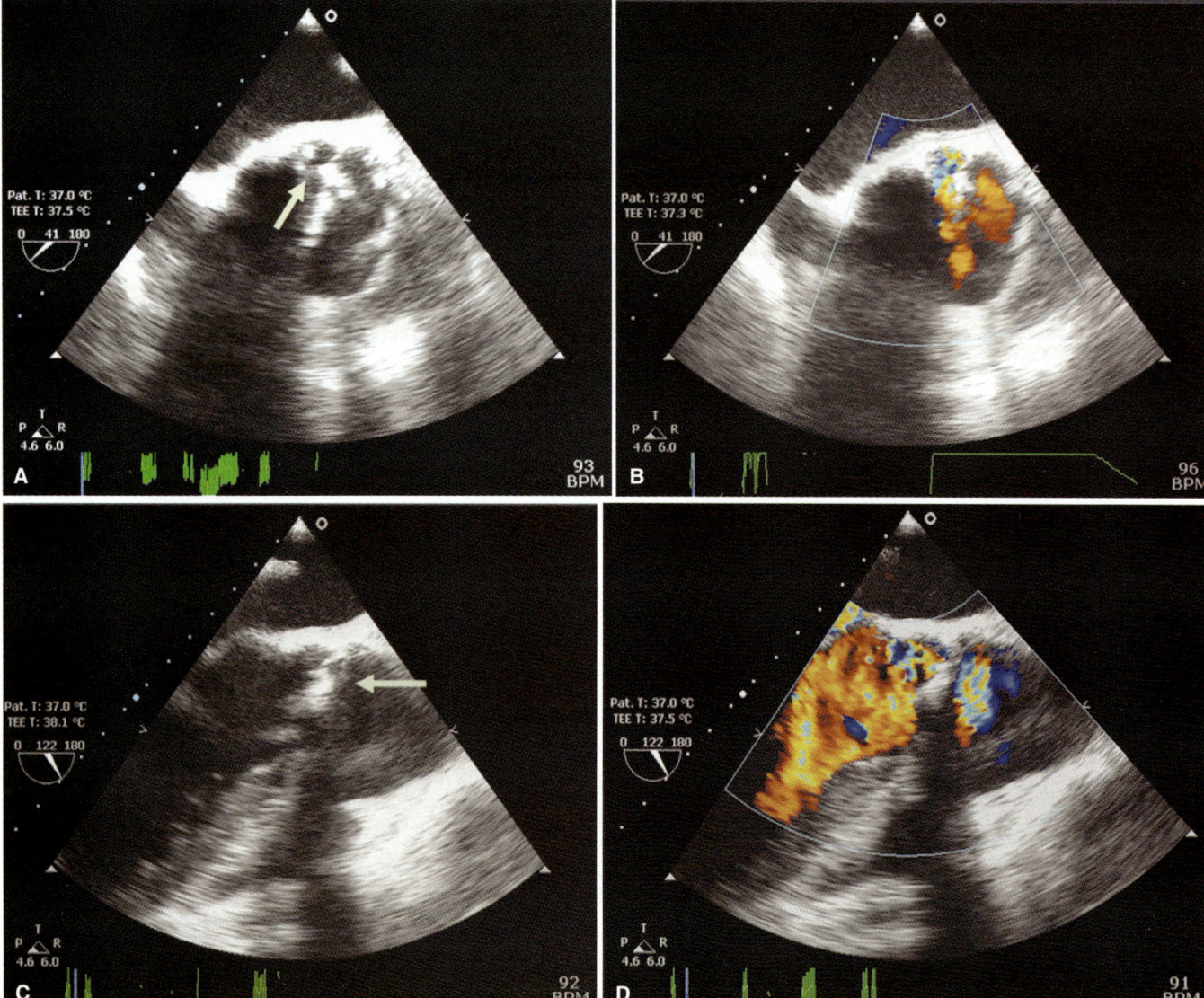

Fig. 5.22: Midesophageal aortic valve short-axis view (A) and long-axis view (C) showing thickening of the aortic leaflets and perforation on the non-coronary cusp (arrow) due to infective endocarditis. A small regurgitant jet is seen through it on color flow Doppler (B and D).

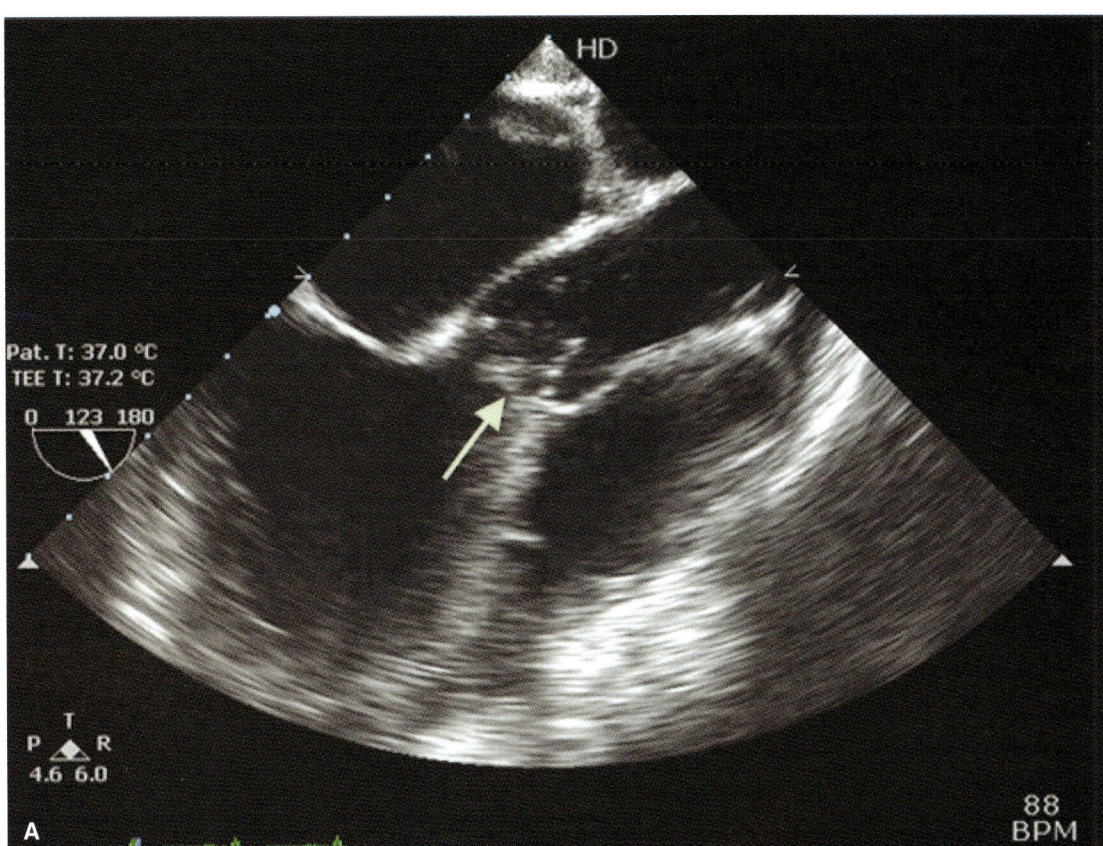

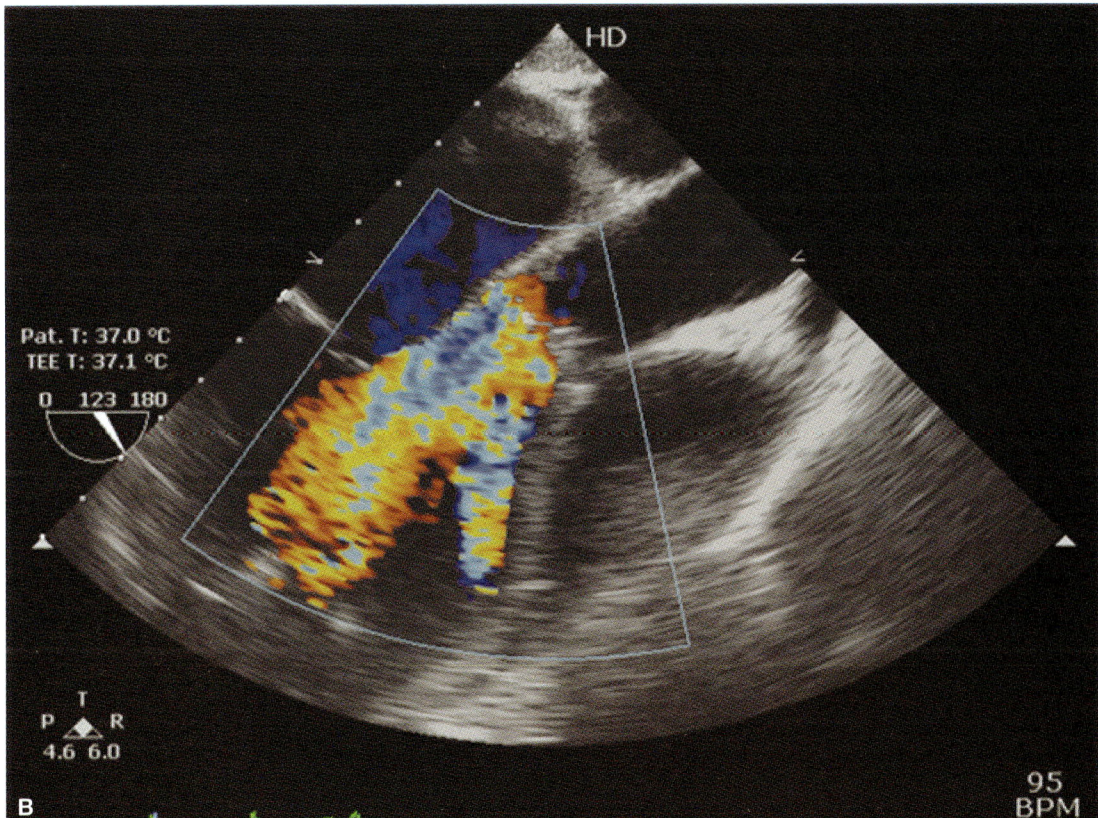

Fig. 5.23: A vegetation on the right coronary cusp (arrow, A) causing distortion of the leaflet and leading to severe aortic regurgitation (B).

JET WIDTH vs LVOT WIDTH

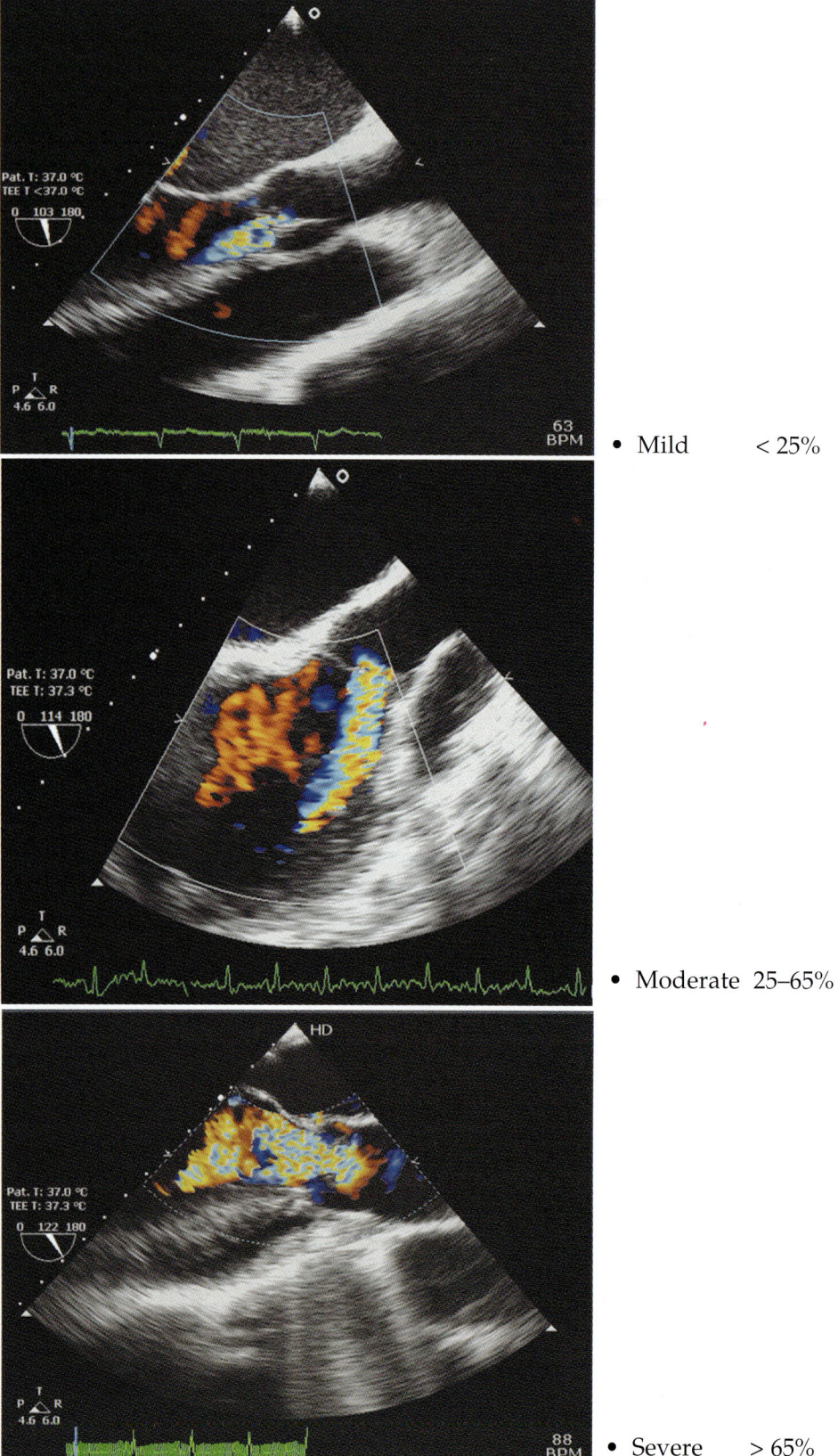

- Mild   < 25%

- Moderate 25–65%

- Severe   > 65%

Fig. 5.24: Grading of aortic regurgitation according to the jet width as a fraction of the left ventricular outflow tract width.

CONTINUOUS WAVE DOPPLER

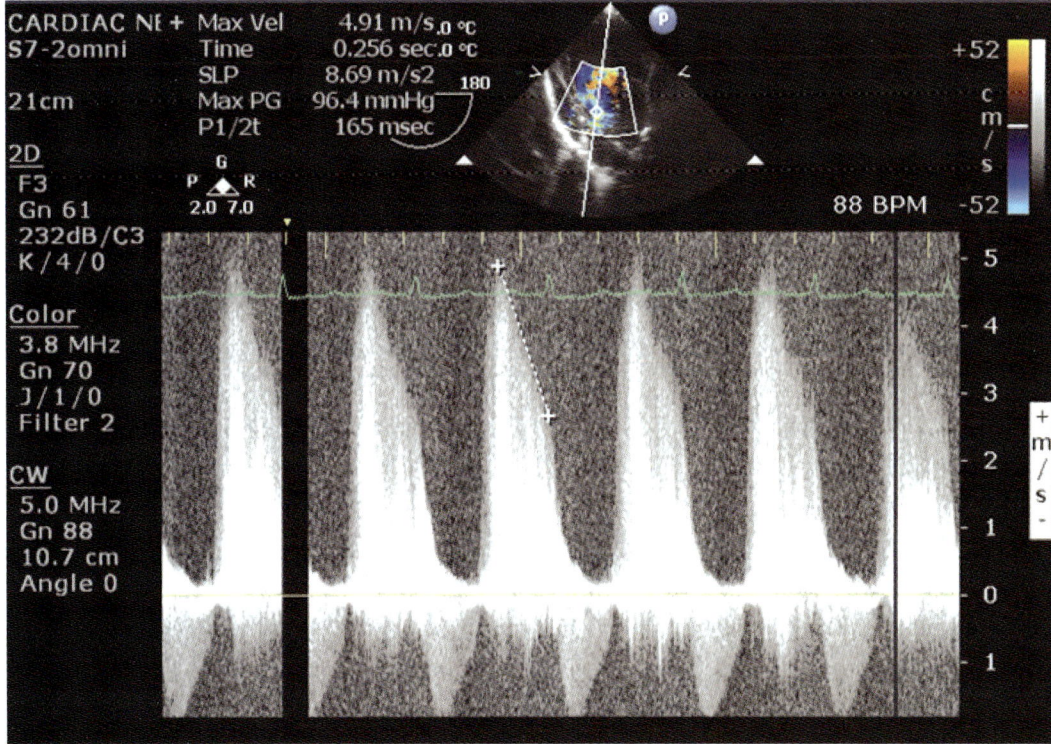

Fig. 5.25: Deep transgastric long-axis view in a patient with severe aortic regurgitation showing a dense flow tracing with a steep decay slope ~ 8.69 m/s^2 and pressure half-time ~ 165 ms.

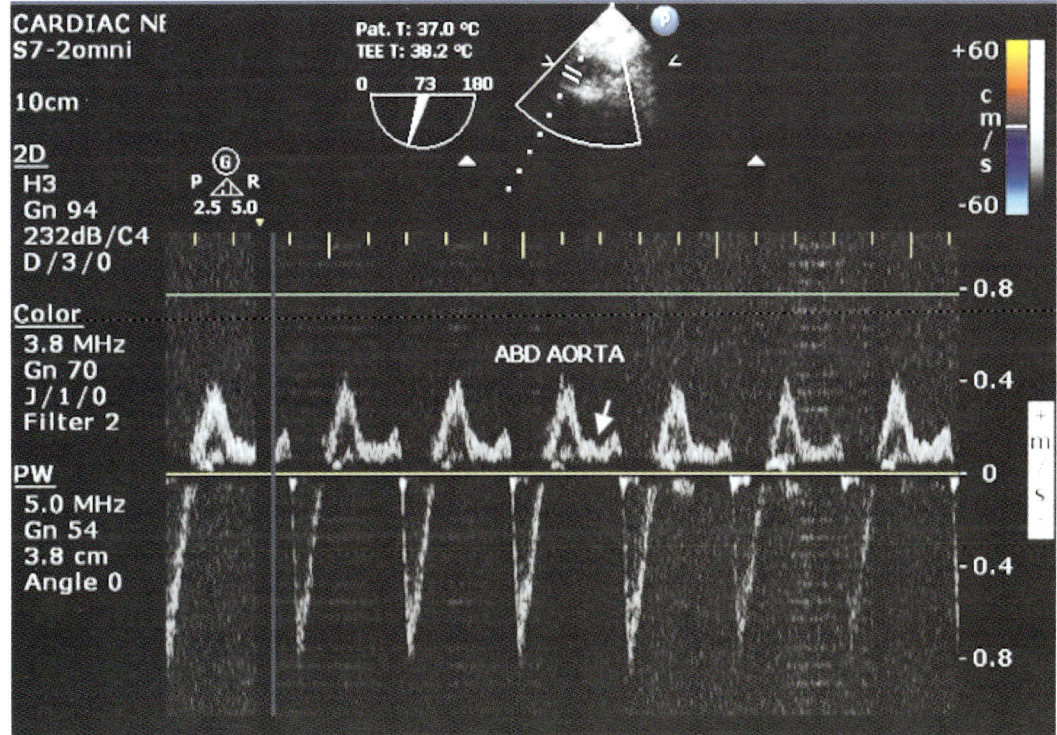

Fig. 5.26: Holodiastolic flow reversal can be appreciated in the abdominal aorta in severe aortic regurgitation (arrow).

Evaluation of the Right Side of the Heart

6

• Deepak K. Tempe • Suruchi Hasija

The right side of the heart is perhaps the most neglected area of assessment during transesophageal echocardiographic (TEE) examination. The tricuspid valve, right ventricle (RV) and pulmonary valve can be accurately studied by TEE. In India, rheumatic heart disease is still common, so that a large proportion of patients undergo valve surgery. Mitral valve surgery is the commonest operation in these patients. Assessment of the tricuspid valve is particularly important in these patients. Tricuspid regurgitation is a common accompaniment of the lesions of mitral valve. An accurate assessment of tricuspid regurgitation can be made with the help of TEE, thereby assisting the decision regarding the need to carry out tricuspid valve repair. Likewise, the assessment of RV function can guide the need for fluid requirement and pharmacological hemodynamic support. In this chapter, some interesting TEE pictures related to the evaluation of the right side of the heart have been depicted.

ANATOMY

The RV is asymmetrical crescent-shaped structure. It consists of a free wall and the interventricular septum. The RV free wall can be divided into basal, mid and apical segments. The interventricular septum can be considered functionally as part of the left ventricle (LV). The RV can be divided into a trabeculated posteroinferior inflow tract, consisting of the tricuspid valve, papillary muscles, chordae tendinea and chamber walls, and a smooth walled anterosuperior outflow tract (infundibulum). The inflow and outflow portions are separated by an encircling muscular band consisting of the parietal band, crista supraventricularis, septal band and the moderator band. The moderator band is frequently seen during TEE examination extending from the lower ventricular septum to the RV free wall.

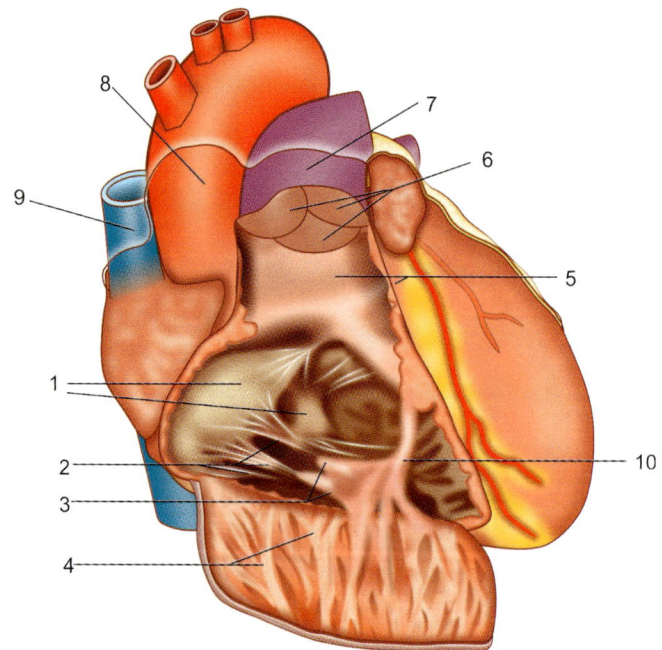

Fig. 6.1: Right ventricular anatomy: (1) Tricuspid valve leaflets, (2) chordae tendinea, (3) papillary muscles, (4) trabeculae carnea, (5) infundibulum, (6) pulmonary valve, (7) pulmonary artery, (8) aorta, (9) superior vena cava, (10) moderator band.

TEE VIEWS

Since the right heart structures are anteriorly located, their TEE examination is difficult. Multiple views are required for assessing the RV as it is crescent shaped and invariably imaged in an oblique plane.

1. Midesophageal Four-chamber (ME 4-ch) View

This is the long axis view of the RV that allows assessment of apical, mid and basal segments of the RV free wall, the interatrial and interventricular septae, and the anterior and septal leaflets of the tricuspid valve.

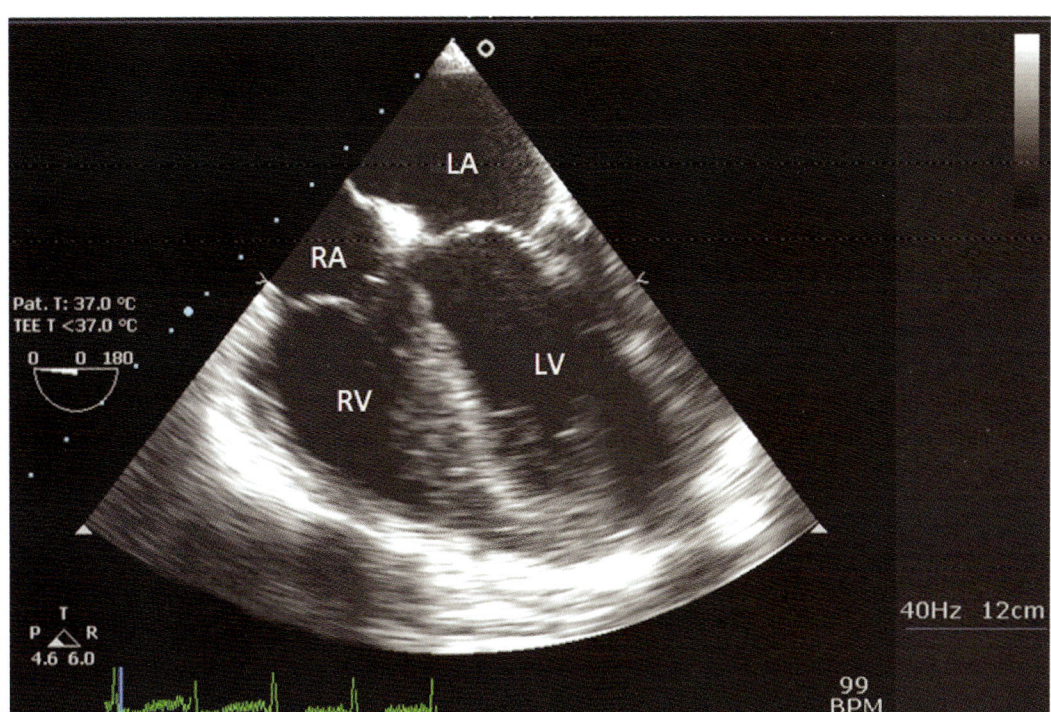

Fig. 6.2: Midesophageal 4-chamber view showing the normal right ventricle. Please note the right ventricle is triangular and smaller than the left ventricle. (LA: left atrium, RA: right atrium, LV: left ventricle, RV: right ventricle).

2. Midesophageal RV Inflow-outflow View

The right atrium (RA), RV and pulmonary artery (PA) subscribe a 270° arc around the aortic valve. It allows assessment of the inferior RV free wall, right ventricular outflow tract (RVOT), the posterior and anterior tricuspid valve leaflets, and the pulmonary valve.

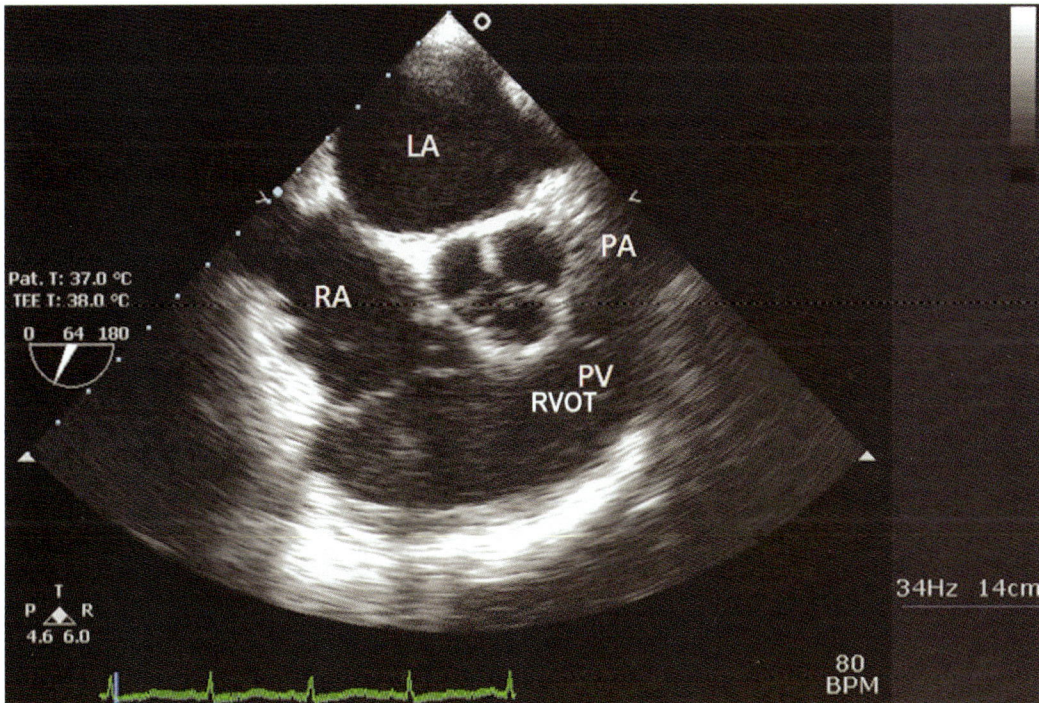

Fig. 6.3: Midesophageal right ventricular inflow-outflow view. (LA: left atrium, RA: right atrium, RVOT: right ventricular outflow tract, PV: pulmonary valve, PA: pulmonary artery).

3. Transgastric Midpapillary Short-axis (TG midpapillary SAX) View

In addition to examining the left ventricle, this view allows the assessment of right ventricular free wall and interventricular septum. The transducer should be rotated to right after obtaining the classical TG midpapillary SAX view.

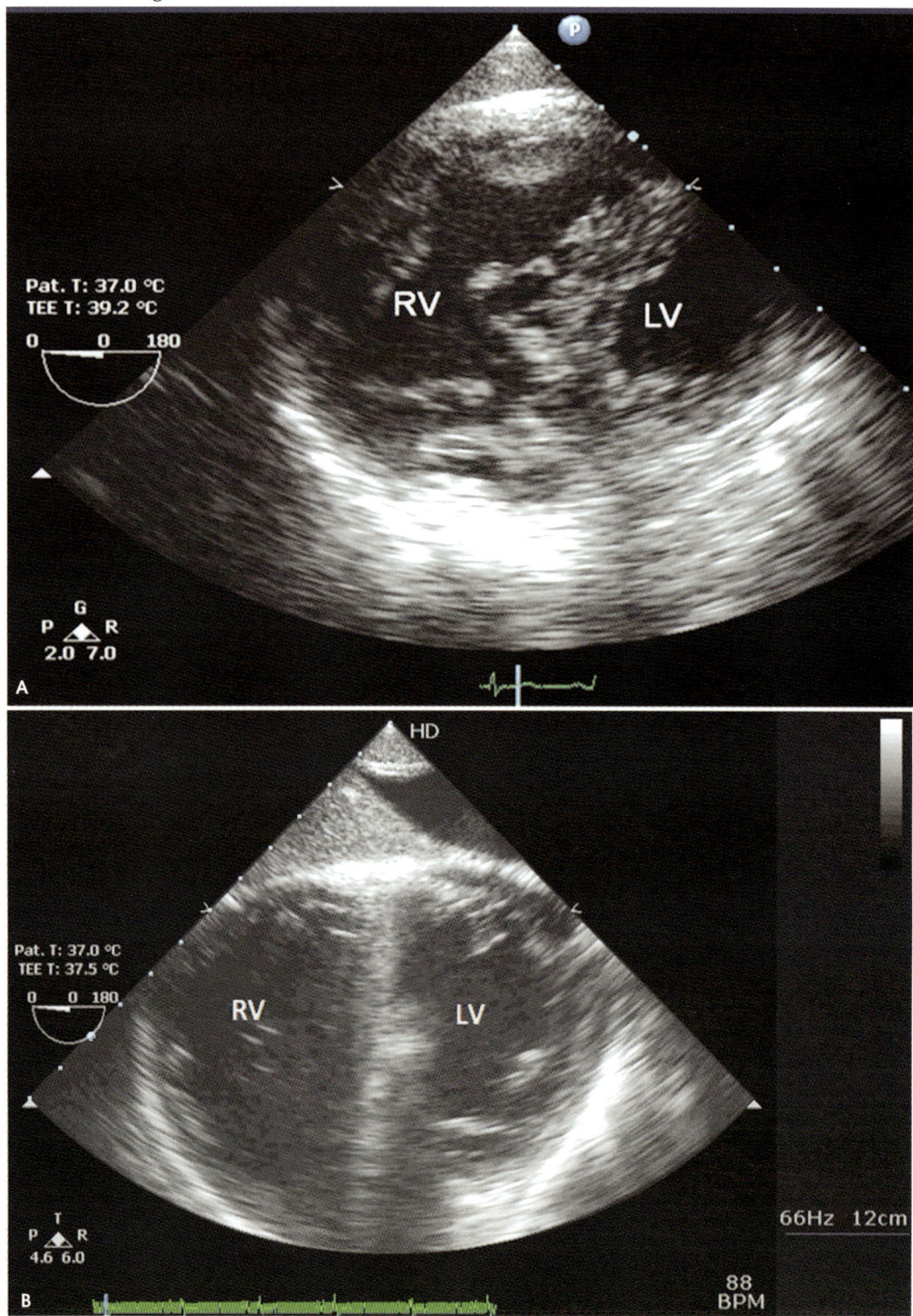

Fig. 6.4: Transgastric midpapillary short-axis view of the right and left ventricles. Note that the interventricular septum (IVS) functions as a part of the left ventricle with convexity towards right ventricle (A). In a failing RV, the IVS becomes flattened (B). (LV: left ventricle, RV: right ventricle).

4. Transgastric RV Inflow View

It is useful for evaluation of the tricuspid valve and subvalvular apparatus.

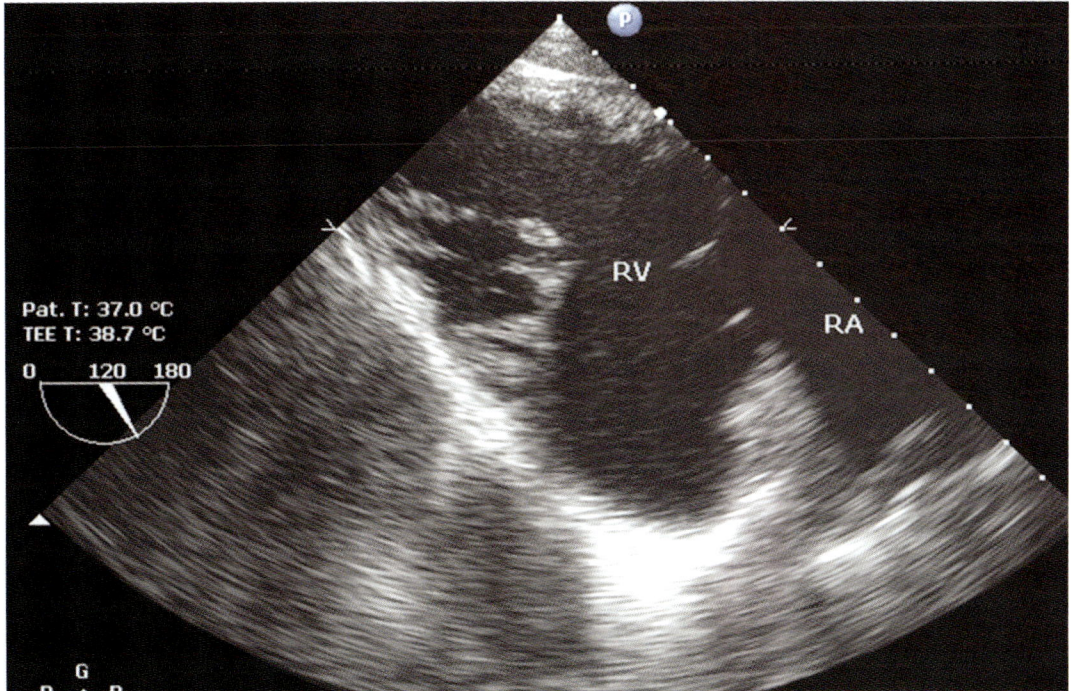

Fig. 6.5: Transgastric right ventricular inflow view at 120° (RV: right ventricle, RA; right atrium).

5. Deep Transgastric View

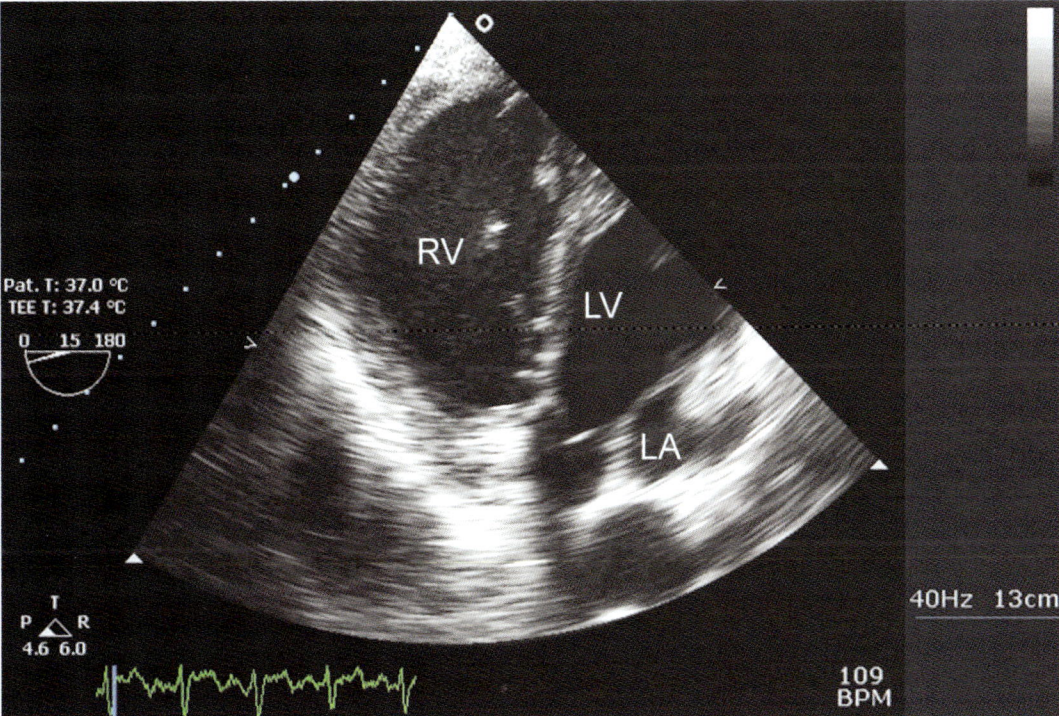

Fig. 6.6: Deep transgastiric view. The normal sized right ventricle (RV) is usually not visible in this view, but an enlarged RV can be easily visualized as in this patient (LA: left atrium, LV: left ventricle, RV: right ventricle).

6. The Midesophageal Long-axis (ME LAX) View

The RVOT and the pulmonary valve are seen anterior to the aortic valve.

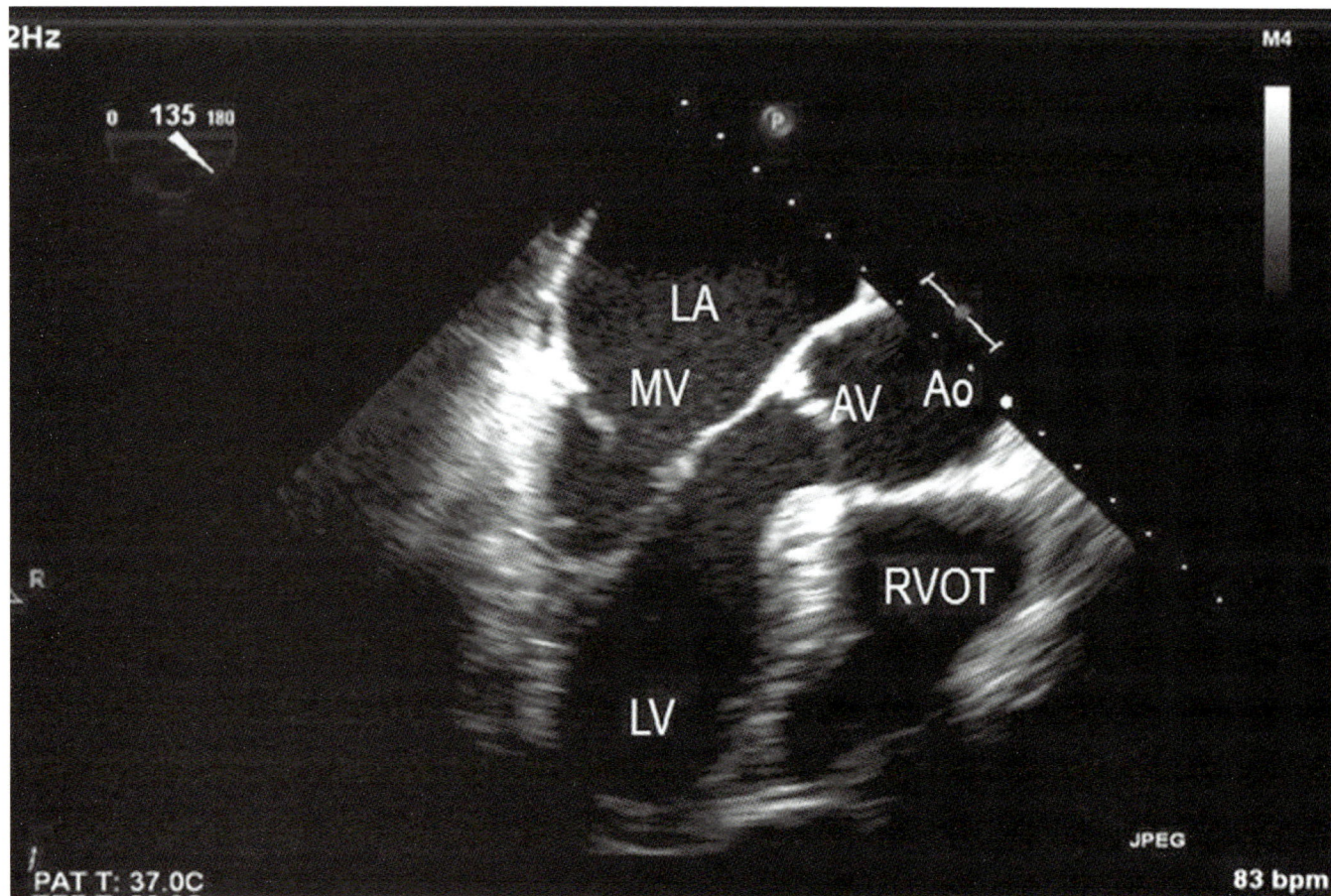

Fig. 6.7: Midesophageal long-axis view showing the right ventricular outflow tract anterior to the aortic valve (LA: left atrium, MV: mitral valve, AV: aortic valve, Ao: aorta, LV: left ventricle, RVOT: right ventricular outflow tract).

7. The Transgastric RV Inflow-outflow View

The transgastric RV inflow-outflow view provides an image of the RA, RV, PA, tricuspid and pulmonary valves. It allows calculation of the cardiac output and RVOT tract dimensions.

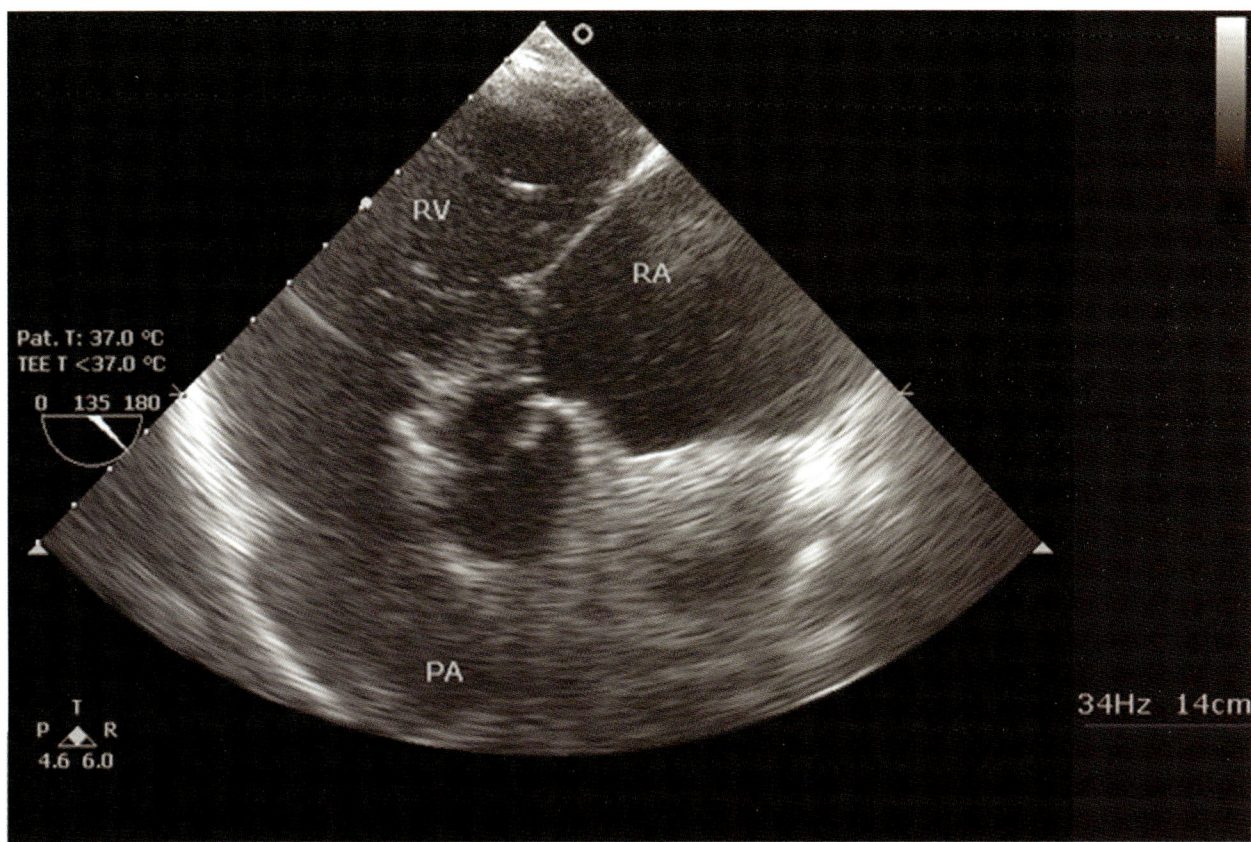

Fig. 6.8: Transgastric right ventricular inflow-outflow view. (RA: right atrium, RV: right ventricle, PA: pulmonary artery).

ASSESSMENT OF GLOBAL RV FUNCTION

Hypertrophy

The normal thickness of the RV free wall is less than 5 mm at end-diastole, which is less than half of that of LV. RV free wall thickness of > 5 mm indicates RV hypertrophy and is suggestive of elevated PA pressure or pulmonary stenosis. In addition, the intracavitary trabecular pattern becomes more prominent, particularly at the apex. RV pressure overload is characterized by hypertrophy of the RV free wall. The septum hypertrophies in chronic pressure overload. In contrast to RV volume overload, RV pressure overload produces maximal septal distortion at end-systole and early diastole.

Dilatation

RV dilatation occurs most commonly with RV volume overload or chronic pressure overload. The normal RV end-diastolic cross-sectional area is about 60% of the area of LV, and RV length extends up to two-thirds the length of the LV. With mild RV dilatation, RV end-diastolic area is 60–100% of LV area; with moderate RV

dilatation, RV area equals LV area; and with severe RV enlargement, the RV area often exceeds the LV area. The shape of the RV changes from triangular to round as the RV dilates. In addition, RV forms part of the cardiac apex in the four-chamber view (Fig. 6.9). The examination of interventricular septal motion can help to differentiate between RV volume overload and pressure overload. RV volume overload produces RV dilatation. The interventricular septum that normally maintains a convex curvature towards RV throughout the cardiac cycle, flattens when the RV mass equals that of LV (LV appears D-shaped in cross-section). The paradoxical septal motion appears when the RV mass exceeds LV mass. With RV volume overload, septal distortion is maximal at end-diastole. During systole, the end-diastolic septal flattening reverses, with paradoxical septal motion towards the RV cavity.

Systolic Function

The asymmetric shape of the RV complicates assessment of the global RV function and necessitates

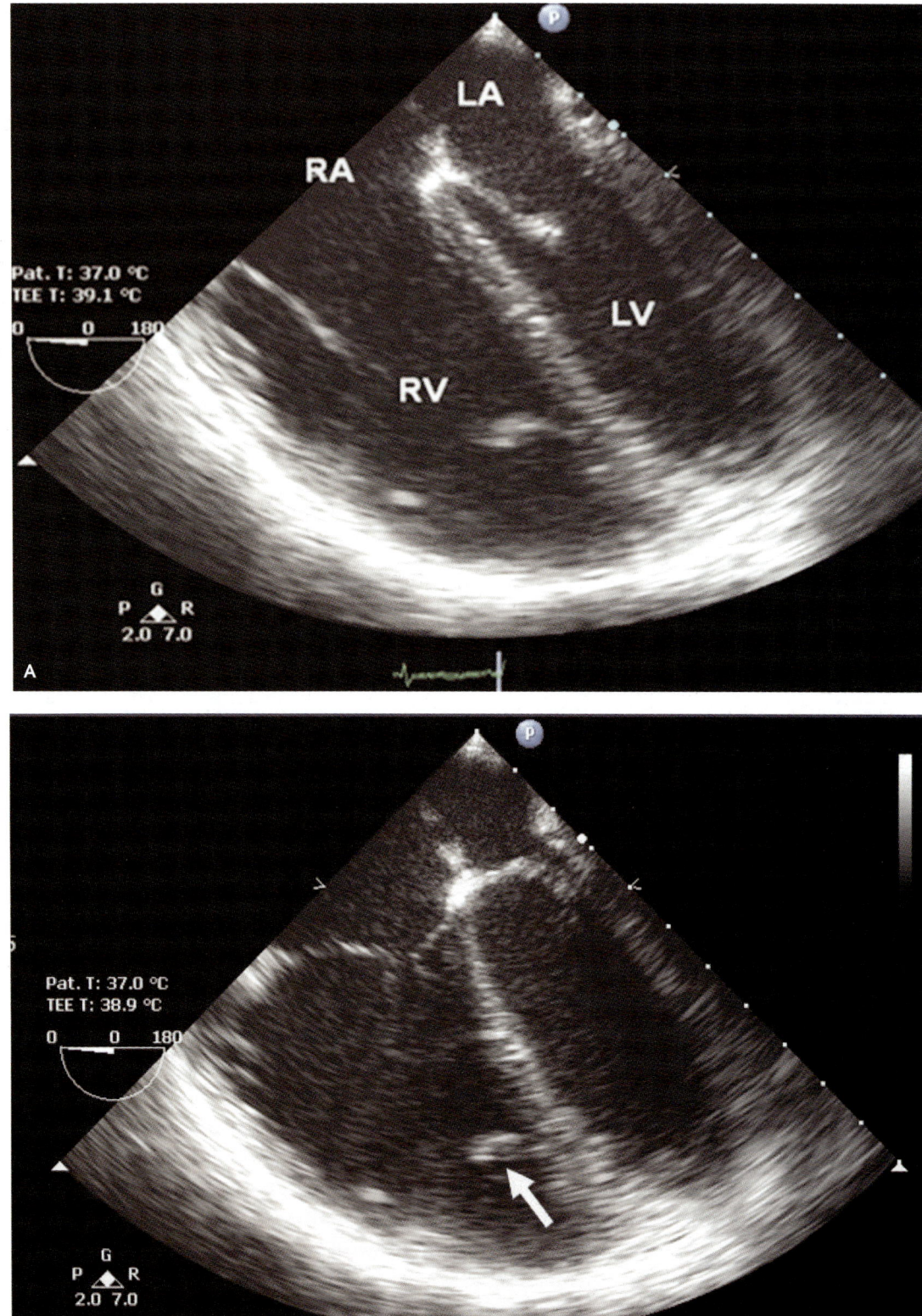

Fig. 6.9: Midesophageal 4-chamber view showing the right ventricular dilatation. Note that the right ventricular area far exceeds that of the left ventricle and the apex is formed by the right ventricle. (LA: left atrium, RA: right atrium, LV: left ventricle, RV: right ventricle). Note the moderator band in B (arrow).

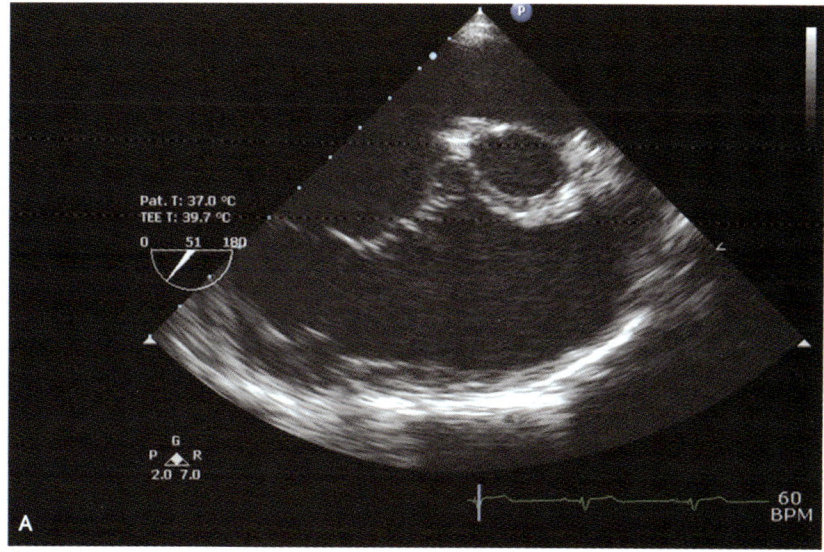

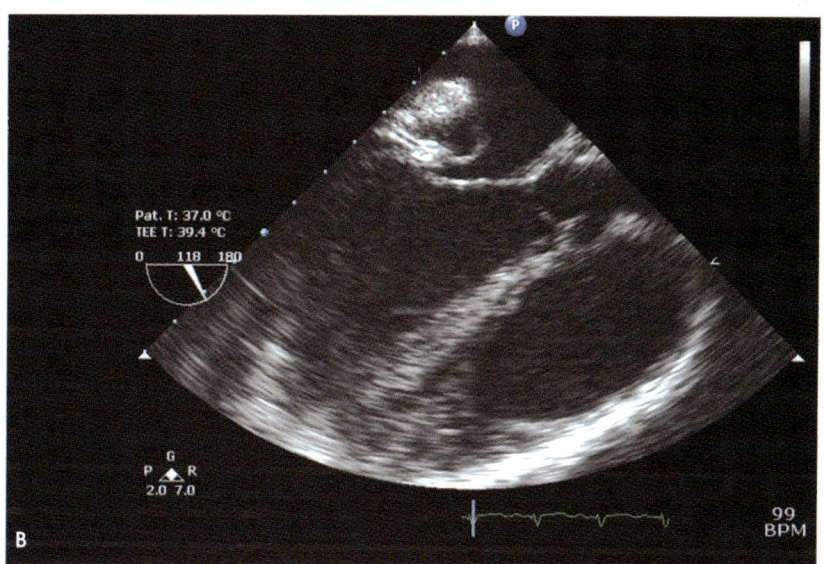

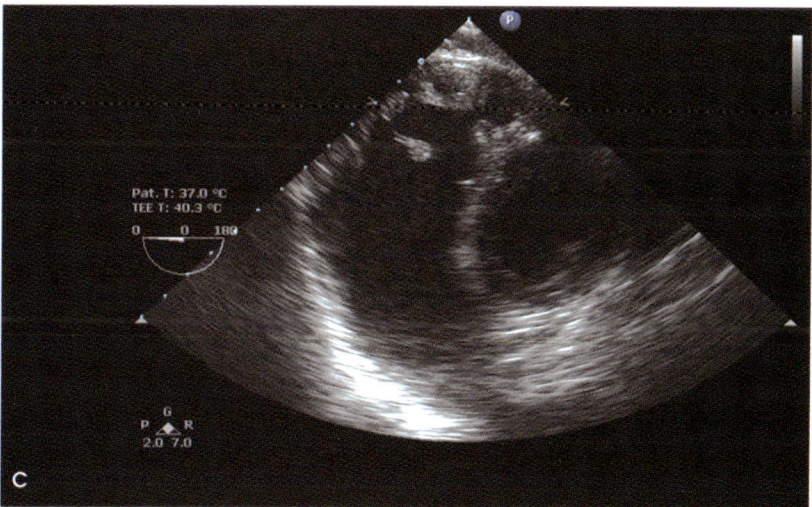

Fig. 6.10: Right ventricular dilatation in the midesophageal right ventricular inflow-outflow view (A), midesophageal long-axis view (B) and transgastric mid-papillary short-axis view (C).

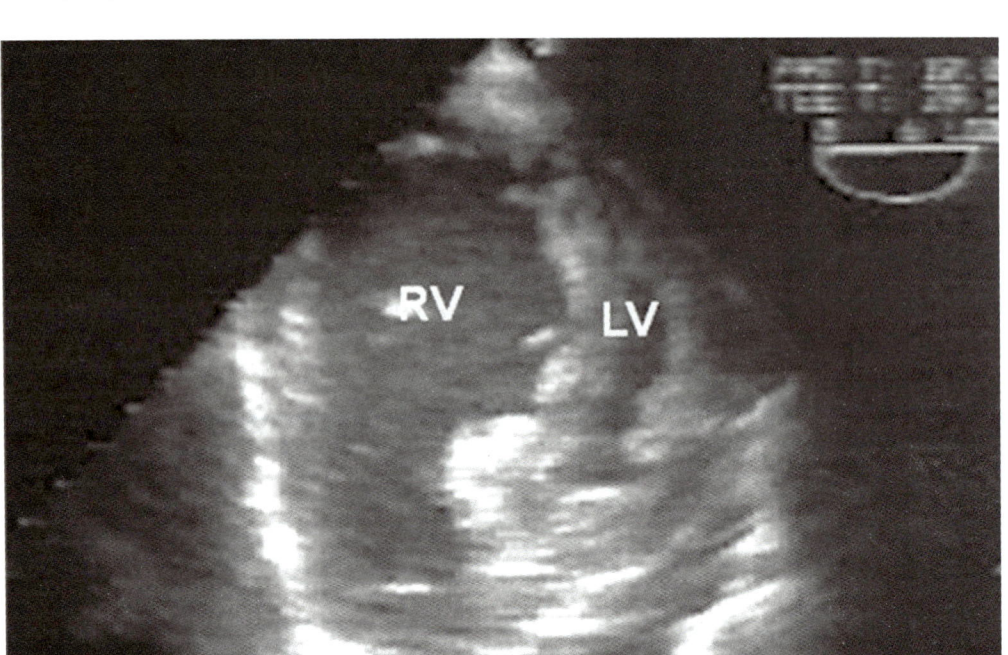

Fig. 6.11: Transgastric short-axis view showing hugely dilated right ventricle. Note the deviation of the interventricular septum to the left with a small size left ventricle. (RV: right ventricle, LV: left ventricle).

acquisition of multiple images for estimation of chamber size and shape. The signs of RV dysfunction include, severe hypokinesis or akinesis of the RV free wall, RV enlargement, change in shape of the RV from crescent to round, and flattening or bulging of the interventricular septum from right to left. RV free wall excursion and extent of systolic obliteration of the RV cavity help to estimate RV ejection fraction.

Quantification of RV volume and function can be performed by one of the following methods:

1. Maximal short-axis and mid short-axis measurements of RV chamber in a single plane measured perpendicular to the long axis of the RV in the midesophageal four-chamber view (normal: 3.5 ± 0.2 cm and 2.8 ± 0.2 cm, respectively).
2. Calculation of volumes and ejection fraction using multiplane method or modified Simpson's rule.
3. Summation of smaller geometric volumes using models of an ellipsoid/prism/pyramid.
   Stroke volume measured across the pulmonary artery (cm³) = cross-sectional area (cm²) × velocity time integral (cm)
   Cardiac output (L/min) = stroke volume (L) × heart rate,
4. Using planimetry,

Fractional area change (FAC)

$$= \frac{\text{end-diastolic area} - \text{end-systolic area}}{\text{end-diastolic area}} \times 100$$

Normal value: 32–60%.

5. Automated border detection. The presence of trabeculations renders endocardial tracing difficult.
6. RV dP/dt: The rate of rise of tricuspid jet velocity (dP/dt) > 250 mm Hg/sec is indicative of normal RV contractility.
7. RV myocardial performance index or Tei index = (ICT + IRT)/ET
   where, ICT is isovolumic contraction time, IRT is isovolumic relaxation time and ET is ejection time. Tei index > 0.3 indicates poor ventricular function.
8. Tricuspid annular plane systolic excursion (TAPSE): systolic excursion of the lateral aspect of the tricuspid annulus can be used as an indicator of RV systolic function. The normal systolic excursion is 20–25 mm towards the cardiac apex or 35% of the RV length (Fig. 6.12).
9. *Tissue Doppler*: Tricuspid annular plane maximal systolic velocity, isovolumic acceleration, myocardial strain and strain rate are tissue Doppler derived indices of RV function.

Diastolic Function

1. *RA pressure*: Inferior vena cava size < 2 cm and inspiratory collapse > 50% corresponds to RA pressure < 5 mm Hg

2. *RV filling profile*: The normal tricuspid blood flow tracing is M-shaped, similar to mitral inflow pattern. Reduced E/A results from external constraint or RV overload causing diastolic dysfunction (Fig. 6.13).

3. *Hepatic venous flow pattern*: The examination of the patterns of flow velocity in the hepatic vein during the different phases of cardiac cycle can reveal important information about RV function. The normal hepatic venous flow has four components. The initial forward flow towards the RA occurs during systole and is caused by the decrease in atrial pressure due to atrial relaxation and apical movement of tricuspid valve during RV systole. (corresponds to x-descent in atrial pressure). Forward flow in diastole is caused by a decrease in atrial pressure during early ventricular filling and corresponds to y-descent in atrial pressure. The two small retrograde flows may be observed; one corresponding to atrial contraction (end-diastole) and one appearing at end-systole, before the y-descent in atrial pressure. When the RV function is impaired, the systolic inflow wave of hepatic venous flow is attenuated. The reversal of systolic flow represents severe tricuspid regurgitation (Figs 6.14 and 6.15).

ASSESSMENT OF REGIONAL RIGHT VENTRICULAR FUNCTION

Regional RV ischemia is difficult to detect, especially the mild changes. However, akinesia or dyskinesia can be easily identified and is a sensitive indicator of RV infarction. RA enlargement, RV dilatation, papillary muscle dysfunction, tricuspid regurgitation and paradoxical interventricular septal motion are other indicators of RV infarction.

Estimation of Right Ventricular Systolic Pressure (RVSP)

$$RVSP = 4v^2 + RA$$

The RVSP is calculated by adding the tricuspid transvalvular gradient to the RA pressure (Fig. 6.16). In the absence of any obstruction to the RV outflow, the RVSP provides a good estimate of the PA systolic pressure. Similarly, in the presence of pulmonary regurgitation, the diastolic PA pressure can be estimated by adding the diastolic gradient between the PA and the RV to the RA pressure.

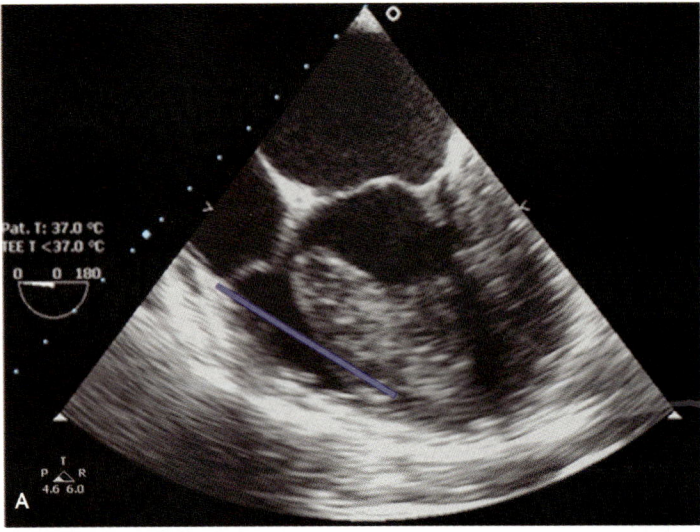

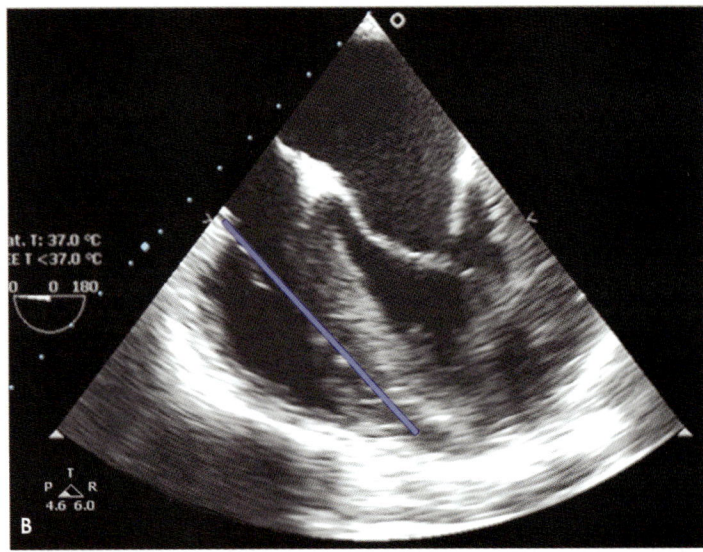

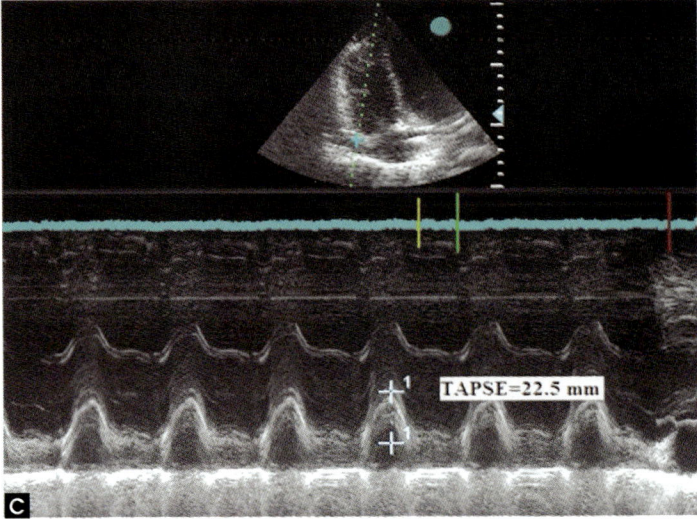

Fig. 6.12: Triuspid annular plane systolic excursion: The difference between the end-systolic and the end-diastolic distance from the tricuspid annulus to the apex is obtained by placing the cursor on the lateral aspect of the tricuspid annulus in the midesophageal four-chamber view (A,B) or the deep transgastric view. Alternately, the same can be obtained using M-mode echocardiography (C).

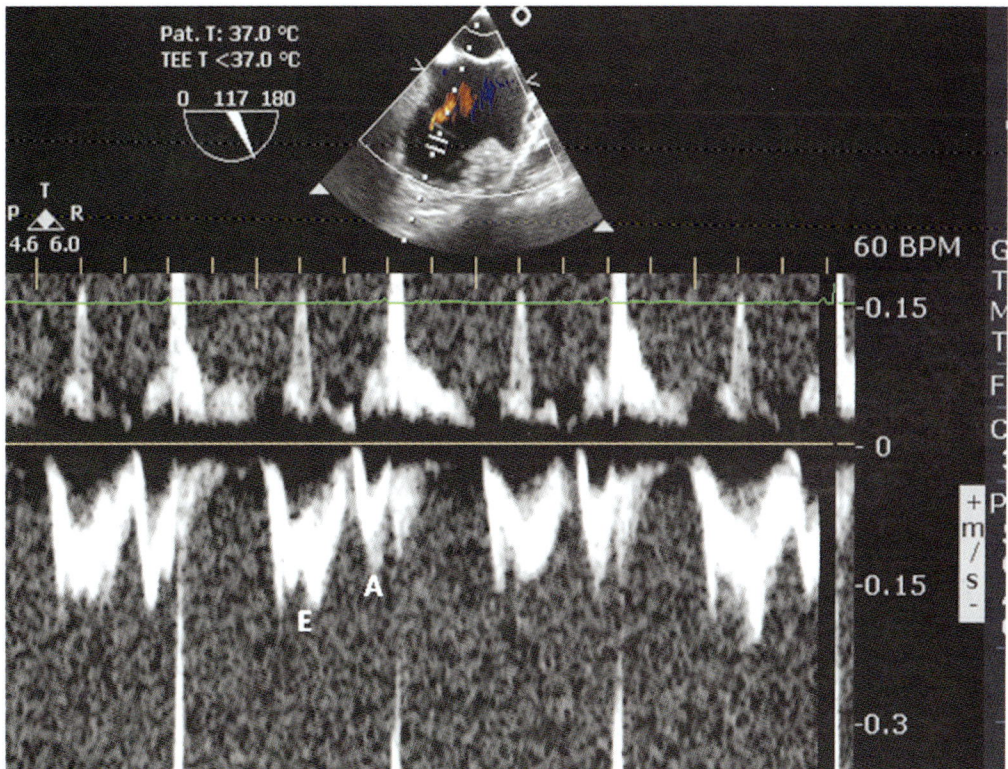

Fig. 6.13: Normal tricuspid inflow pattern. Normally, E > A. (E: early atrial filling, A: late atrial filling).

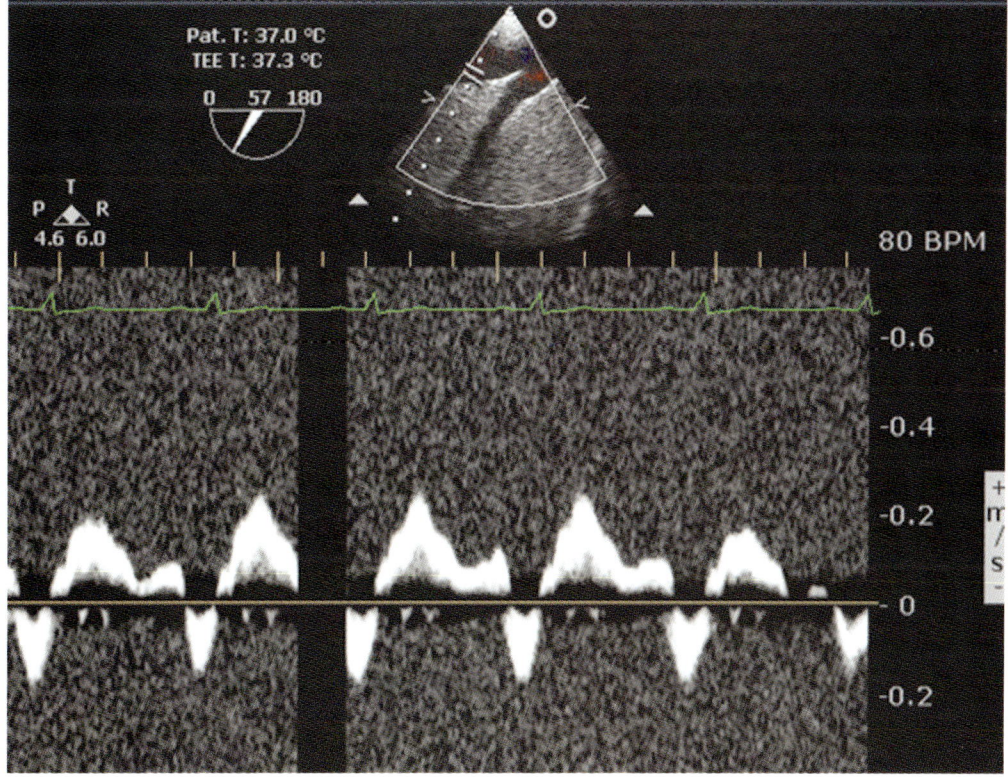

Fig. 6.14: Pulsed wave Doppler image of normal hepatic venous flow with forward flow in systole and diastole.

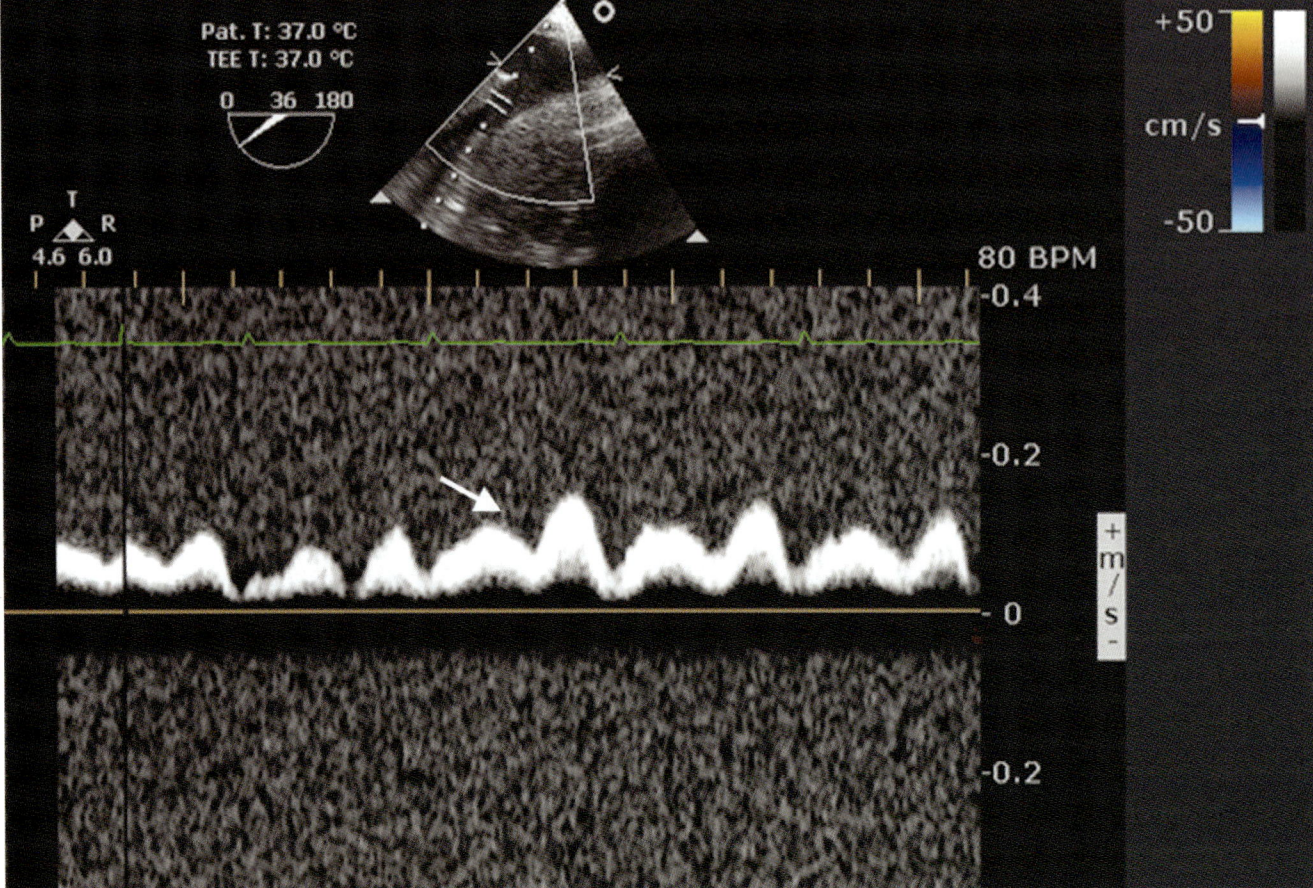

Fig. 6.15: The systolic inflow wave of hepatic venous flow is attenuated (arrow) in impaired right ventricular function.

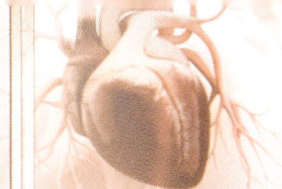

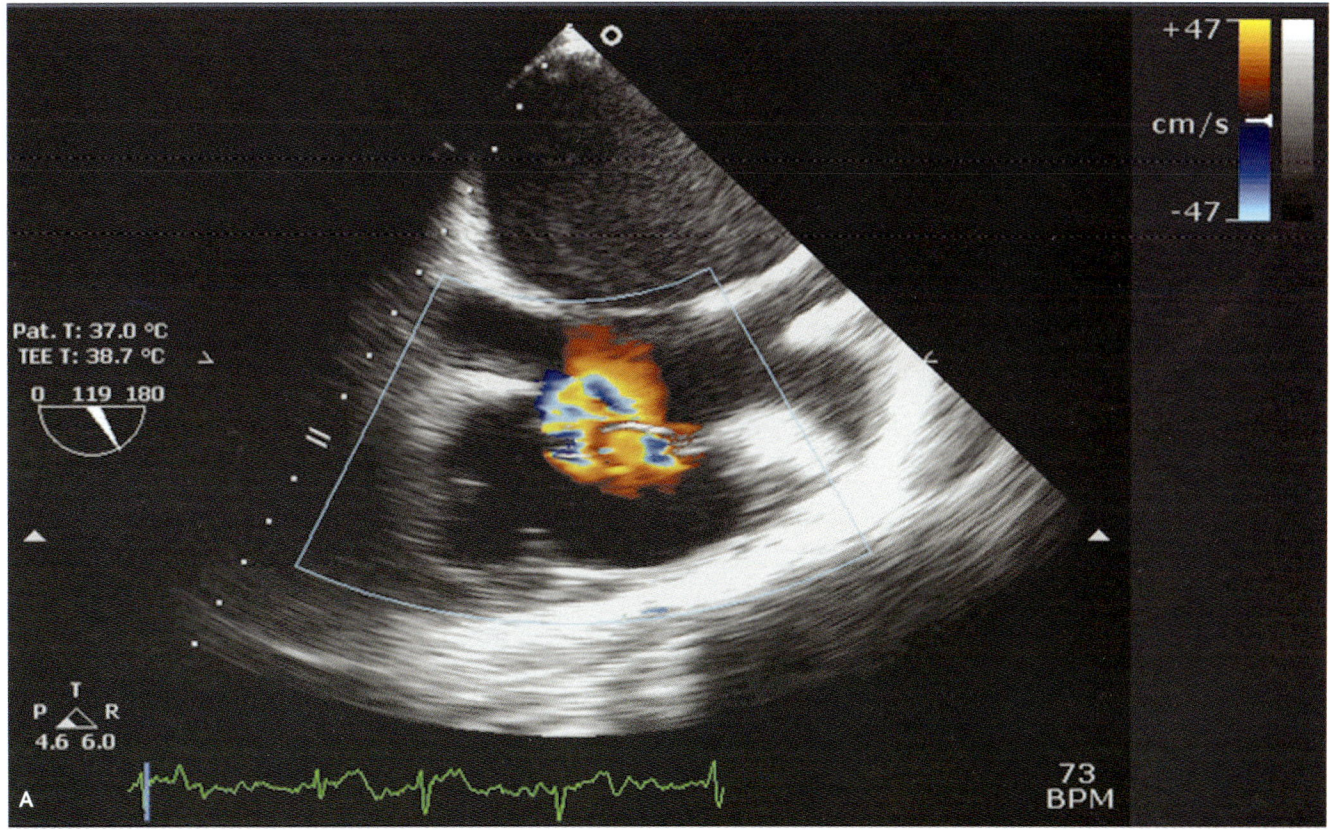

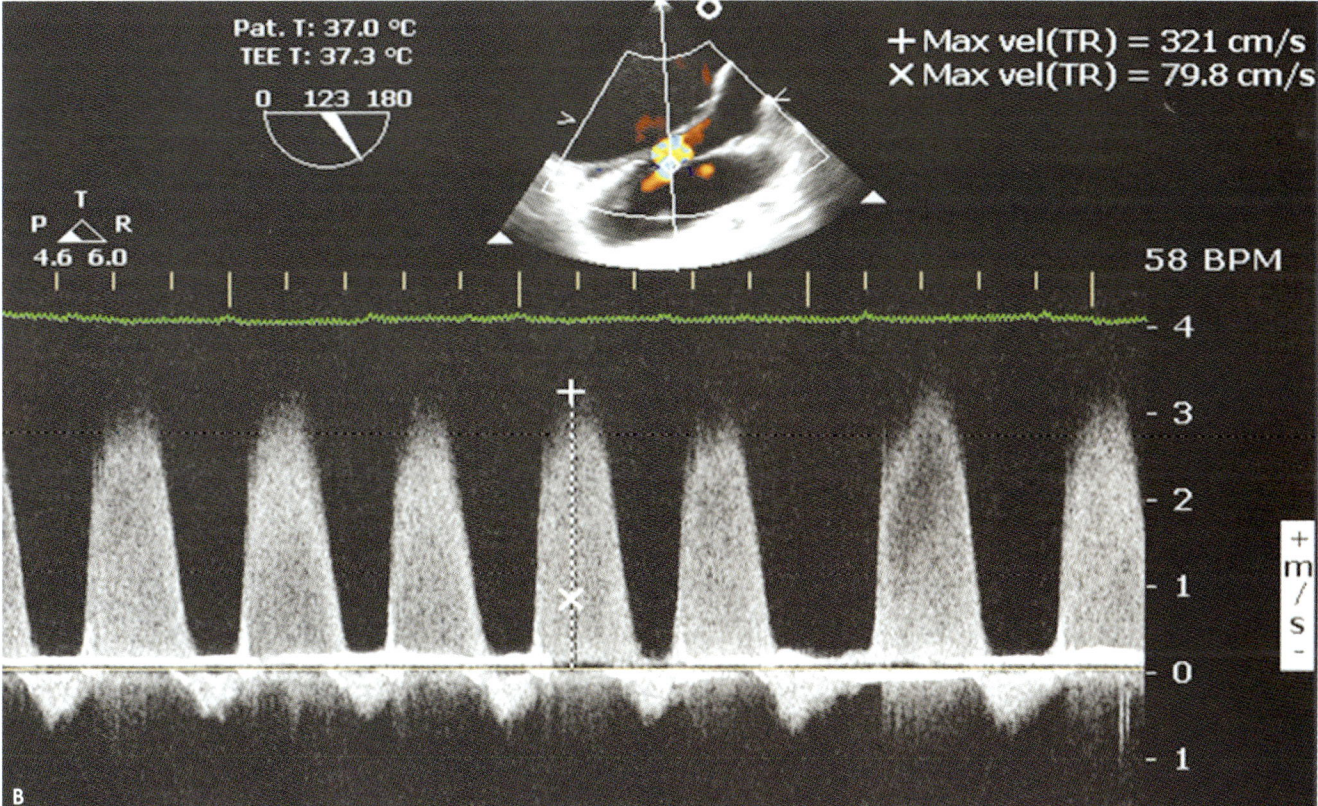

Fig. 6.16: Modified bicaval view with color flow Doppler interrogation of the tricuspid valve (A). The tricuspid regurgitation jet can be interrogated with continuous wave Doppler to measure the peak velocity of the regurgitant jet (B).

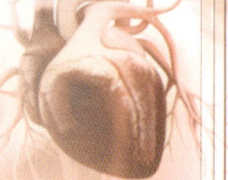

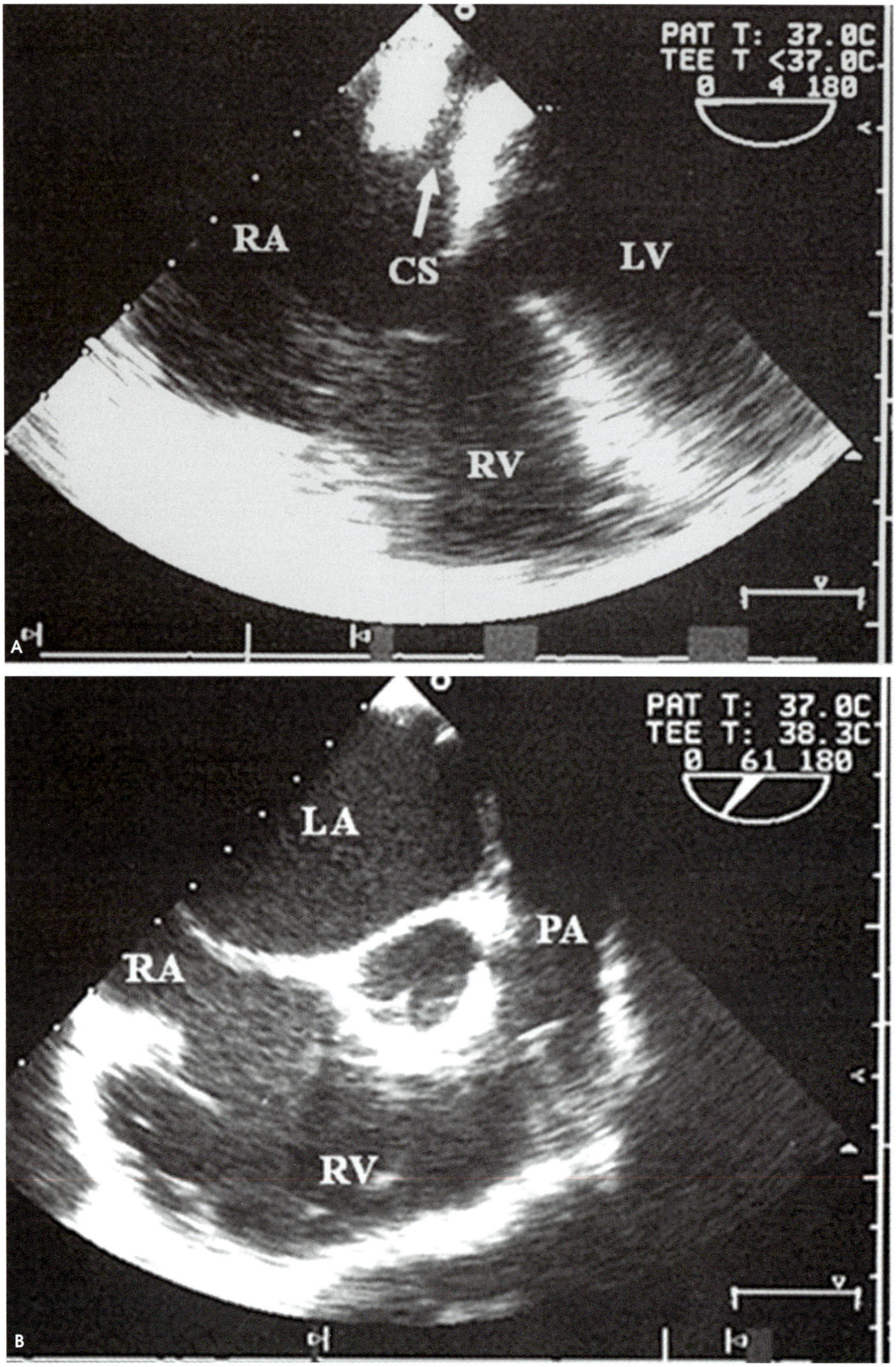

Fig. 6.17: Views for evaluation of the right ventricular function. Note the appearance of RV in a normal individual. A: Modified 4-chamber view; B. Midesophageal RV inflow-outflow view (RA: right atrium, RV: right ventricle, LV: left ventricle, CS: coronary sinus, LA: left atrium, PA: pulmonary artery).

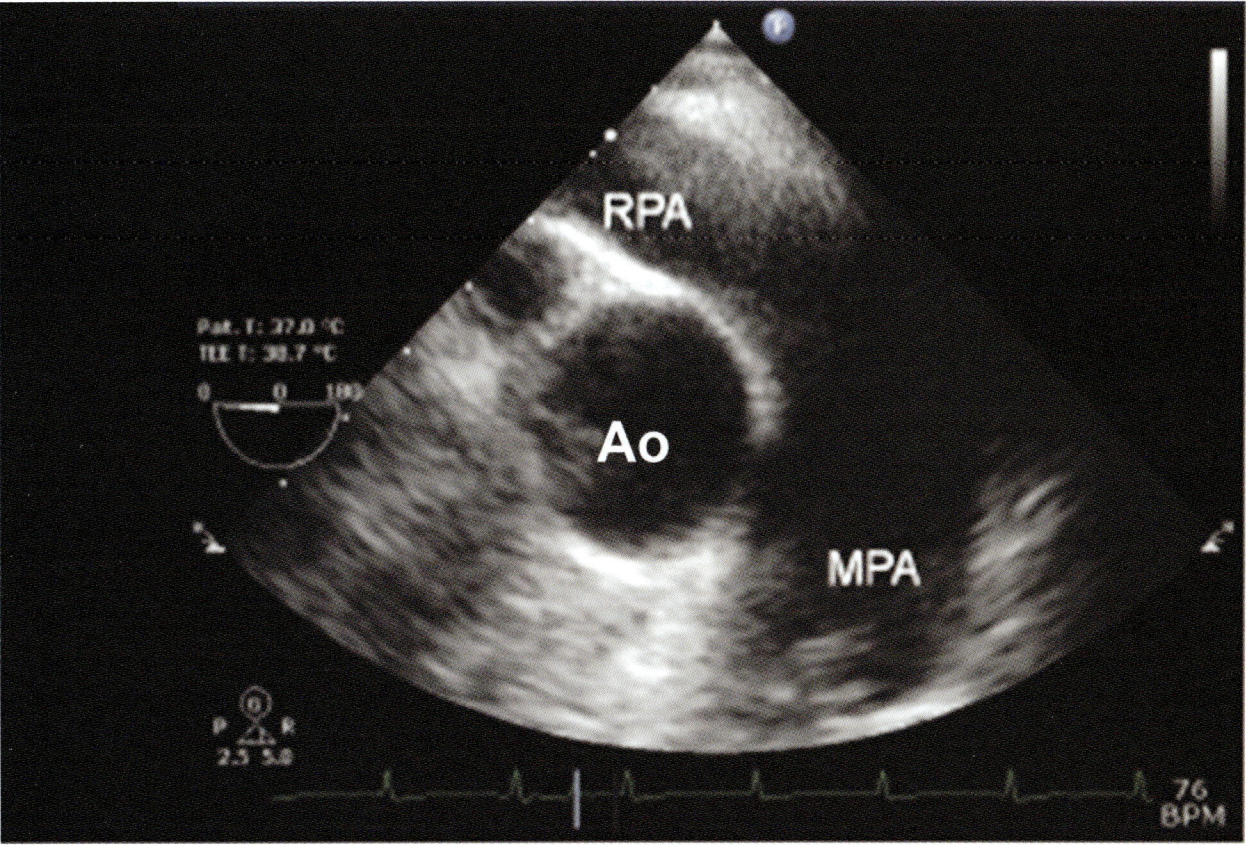

Fig. 6.18: Midesophageal ascending aorta short-axis view for evaluating the main pulmonary artery and its branches. (RPA: right pulmonary artery, Ao: aorta, MPA: main pulmonary artery).

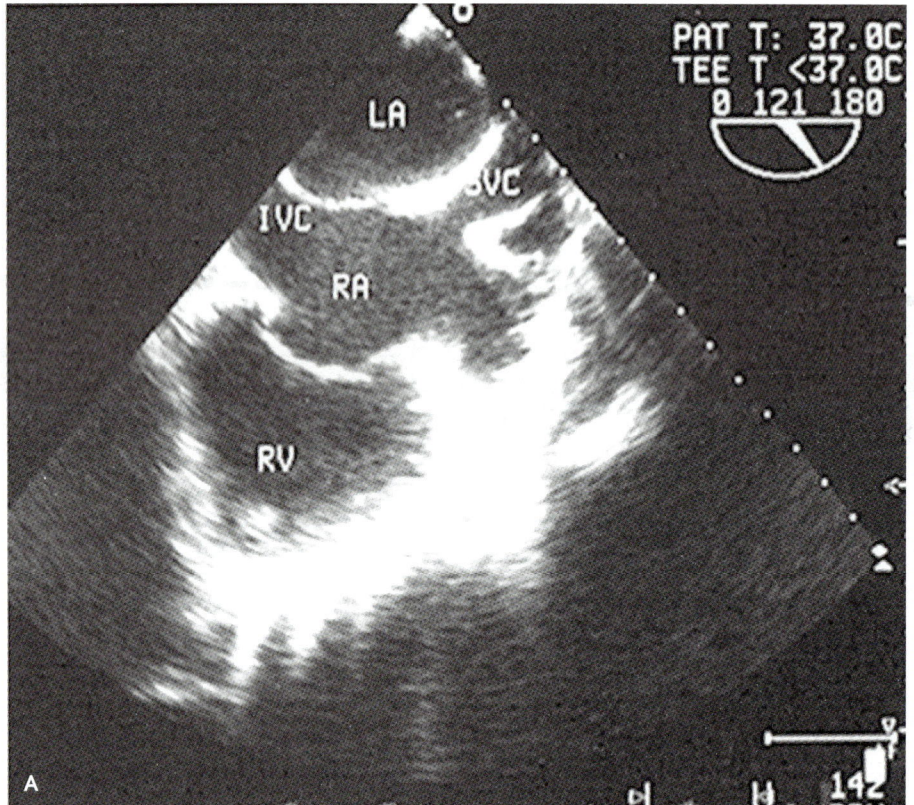

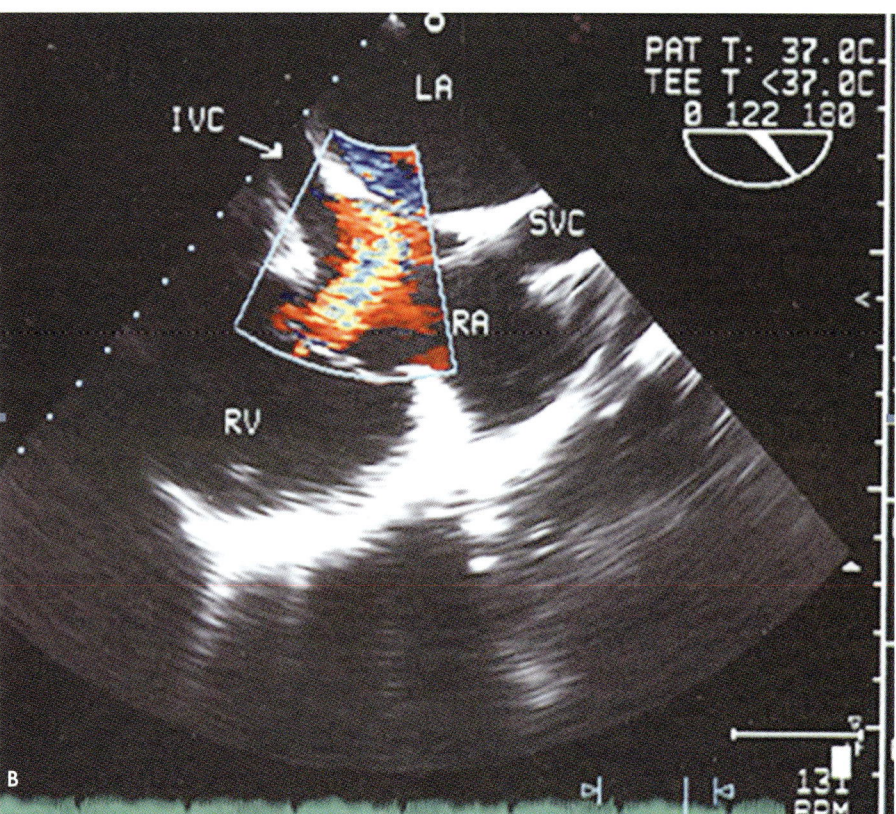

Fig. 6.19: Appearance of the tricuspid valve (A) in modified bicaval view. Note the appearance of tricuspid regurgitation jet on color flow study (B). (LA: left atrium, RA: right atrium, SVC: superior vena cava, IVC: inferior vena cava, RV: right ventricle)

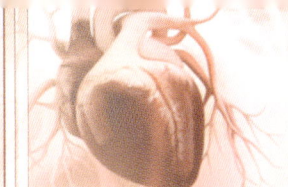

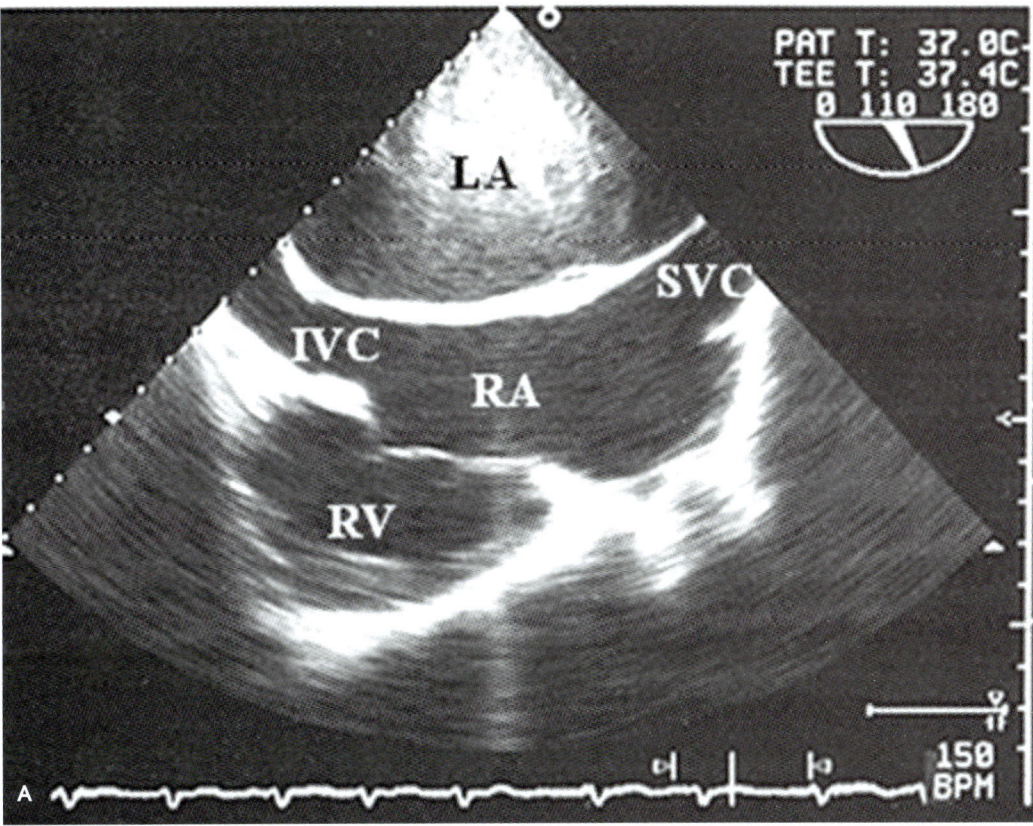

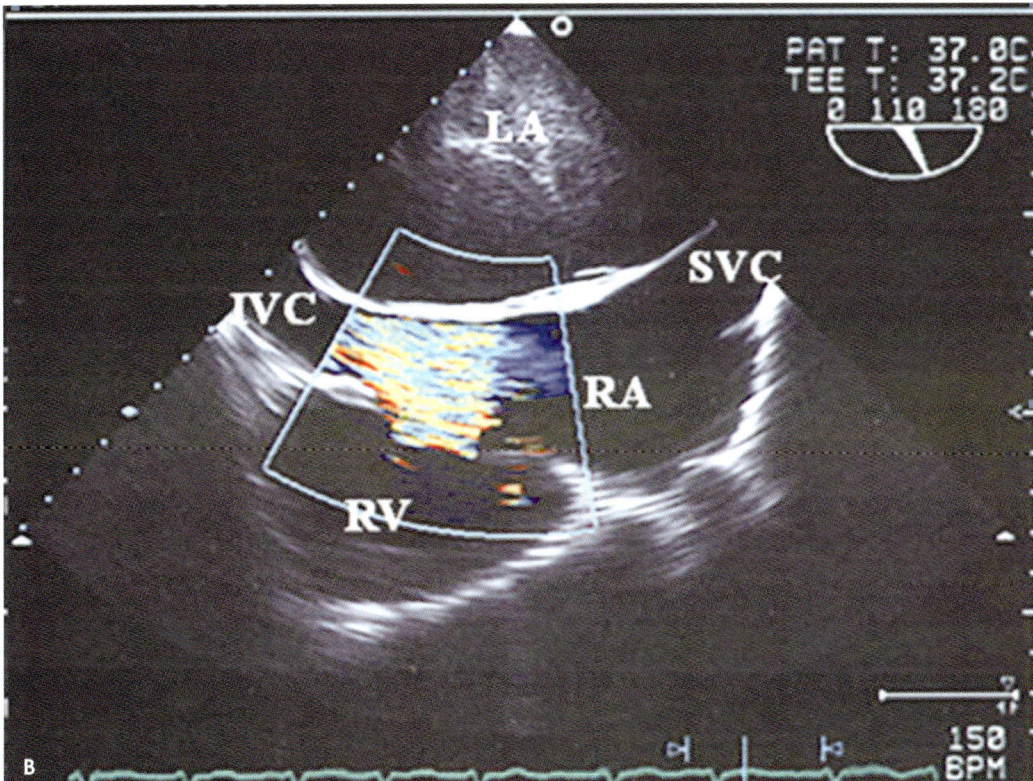

Fig. 6.20: Panel A: Appearance of the tricuspid valve in a patient with rheumatic mitral stenosis (note the large left atrium with dense spontaneous echo contrast). Panel B shows the color flow across the tricuspid valve showing severe tricuspid regurgitation. (LA: left atrium, RA: right atrium, RV: right ventricle, SVC: superior vena cava, IVC: inferior vena cava).

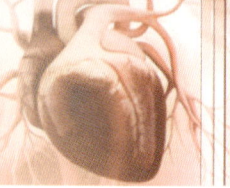

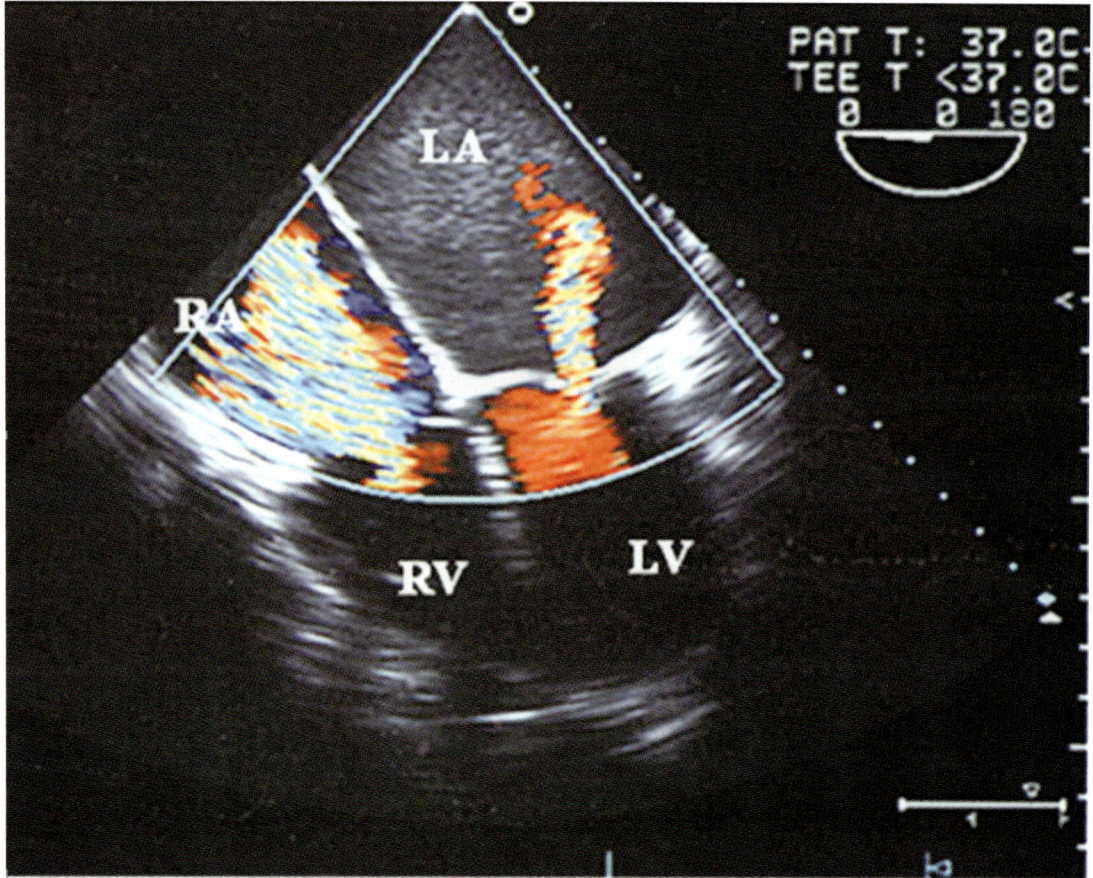

Fig. 6.21: Appearance of severe hypertensive tricuspid regurgitation in a patient with rheumatic mitral valve disease. Note the enlarged left atrium with dense spontaneous echo contrast. The patient also has mild mitral regurgitation (LA: left atrium, RA: right atrium, LV: left ventricle, RV: right ventricle).

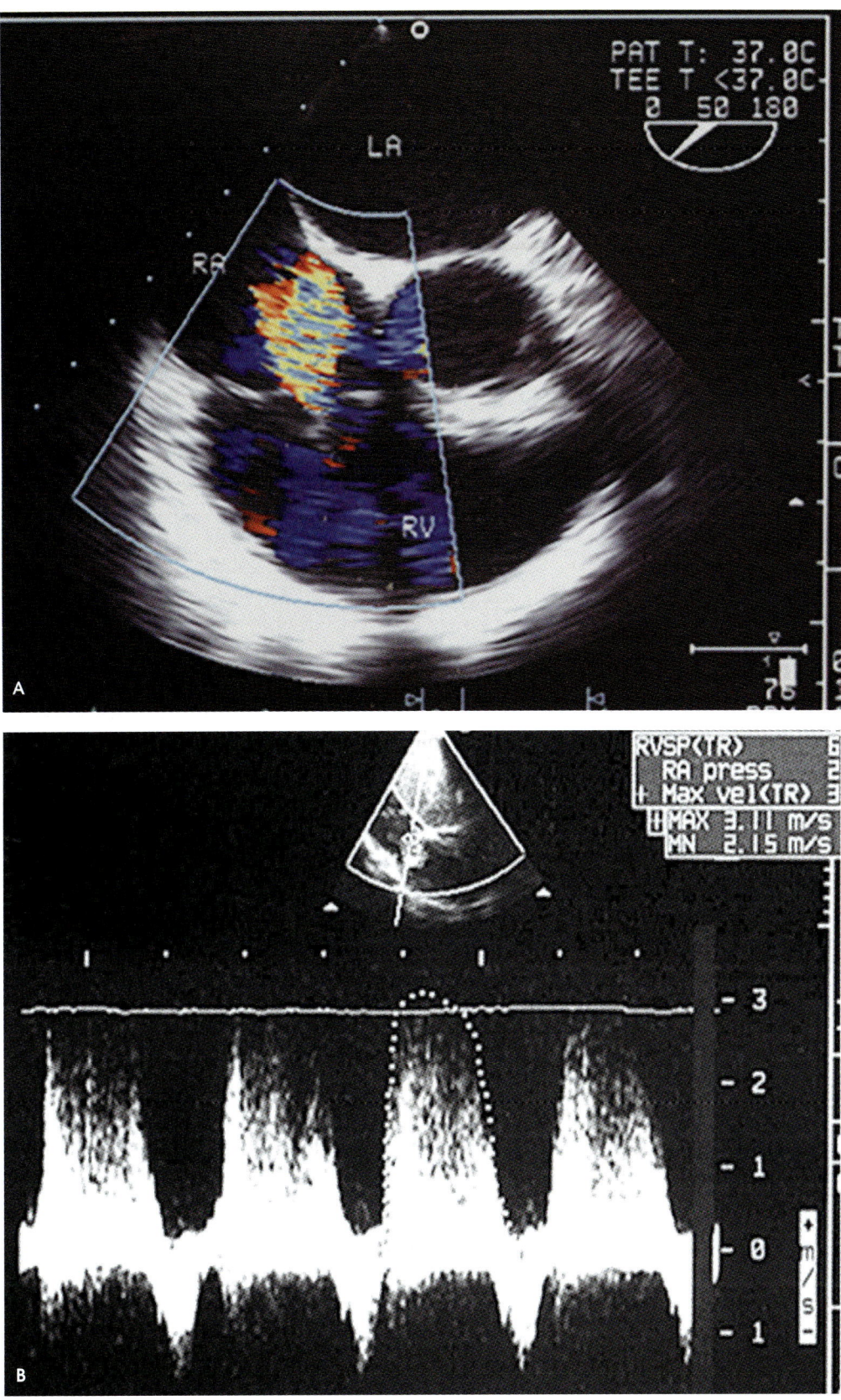

Fig. 6.22: Appearance of the tricuspid regurgitation in midesophageal right ventricular inflow-outflow (A) view. Continuous wave Doppler can be used for estimating the right atrioventricular gradient ($4 V^2 = 4 \times 3^2 = 36$ mm Hg) (B) (LA: left atrium, RA: right atrium, RV: right ventricle).

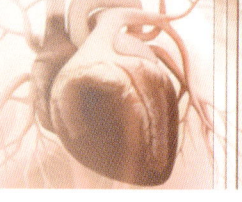

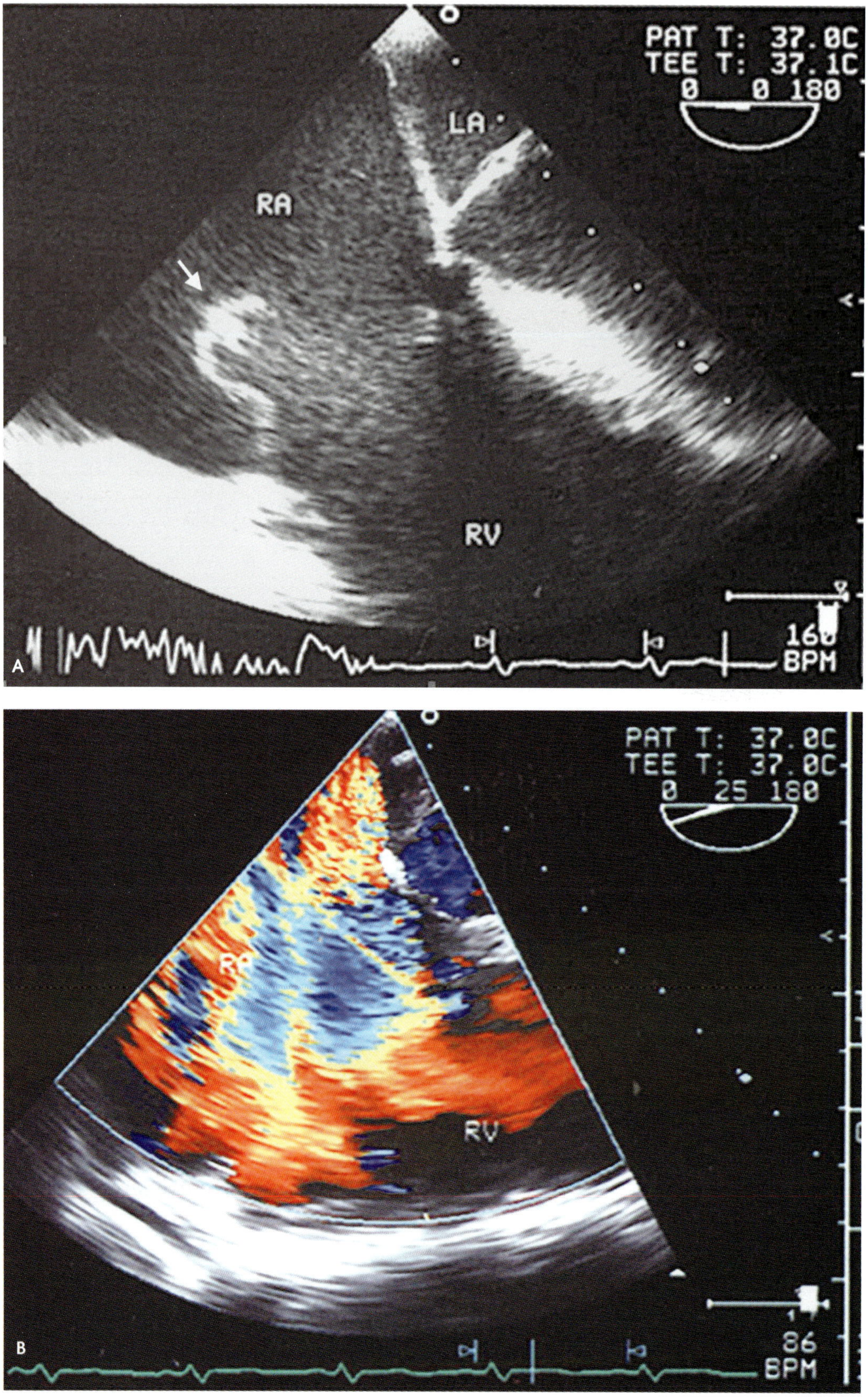

Fig. 6.23: Panel A: A patient with congenital dysplastic tricuspid valve. Note the flail tricuspid leaflet (arrow) and Panel B: The severe normotensive tricuspid regurgitation on color flow. (RA: right atrium, LA: left atrium, RV: right ventricle).

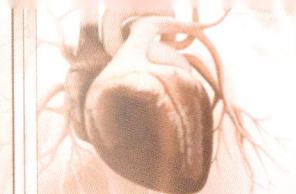

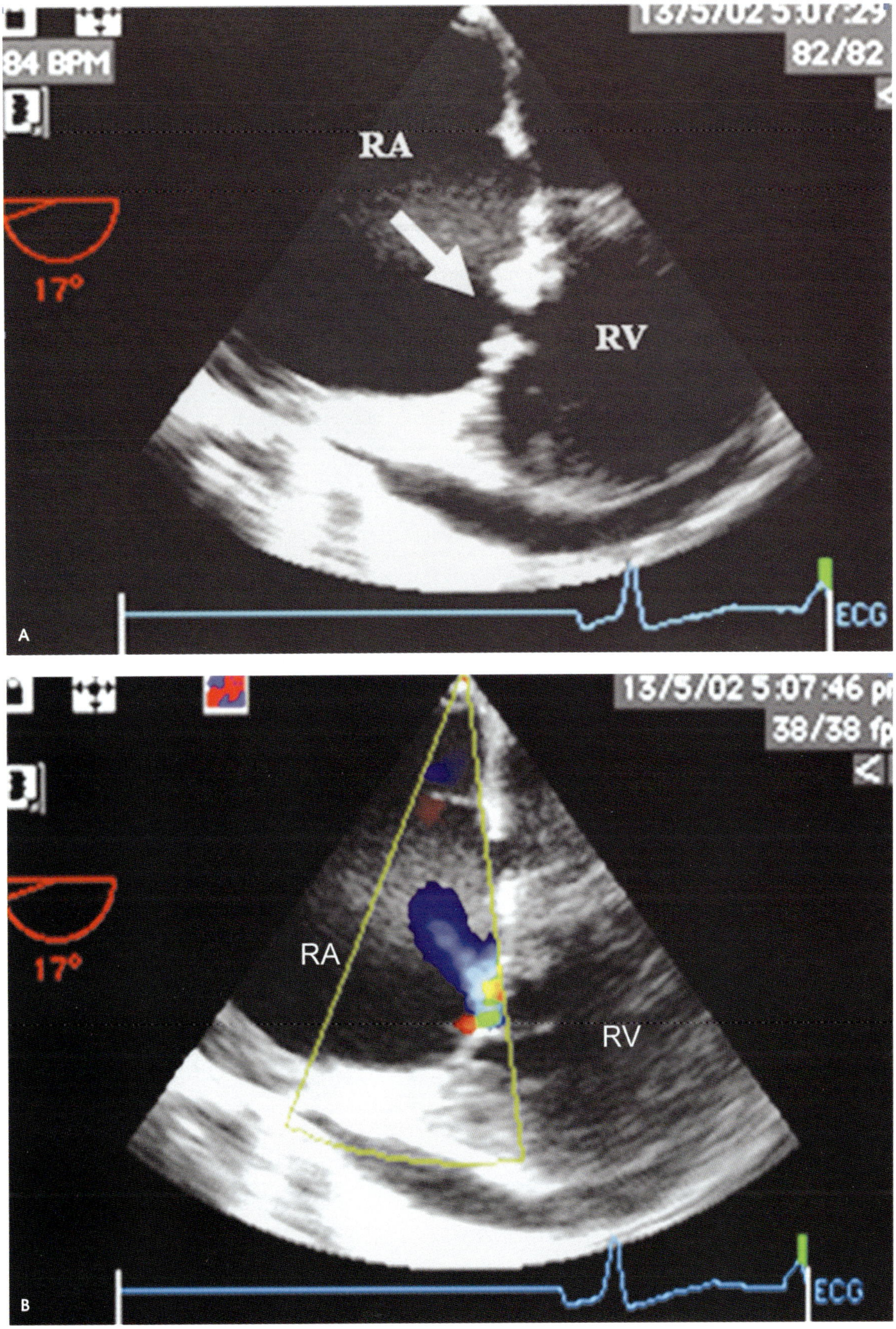

Fig. 6.24: Panel A: Appearance of the tricuspid valve (arrow). Note the marked thickening, calcification and doming of tricuspid leaflets. Panel B: Color flow across the tricuspid valve shows mild tricuspid regurgitation. (RA: right atrium, RV: right ventricle).

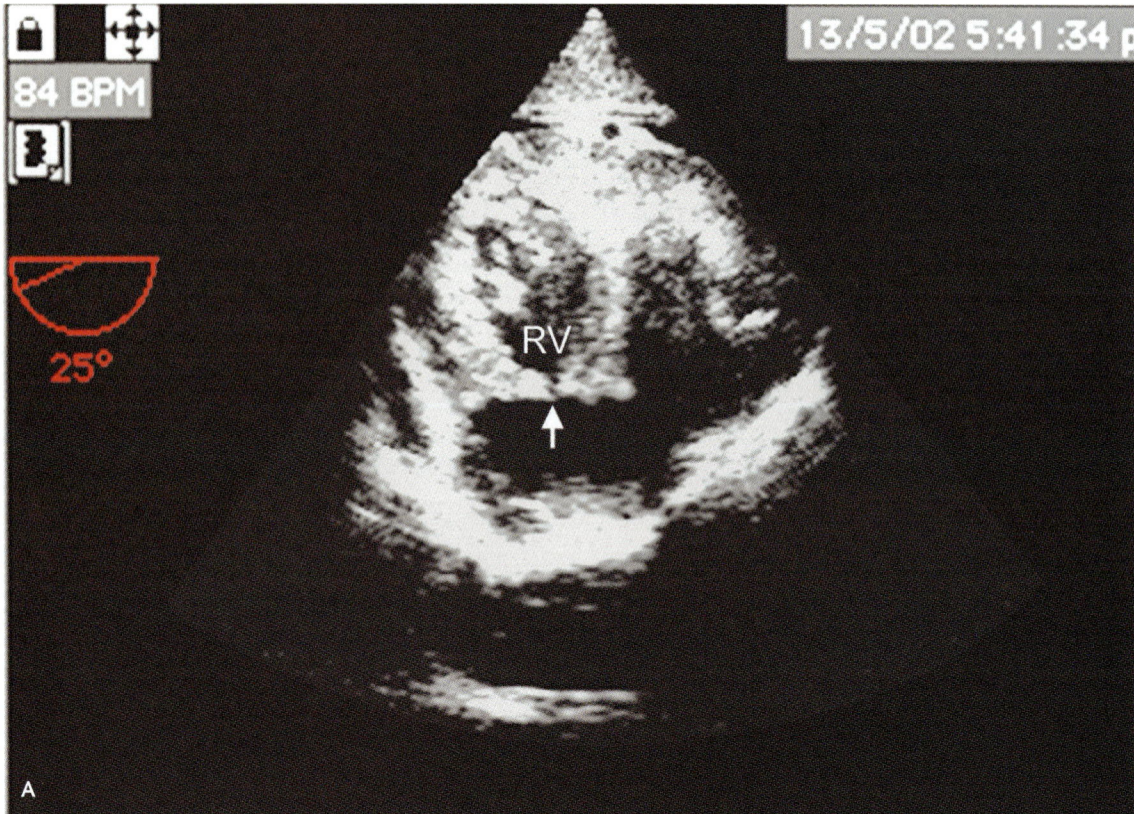

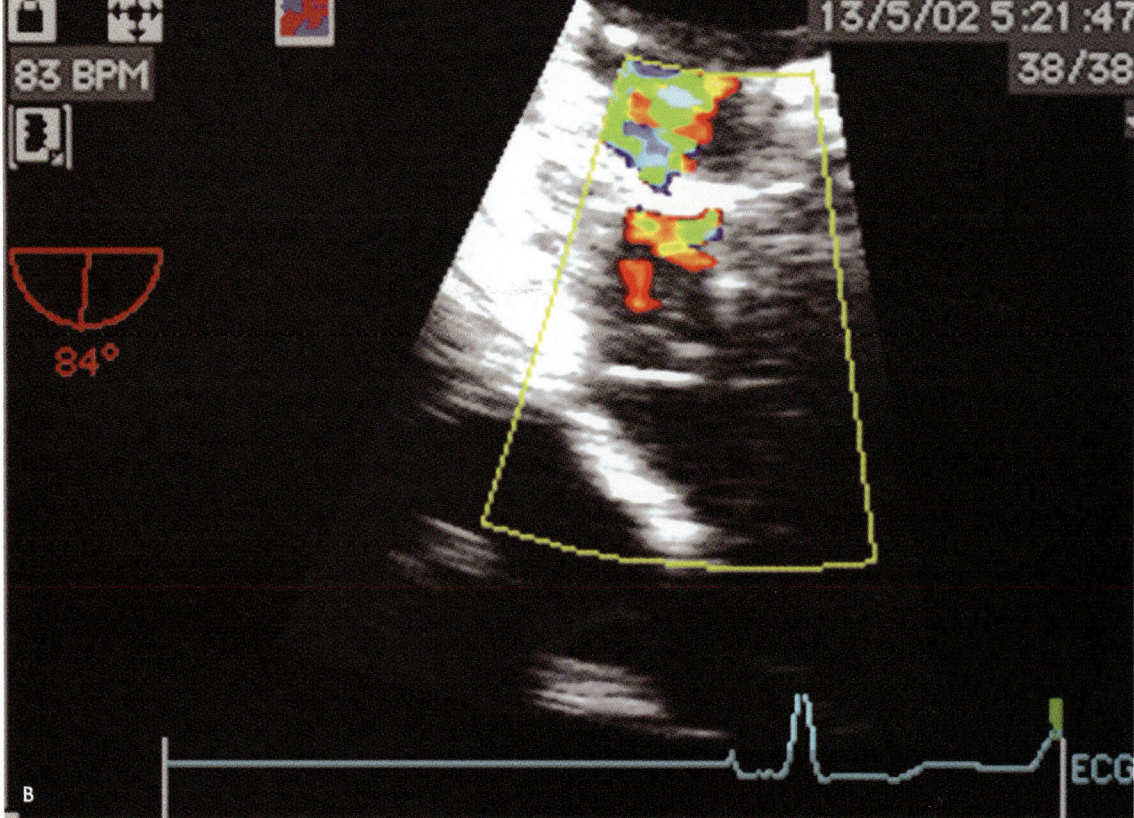

Fig. 6.25: Appearance of subpulmonary membrane (arrow, A) in deep transgastric view of the right ventricular outflow tract. Color flow (B) revealed marked turbulence caused by severe right ventricular outflow tract obstruction (RV: right ventricle).

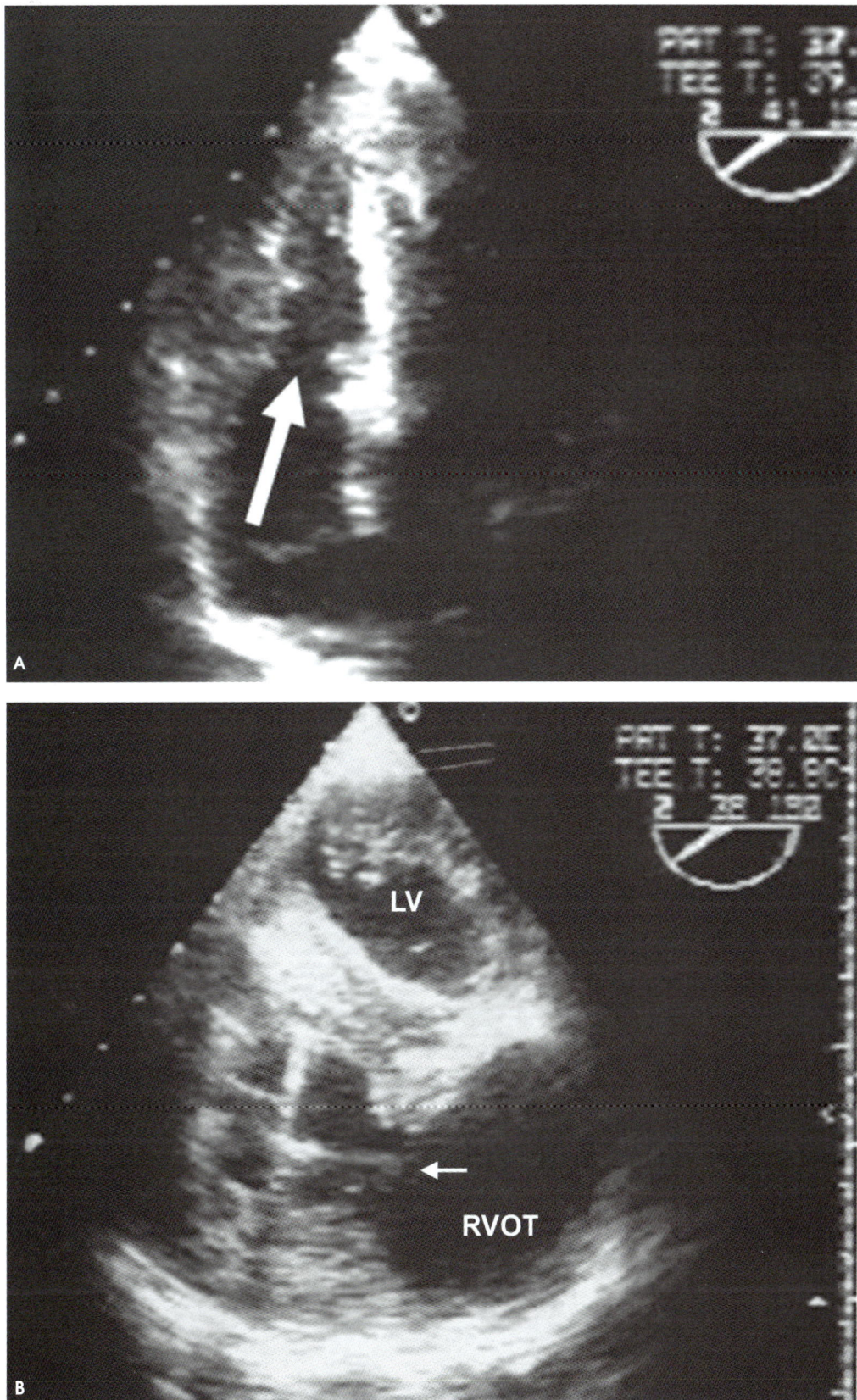

Fig. 6.26: Postoperative appearance of the resected portion of the right ventricular outflow tract seen in deep transgastric view (arrow, A) and modified transgastric view showing Starr-Edwards prosthesis (arrow) in tricuspid position (B). (LV: Left ventricle, RVOT: Right ventricular outflow tract).

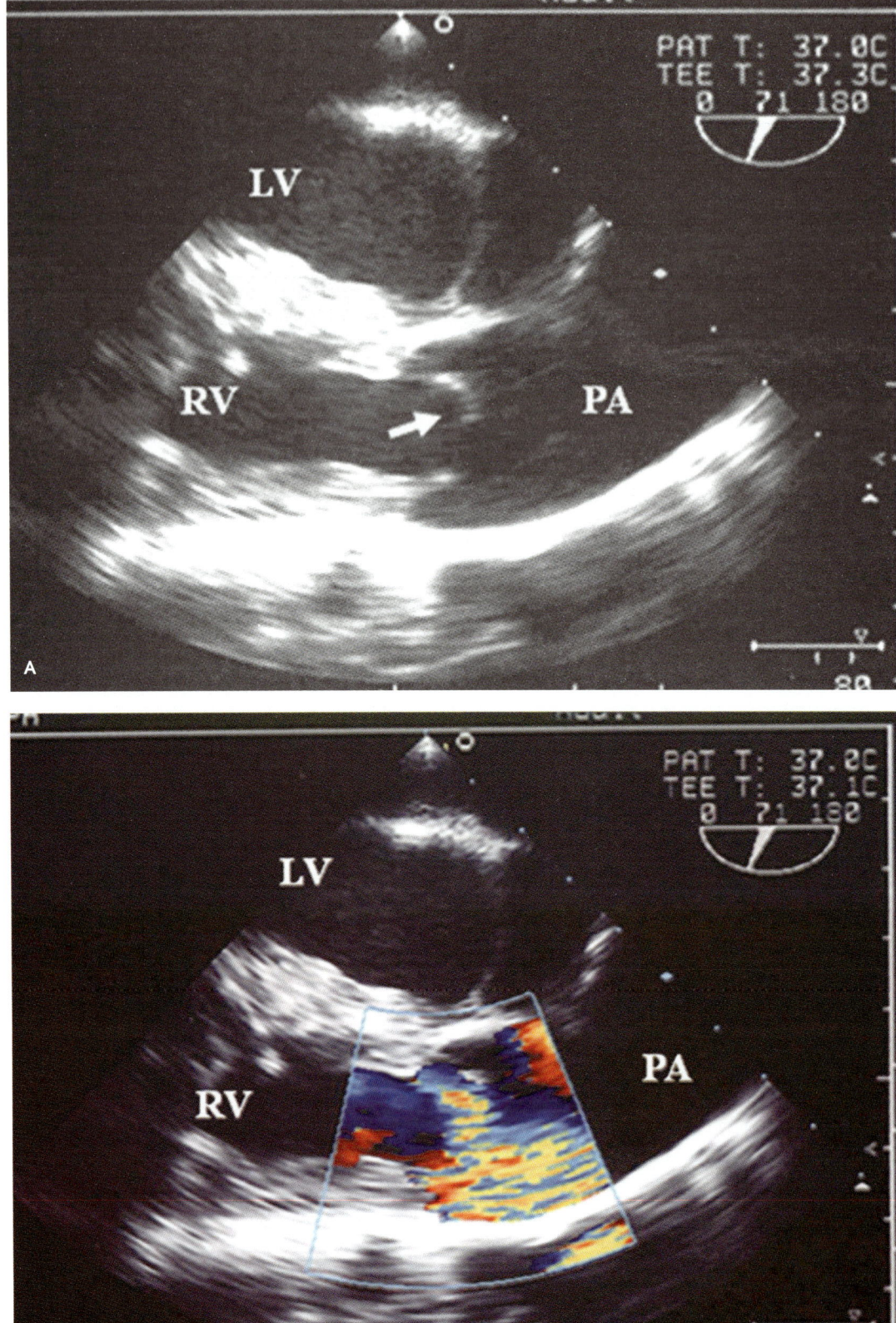

Fig. 6.27: Appearance of congenital pulmonary valve stenosis. Note the doming pulmonary valve (arrow, A) and the turbulent stenotic jet across it on color flow (B) (LV: left ventricle, RV: right ventricle, PA: pulmonary artery).

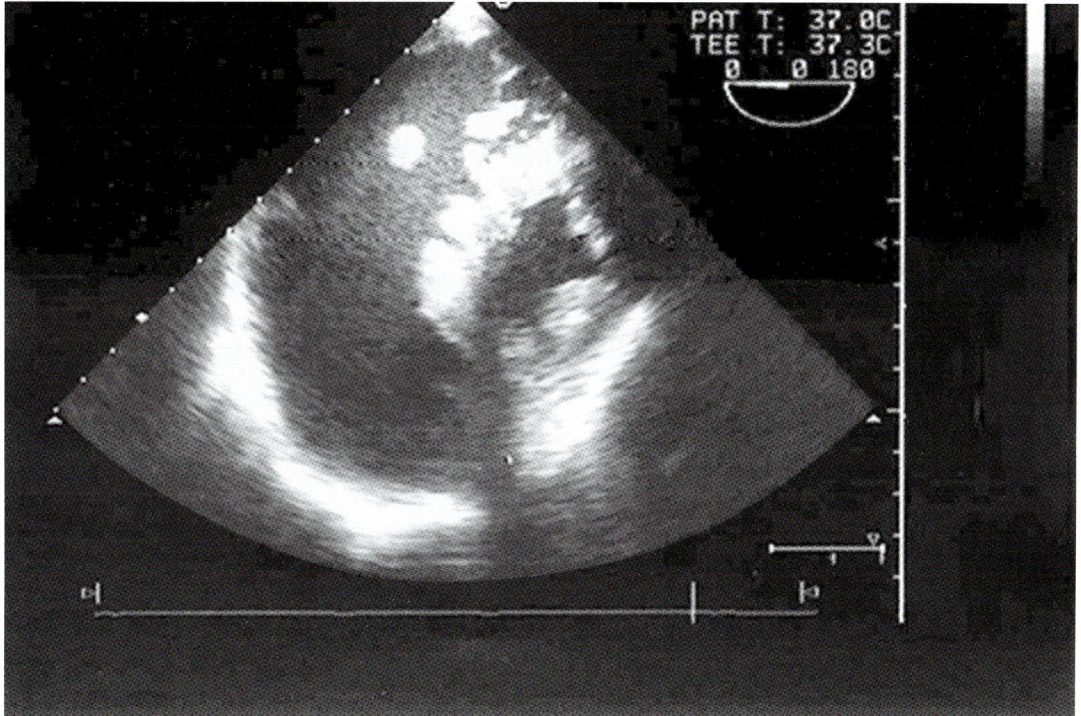

Fig. 6.28: Transgastric view showing dilated right ventricle in a patient with a large atrial septal defect.

Evaluation of Left Ventricular Function

7

• Deepak K. Tempe • Suruchi Hasija

Transesophageal echocardiography (TEE) has been used extensively for the evaluation of hemodynamic, and global and regional ventricular function. Standard hemodynamic variables, e.g. filling pressures and cardiac output that are normally obtained by other invasive techniques such as pulmonary artery catheterization have been estimated with TEE. In addition, it has also been used to quantify cardiac dimensions, intracardiac flow rates and overall cardiac performance.

Hemodynamic and other physiologic stresses during the perioperative period increase the risk of perioperative myocardial ischemia. This is particularly true for patients with coronary artery disease or those who have multiple risk factors for coronary artery disease. The role of TEE in detecting ischemia during both cardiac and noncardiac surgery is being increasingly recognized, since traditional methods such as ECG have a limited diagnostic accuracy. Detection of regional ventricular dysfunction can be useful for making therapeutic decisions like graft revision and instituting hemodynamic support in these patients. Such interventions improve the overall surgical success and outcome. TEE evaluation in multiple planes is required for delineating the area at risk. Interpretation of wall motion abnormalities however, requires expertise. TEE provides a more accurate estimate of changes in preload and left ventricular filling pressures. The diagnosis of hemodynamic problem such as hypovolemia or myocardial dysfunction as a cause of decreased cardiac output can be easily differentiated for choosing the right therapeutic options in the postoperative period.

Anesthesiologists with basic TEE training should be able to make qualitative assessment of the hemodynamic status and myocardial function. This chapter illustrates the images that are utilized for the assessment of left ventricular (LV) function.

SYSTOLIC FUNCTION

The following are the echocardiographic methods of assessing global LV systolic function:

1. Fractional Shortening (FS)

The end-diastolic and end-systolic diameters of the LV are obtained from the transgastric midpapillary short-axis view using M-mode echocardiography.

$$FS = \{(LVIDd - LVIDs)/LVIDd\} \times 100$$

where, LVIDd and LVIDs are left ventricular internal diameter at end-diastole and end-systeole, respectively.

Normal: Men 25 to 43%, women 27 to 45%

2. Fractional Area Change (FAC)

Images are collected from the transgastric midpapillary short-axis view. Using the freeze and scroll functions the largest [end-diastolic area (EDA)] and smallest [end-systolic area (ESA)] frames of a cardiac cycle are identified and the endocardial surfaces are traced.

$$FAC = \frac{(EDA - ESA)}{EDA} \times 100$$

Normal values: Men: 56 to 62%; women: 59 to 65%

3. Ejection Fraction (EF)

The endocardial borders are traced from the end-diastolic and end-systolic frames from a single midesophageal four-chamber loop. Assuming the shape of the LV to be ellipsoid, volume ($8A^2/3pL$) is calculated from the area (A) and length (L) of the cavity.

$$EF = \frac{(EDV - ESV)}{EDV} \times 100$$

4. Stroke Volume (SV) and Cardiac Output (CO)

$$SV = CSA \times VTI$$
$$CO = SV \times HR$$

Where, CSA is cross-sectional area
VTI is velocity time integral
$CSA = \pi D^2/4$
HR is heart rate
The left ventricular outflow tract (LVOT) diameter (D) is obtained from the midesophageal long-axis view or deep transgastric long-axis view.

VTI is calculated from the LVOT continuous wave Doppler spectrum in the transgastric long-axis or deep transgastric long-axis view.

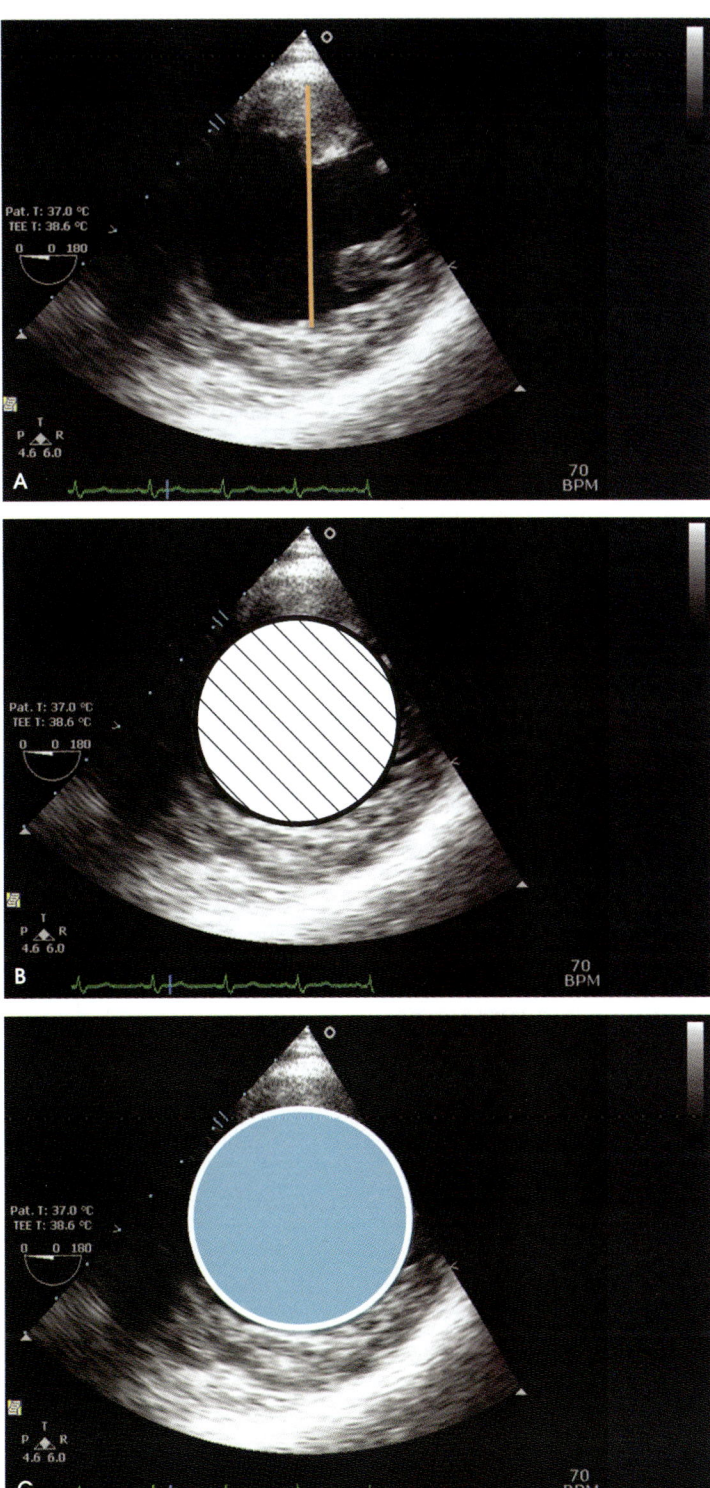

Fig. 7.1: Transgastric midpapillary short-axis view showing the method of measurement of left ventricular internal diameter (A), area (B) and volume (C).

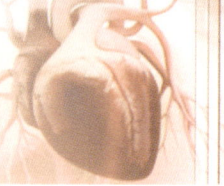

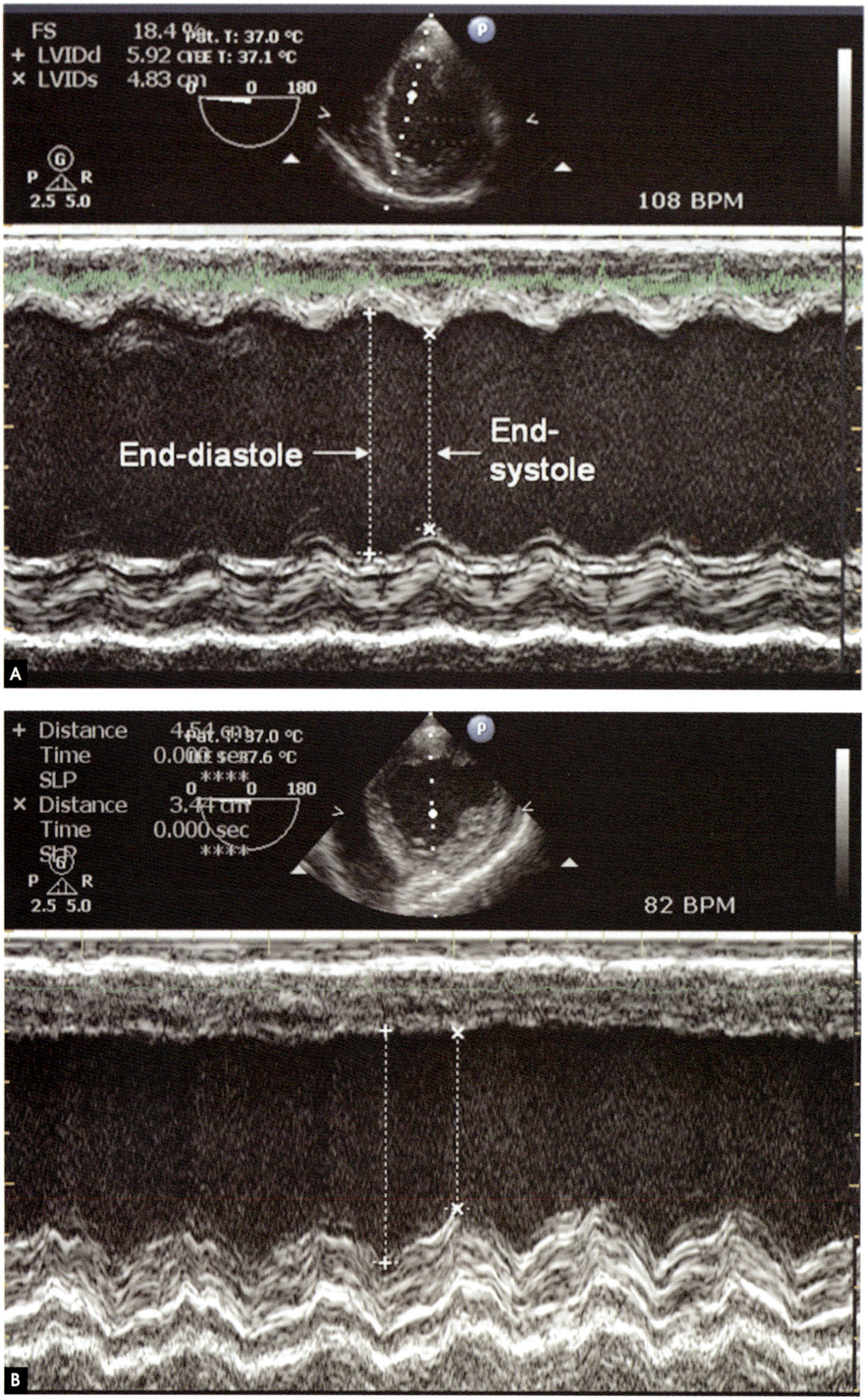

Fig. 7.2: Transgastric midpapillary short-axis view is utilized by M-mode for calculation of left-ventricular internal diameter in diastole and systole. Panel A: Fractional shortening (FS) = (5.92 – 4.83) × 100/5.92 = 18.4%, Panel B: FS = (4.54 – 3.44) × 100/4.54 = 24.2%.

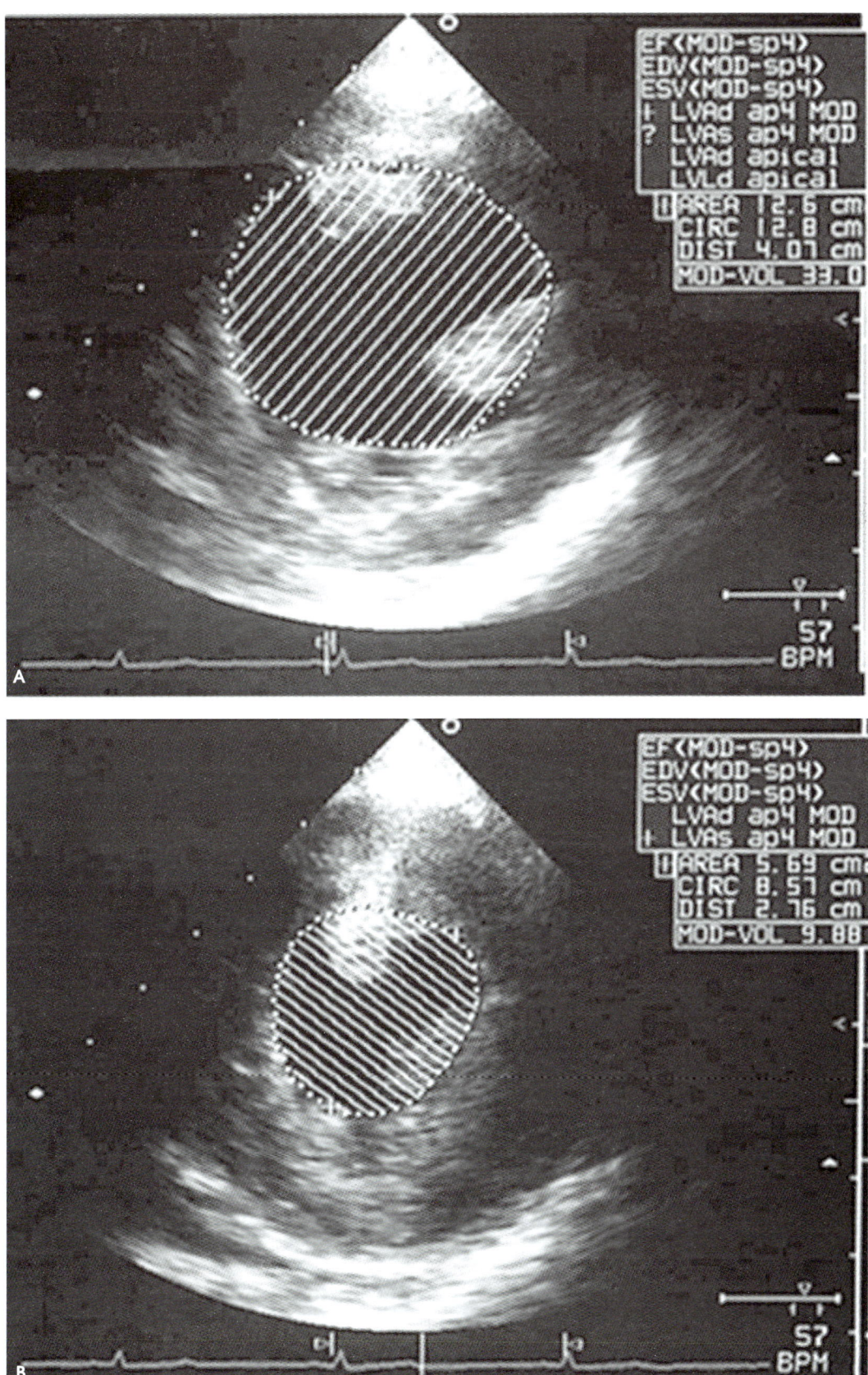

Fig. 7.3: Transgastric midpapillary short-axis view displaying the calculation of fractional area change (FAC) from end-diastolic area (A) and end-systolic area (B): FAC = (12.60 – 5.69) × 100/12.60 = 54.8%.

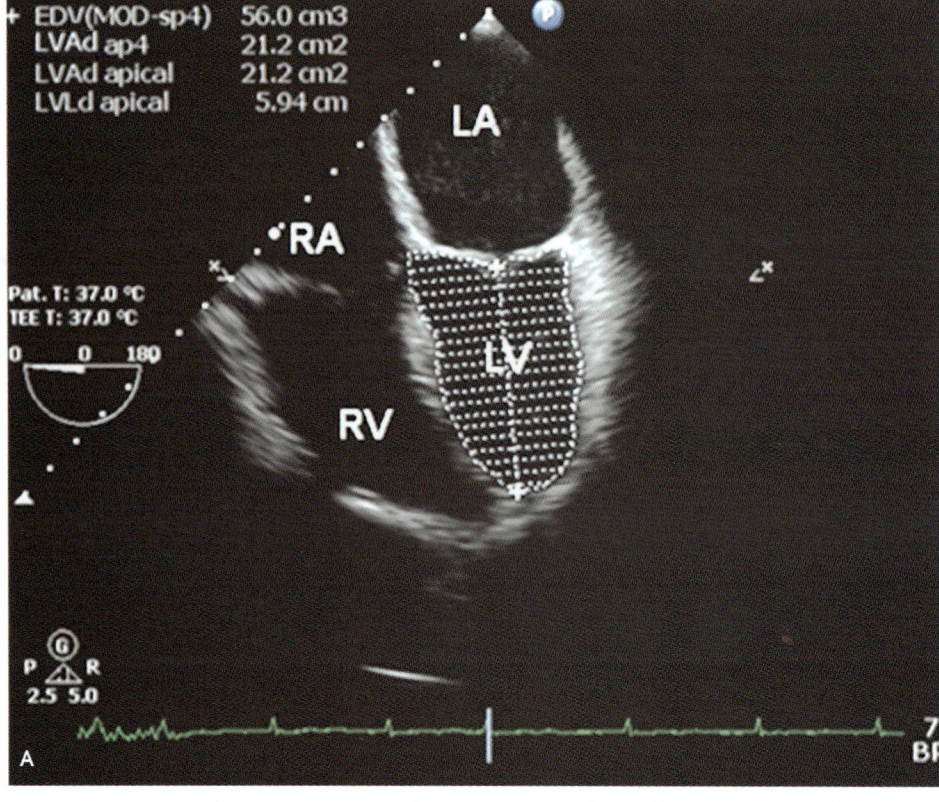

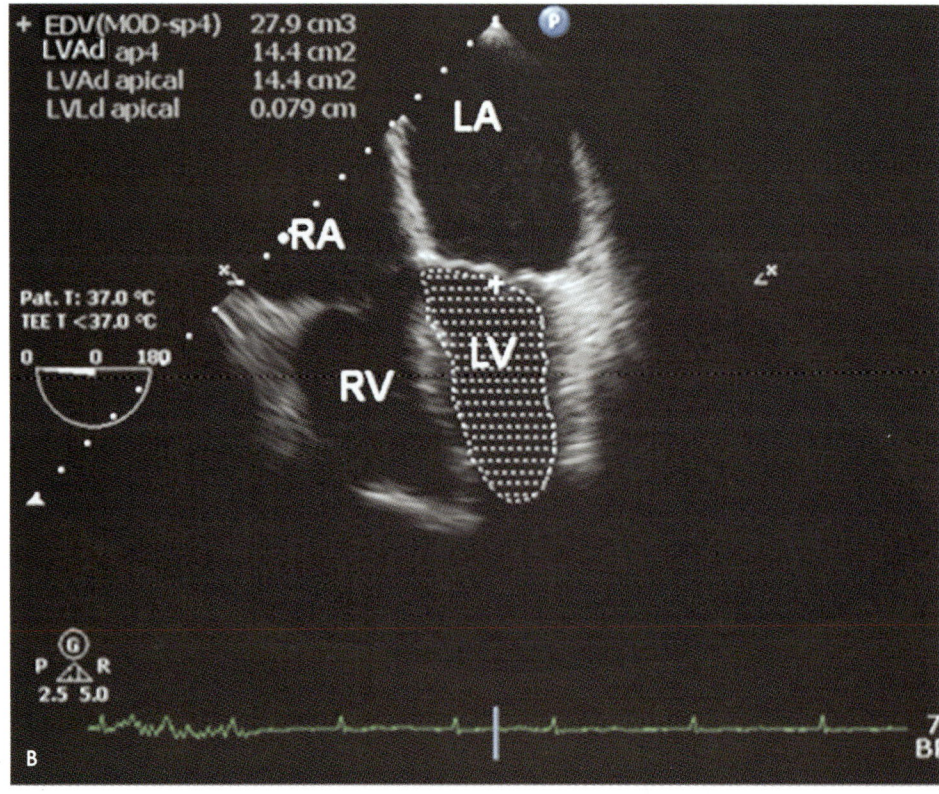

Fig. 7.4: Midesophageal four-chamber view showing the application of the Simpson's rule to determine the left ventricular end-diastolic (A) and end-systolic volumes (B). According to this rule, planimetry (computer assisted) is used to outline the endocardial border in longitudinal view. The software subsequently dissects the outlined area into a series of 20 ellipsoid cylinders of equal height. The sum of volumes of the individual slices gives the total chamber volume. Ejection fraction = (56.0 – 27.9) × 100/56.0 = 50.2% (LA: left atrium, LV: left ventricle, RA: right atrium, RV: right ventricle).

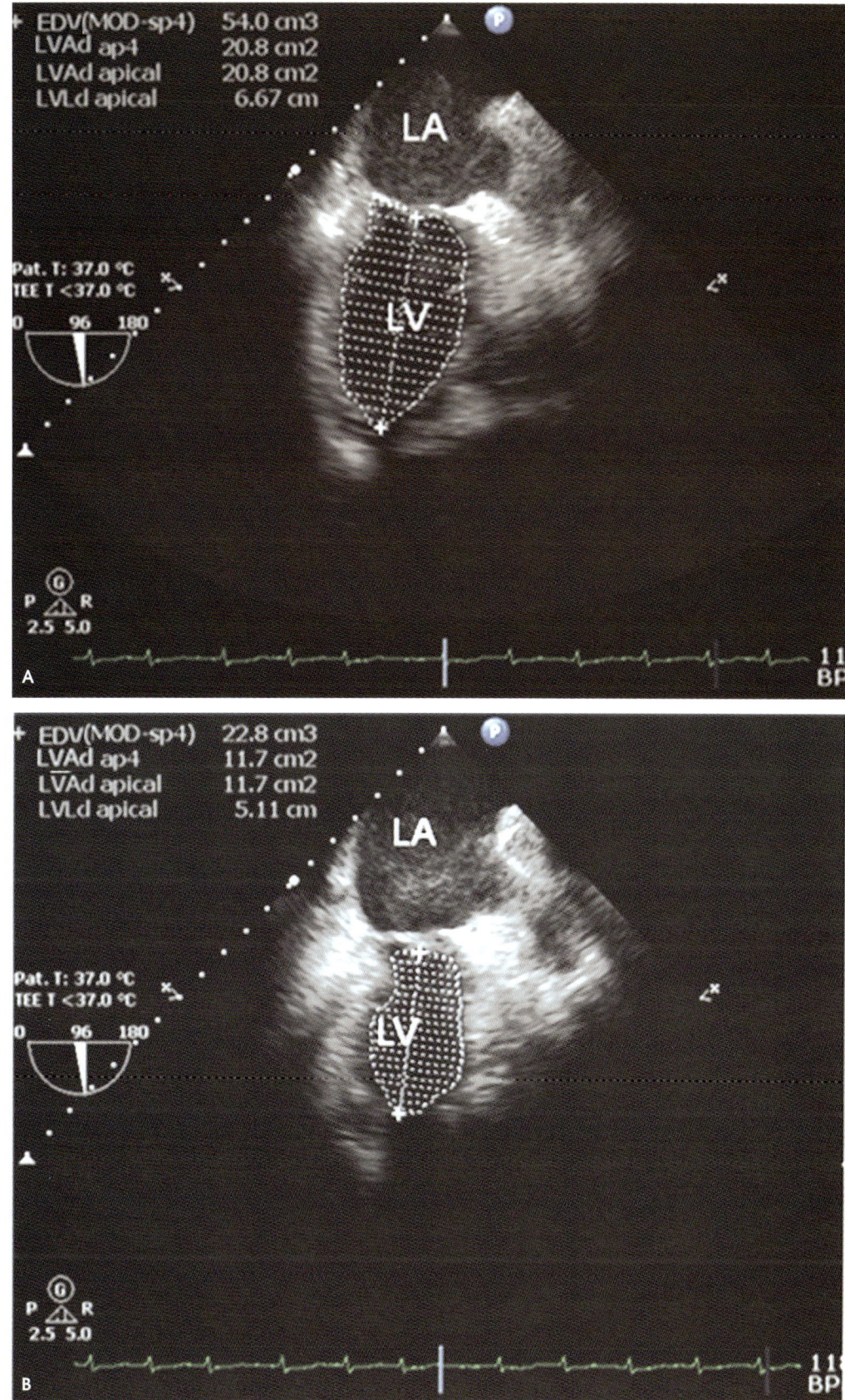

Fig. 7.5: Midesophageal two-chamber view showing the application of the Simpson's rule to determine the left ventricular end-diastolic (A) and end-systolic volumes (B). Ejection fraction = (54.0 – 22.8) x 100 / 54.0 = 57.8%. (LA: left atrium, LV: left ventricle).

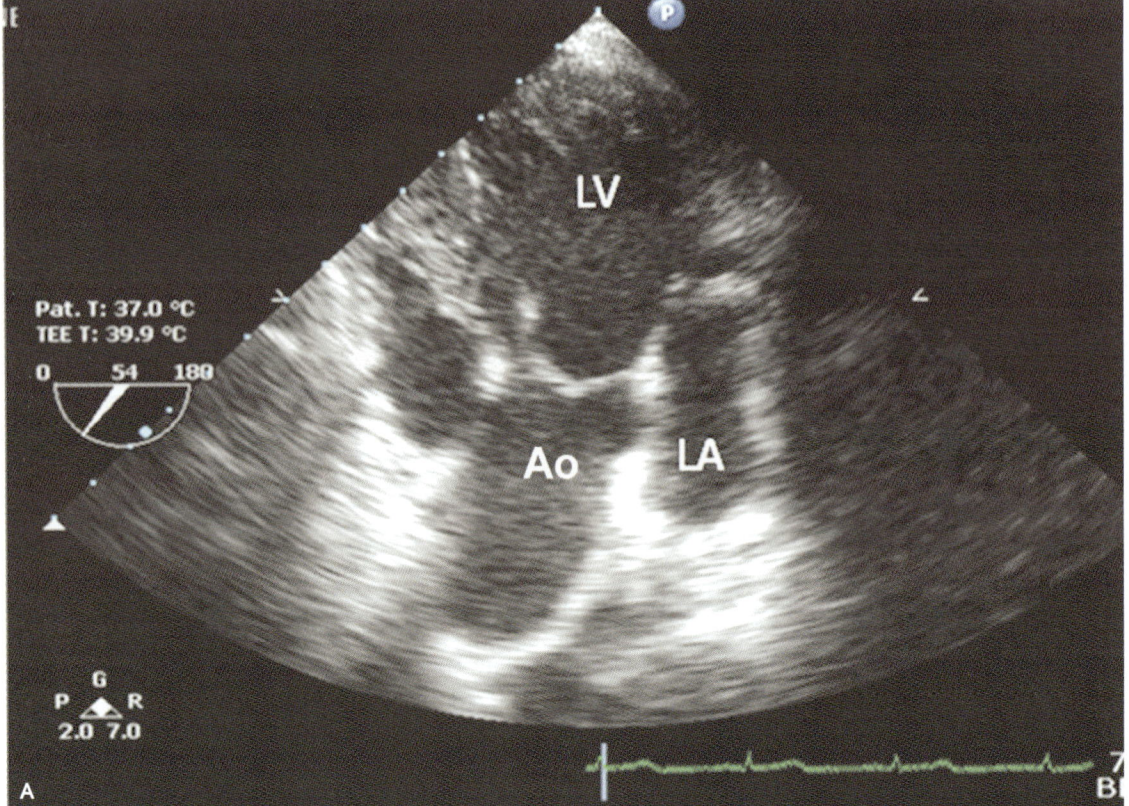

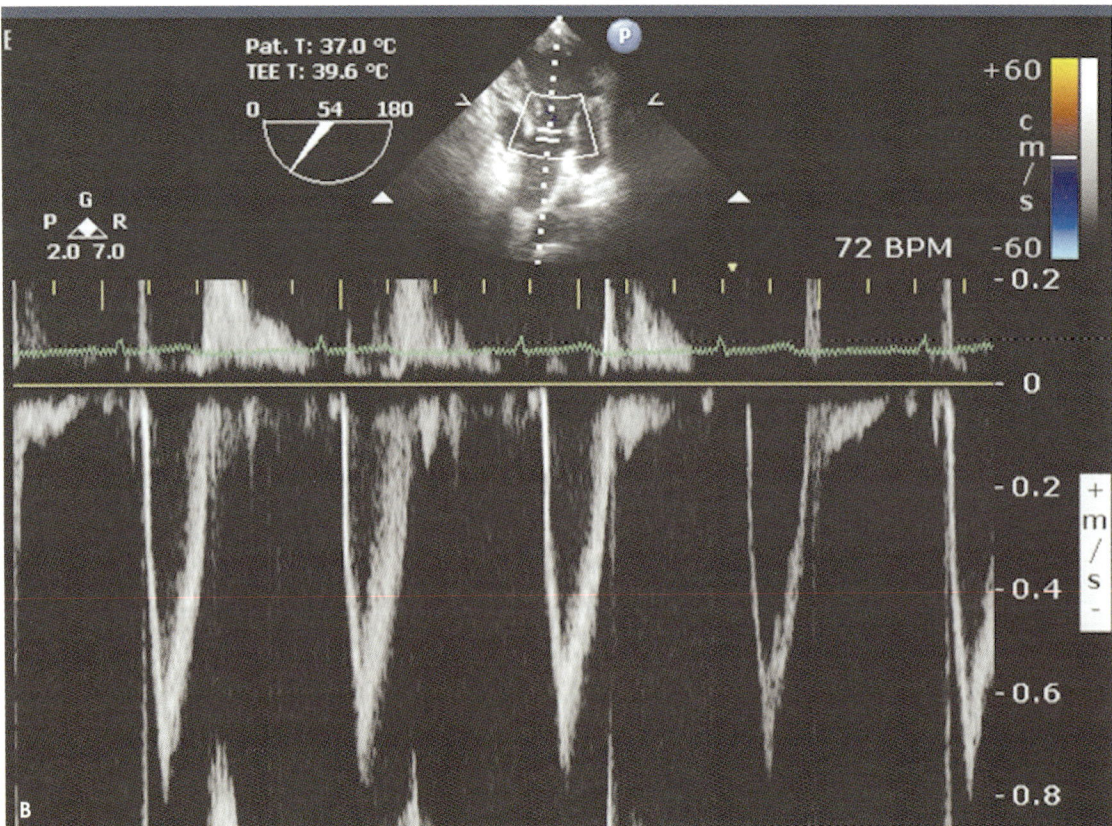

Fig. 7.6: Deep transgastric view can be utilized to measure the stroke volume and cardiac output from the left ventricular outflow tract diameter (Panel A), and pulsed wave Doppler velocity time integral and heart rate (Panel B) (LV: left ventricle, LA: left atrium, Ao: aorta).

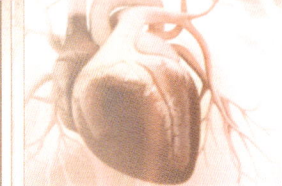

5. dP/dt

The rate of rise of intraventricular pressure (dP/dt) is the ratio of the increase in transmitral pressure gradient from 4 to 36 mm Hg (dP) to the time taken for the transmitral flow velocity to increase from 1 to 3 m/s (dt).

Normal: > 1200 mm Hg/s (dt < 26 ms)

Ventricular dysfunction: < 800 mm Hg/s (dt > 40 ms)

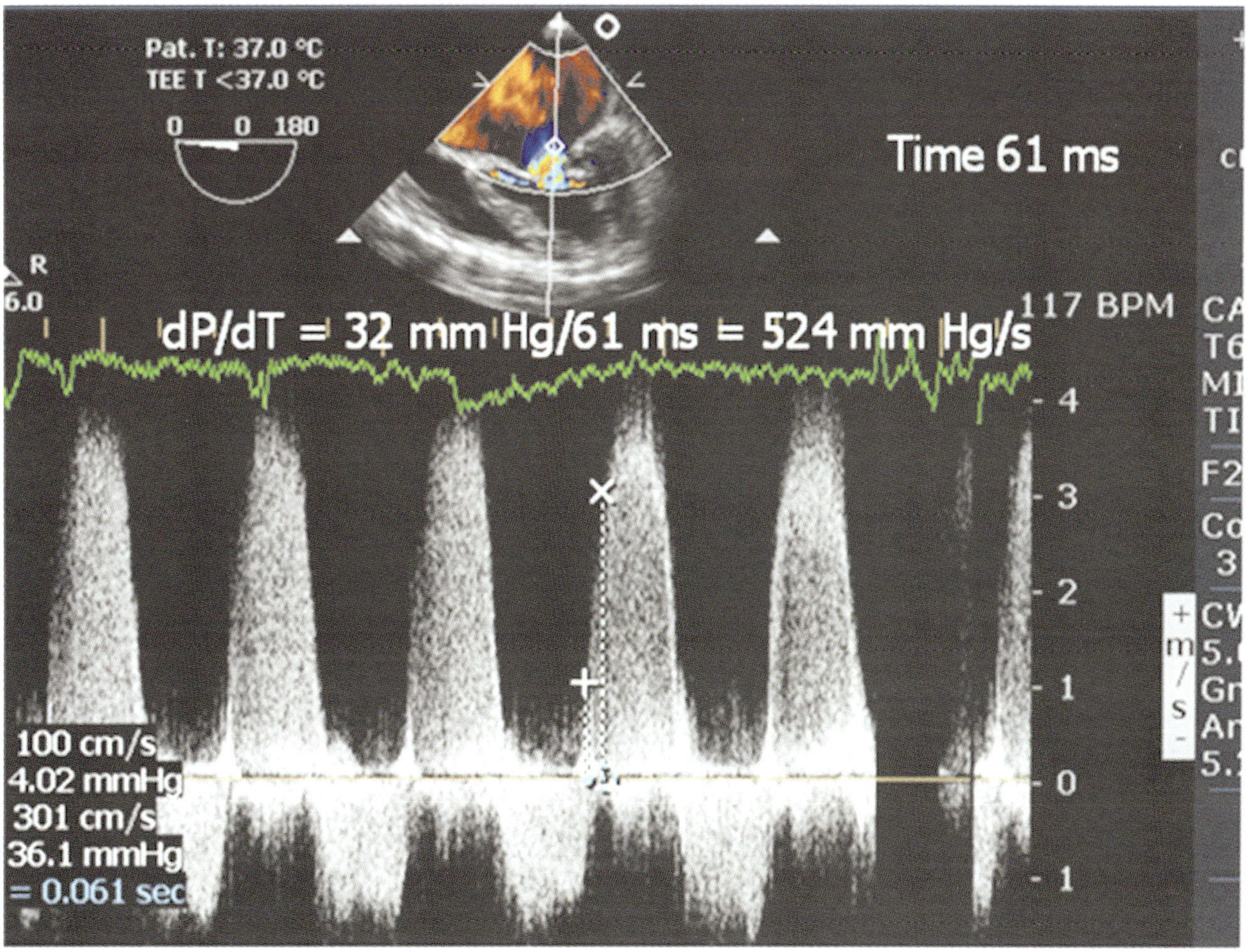

Fig. 7.7: The rate of rise of intraventricular pressure is calculated from the continuous wave Doppler envelope of a mitral regurgitant jet in the midesophageal four-chamber view.

6. Descent of Mitral Annulus/Mitral Annular Plane Systolic Excursion (MAPSE)

In the midesophageal four-chamber view, the M mode beam is positioned along the lateral mitral annulus parallel to the long-axis of LV. The difference in the end-diastolic and end-systolic frames gives the magnitude of the mitral annular descent. It should be at least 8 mm.

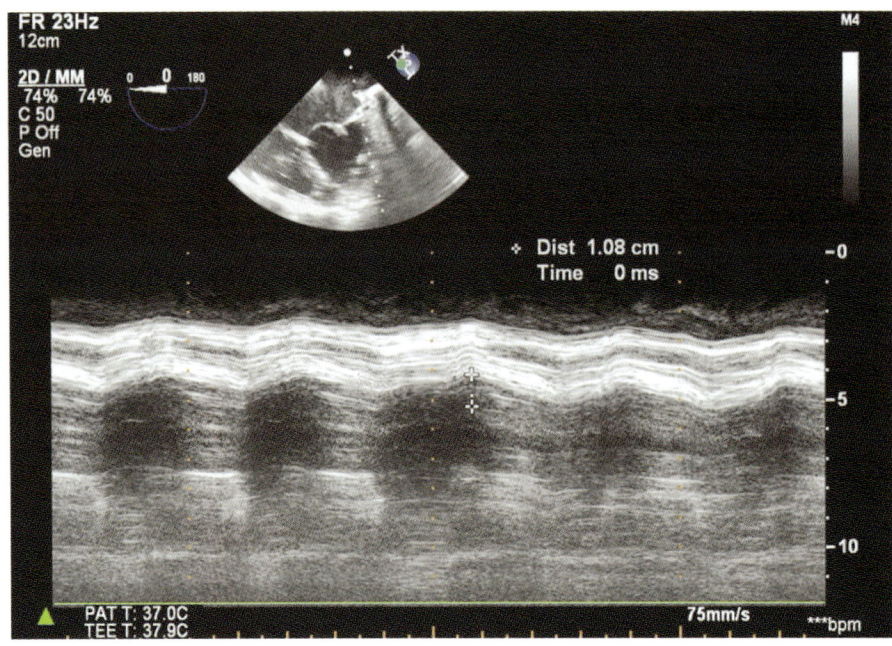

Fig. 7.8: Midesophageal four-chamber view with M-mode beam positioned along the lateral mitral annulus showing the calculation of descent of mitral annulus (MAPSE = 10.8 mm).

7. Myocardial Performance Index

This is calculated by the formula:

$$ICT + IRT/ET$$

(ICT—isovolemic contraction time, IRT—isovolemic relaxation time, ET—ejection time)

Normal value: < 0.4.

Since isovolemic contraction time and isovolemic relaxation time are a part of the calculation of this index, it indicates systolic as well as diastolic function.

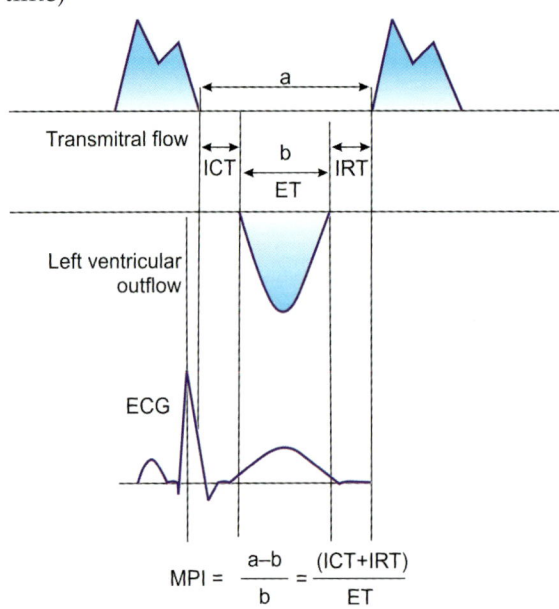

Fig. 7.9: Demonstrating the calculation of the myocardial performance index (MPI) (ICT: isovolemic contraction time, IRT: isovolemic relaxation time, ET: ejection time).

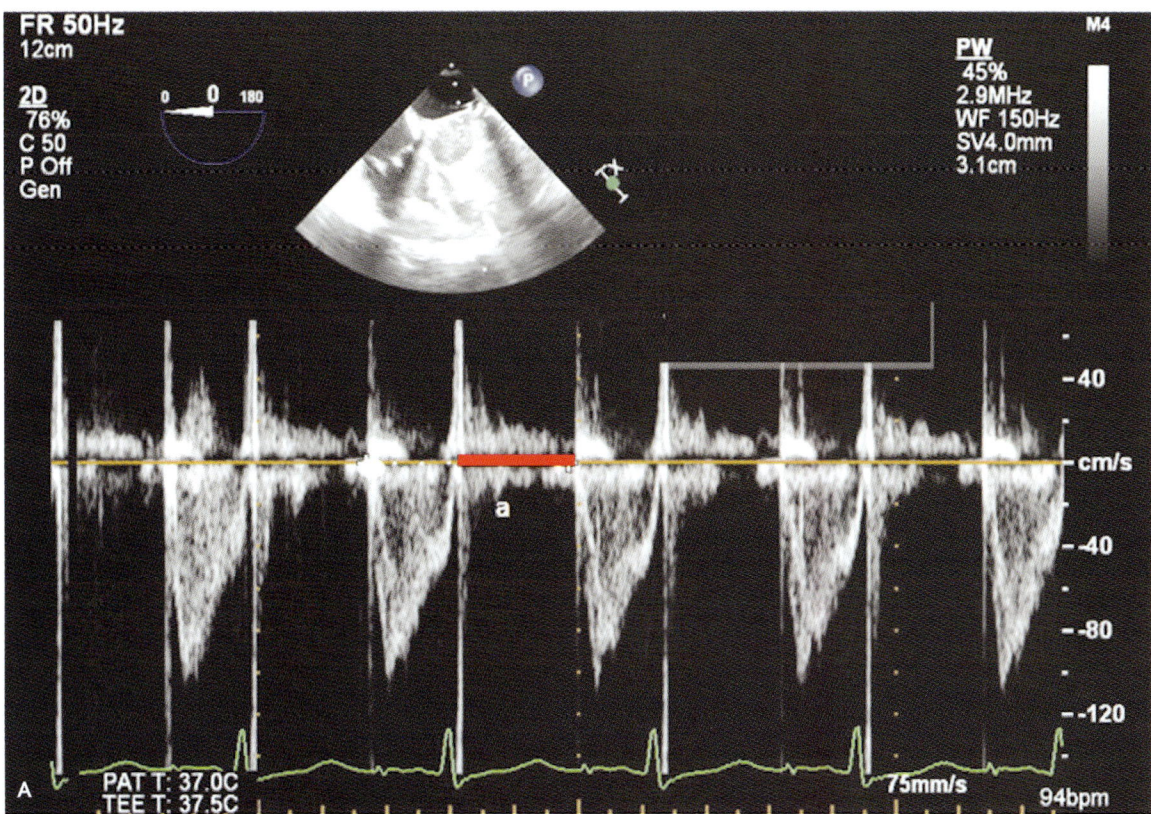

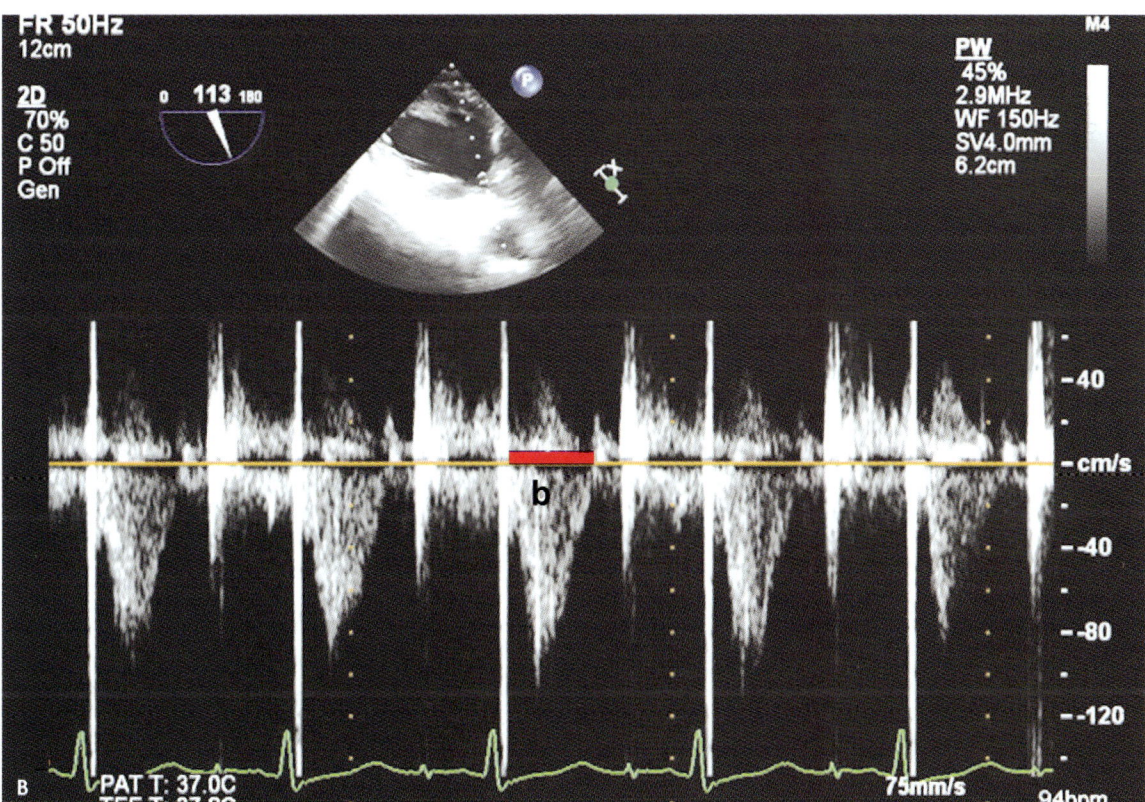

Fig. 7.10: Calculation of the left ventricular (LV) myocardial performance index from the LV inflow (four-chamber view, A) and the LV outflow (transgastric long-axis view, B) pulsed wave Doppler profiles. Tei index $= \dfrac{a-b}{b}$.

8. Tissue Doppler—Mitral Annular Systolic Velocity

Tissue Doppler echocardiography measures the velocity of myocardial tissue using low-pass filters to screen out higher velocities generated by blood flow. Tissue motion creates Doppler shifts and the velocities rarely exceed 20 cm/s. During image acquisition, the

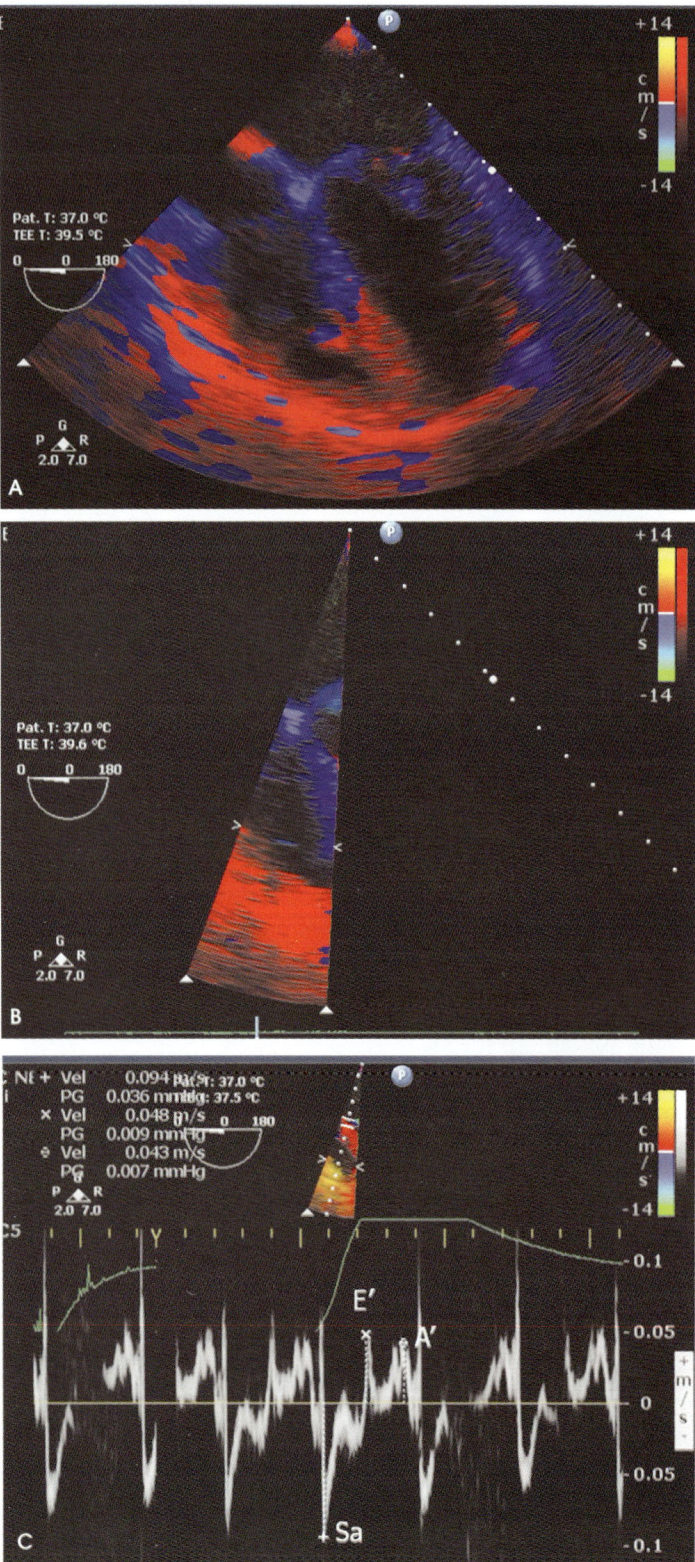

Fig. 7.11: Midesophageal four-chamber view with tissue Doppler imaging (A), the sector is narrowed to the medial mitral annulus (B), application of pulsed wave Doppler for calculation of mitral annular systolic velocity Sa (C: Here, it equals 9.4 cm/s).

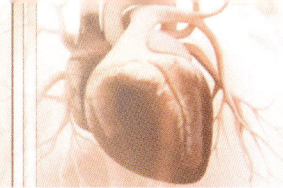

temporal resolution is optimized by selecting as narrow an image sector as possible, which increases the frame rate. The mitral annular motion is utilized for assessing the ventricular function. A typical Doppler velocity profile of the mitral annulus has a systolic wave (Sa), early diastolic wave (E') and late diastolic wave (A').

The velocity of systolic wave is used to evaluate systolic function of the LV as follows:

>7.5 cm/s: Normal global LV function
<5.5 cm/s: LV failure
<3 cm/s: Significant risk of cardiac death within 2 years.

REGIONAL WALL MOTION ABNORMALITY

Table 7.1: Classification of left ventricular regional wall motion abnormality

LV function	Wall motion	Endocardial excursion (%)	Wall thickening (%)
Normal	Inward	>30%	30–50%
Mild hypokinesia	Inward	10–30%	30–50%
Severe hypokinesia	Inward	<10%	<30%
Akinesia	None	None	<10%
Dyskinesia	Outward	None	None

Table 7.2: Nomenclature of left ventricular segments for assessing regional wall motion abnormality

Basal segments	Mid segments	Apical segments
1. Basal anterior	7. Mid-anterior	13. Apical anterior
2. Basal anteroseptal	8. Mid antero-septal	14. Apical septal
3. Basal inferoseptal	9. Mid infero-septal	15. Apical inferior
4. Basal inferior	10. Mid-inferior	16. Apical lateral
5. Basal inferolateral	11. Mid infero-lateral	17. Apex
6. Basal anterolateral	12. Mid antero-lateral	

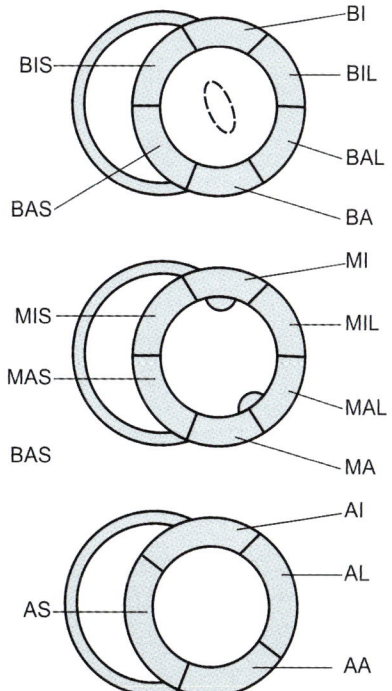

Fig. 7.12: Diagrammatic representation of the various myocardial segments (BA: basal anterior, BAL: basal anterolateral, BIL: basal inferolateral, BI: basal inferior, BAS: basal anteroseptal, BIS: basal inferoseptal, MA: mid-anterior, MAL: mid anterolateral, MIL: mid inferolateral, MI: mid-inferior, MAS: mid-antero-septal, MIS: mid-inferoseptal, AA: apical anterior, AL: apical lateral, AI: apical inferior, AS: apical septal).

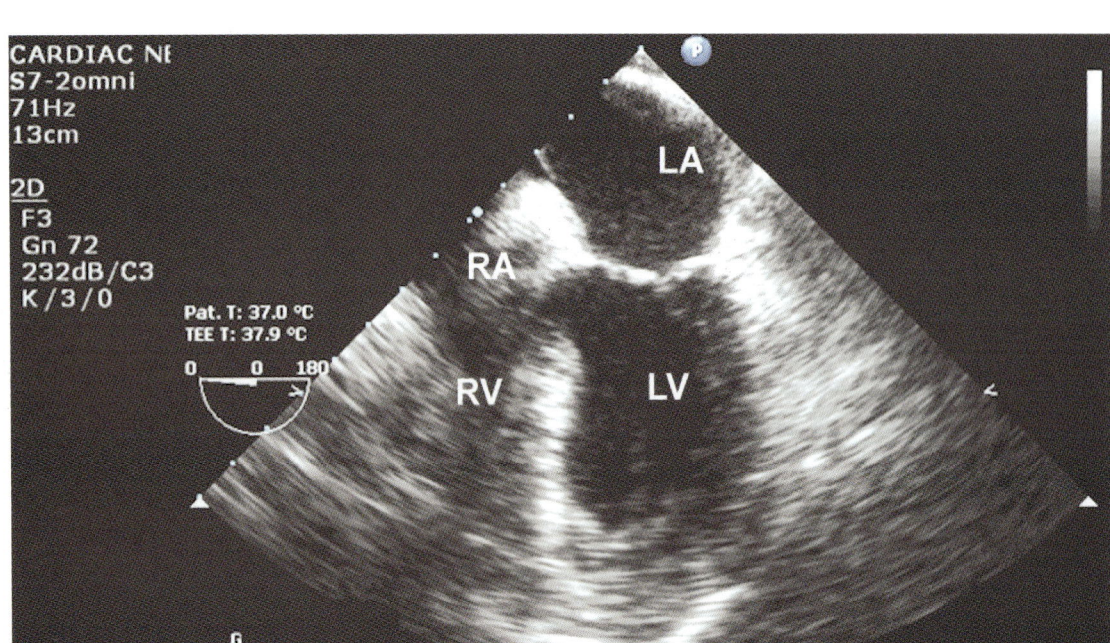

Fig. 7.13: Midesophageal four-chamber view allows the assessment of the anterolateral and inferoseptal walls of the left ventricle. (LA: Left atrium, LV: left ventricle, RA: right atrium, RV: right ventricle).

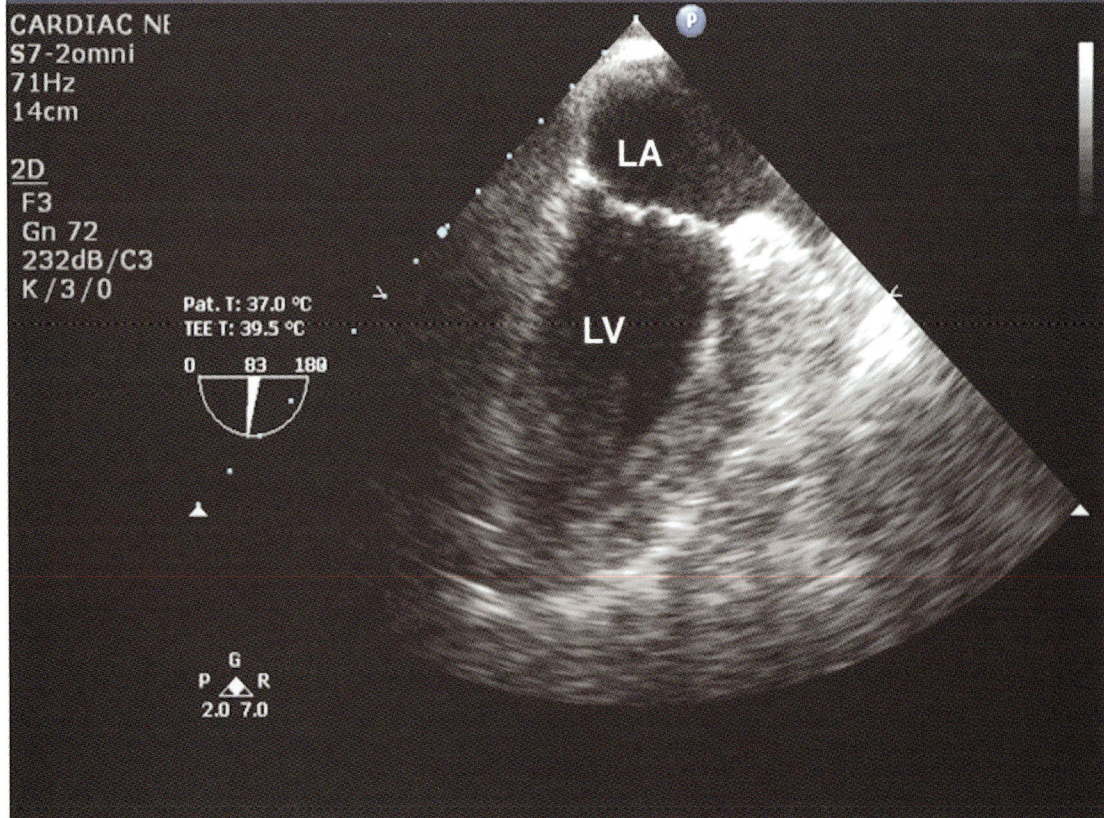

Fig. 7.14: Midesophageal two-chamber view allows the assessment of the anterior and inferior walls of the left ventricle (LA: left atrium, LV: left ventricle).

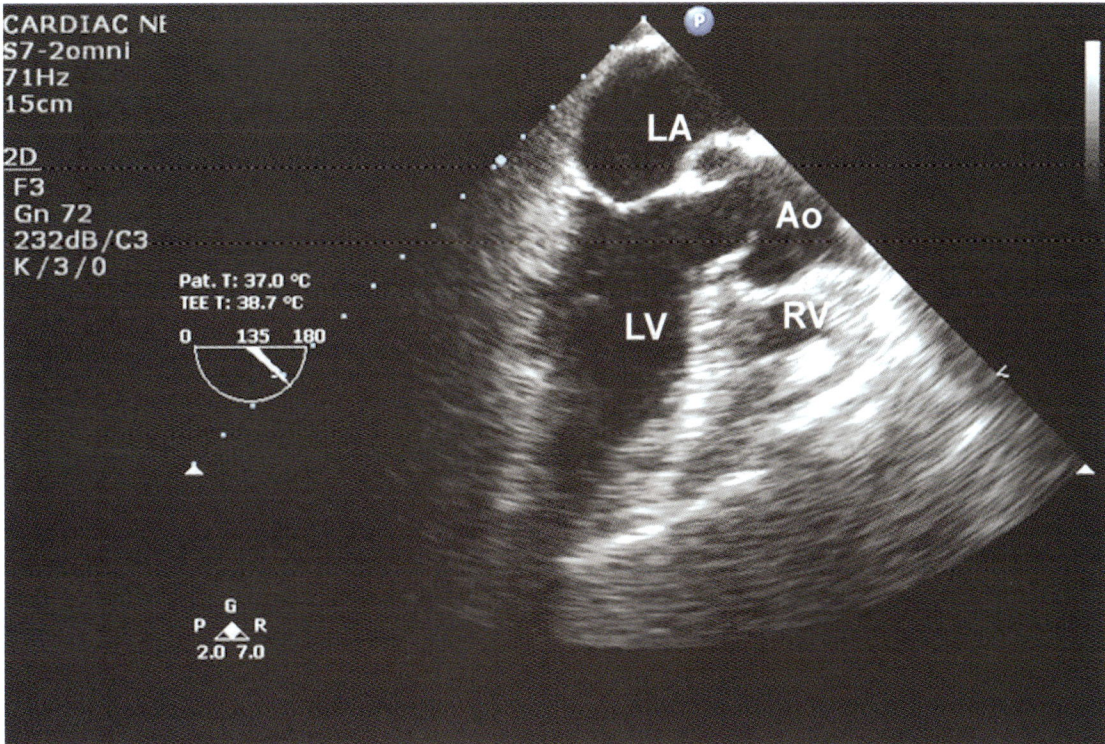

Fig. 7.15: Midesophageal long-axis view allows the assessment of the anteroseptal and inferolateral walls of the left ventricle. (LA: left atrium, LV: left ventricle, RV: right ventricle, Ao: aorta).

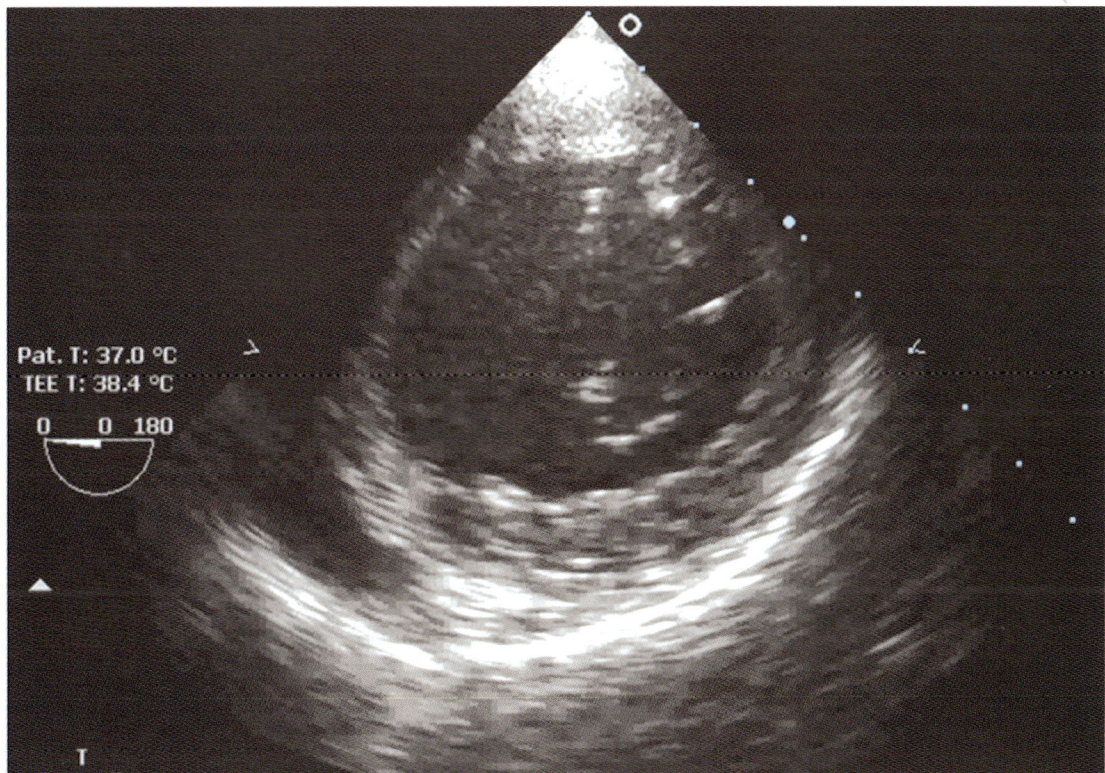

Fig. 7.16: Transgastric basal short-axis view allows the assessment of all the six basal segments of the left ventricle. Correlate with Fig. 7.12.

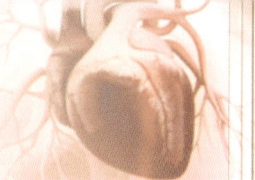

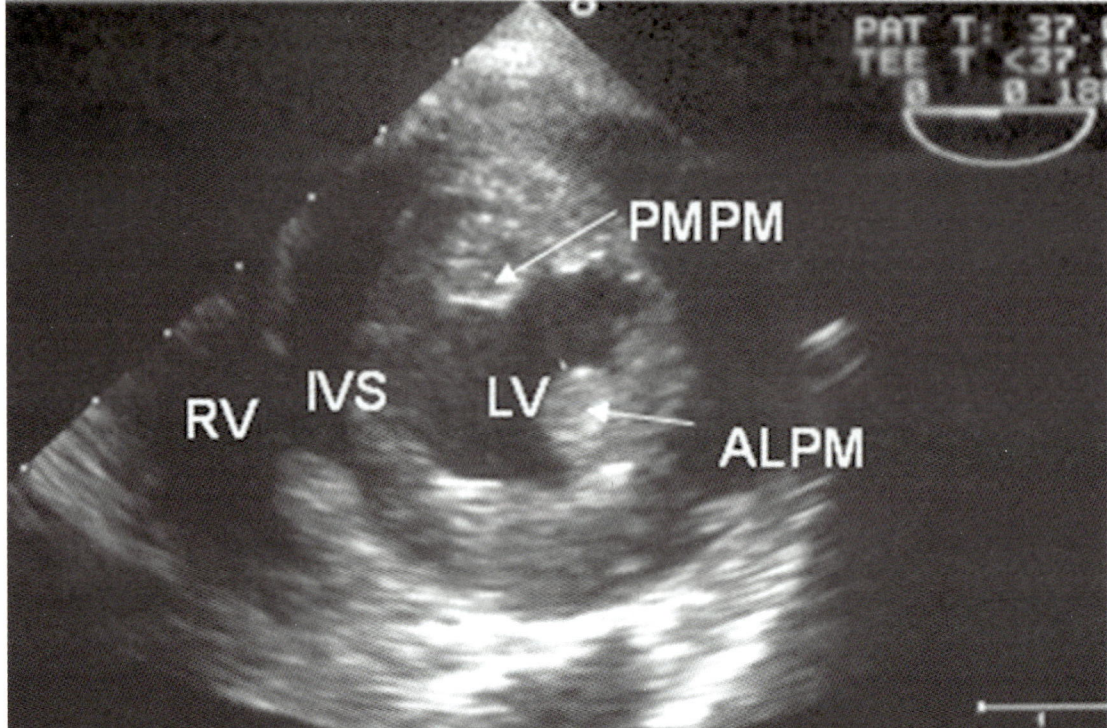

Fig. 7.17: Transgastric midpapillary short-axis view allows the assessment of all the six mid segments of the left ventricle. (LV: left ventricle, RV: right ventricle, IVS: interventricular septum, ALPM: anterolateral papillary muscle, PMPM: posteromedial papillary muscle). Correlate with Fig. 7.12.

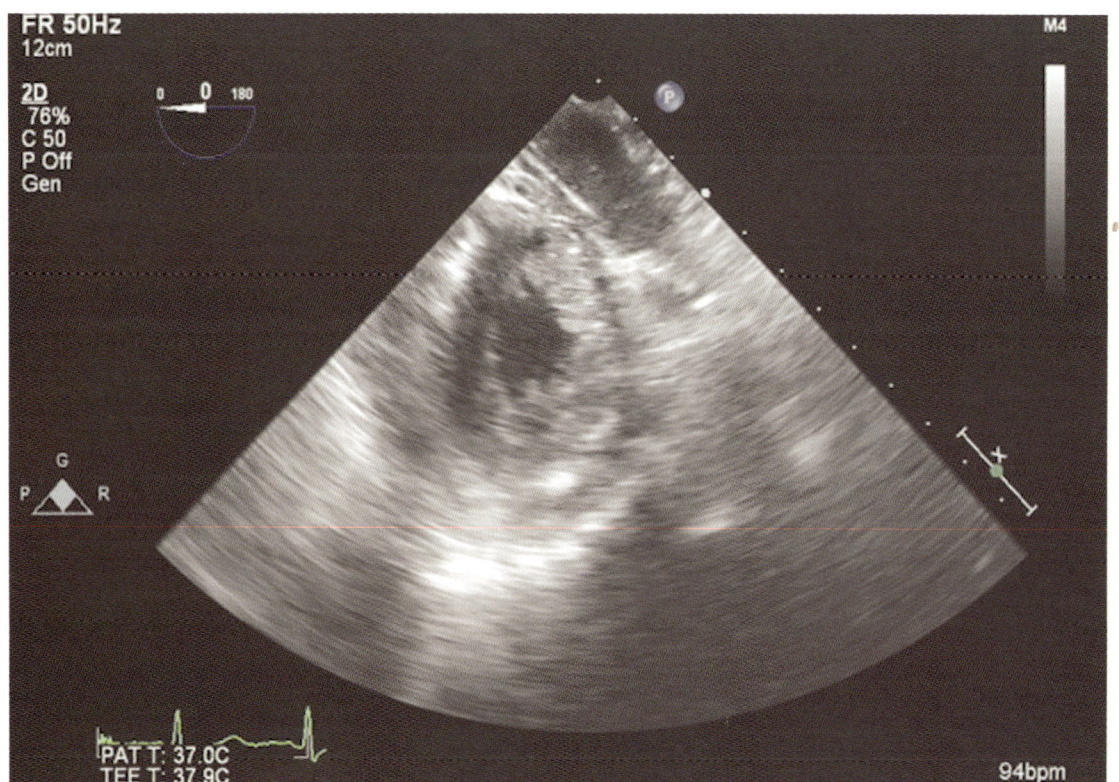

Fig. 7.18: Transgastric apical view allows the assessment of all the four apical segments of the left ventricle. Correlate with Fig. 7.12.

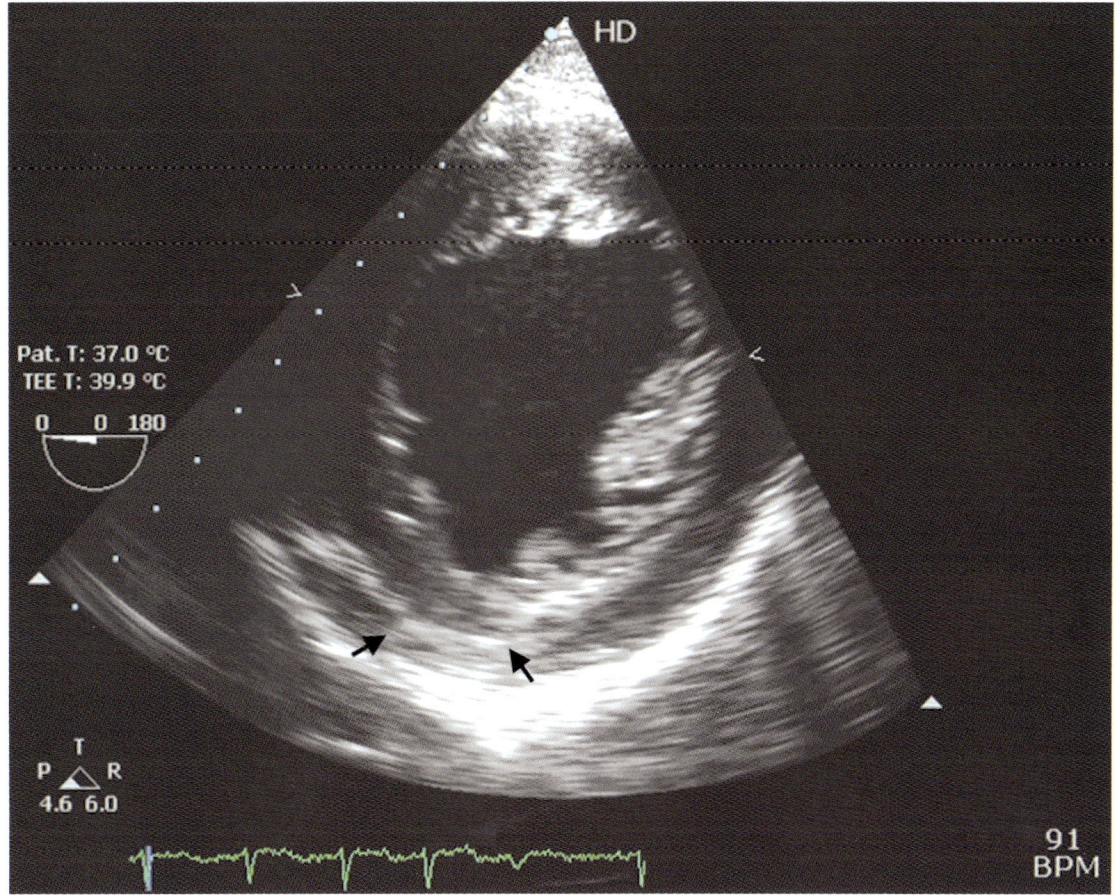

Fig. 7.19: Transgastric midpapillary short-axis view showing hypokinetic anterior and anteroseptal segments of the left ventricle (arrows).

DIASTOLIC FUNCTION

The diastolic function of the LV is determined by the pulsed wave Doppler (PWD) recording of the transmitral diastolic flow velocity and the pulmonary venous flow velocity. In addition, the E wave deceleration time, isovolumetric relaxation time and color M-mode flow propagation velocity are also used. The following grades of diastolic dysfunction are described as it progresses.

Grade I (Impaired relaxation)
Grade II (Pseudonormalisation)
Grades III and IV (Restrictive filling pattern)

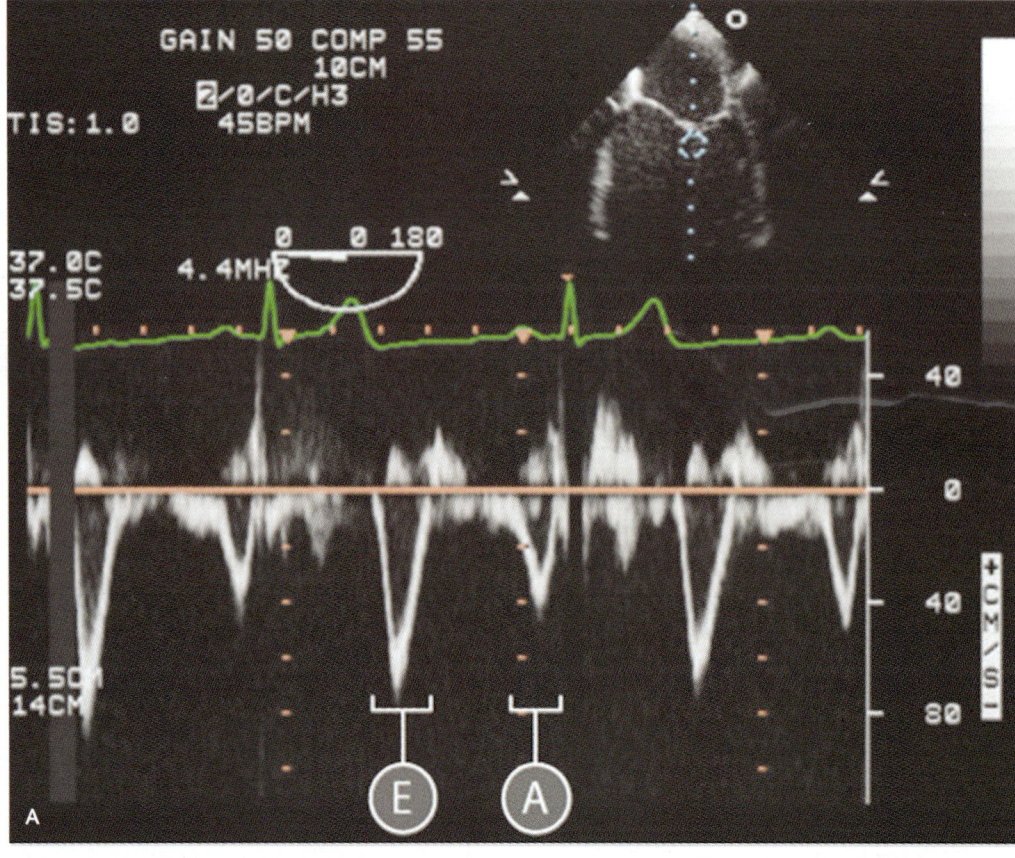

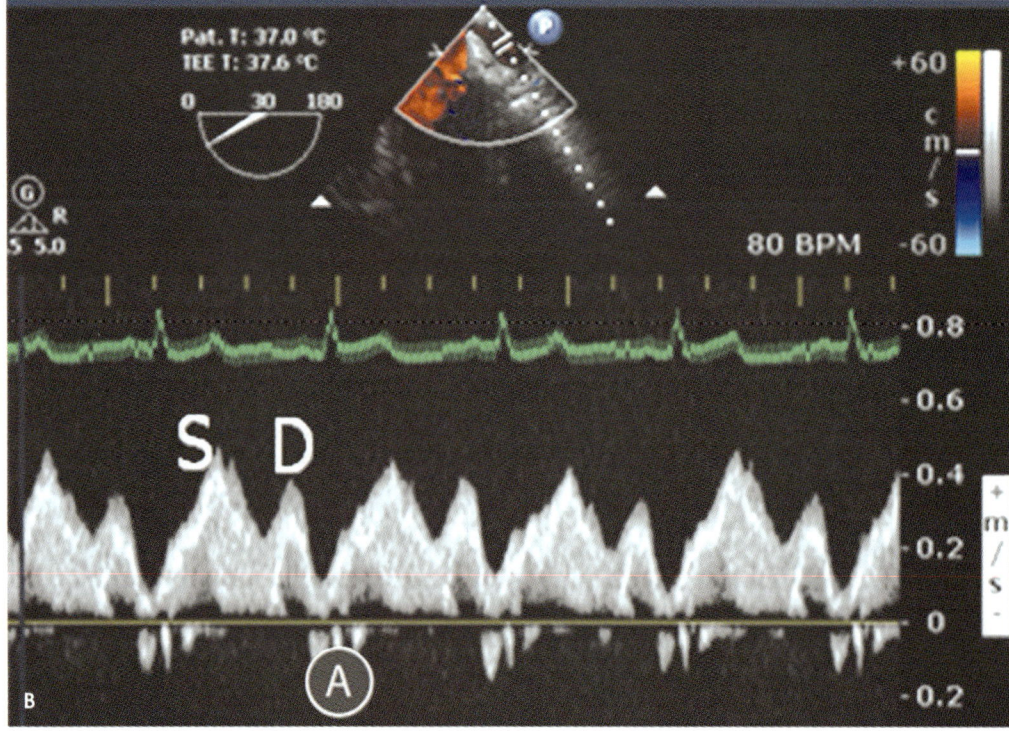

Fig. 7.20: Panel A: Normal appearance of the transmitral flow on pulsed wave Doppler. A typical velocity pattern is biphasic, an initial peak flow velocity (E wave) occurs during early diastolic filling and a later peak flow velocity (A wave) occurs during the atrial systole. The normal E/A ratio is > 1. Panel B: Pulsed wave Doppler from pulmonary vein for estimating the left ventricular filling pressures. The pulmonary venous flow velocity is obtained by placing the sample volume within 1 cm of the opening of the pulmonary vein into the left atrium. Note the normal waveforms (antegrade systolic—S, diastolic—D and retrograde A wave).

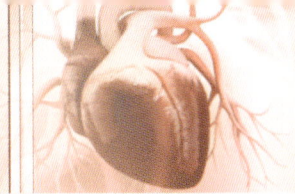

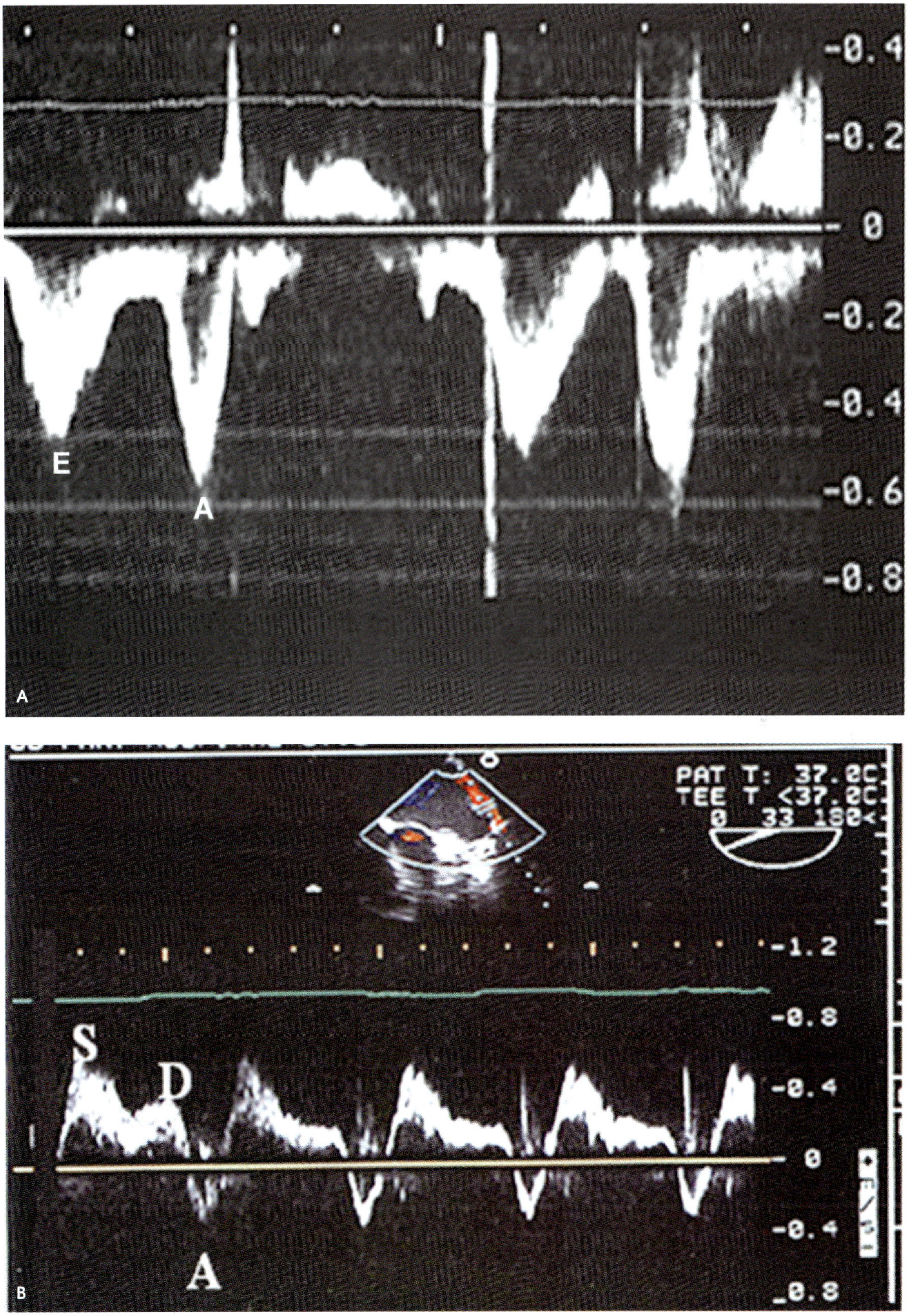

Fig. 7.21: Panel A: Mitral inflow pulsed wave Doppler in a patient with Grade 1 diastolic dysfunction (impaired relaxation). Note the taller late diastolic filling wave (A) caused by the exaggerated atrial contraction (E/A ratio < 1). Panel B: Pulsed wave pulmonary venous Doppler waveform maintains the normal appearance (systolic flow > diastolic flow).

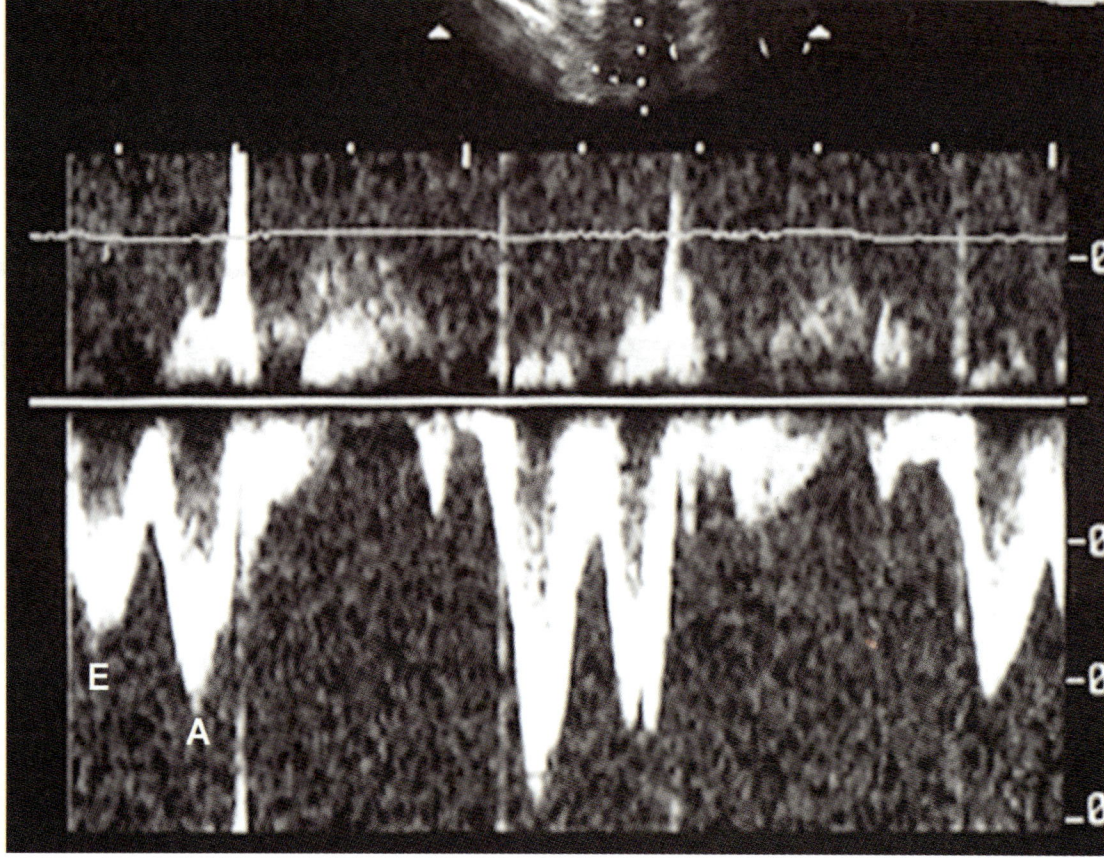

Fig. 7.22: Transmitral pulsed wave Doppler flow pattern in a patient with diastolic dysfunction. E/A ratio in the first beat shows grade I dysfunction (E/A < 1). With increase in the left atrial preload, at the onset of expiration, there is a change to a pseudonormal pattern/ Grade II dysfunction (E/A > 1) in the subsequent beat.

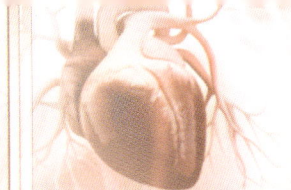

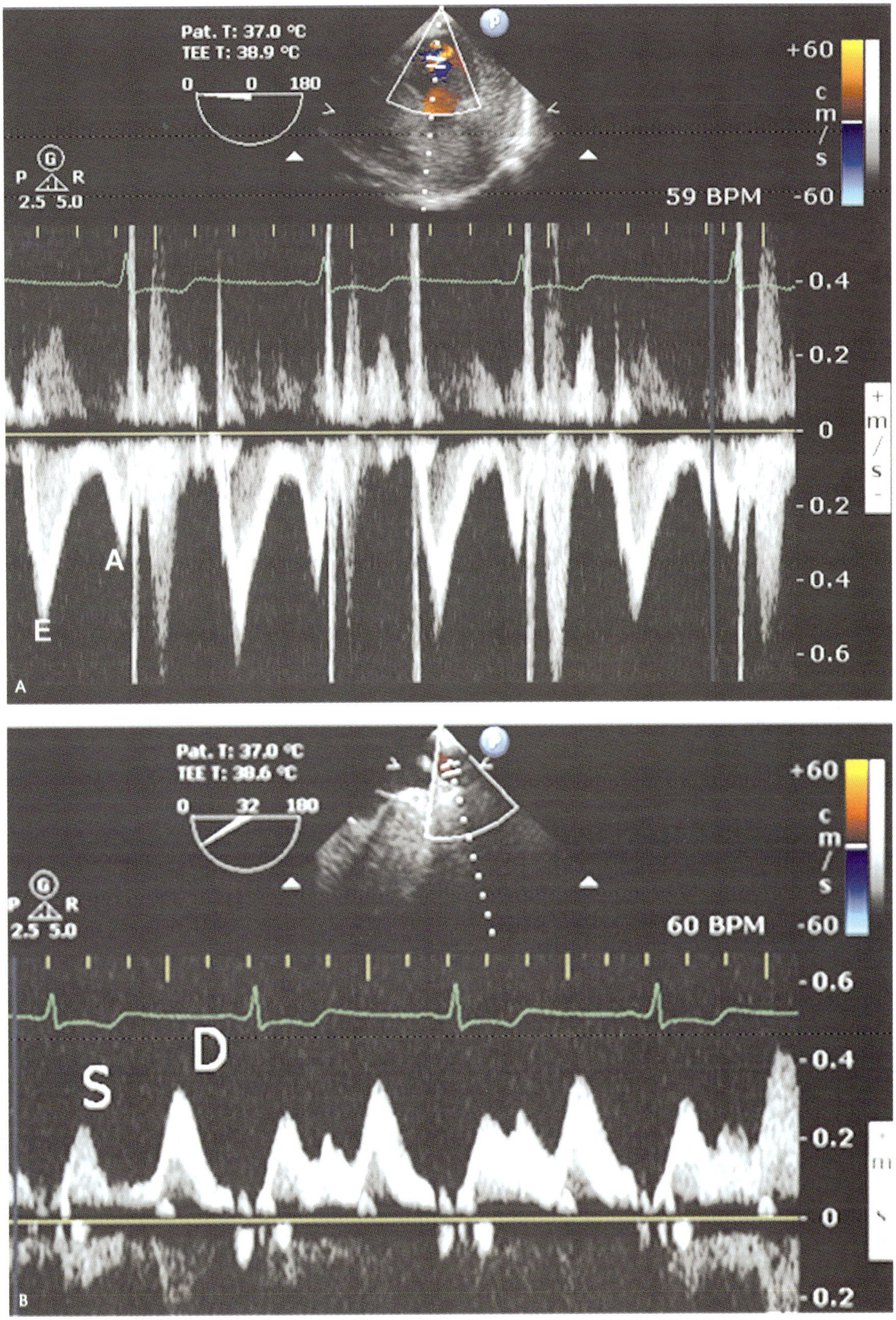

Fig. 7.23: Panel A: Transmitral pulsed wave Doppler waveform in a patient with Grade II diastolic dysfunction (pseudonormal filling, E/A > 1). Panel B: Pulsed wave Doppler pulmonary venous waveform in the same patient showing the attenuated flow in systole that confirms the grade II diastolic dysfunction.

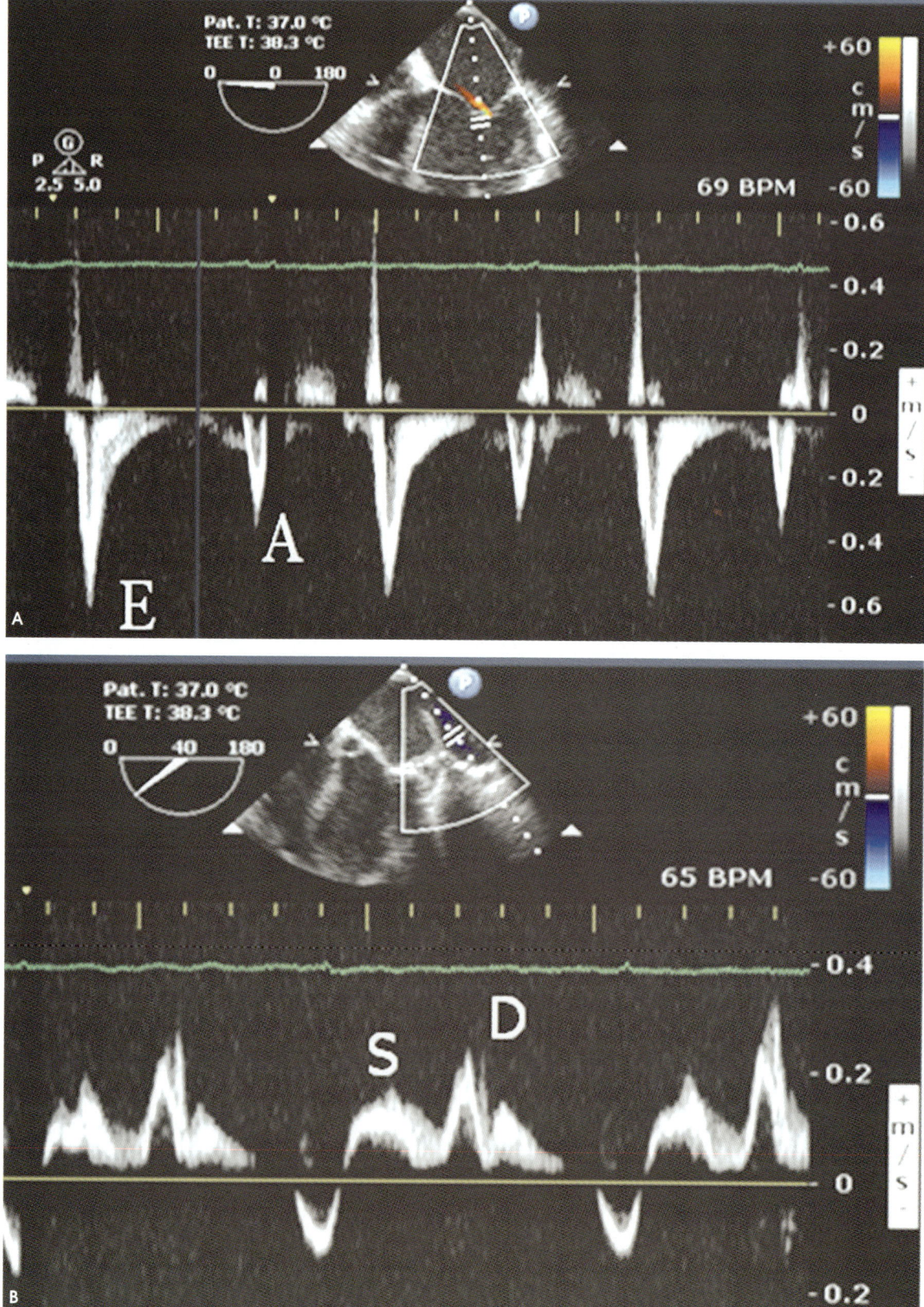

Fig. 7.24: Panel A: Transmitral pulsed wave Doppler waveform in a patient with Type III diastolic dysfunction (restrictive filling, E >> A). Panel B: Pulsed wave Doppler pulmonary venous waveform in the same patient showing the attenuated forward flow in systole and exaggerated flow in diastole.

ISOVOLUMIC RELAXATION TIME (IVRT)

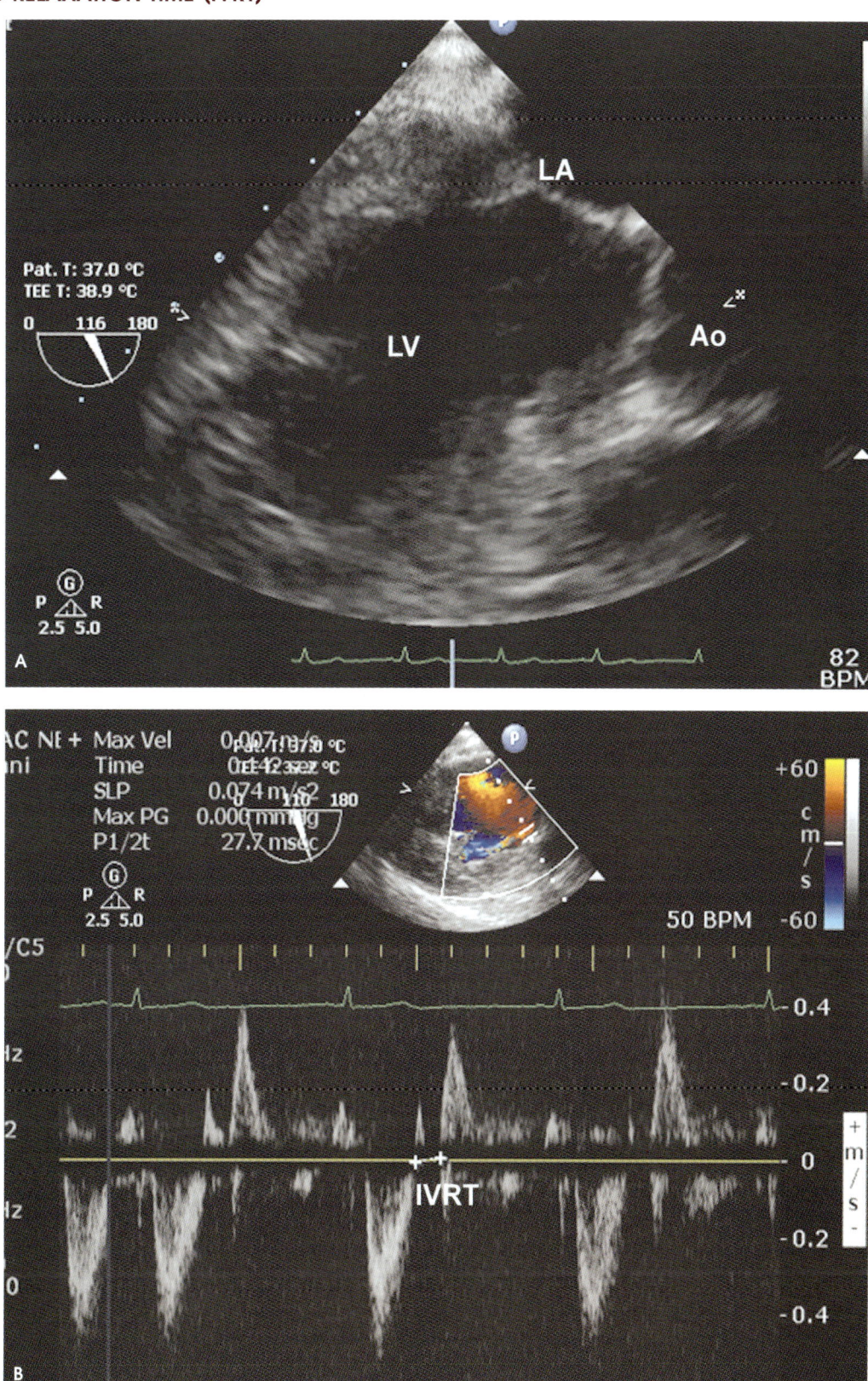

Fig. 7.25: Transgastric long-axis view (A) with pulsed wave Doppler profile (B) showing the sample volume placed at the junction of left ventricular inflow and outflow. The time lag between the outflow profile and the inflow profile is the isovolumetric relaxation time (IVRT). (LA: left atrium, LV: left ventricle, Ao: aorta)

Color M-mode Flow Propagation Velocity (Vp)

In the midesophageal four-chamber view, M-mode cursor is placed through the mitral valve directed towards the LV apex. By applying color M-mode, Vp is calculated from the slope of an isovelocity line on the color E wave. The slope is measured from the mitral annulus to a point 4 cm into the LV. Vp < 50 cm/s signifies impaired LV systolic function.

Tissue Doppler Imaging

The PWD sample volume is positioned at the lateral mitral annulus to obtain the tissue Doppler profile, which has a biphasic diastolic component that includes an initial early (E') and a late (A') diastolic tissue velocity (Fig. 7.27). The diastolic component thus obtained appears as a mirror image of the transmitral diastolic blood flow velocity except that the tissue velocities are much lower in magnitude (8–15 cm/s). In healthy patients, the peak E' is greater than A'. E' and E'/A' decline with age and are reduced in LV hypertrophy. E' remains reduced in impaired ventricular relaxation and pseudonormalization, suggesting relative preload independence. E' velocity is reduced (<8 cm/s) in all types of diastolic dysfunction and, therefore, can be used to differentiate between normal and pseudonormal mitral inflow pattern. Thus, E' can be used as a discriminator between normal and pseudonormal patterns of diastolic dysfunction.

E : E' ratio < 8 indicates normal LA pressure

E : E' ratio > 15 indicates raised LA pressure

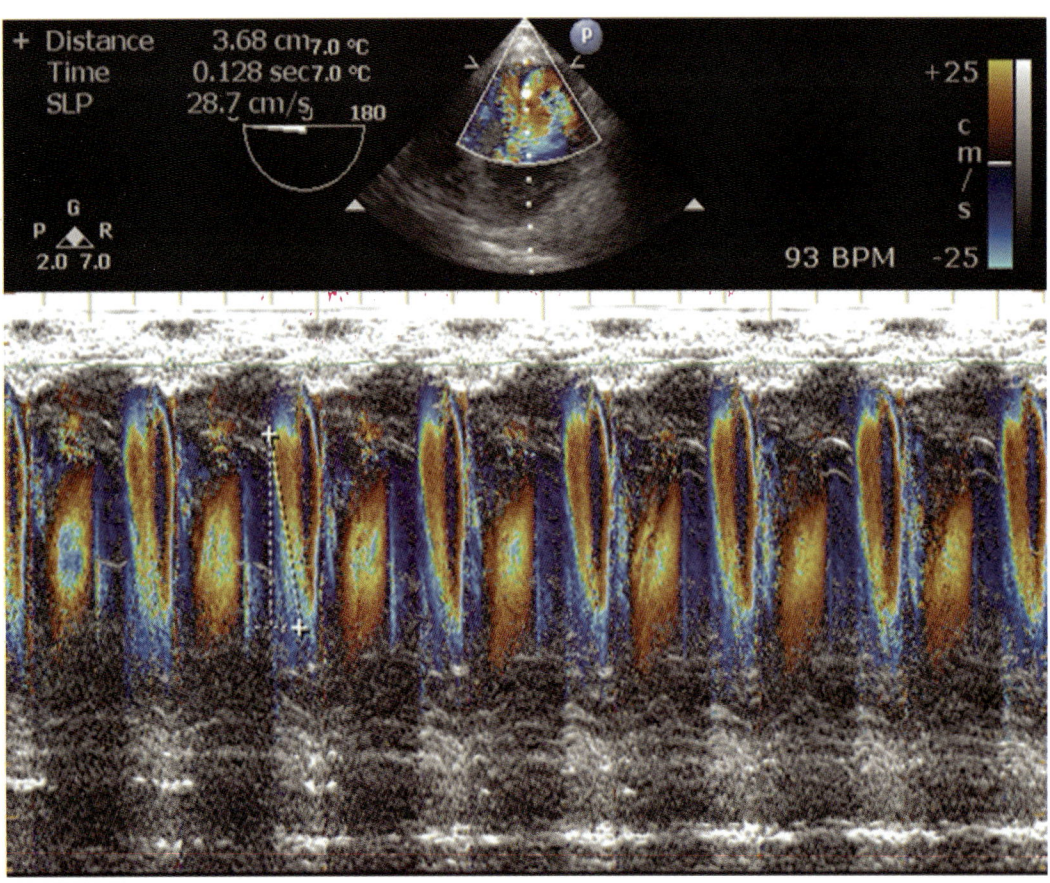

Fig. 7.26: Midesophageal four-chamber view with color M-mode showing the calculation of transmitral flow propagation velocity. In this case, it is 28.7 cm/s indicating impaired left ventricular diastolic function.

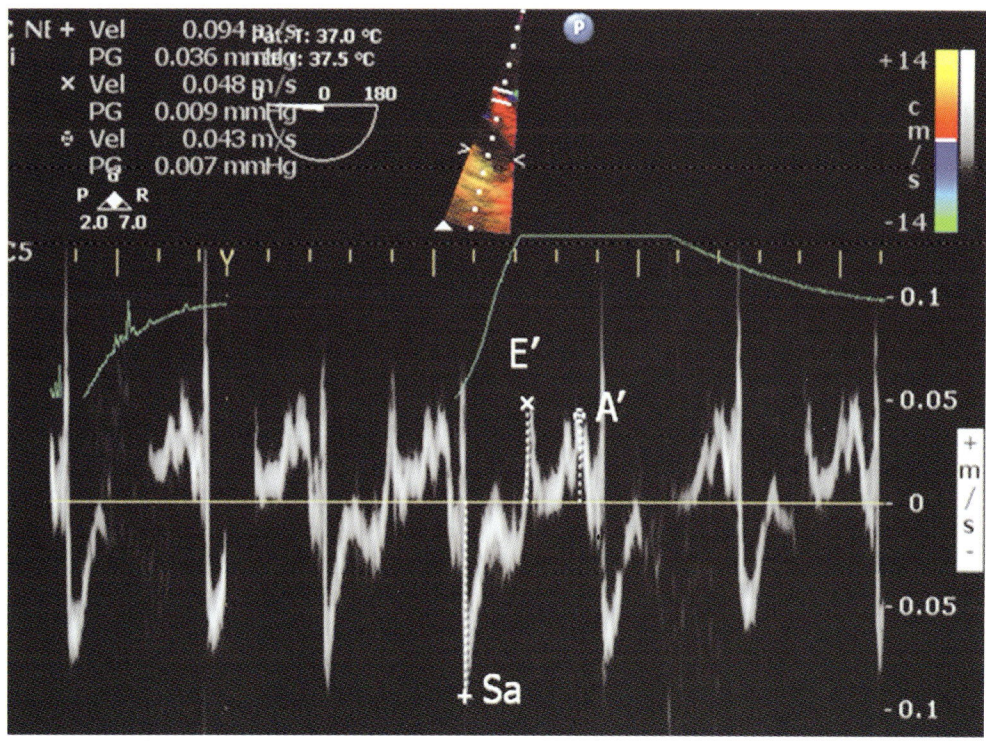

Fig. 7.27: Tissue Doppler imaging of the lateral mitral annulus (Sa: mitral annular velocity during left ventricular systole, E': early annular diastolic velocity, A': late annular diastolic velocity during atrial contraction, note that the E'/A' is more than 1, which gets reversed in diastolic dysfunction).

The mitral annual tissue Doppler imaging can also be used to measure the isovolumic contraction and relaxation times which can be utilised to calculate the myocardial performance index.

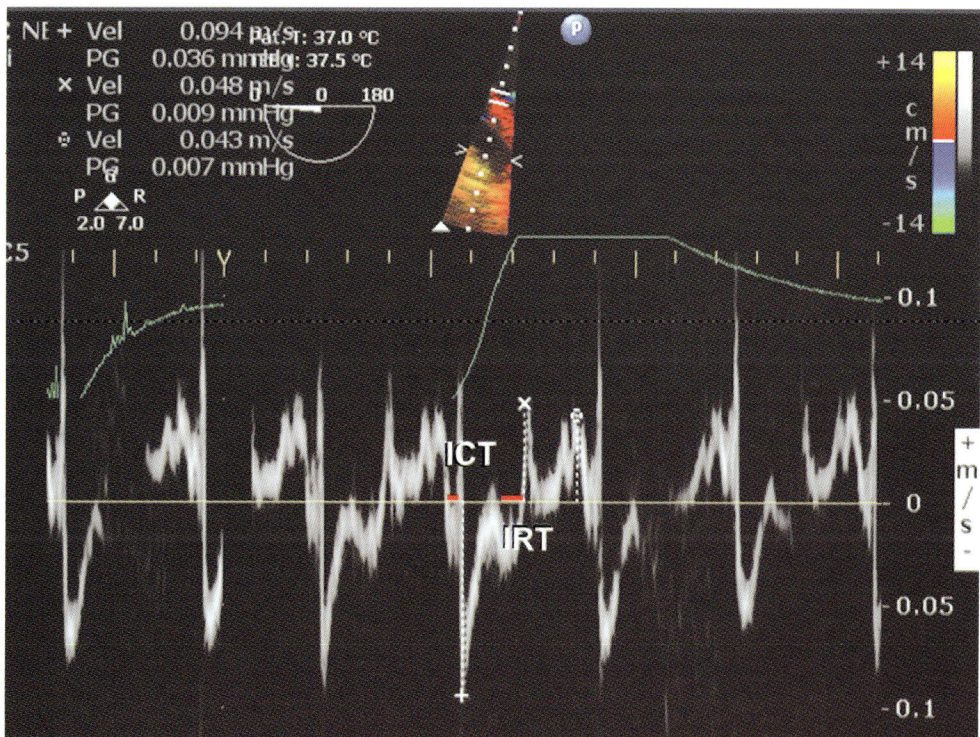

Fig. 7.28: The mitral annular tissue Doppler image showing measurement of isovolumic contraction time (ICT) and relaxation time (IRT).

Table 7.3: Phases of diastolic dysfunction as determined by the echocardiography

Parameter	Normal	Impaired relaxation	Pseudo normal filling	Restrictive filling
E wave DT (ms)	160–240	> 240	160–200	< 160
IVRT (ms)	70–90	< 90	< 90	< 70
E : A	1–2	< 1	1–1.5	> 1.5
Am : Ap duration	Am $\geq$ AP	Am > Ap	Am < Ap	Am << Ap
$PV_S : PV_D$	$PV_S > PV_D$	$PV_S > PV_D$	$PV_S < PV_D$	$PV_S << PV_D$

DT: deceleration time, ms: milli second, IVRT: isovolumetric relaxation time, Am : Ap duration: ratio of mitral (Am) and pulmonary venous inflow (Ap) "A" wave duration, PV_S: Pulmonary venous systolic flow, PV_D: Pulmonary venous diastolic flow, E:A: ratio of early (E) and late (A) wave velocities

Artifacts and Diagnostic Dilemma

8

• Deepak K. Tempe • Suruchi Hasija

ARTIFACTS

In the routine practice of transesophageal echocardiography, errors commonly occur due to inherent properties of ultrasound technology.

Acoustic Shadowing

Ultrasound beams are reflected or refracted whenever they encounter an object of different acoustic impedance. Dense objects like calcium and prosthetic valves cause acoustic shadowing due to near complete reflection of ultrasound beams (Figs 8.1 and 8.2).

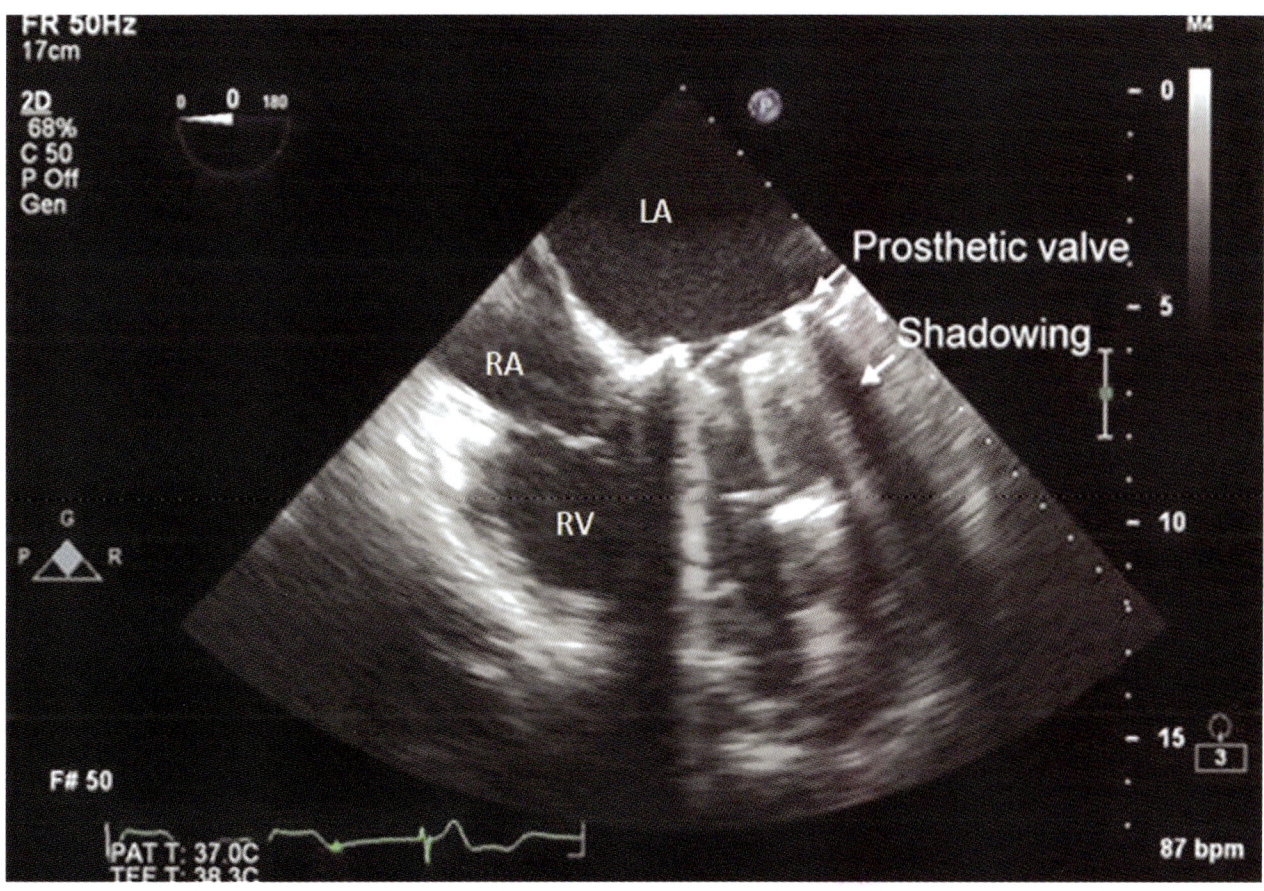

Fig. 8.1: Midesophageal four-chamber view showing shadowing (arrow) beyond the metallic leaflets and struts of the prosthetic valve (LA: left atrium, RA: right atrium, RV: right ventricle).

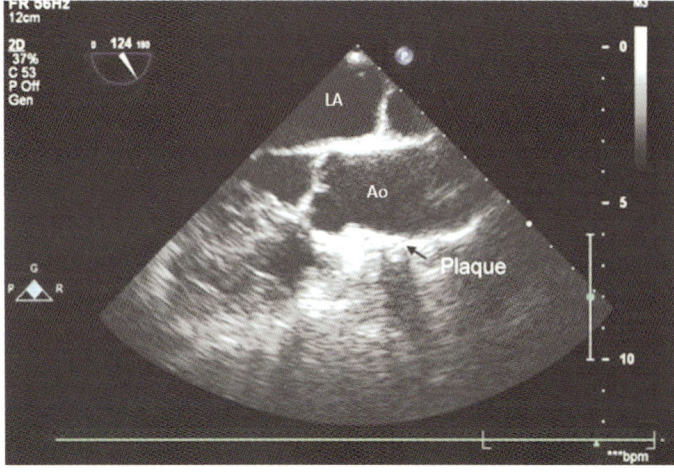

Fig. 8.2: Midesophageal aortic valve long-axis view showing shadowing due to calcific atheromatous plaque in the ascending aorta (LA: left atrium, Ao: ascending aorta).

Mirror Image Artifact

The presence of a strong reflector such as a flat surface leads to the formation of a duplicate mirror image (Figs 8.3 and 8.6).

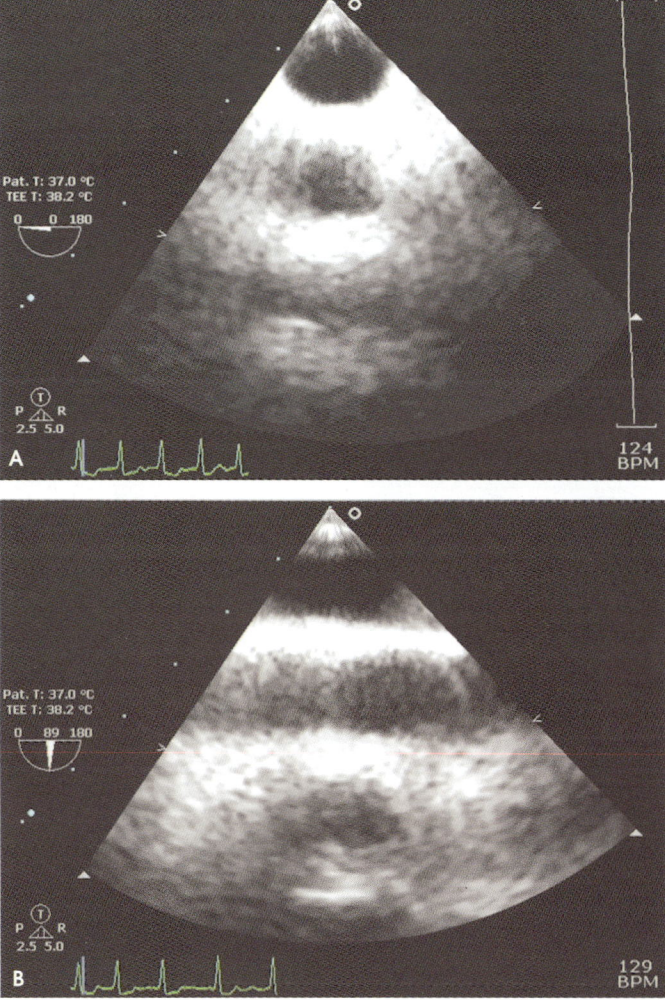

Fig. 8.3: Midesophageal descending aorta short-axis (A) and long-axis (B) views showing double descending thoracic aorta (mirror image artifact).

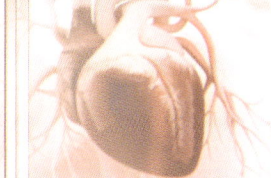

Reverberation Artifact

It is opposite of shadowing. Instead of absence of an echo, reverberations appear as one or multiple echos directly behind the reflector surface (Figs 8.4 and 8.5).

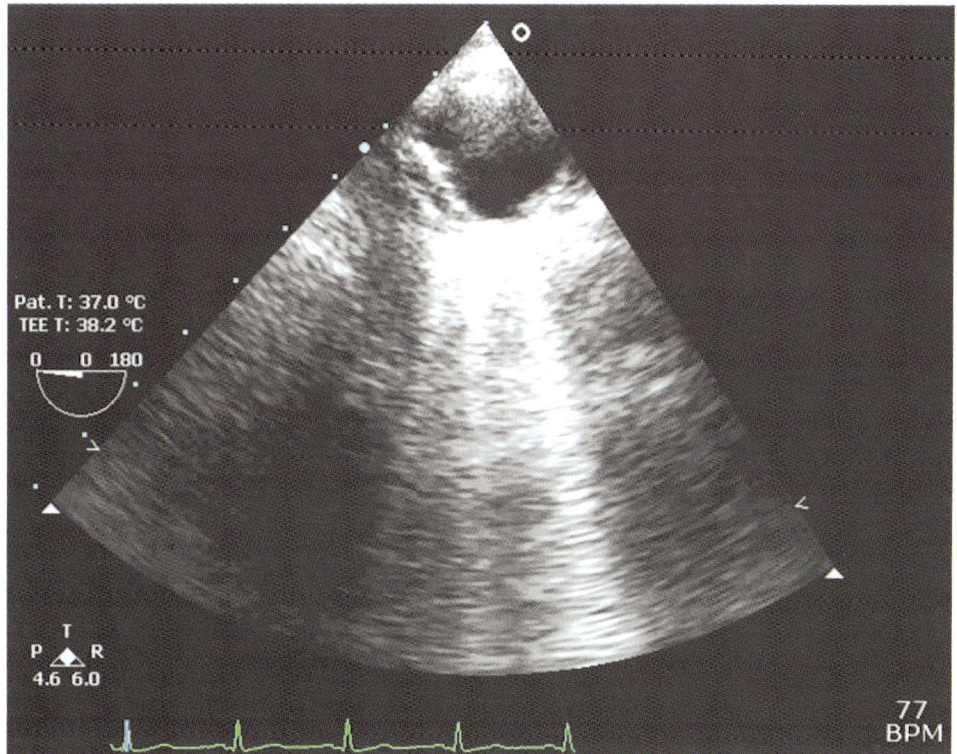

Fig. 8.4: Midesophageal descending aorta short-axis view showing a reverberation artifact in the far field.

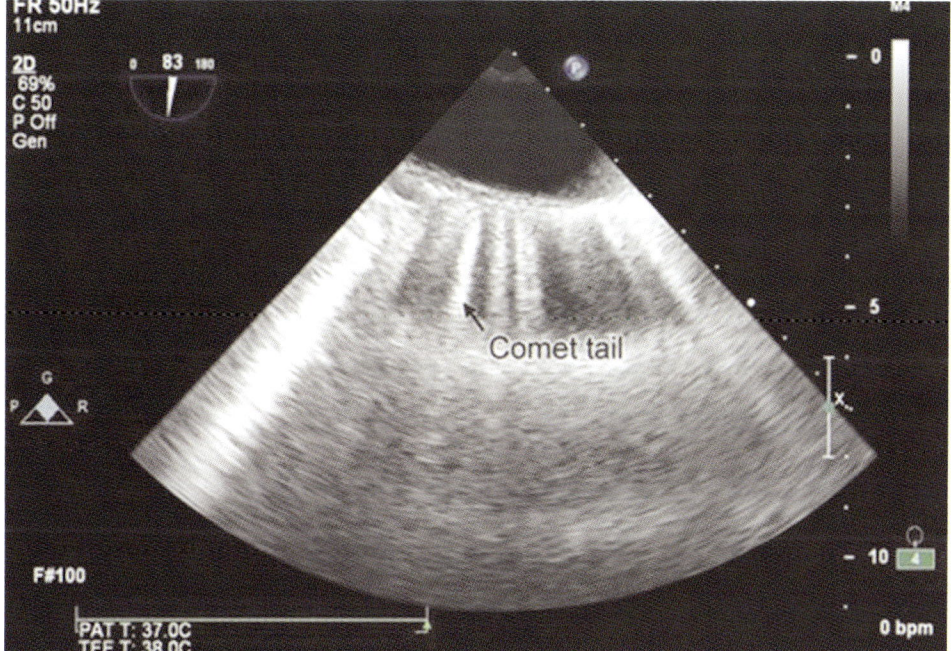

Fig. 8.5: Midesophageal descending aorta long-axis view showing the merging of multiple reverberation artifacts to produce a solid line away from the distal aortic wall giving appearance of a comet tail (ringdown artifact).

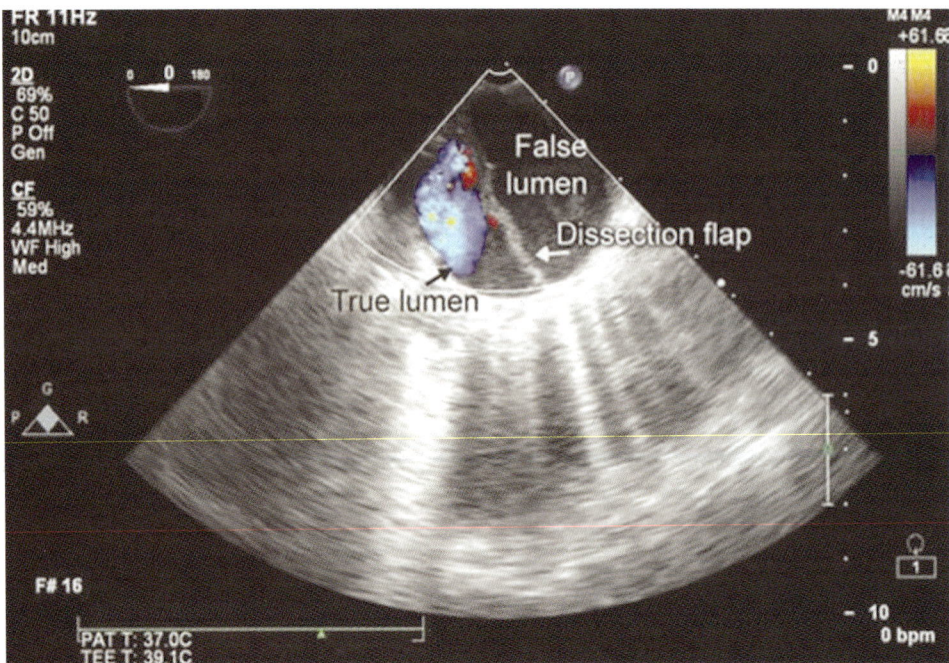

Fig. 8.6: Midesophageal descending aorta short-axis view showing a dissection flap between the large false lumen and the small true lumen. Aortic dissection is differentiated from mirror image artifact by the different color-flow pattern in the two lumen of aortic dissection. Mirror image artifact is formed at a predictable distance and has the same width as the aorta.

Side-lobe Artifact/Edge Effect

The echo images produced from off-side ultrasound beams on striking an object are displayed in the center, similar to an image generated from the main beam. This is referred to as side-lobe artifact. The side-lobes are weaker and differentiated by imaging in multiple planes (Figs 8.7 and 8.8).

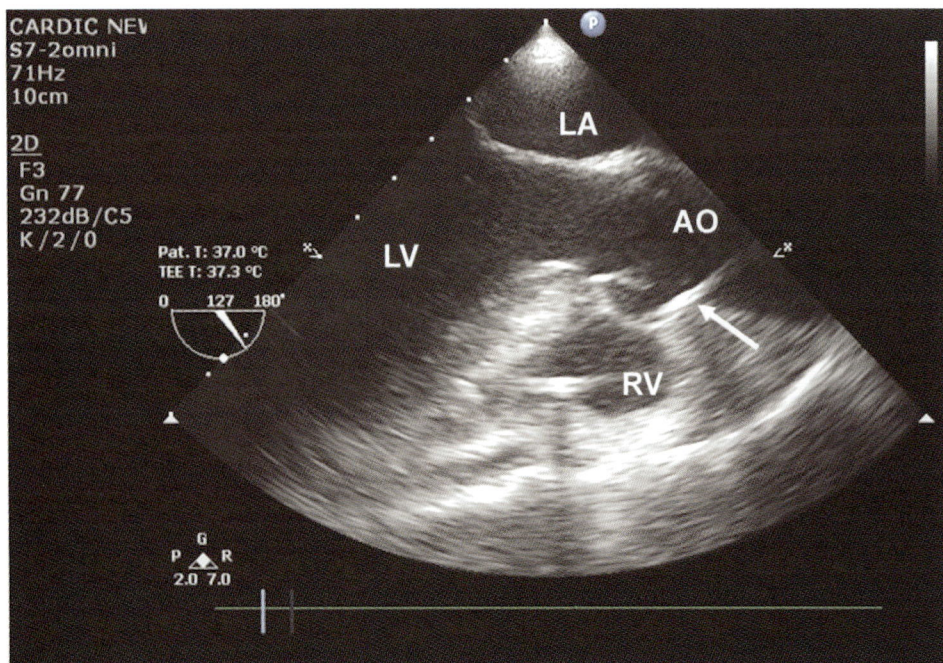

Fig. 8.7: Midesophageal aortic valve long-axis view showing a side-lobe artifect produced by the pulmonary artery cetheter in the right ventricle. A thin flap-like structure (arrow) in the ascending aorta is seen giving an impression that the pulmonary artery catheter is in the aorta (LA: left atrium, LV: left ventricle, AO: aorta, RV: right ventricle).

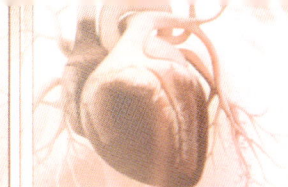

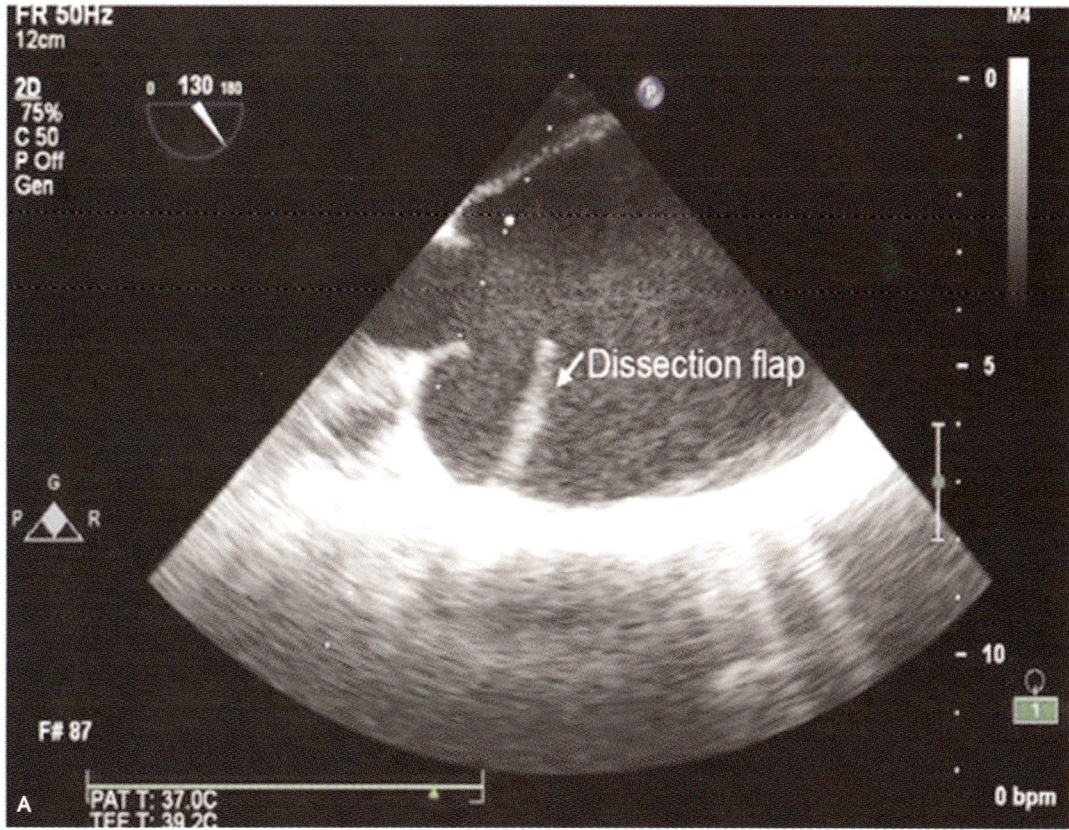

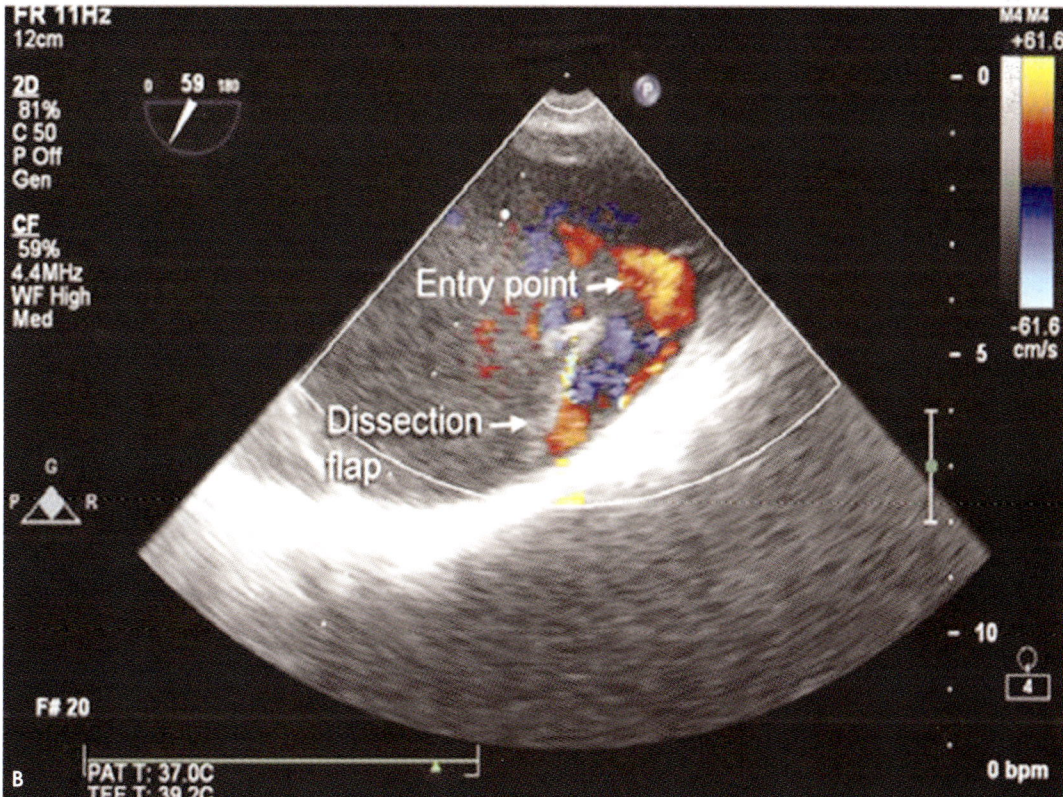

Fig. 8.8: Modified midesophageal ascending aorta long-axis view showing a dissection flap in the dilated ascending aorta. A dissection flap, in contrast to a side-lobe artifact, has homogenous echo intensity along its course (A), has random mobility and causes margination of flow on color flow imaging (B).

Aliasing

Aliasing refers to the wrap-around of the pulsed wave spectral display observed when the Nyquist limit (Doppler frequency corresponding to half of pulse repetition frequency) is exceeded. This phenomenon is misleading about the direction of blood flow. It may also be observed on color flow Doppler as change in color of sample volume from red to blue, or vice versa (Fig. 8.9).

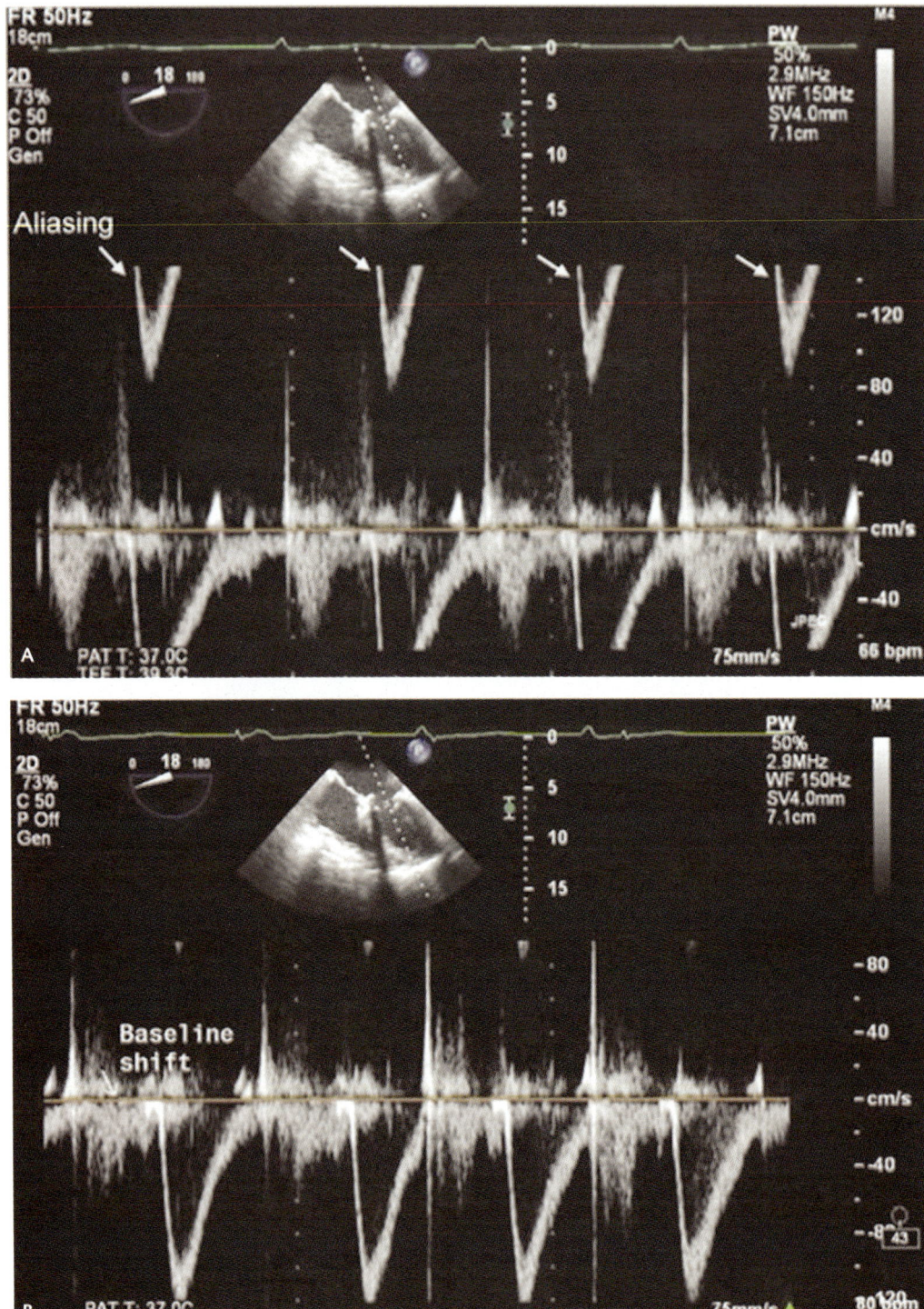

Fig. 8.9: Pulsed wave Doppler across the mitral valve showing the maximum velocity detected as 60 cm/sec, velocity beyond this limit wrapped around and presented above the line (arrow) giving an appearance of flow towards the transducer (A), Aliasing disappeared after shifting the baseline above as it could detect velocity up to 80 cm/sec (B).

Ghosting

Ghosting refers to the appearance of brief flashes of color outside the expected flow areas, i.e., in the tissue area of the image produced by mobile strong reflector such as prosthetic valves (Fig. 8.10).

Shadowing

Shadowing refers to the loss of information beyond a strong reflector on color flow imaging (Figs 8.11 and 8.12).

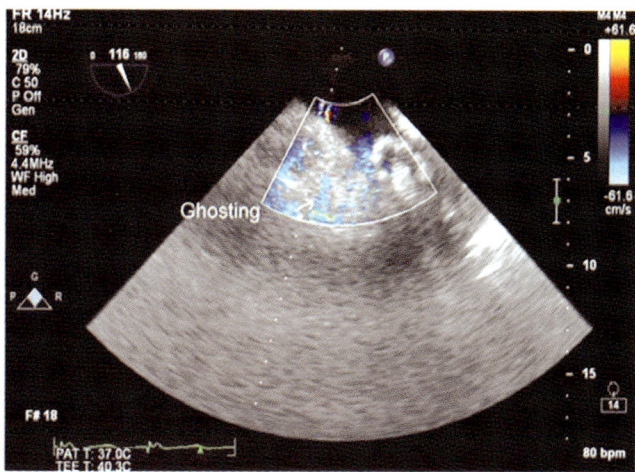

Fig. 8.10: Modified midesophageal two-chamber view showing blue color in the tissue area (ghosting).

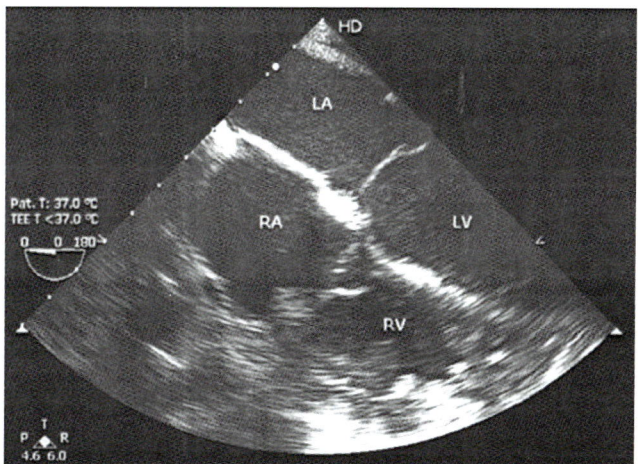

Fig. 8.11: Midesophageal four-chamber view showing a hyperechoic PTFE patch positioned at the interatrial septum and an anechoic right atrium due to shadowing cast by the patch (LA: left atrium, RA: right atrium, LV: left ventricle, RV: right ventricle).

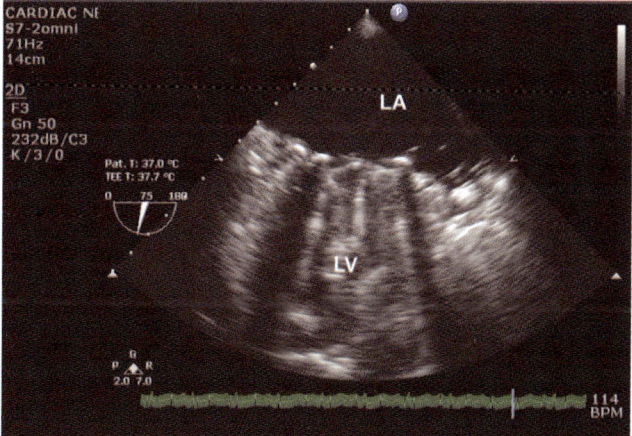

Fig. 8.12: Midesophageal two-chamber view showing the formation of acoustic shadowing beyond the prosthetic mitral ring (LA: Left atrium, LV: Left ventricle).

PITFALLS

Pitfalls refer to misdiagnosis of normal structures as pathological entities.

Eustachian Valve

The Eustachian valve is a remnant of the right horn of sinus venosus. It is located at the junction of the inferior vena cava and right atrium. It may be mistaken for an intracardiac tumor or thrombus (Fig. 8.13).

Crista Terminalis

Crista terminalis is a muscular ridge demarcating the smooth and trabeculated parts of the right atrium. It is formed by the junction of sinus venosus and primitive right atrium. It may also be mistaken for an intracardiac tumor or thrombus (Fig. 8.14).

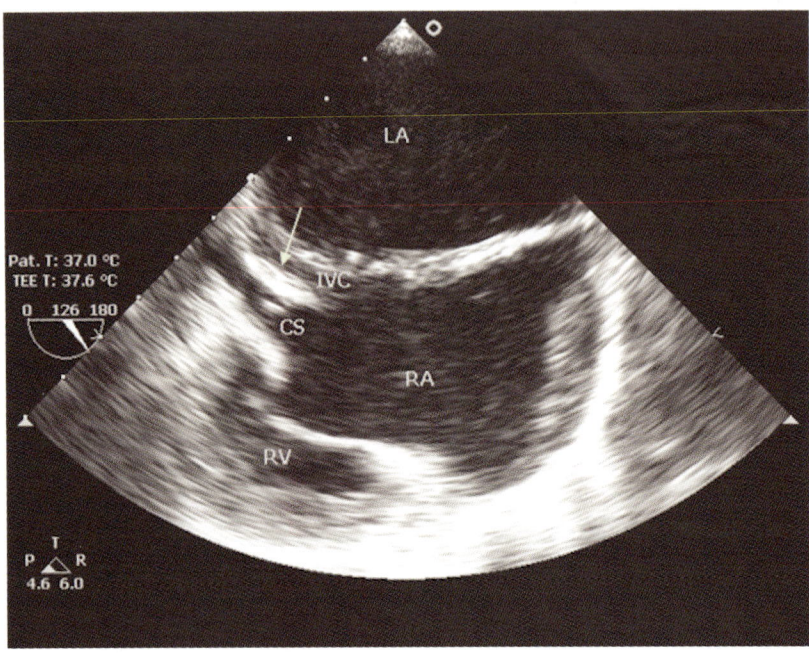

Fig. 8.13: Midesophageal modified bicaval view showing the Eustachian valve as a membranous structure at the opening of the inferior vena cava (arrow). (LA: left atrium, RA: right atrium, RV: right ventricle, IVC: inferior vena cava, CS: coronary sinus).

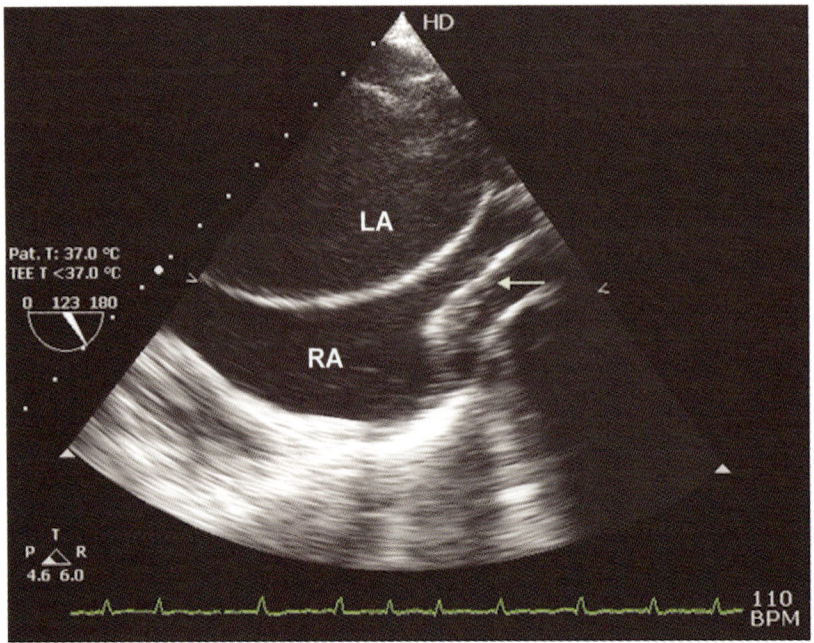

Fig. 8.14: Midesophageal modified bicaval view showing crista terminalis as a muscular ridge at superior vena cava-right atrial junction (arrow) (LA: left atrium, RA: right atrium).

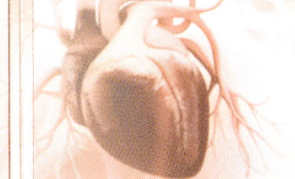

Chiari Network

Chiari network is a remnant of the right horn of sinus venosus. It is attached above to the Eustachian or Thebesian valve and below to the crista terminalis or the floor of the right atrium. It is seen as a large thread or whip like structure on echocardiography. It may be confused with an intracardiac tumor, thrombus or vegetation (Fig. 8.15).

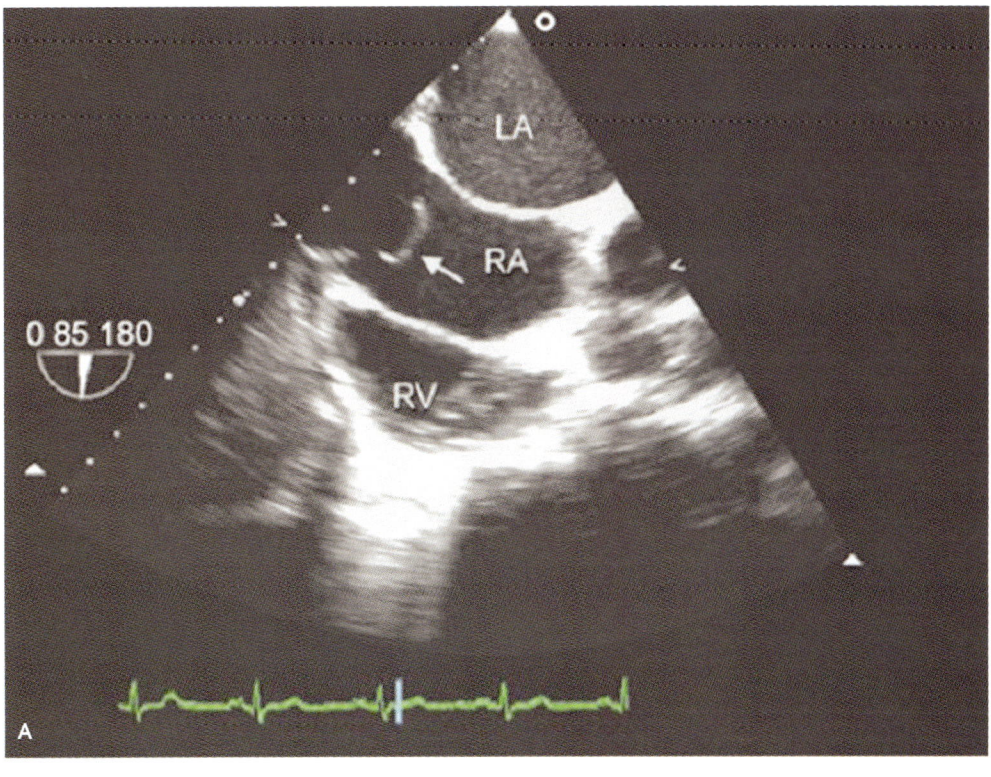

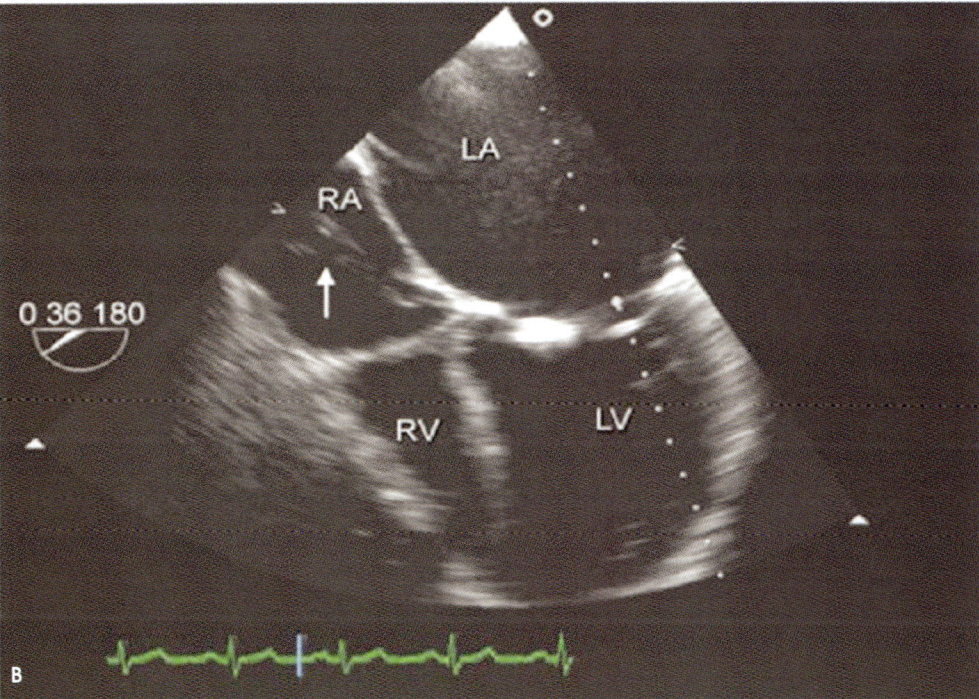

Fig. 8.15: Midesophageal bicaval view (A) and midesophageal four-chamber view (B) showing the Chiari network as a thin flap-like structure attached to the Eustachian valve and to lower portion of the interatrial septum. (RA: right atrium, RV: right ventricle, LA: left atrium, LV: left ventricle).

Thebesian Valve

The opening of the coronary sinus is guarded by the Thebesian valve (Fig. 8.16).

Lipomatous Hypertrophy of the Interatrial Septum

Fatty infiltration of the interatrial septum sparing the region of fossa ovalis imparts it a dumbbell shape (Fig. 8.17).

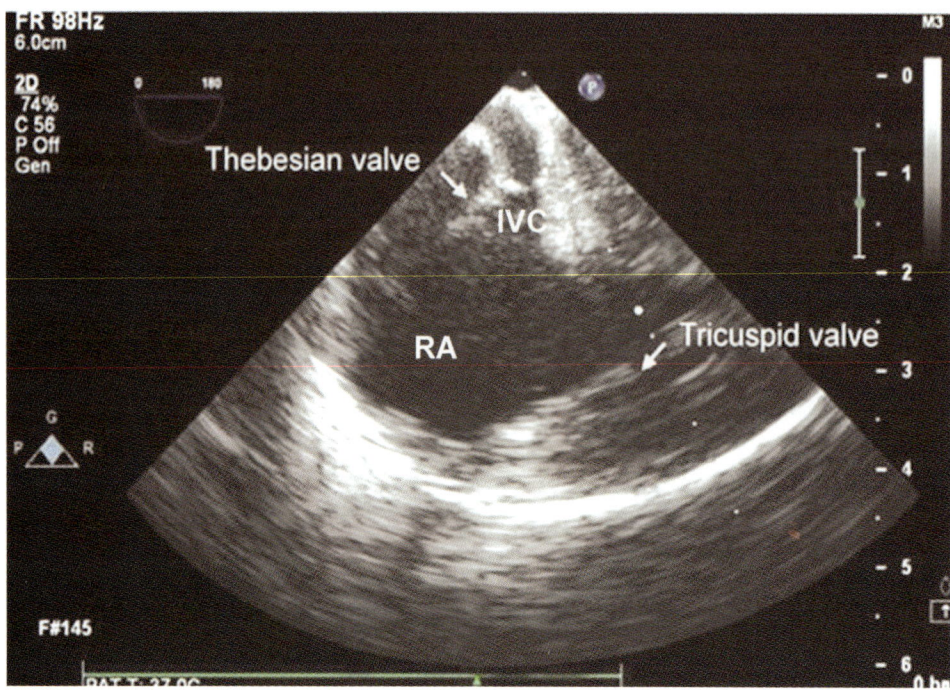

Fig. 8.16: Modified midesophageal four-chamber view showing the Thebesian valve as a leaf-like structure (arrow) at the opening of coronary sinus (RA: right atrium, IVC: inferior vena cava).

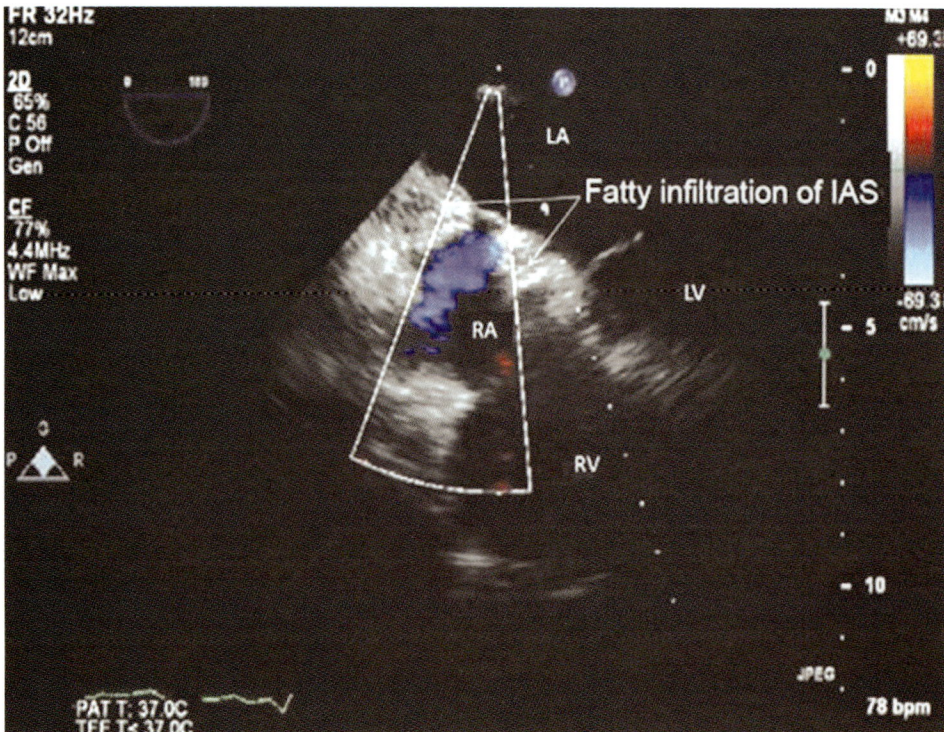

Fig. 8.17: Midesophageal four-chamber view, showing a thickened dumbbell shaped inter-atrial septum (IAS) due to lipomatous hypertrophy. (LA: left atrium, RA: right atrium, RV: right ventricle, LV: left ventricle).

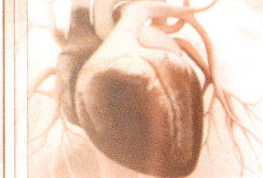

Aneurysm of the Interatrial Septum

An interatrial septal aneurysm appears as a localized outpouching more than 1.5 cm from the plane of the interatrial septum towards the right atrium or the left atrium. It is often implicated as a cause of cryptogenic stroke (Fig. 8.18).

Enlarged Coronary Sinus

Coronary sinus diameter greater than 1 cm may be seen in the presence of a persistent left superior vena cava or cardiac type of total anomalous pulmonary venous connection. It can be confused with an abscess or cyst in relation to the mitral valve or an enlarged left circumflex artery (Fig. 8.19).

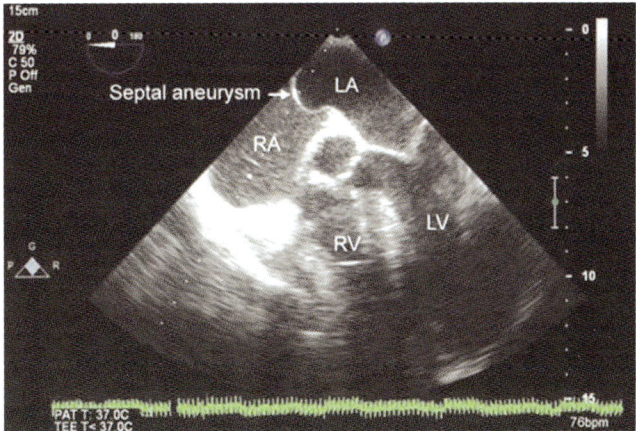

Fig. 8.18: Midesophageal five-chamber view showing an aneurysmal interatrial septum as a thin membrane outpouching towards the right atrium. (RA: right atrium, LA: left atrium, RV: right ventricle, LV: left ventricle).

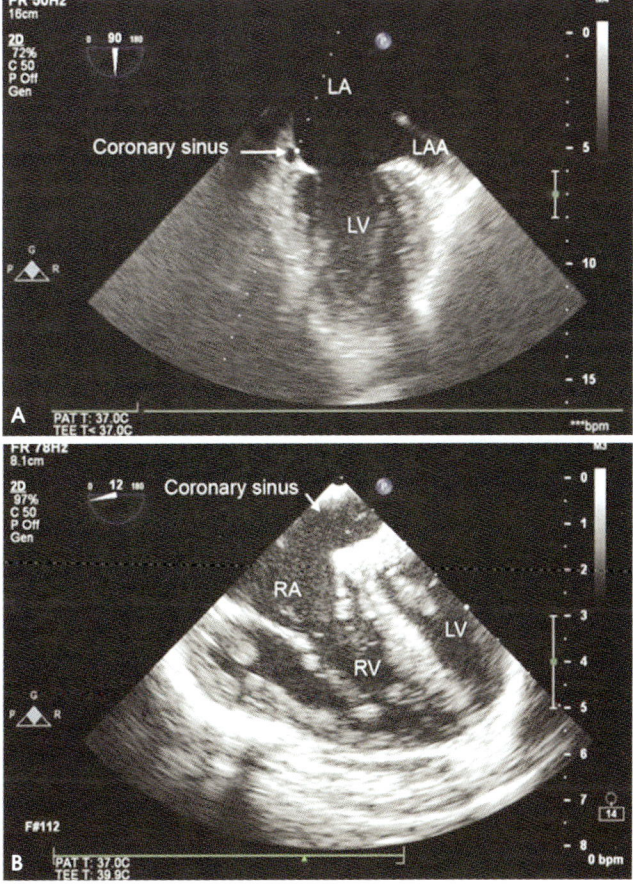

Fig. 8.19: (A) Midesophageal two-chamber view showing the coronary sinus in short-axis as a circular structure. (B): Modified midesophageal four-chamber view obtained by retroflexing the probe from the four-chamber view showing the coronary sinus in long-axis. (LA: left atrium, LAA: left atrial appendage, LV: left ventricle, RA: right atrium, RV: right ventricle).

Catheters and Wires

Invasive lines such as the central venous catheter, pulmonary artery catheter and pacing wires can frequently be seen in the right side of the heart (Figs 8.20 and 8.21).

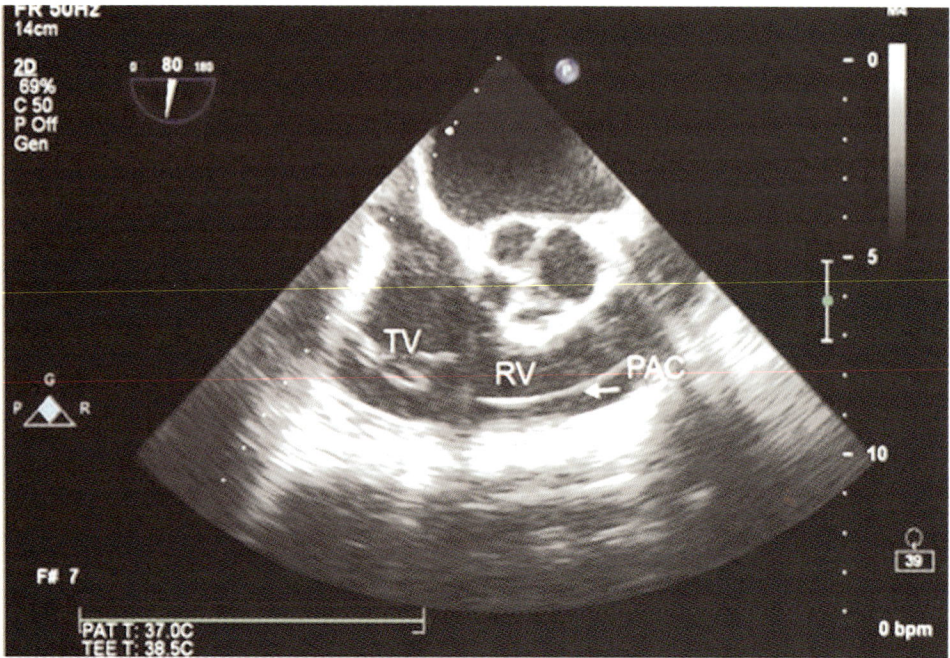

Fig. 8.20: Midesophageal right ventricular inflow-outflow view showing the course of a pulmonary artery catheter across the tricuspid valve coursing along the free wall of the right ventricle to enter the pulmonary artery. (TV: tricuspid valve, RV: right ventricle, PAC: pulmonary artery catheter).

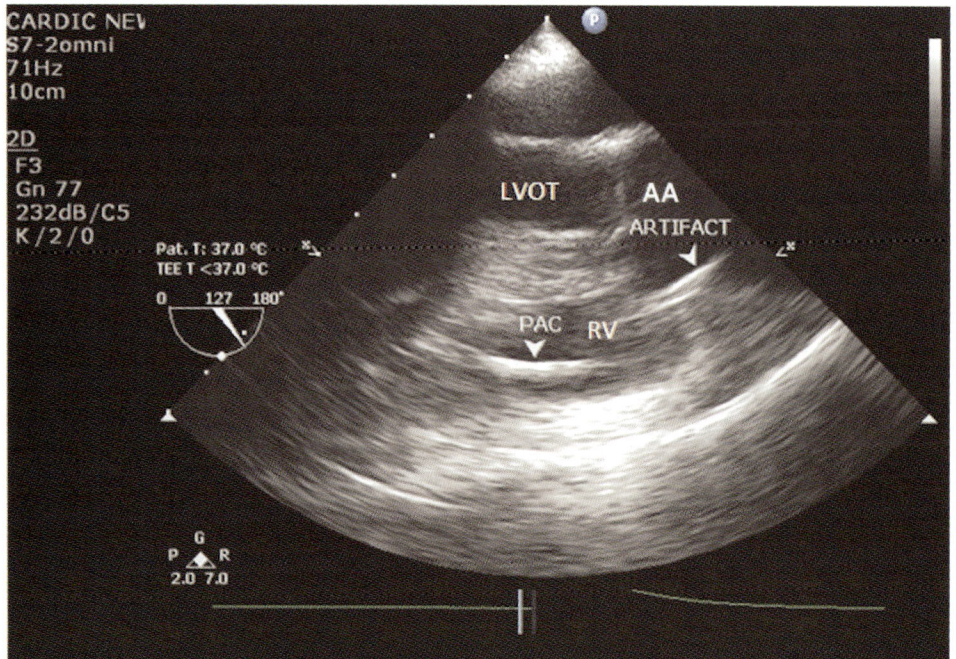

Fig. 8.21: Midesophageal long-axis view showing the course of the pulmonary artery catheter in the right ventricle and an artifact formed by it in the ascending aorta (LVOT: left ventricular outflow tract, RV: right ventricle, AA: ascending aorta, PAC: pulmonary artery catheter).

Pectinate Muscle

The left atrial appendage is lined with parallel muscular ridges of the pectinate muscle. It must be differentiated from a thrombus as it is like a strand; unlike a thrombus which is round, pedunculated, and usually associated with spontaneous echo contrast (Fig. 8.22).

Warfarin (Coumadin) Ridge

A globular mass of atrial tissue may sometimes be seen separating the left atrial appendage from the left upper pulmonary vein. Since it protrudes into the lumen of the left atrium, it must be differentiated from a tumor or thrombus (Fig. 8.23).

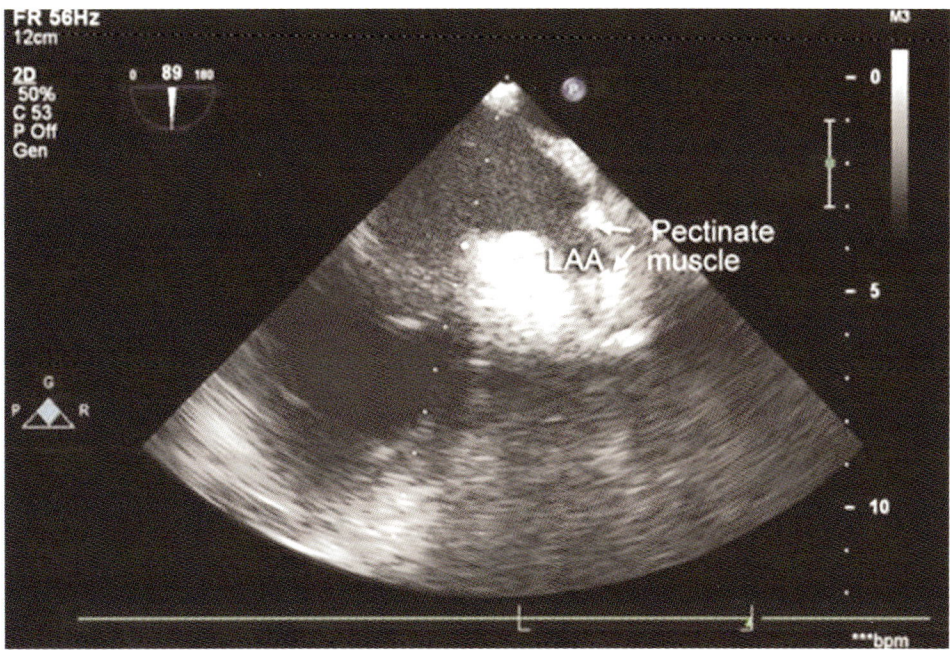

Fig. 8.22: Midesophageal two-chamber view showing the pectinate muscle as a triangular bulge in the wall of left atrial appendage (LAA).

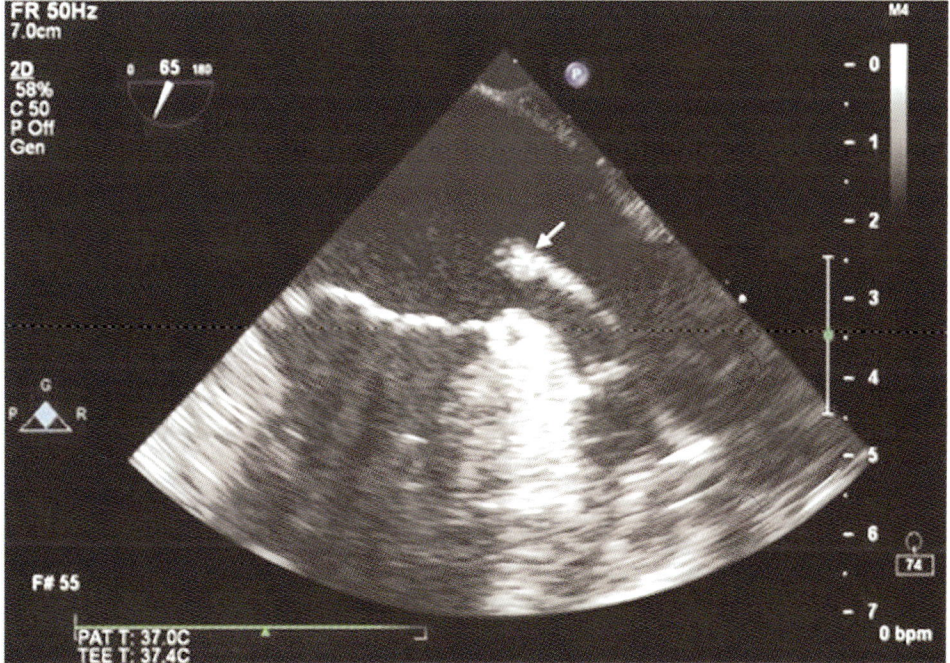

Fig. 8.23: Modified midesophageal two-chamber view showing the Coumadin ridge as a globular mass between the left atrial appendage and the left upper pulmonary vein (arrow).

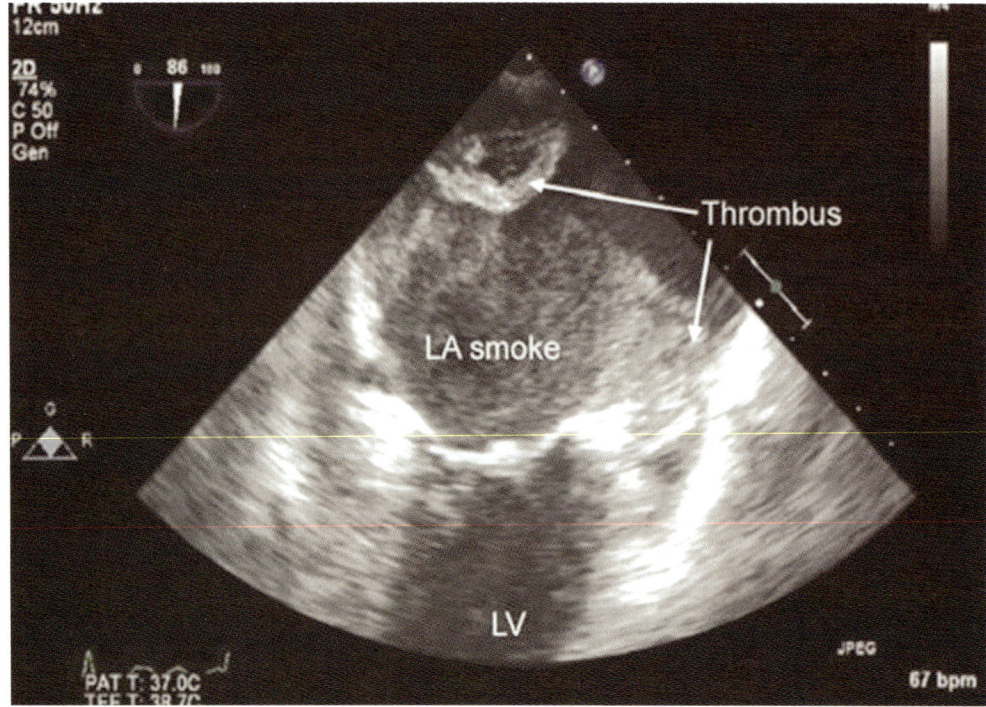

Fig. 8.24: Midesophageal two-chamber view showing the left atrial appendage filled by a thrombus, also notice the smoke in the left atrium. (LA: left atrium, LV: left ventricle).

Inverted Left Atrial Appendage

The left atrial appendage may get inverted following cardiac surgery and appear as a homogenous, freely mobile structure mimicking a mass. Likewise any other purse-string suture may project into the chamber and mimic a mass/thrombus (Figs 8.24 and 8.25).

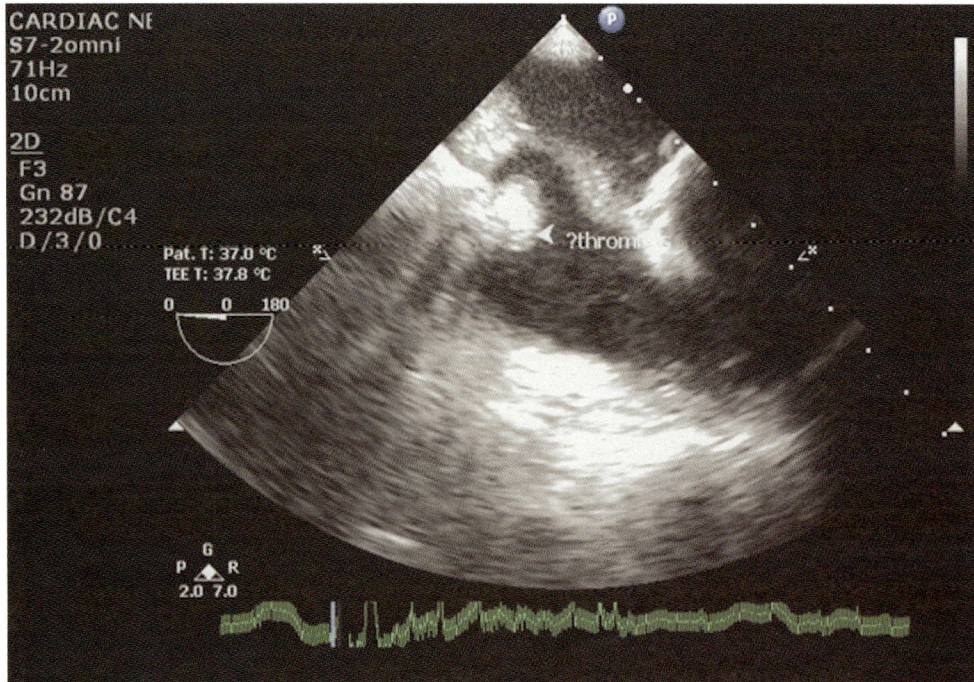

Fig. 8.25: Midesophageal four-chamber view showing a tied purse string suture invaginating in the right atrium and mimicking a thrombus. In this patient, cardiopulmonary bypass was established and the right atrium was opened to confirm the diagnosis.

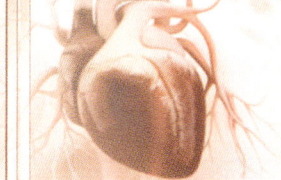

Left Atrial Membrane

An incomplete membrane is sometimes seen extending from the region of the Coumadin ridge to the upper border of fossa ovalis. A left atrial membrane is differentiated from the supramitral ring by its attachment to the left atrial wall above the left atrial appendage (Fig. 8.26).

Moderator Band

The moderator band is a prominent muscle bundle in the right ventricle extending from the apical one-third and basal two-thirds junction of the interventricular septum to the base of the anterior papillary muscle (Fig. 8.27).

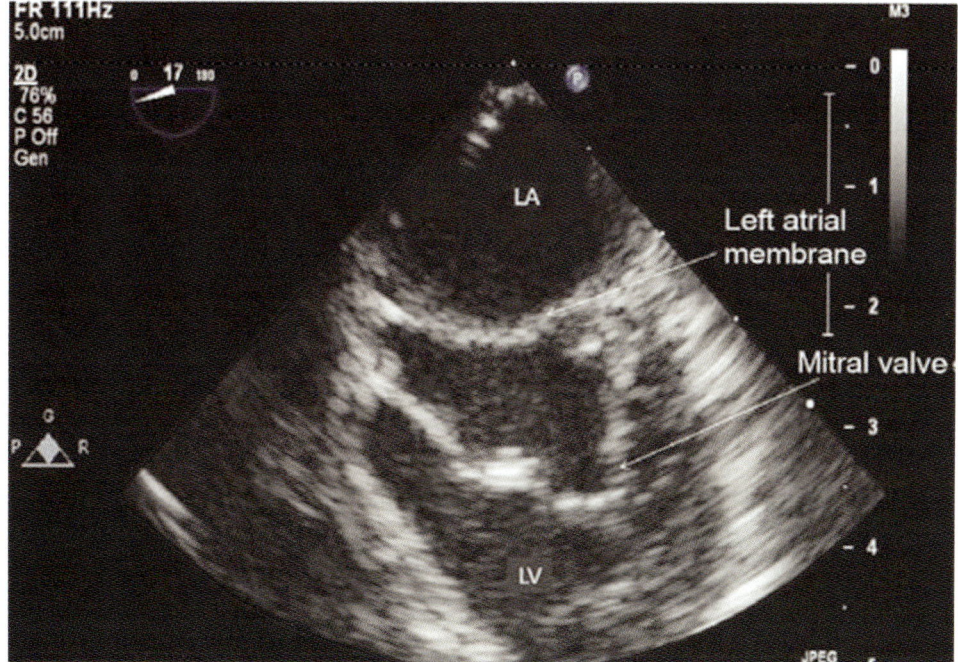

Fig. 8.26: Midesophageal four-chamber view showing a left atrial membrane extending from the lateral wall of left atrium to the interatrial septum (LA: left atrium, LV: left ventricle).

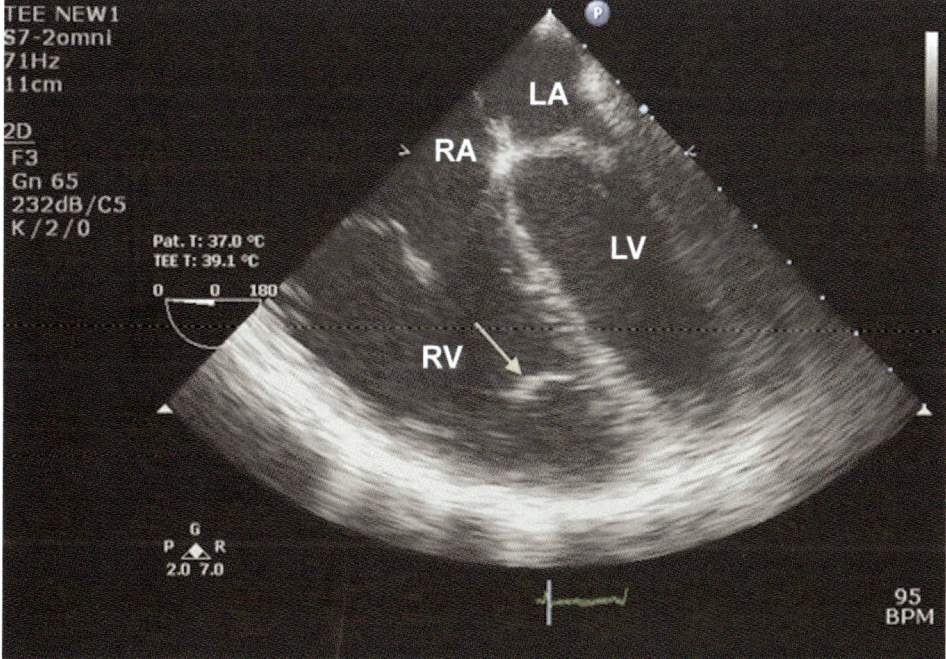

Fig. 8.27: Midesophageal four-chamber view showing the moderator band in the right ventricle (arrow) (RA: right atrium, RV: right ventricle, LA: left atrium, LV: left ventricle).

Bifid Papillary Muscle

The papillary muscles of the left ventricle may rarely be lobulated and confused with a mass or a thrombus (Fig. 8.28).

Lambl's Excrescences

Thin, mobile strands up to 1 cm may be seen attached to the under surface of aortic, mitral or any prosthetic valve (usually seen with aortic valve). They may be confused with vegetations (Fig. 8.29).

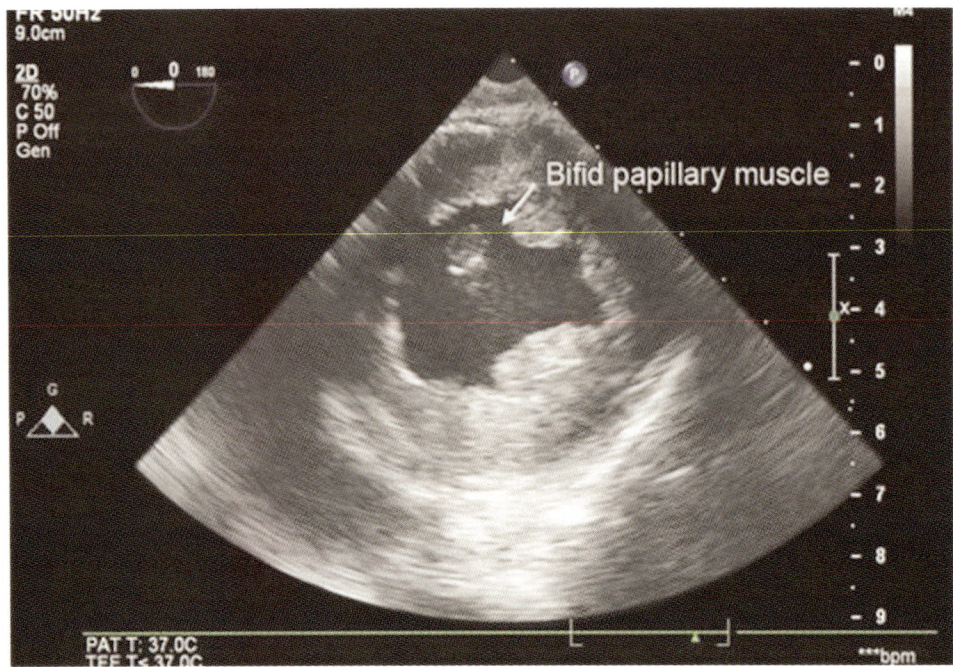

Fig. 8.28: Transgastric midpapillary short-axis view showing a bifid posteromedial papillary muscle giving the appearance of presence of three papillary muscles.

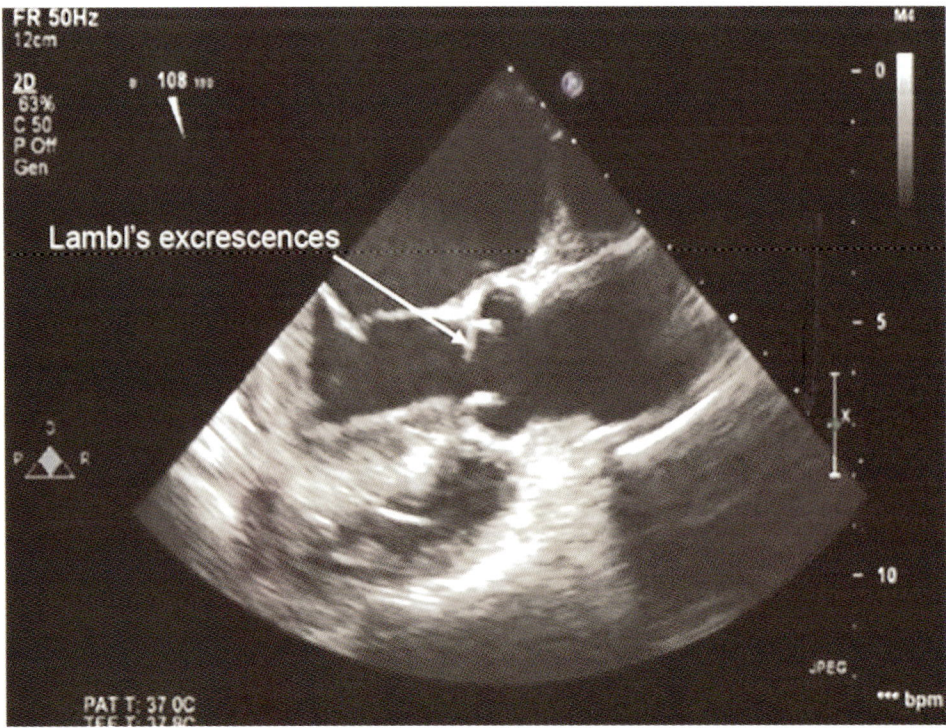

Fig. 8.29: Midesophageal aortic valve long-axis view showing the Lambl's excrescences under the surface of the aortic valve cusp.

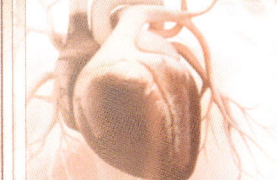

Transverse Sinus

The transverse sinus appears as a crescent shaped echo free space between the aorta and pulmonary trunk anteriorly, and the left atrium posteriorly. It is confused with a cyst, abscess or aneurysm (Fig. 8.30).

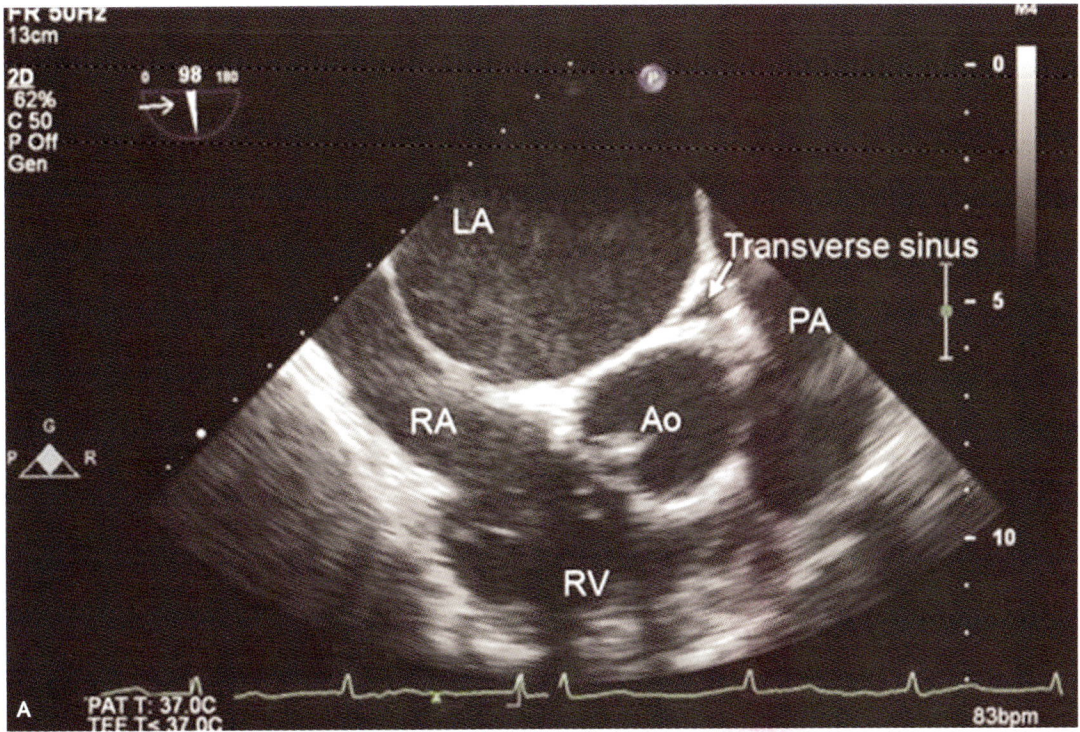

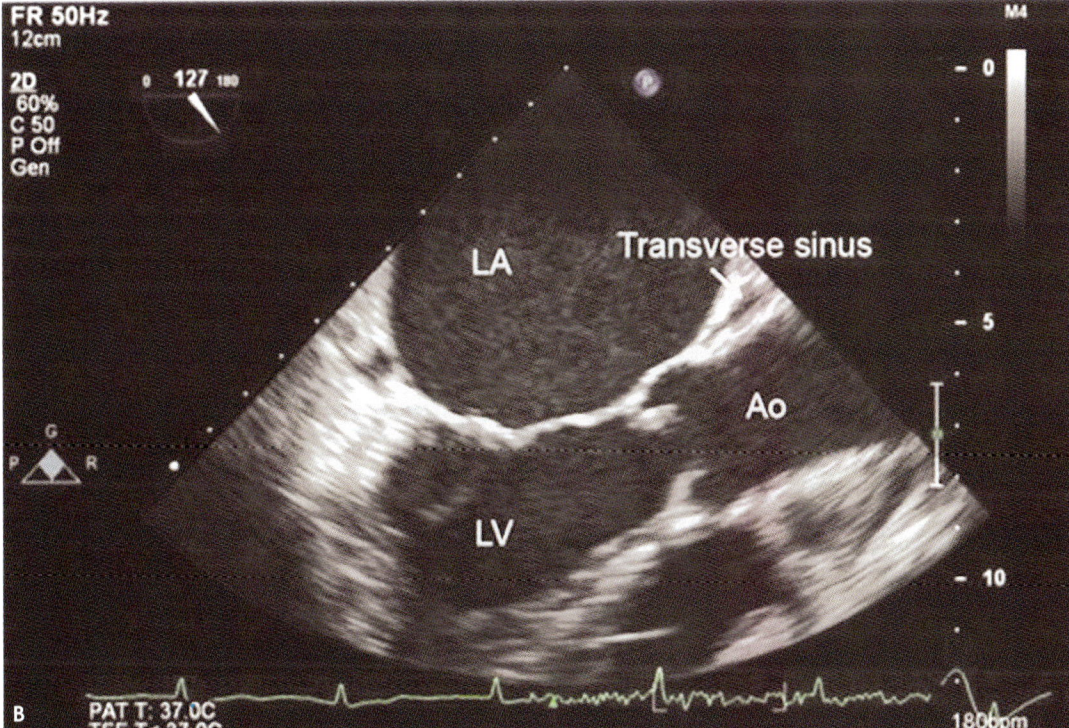

Fig. 8.30: (A) Midesophageal right ventricular inflow-outflow view showing the transverse sinus as a triangular gap between the aorta and the pulmonary artery anteriorly and left atrium posteriorly, (B) Midesophageal aortic valve long-axis view showing the transverse sinus between the aorta anteriorly and left atrium posteriorly. (LA: left atrium, RA: right atrium, RV: right ventricle, Ao: aorta, PA: pulmonary artery, LV: left ventricle).

Oblique Sinus

The oblique sinus is a fold of pericardium between the pulmonary veins and posterior wall of left atrium. It appears as an echo free space or echo dense space depending on whether collected blood is liquid or clotted (Fig. 8.31).

Persistent Left Superior Vena Cava (LSVC)

The LSVC appears as an oval structure between the left atrial appendage and left upper pulmonary vein. Injection of agitated saline into left upper extremity vein leads to opacification of the LSVC. It must be differentiated from an abscess or a cyst (Fig. 8.32).

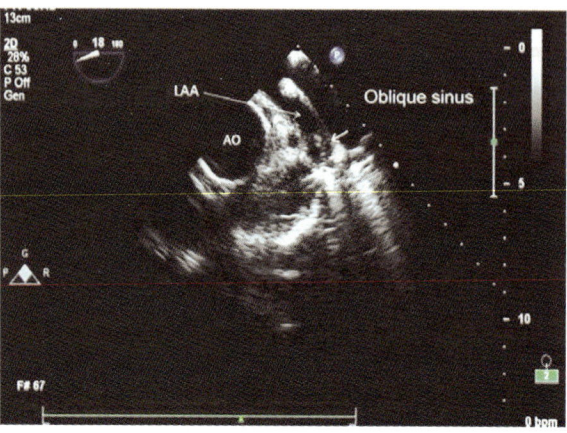

Fig. 8.31: Midesophageal ascending aorta short-axis view showing the oblique sinus between the fold of pericardium of four pulmonary veins and the posterior wall of the left atrium. (Ao: aorta, LAA: left atrial appendage).

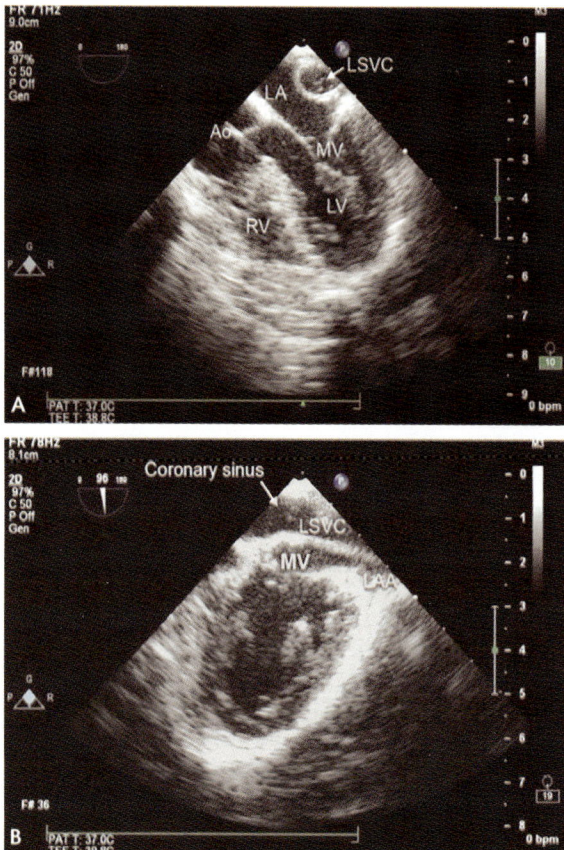

Fig. 8.32: (A) Modified midesophageal four-chamber view showing a persistent left-sided superior vena cava as an echolucent circular space; (B) As an echolucent cavity above the left atrioventricular groove between the left atrial appendage and the left upper pulmonary vein (not shown in picture) opening into the dilated coronary sinus. (Ao: aorta, LA: left atrium, LSVC: left superior vena cava, RV: right ventricle, MV: mitral valve, LV: left ventricle, LAA: left atrial appendage).

Intracardiac Air

Intracardiac air may present as mobile echogenic dots or line at the highest point in a cardiac chamber and accompanied with acoustic shadowing (Fig. 8.33).

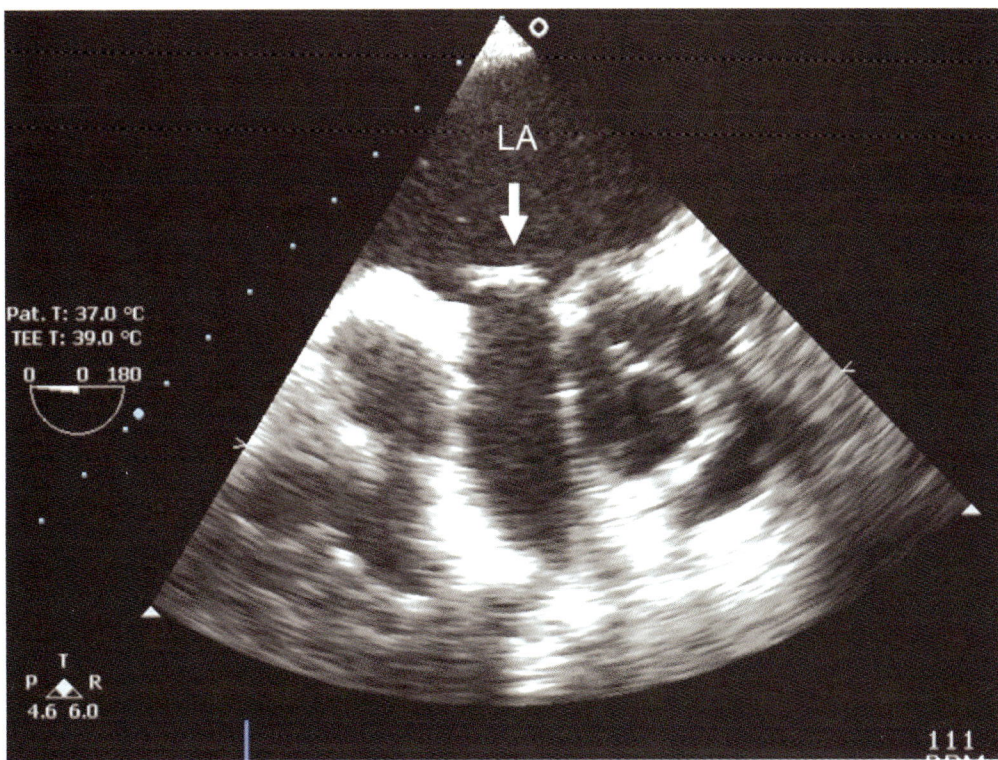

Fig. 8.33: Air bubble: A large air bubble can be entrapeed during open heart surgery and de-airing the cardiac chambers before discontinuning the cardiopulmonary bypass is an important step. Transesophageal echocardiography can be an important tool to detect an air bubble. It can be seen as a linear density (arrow) with a dirty acoustic shadow that occilates (refer to the video). (LA: left atrium).

Evaluation of
Infective Endocarditis

9

• Deepak K. Tempe • Suruchi Hasija

Infective endocarditis can occur in the setting of rheumatic fever, pre-existing abnormality such as bicuspid aortic valve and prosthetic valve implantation. The diagnostic echocardiographic feature of infective endocarditis is the vegetation, a mass that consists of fibrin, blood cells and microorganisms. Vegetations appear as independently mobile echo-dense masses that range in size from microorganisms to several centimeters in length. A vegetation may be confused with a thrombus or calcification and can be differentiated from a thrombus on the basis of its independent mobility that gives it a free floating characteristic. Hence, this differentiation is easily possible on a video rather than a still image. The reader should refer to the video in the enclosed compact disk.

A thrombus on the other hand is generally fixed and the movement if present, is along with the structure to which it is attached. Transesophageal echocardiography (TEE) can identify smaller vegetations that may be missed on transthoracic echocardiography. Vegetations on the valve leaflets can damage it leading to valve regurgitation that can suddenly become severe. The infection can extend to the perivalvular limits forming an abscess or an aneurysm. TEE examination should include careful assessment with short- and long-axis views. Color flow Doppler can be used to detect regurgitation.

This chapter depicts the images showing the vegetations at various positions.

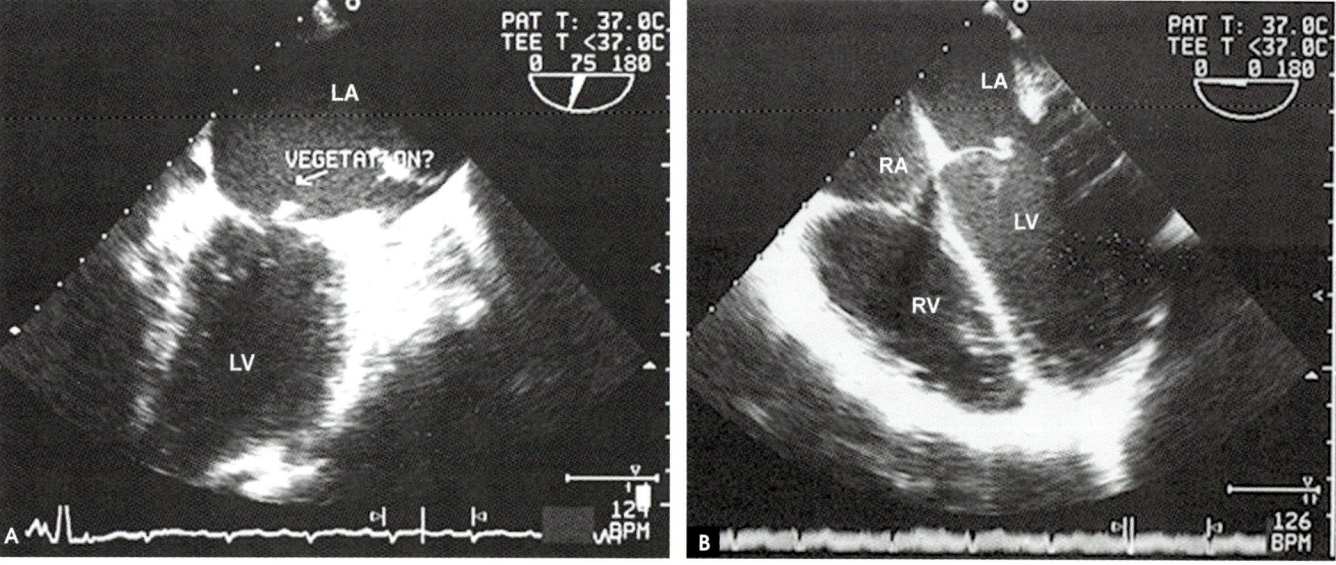

Fig. 9.1: A patient with native valve endocarditis. Note the vegetation (arrow) on the mitral leaflet. (A) Two-chamber view, (B) four-chamber view (LA: left atrium, LV: left ventricle, RA: right atrium, RV: right ventricle).

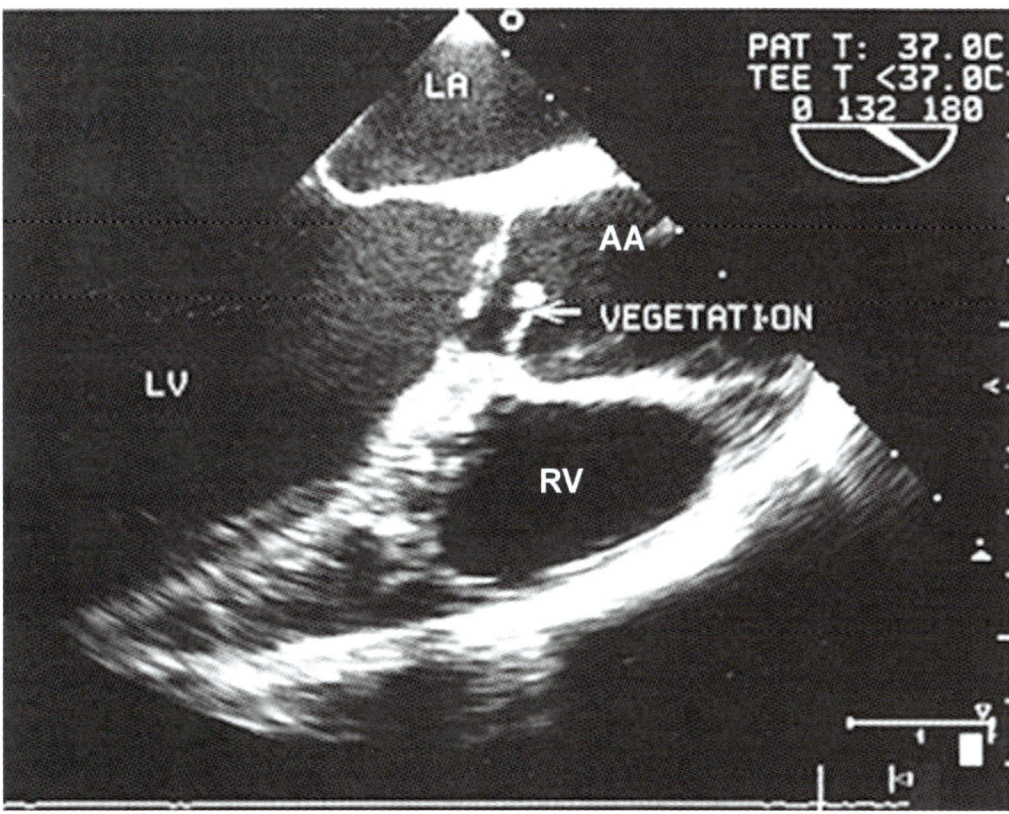

Fig. 9.2: Midesophageal aortic valve long-axis view showing multiple vegetations (arrow) over aortic valve in a patient with native aortic valve endocarditis (LA: left atrium, LV: left ventricle, RV: right ventricle, AA: ascending aorta).

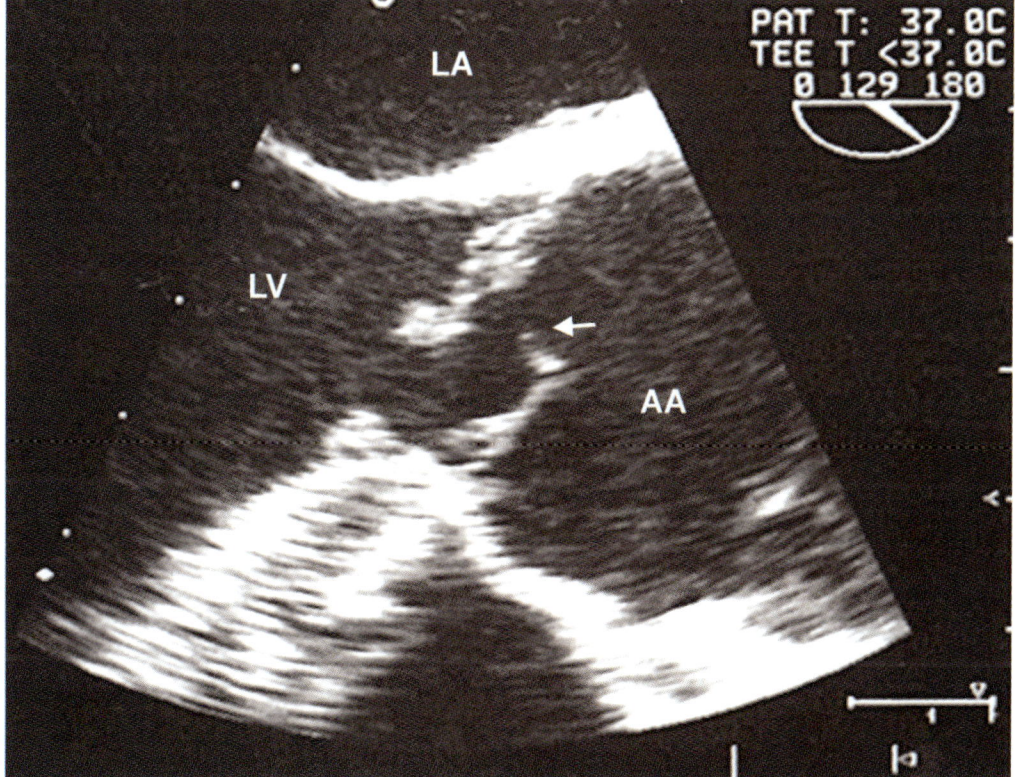

Fig. 9.3: Midesophageal aortic valve long-axis view showing vegetations (arrow) over the aortic leaflets. Note the abnormal appearance of the incompetent aortic leaflets. (LA: left atrium, LV: left ventricle, AA: ascending aorta).

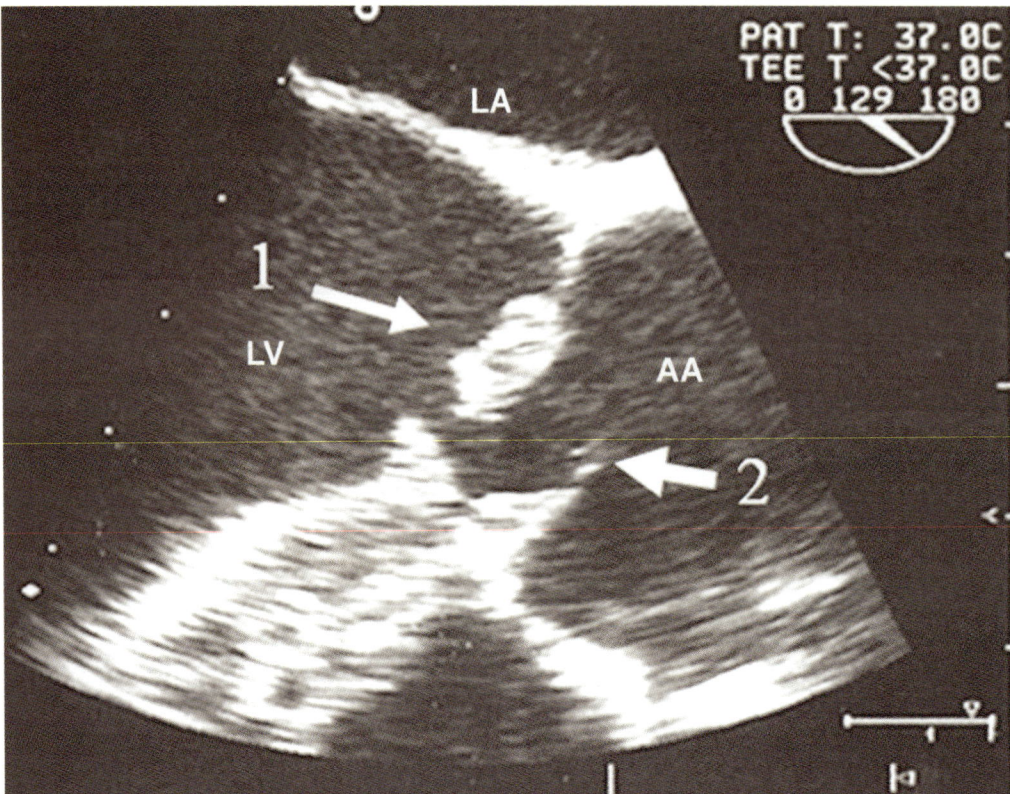

Fig. 9.4: Midesophageal aortic valve long-axis view showing vegetations (arrow 1) over the aortic valve in a patient with aortic valve endocarditis. Note the complete destruction of the other aortic leaflet (arrow 2) (LA: left atrium, LV: left ventricle, AA: ascending aorta).

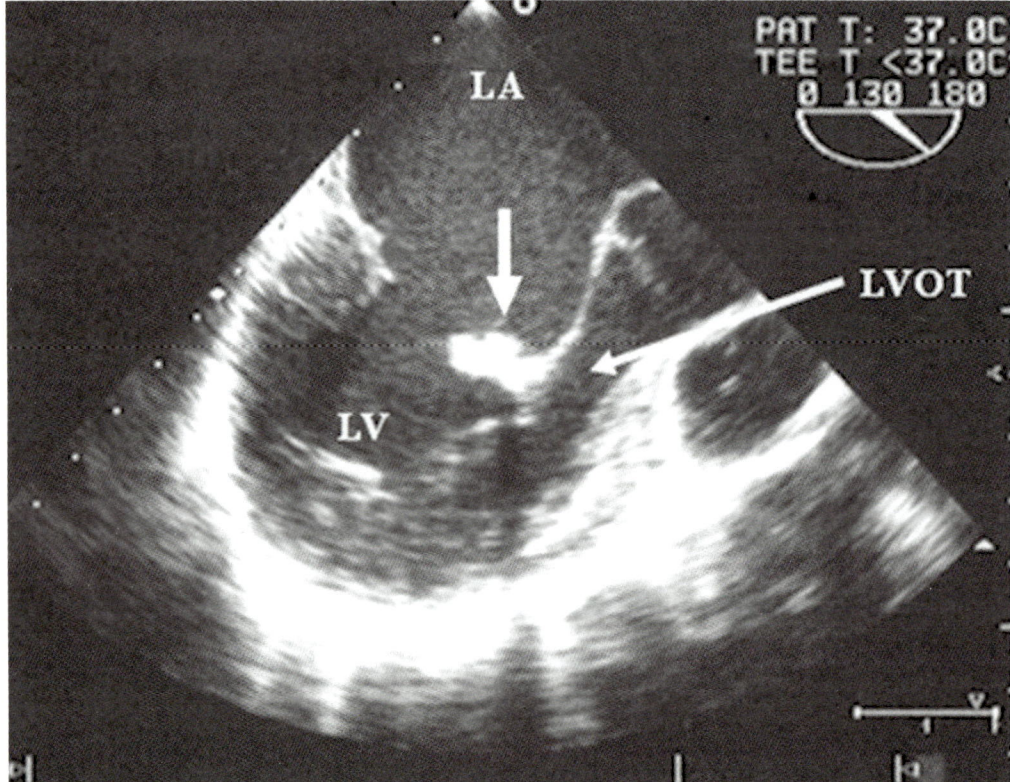

Fig. 9.5: Midesophageal long-axis view showing a large vegetation (arrow) over the anterior mitral leaflet (arrow). (LA: left atrium, LV: left ventricle, LVOT: left ventricular outflow tract).

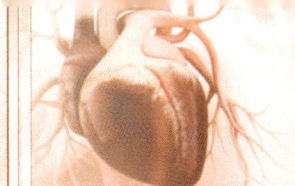

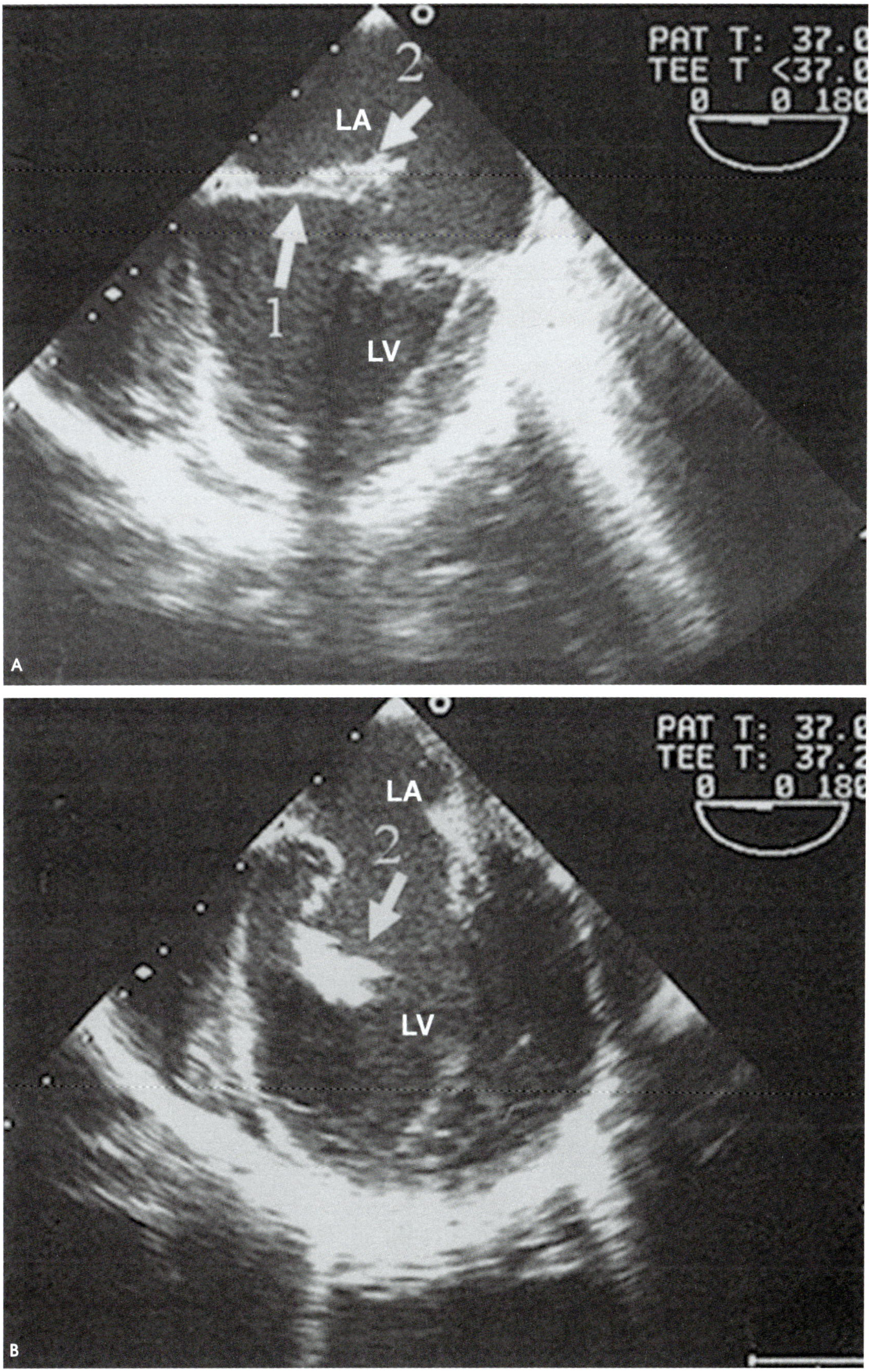

Fig. 9.6 (A and B): Prolapse of the anterior mitral leaflet (arrow 1) in a patient with a large vegetation over the anterior mitral leaflet (arrow 2) (A and B) (LA: left atrium, LV: left ventricle).

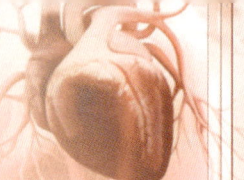

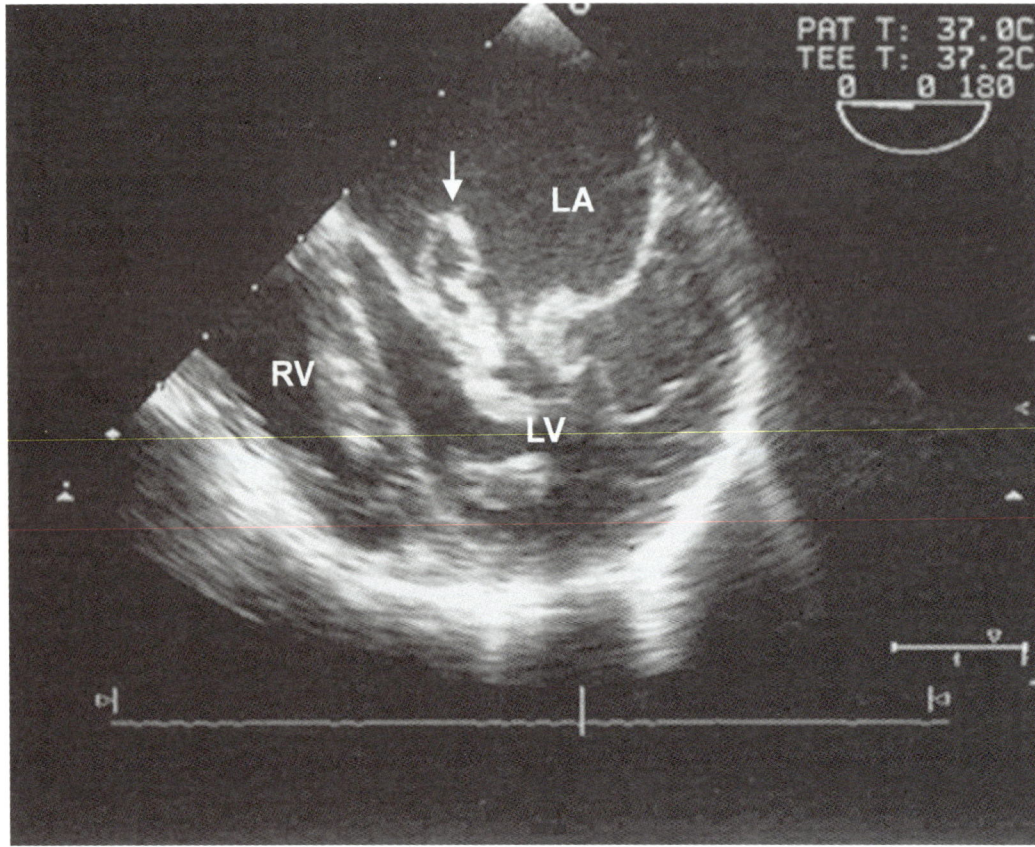

Fig. 9.7: A large vegetation on the anterior mitral leaflet (arrow) (LA: left atrium, LV: left ventricle, RV: right ventricle).

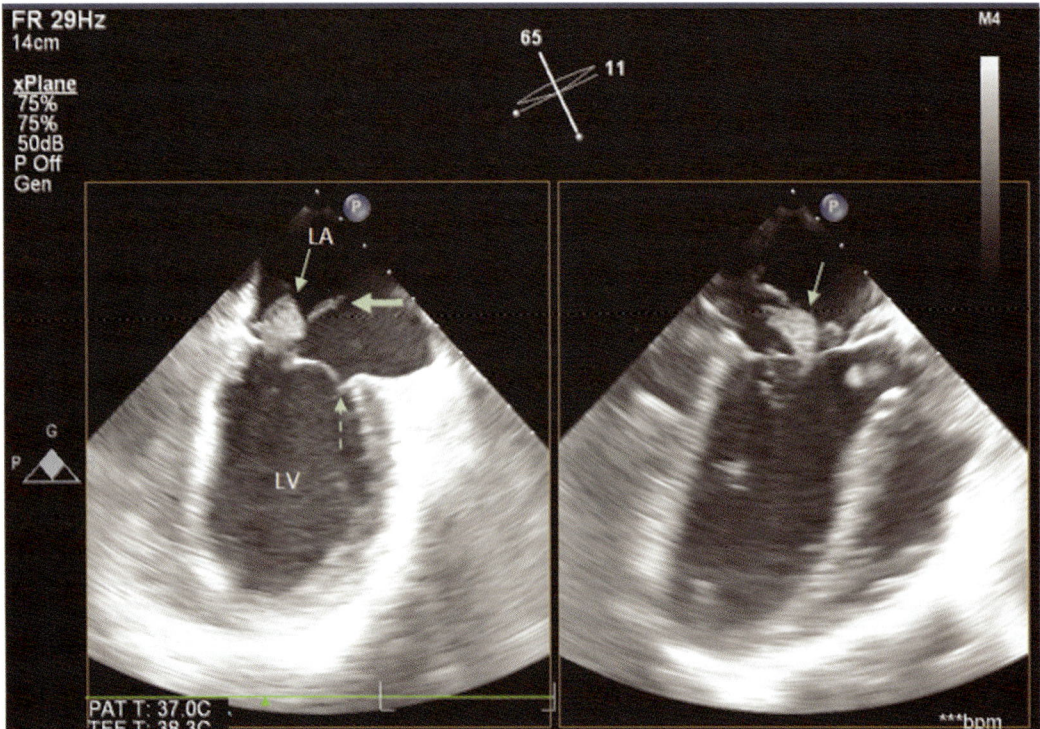

Fig. 9.8: Midesophageal views showing a large vegetation on the posterior mitral leaflet (arrow). The free edge of the ruptured chordae is seen in the left atrium (bold arrow). In addition, there is a perforation on the anterior mitral leaflet (dash arrow). (LA: left atrium, LV: left ventricle).

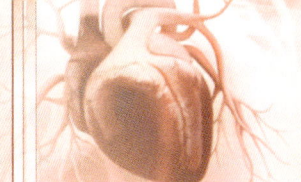

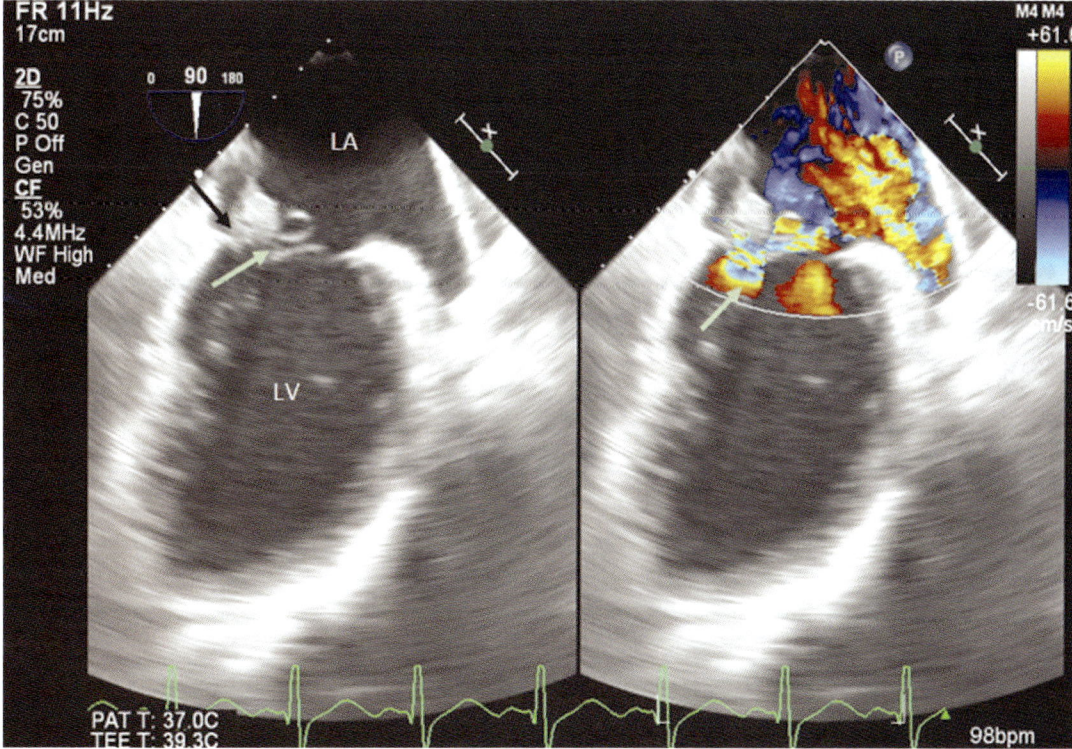

Fig. 9.9: Midesophageal two-chamber view with color showing mitral regurgitation jet through the non coapting leaflets (arrow). There is also a perforation on the posterior mitral leaflet below the vegetation (black arrow). Note the proximal isovelocity area (PISA) formation on the left ventricular side (LA: left atrium, LV: left ventricle).

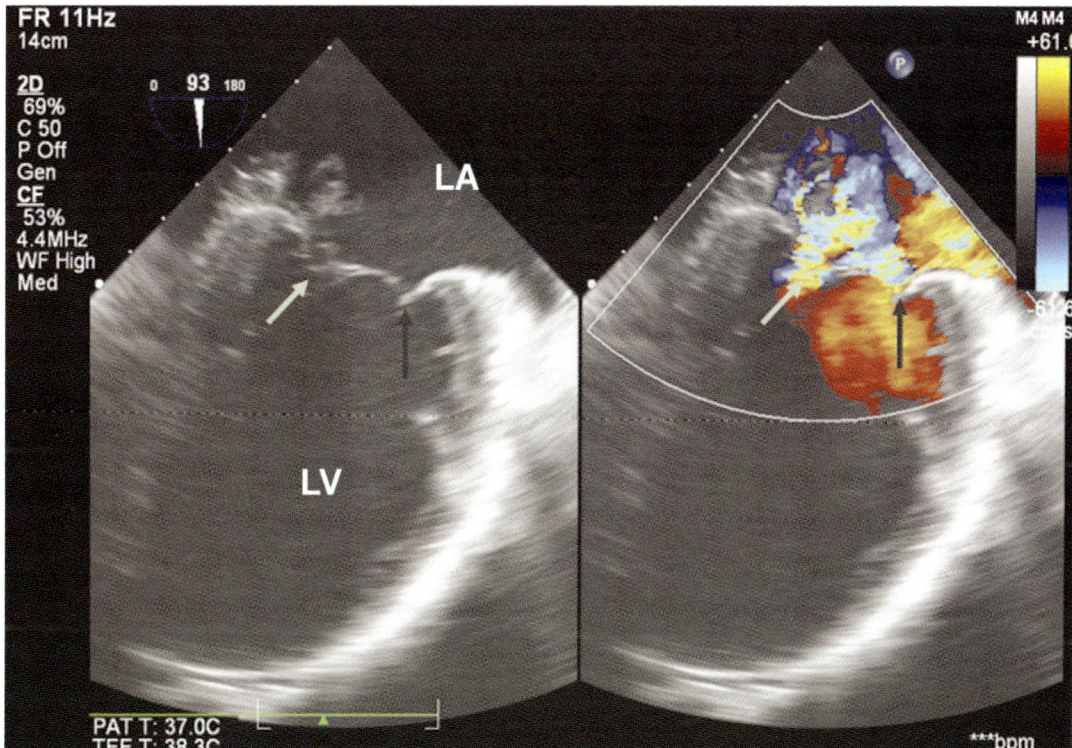

Fig. 9.10: Midesophageal two-chamber view with color showing mitral regurgitation jet through the noncoapting leaflets (white arrow). There is also a perforation on the anterior mitral leaflet (black arrow). (LA: left atrium, LV : left ventricle).

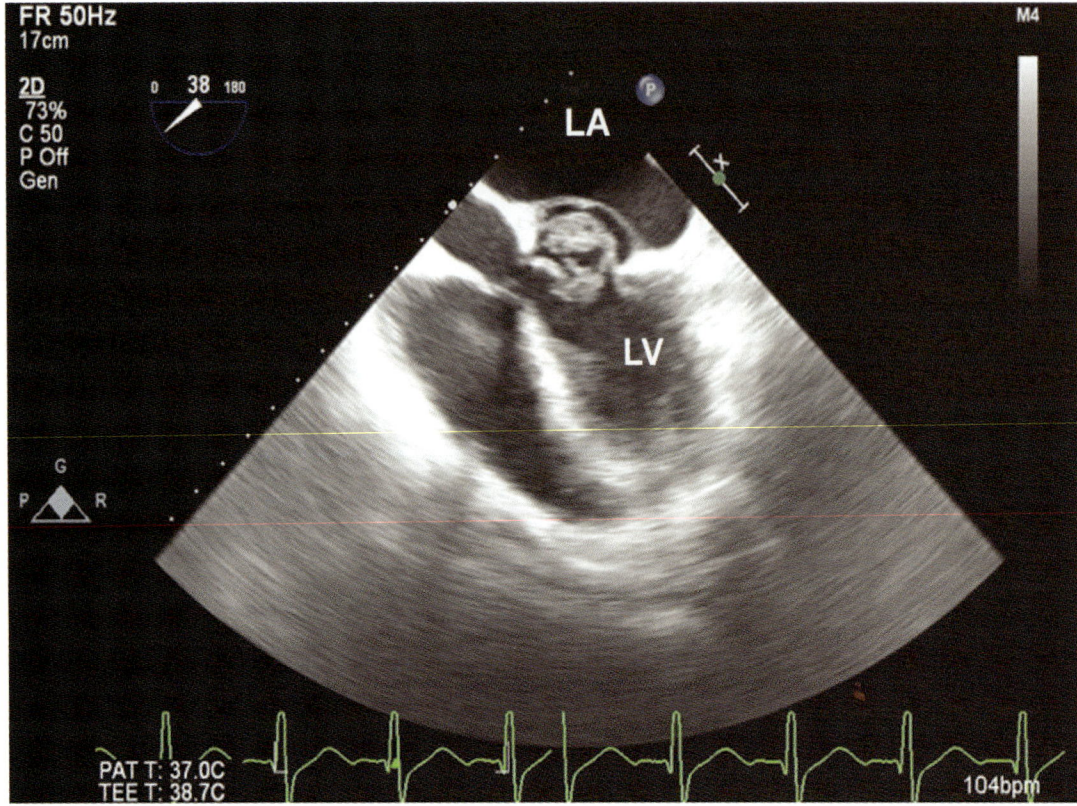

Fig. 9.11: Modified midesophageal ascending aorta short-axis view showing vegetations on both cusps of the bicuspid aortic valve (LA: left atrium, LV: left ventricle).

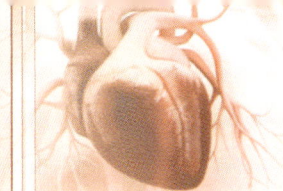

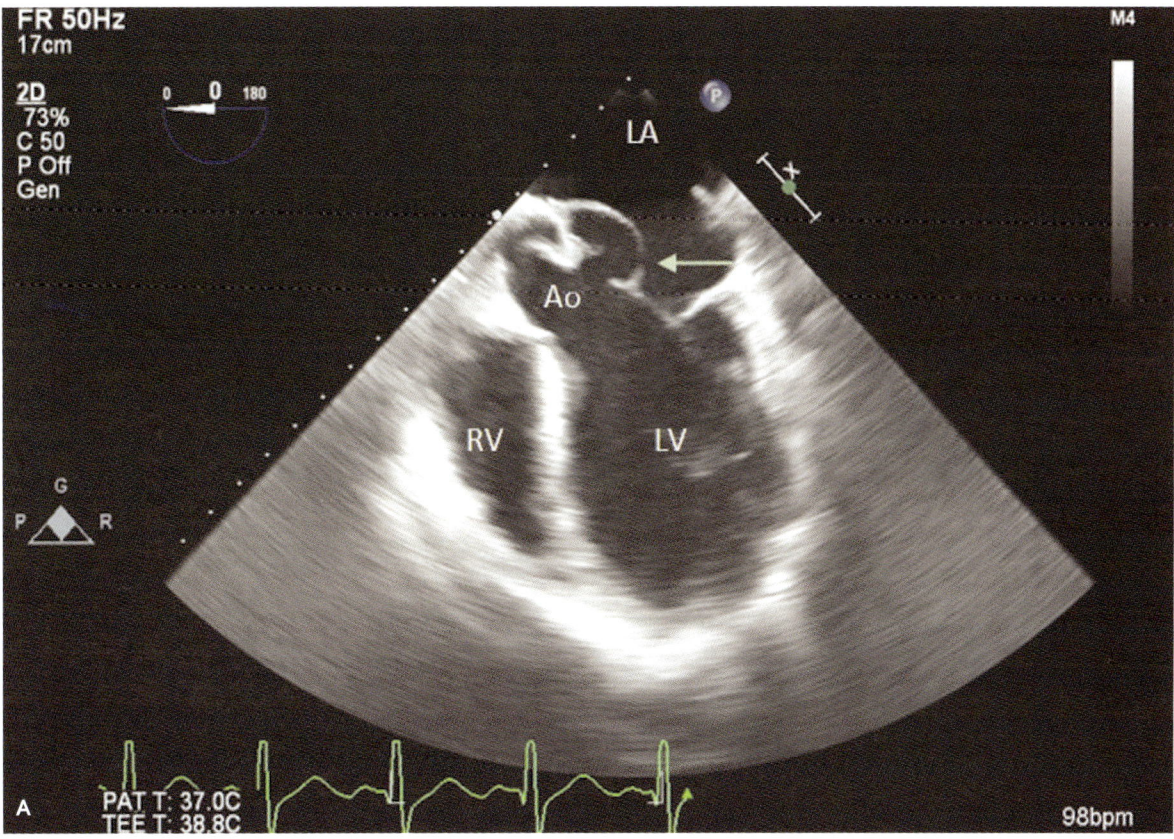

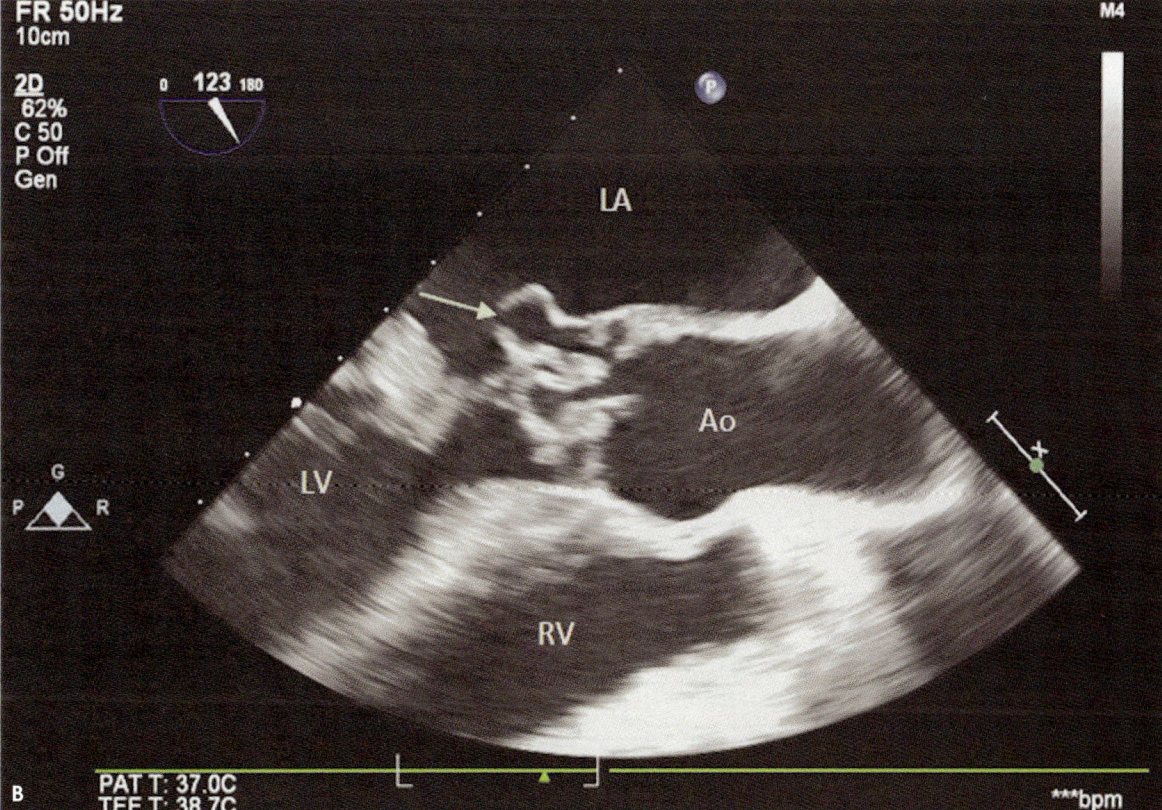

Fig. 9.12: Midesophageal five-chamber view (A) and aortic valve long-axis view (B) showing vegetations on the aortic valve cusps and aortic root abscess perforating into the LA (arrow). (LA: left atrium, LV: left ventricle, RV: right ventricle, Ao: ascending aorta).

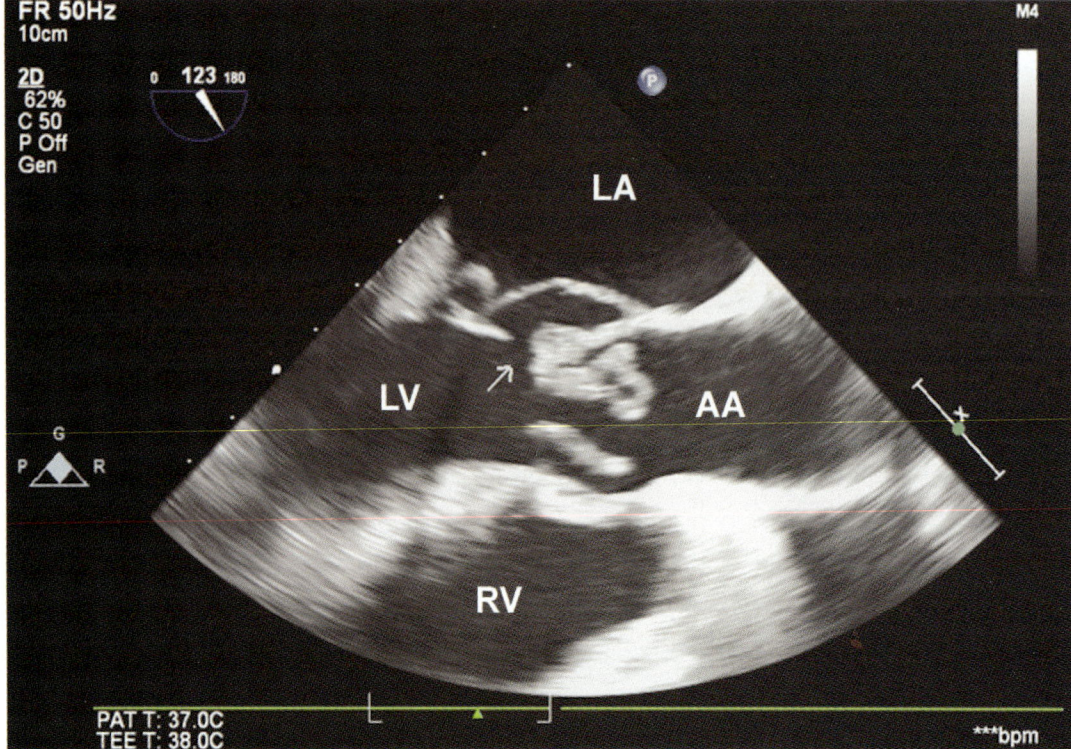

Fig. 9.13: Midesophageal aortic valve long-axis view showing vegetations on the noncoronary cusp, perforation in the aorto-mitral curtain (arrow) and aortic root abscess (LA: left atrium, LV: left ventricle, AA: ascending aorta, RV: right ventricle).

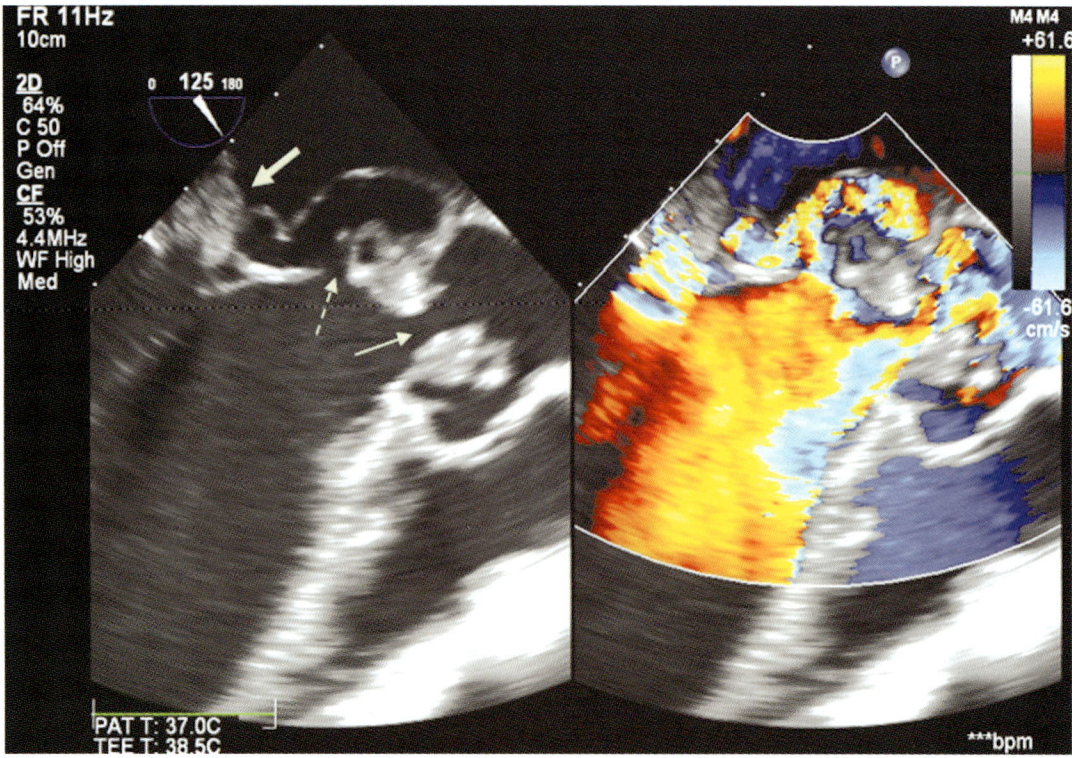

Fig. 9.14: Midesophageal aortic valve long-axis view showing severe aortic regurgitation through the noncoapting aortic leaflets (arrow). Also note the presence of a vegetation on the anterior mitral leaflet (bold arrow) and perforation in the aorto-mitral curtain (dash arrow).

Evaluation of Intracardiac Masses

10

• Deepak K. Tempe • Suruchi Hasija

The important intracardiac masses that can be visualized with transesophageal echocardiography (TEE) include thrombus and tumor. Both are moderately echogenic and can be easily identified on TEE. Thrombus and tumor have different appearances with a common clinical problem of potential embolism. Those present in the venous system can cause pulmonary embolism, while those in the left heart can lead to systemic embolism. Occasionally a right sided thrombus/tumor can embolise into the systemic circulation via intacardiac defects such as atrial or ventricular septal defect.

Thrombus formation is related to the stagnant blood flow, which is depicted by spontaneous echo contrast. Left atrial thrombus is predominantly found in patients with mitral stenosis and/or atrial fibrillation due to stagnation of blood in the left atrium. The spontaneous echo contrast is seen in a dilated left atrium showing

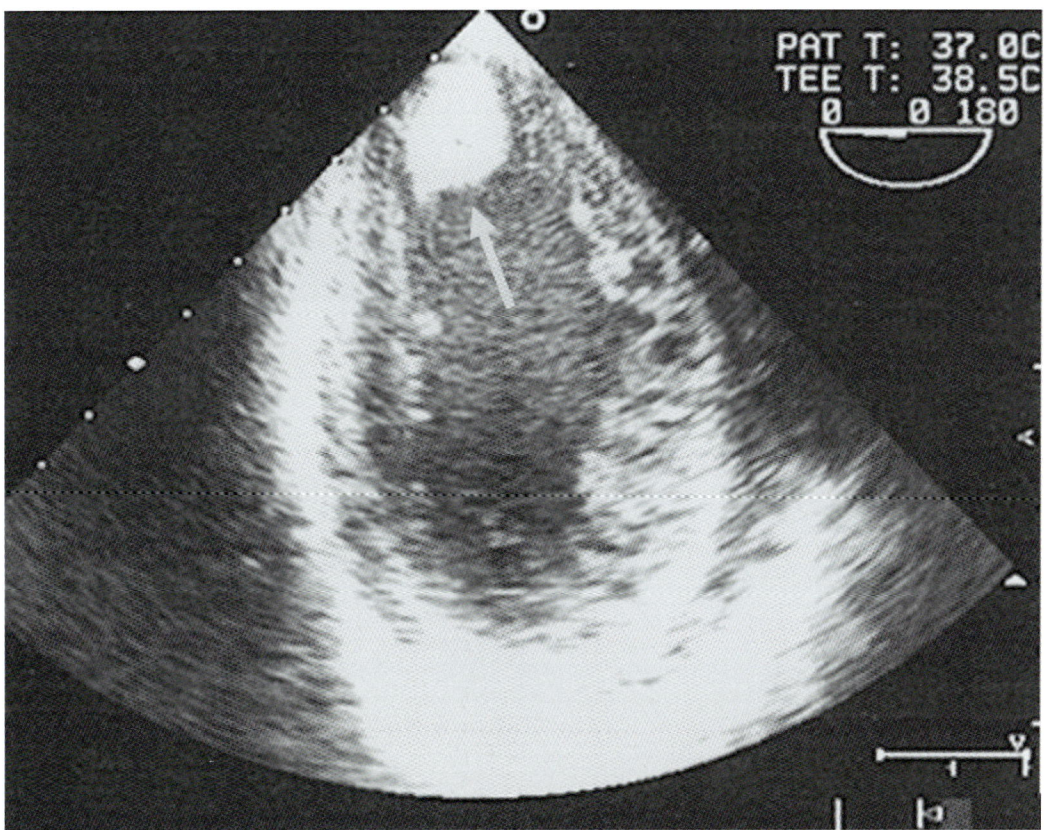

Fig. 10.1: Transgastric short-axis view of the left ventricle in a patient with inferior wall myocardial infarction. Note the aneurysm in inferior wall with a thrombus (arrow).

slow whirling movement. Left atrial appendage is the most common site of thrombus formation, but it can also be found in the body or the posterior wall of the left atrium. Left ventricular thrombus is often associated with myocardial infarction or left ventricular aneurysm. Pulmonary thrombus is generally the result of embolism from the veins of the pelvis and lower extremities.

The most common primary tumor of the heart is myxoma. It is pathologically benign, but is fragile and can cause systemic embolism. It appears as a soft and mobile mass on TEE. The left atrial myxoma is more common than the right atrial myxoma with an attachment to the interatrial septum. The mobile tumor in the left atrium can occlude the mitral valve opening during diastole leading to symptoms of mitral stenosis.

In this chapter, some of the intracardiac masses have been shown.

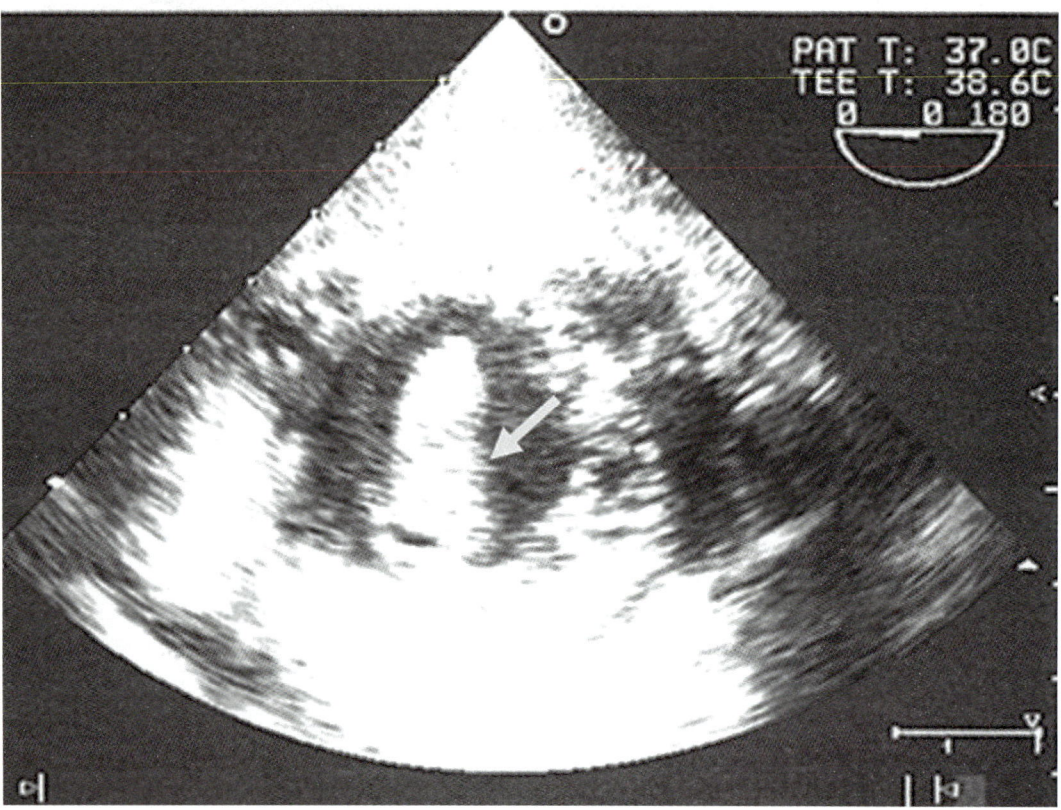

Fig. 10.2: Transgastric short-axis view of the left ventricle in a patient with anterior wall myocardial infarction. Note the apical aneurysm with a thrombus (arrow).

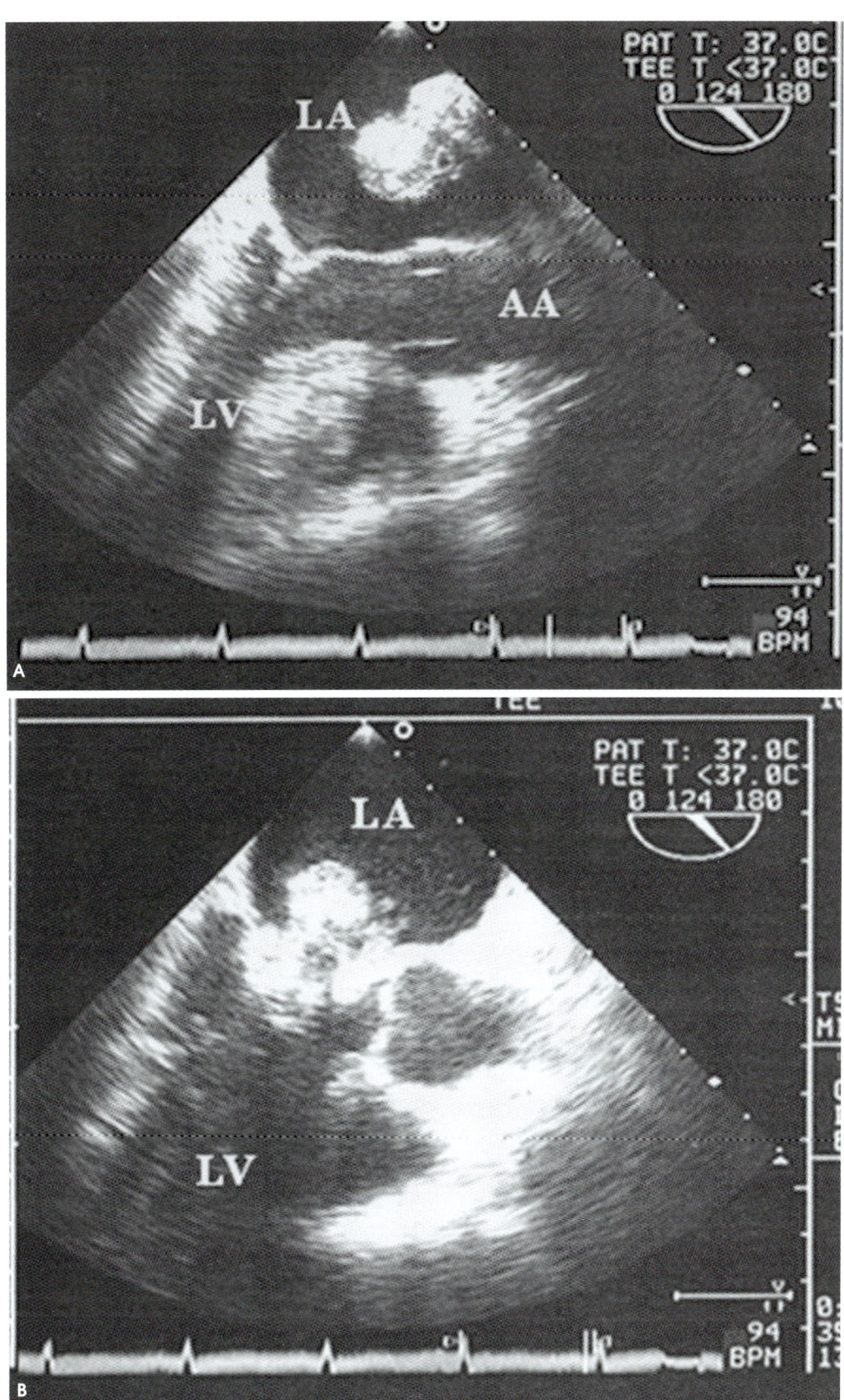

Fig. 10.3: A mobile left atrial myxoma. Note the to and fro movement of the myxoma in the left atrium in systole (A) and diastole (B) causing mitral valve obstruction. (LA: left atrium, LV: left ventricle, AA: ascending aorta).

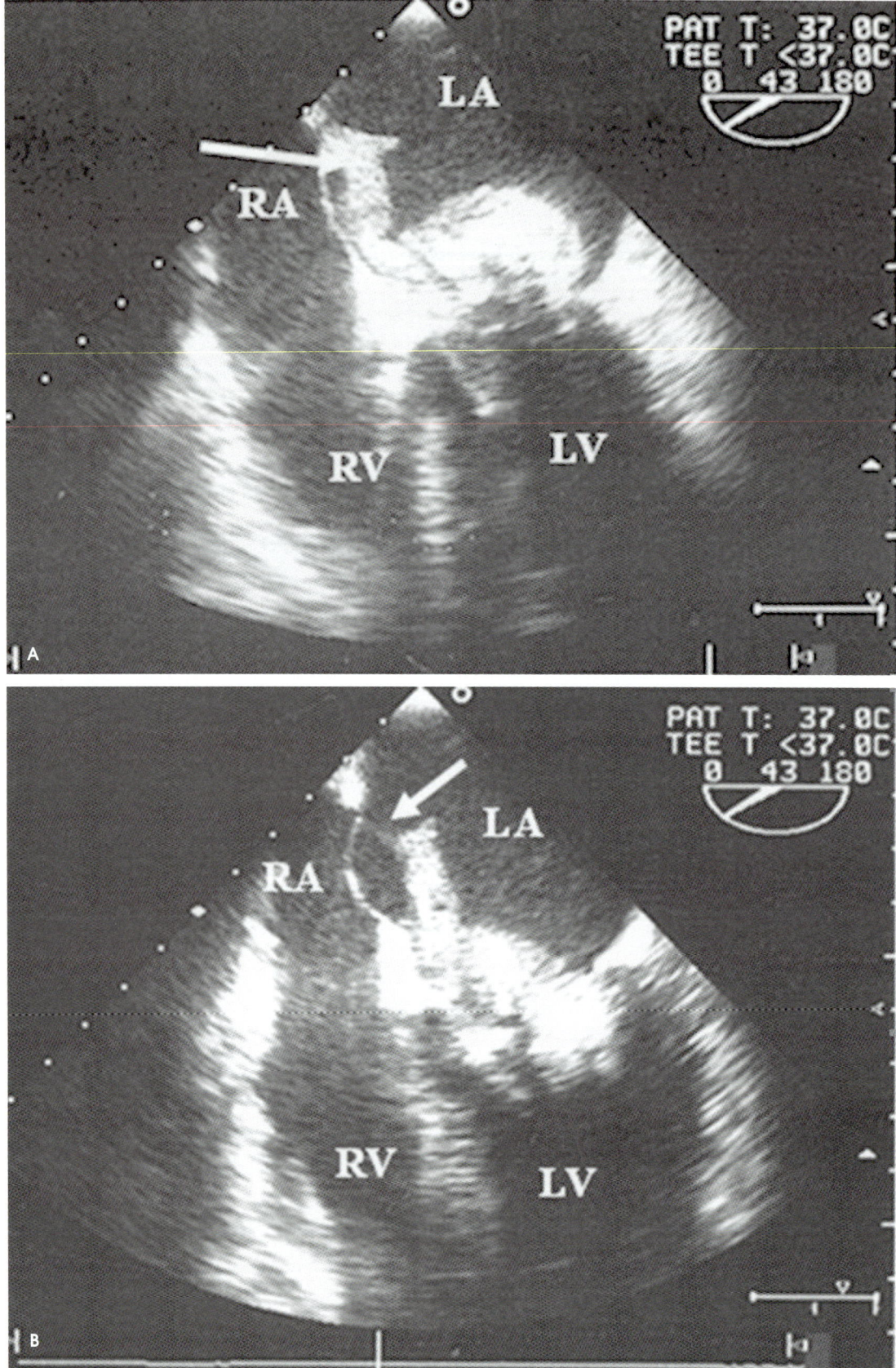

Fig. 10.4: A large left atrial myxoma obstructing the mitral valve. Note the peduncle (arrow) of the myxoma arising from the inter-atrial septum. (LA: Left atrium, LV: left ventricle, RA: right atrium, RV: right ventricle).

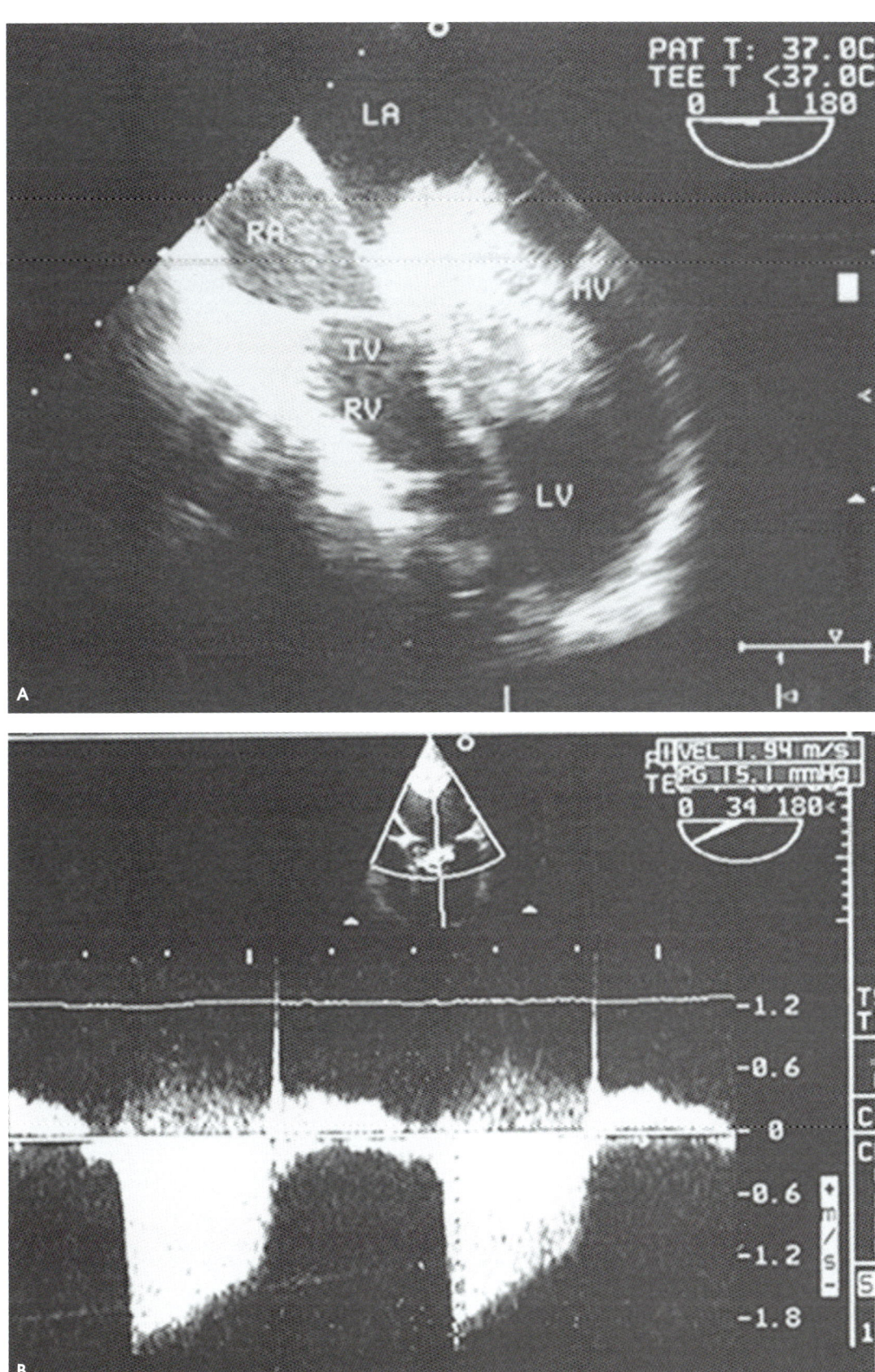

Fig. 10.5: A: A large left atrial myxoma prolapsing across the mitral valve. B: Note the continuous wave Doppler across the mitral valve showing a large transmitral gradient. (LA: left atrium, RA: right atrium, RV: right ventricle, LV: left ventricle, TV: tricuspid valve, MV: mitral valve).

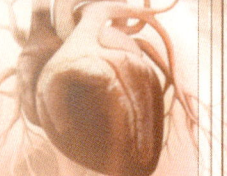

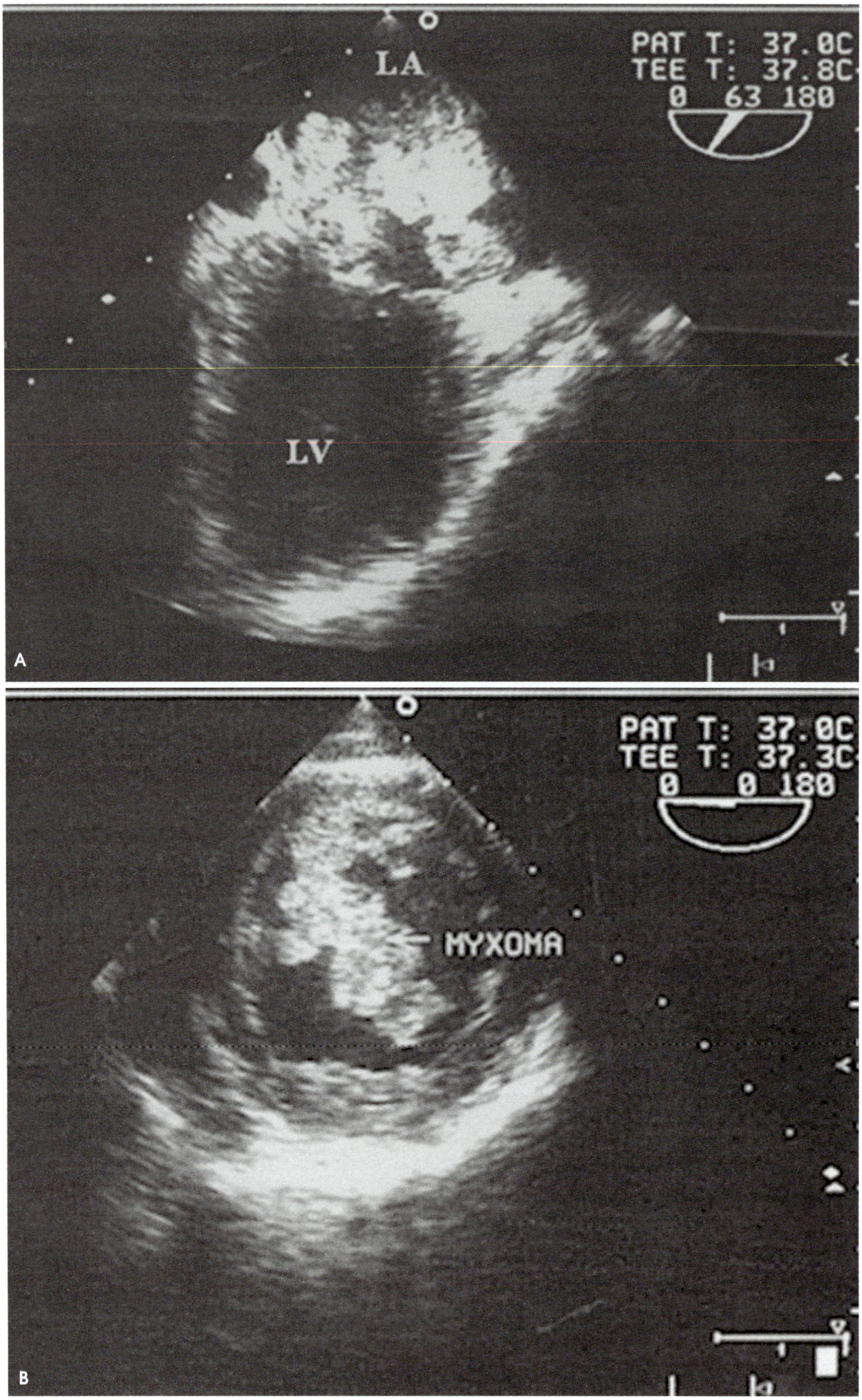

Fig. 10.6: Panel A: Midesophageal two-chamber view showing a fragile left atrial myxoma with a variegated appearance. Panel B is the short-axis transgastric view in the same patient showing a portion of the myxoma prolapsing into the left ventricle. (LA: left atrium, LV: left ventricle).

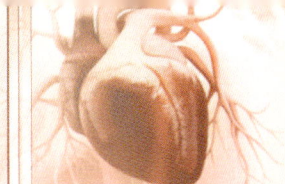

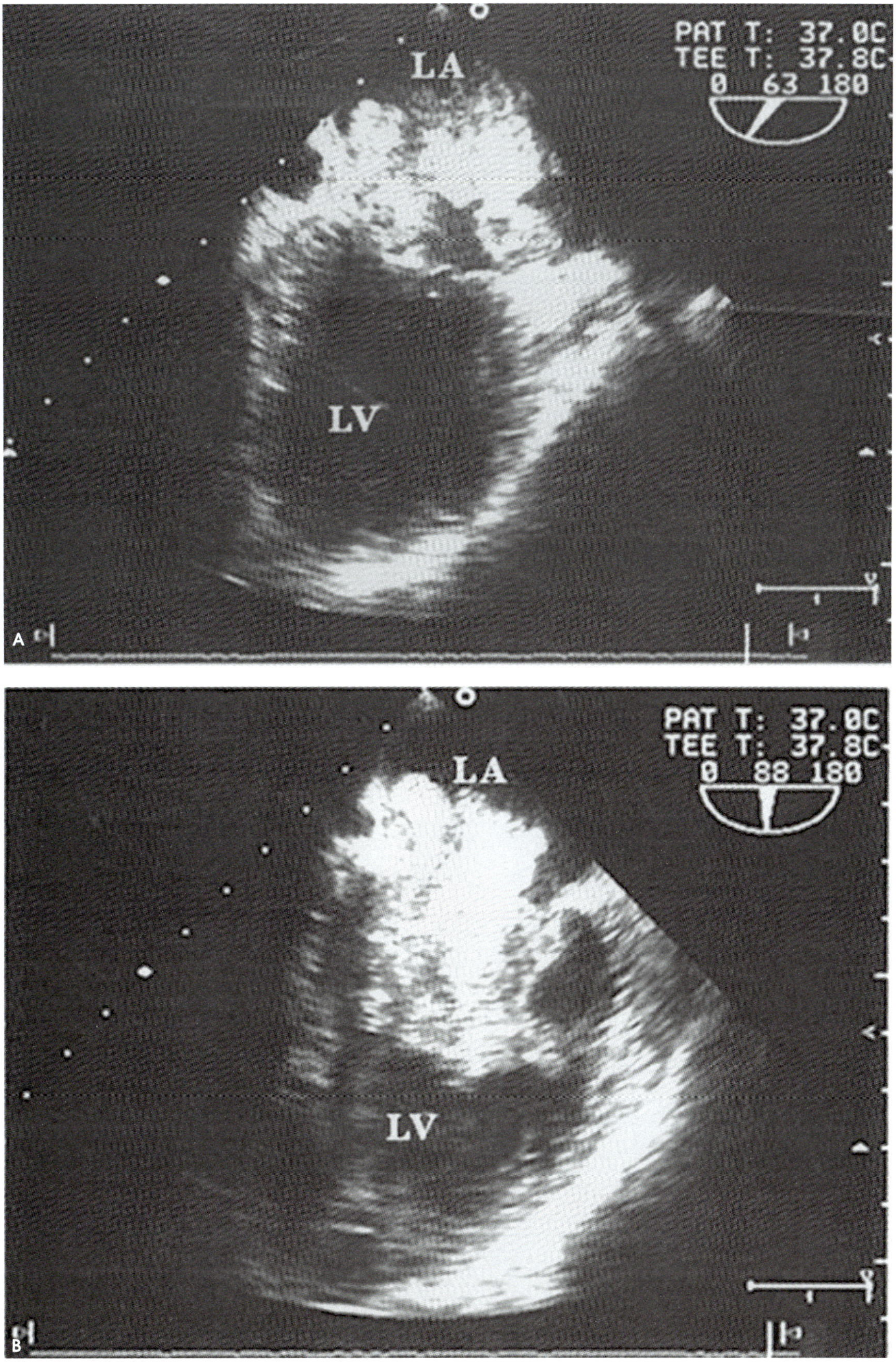

Fig. 10.7: A large mobile left atrial myxoma. Note the variegated appearance and the to and fro motion across the mitral valve in systole (A) and diastole (B). (LA: left atrium, LV: left ventricle).

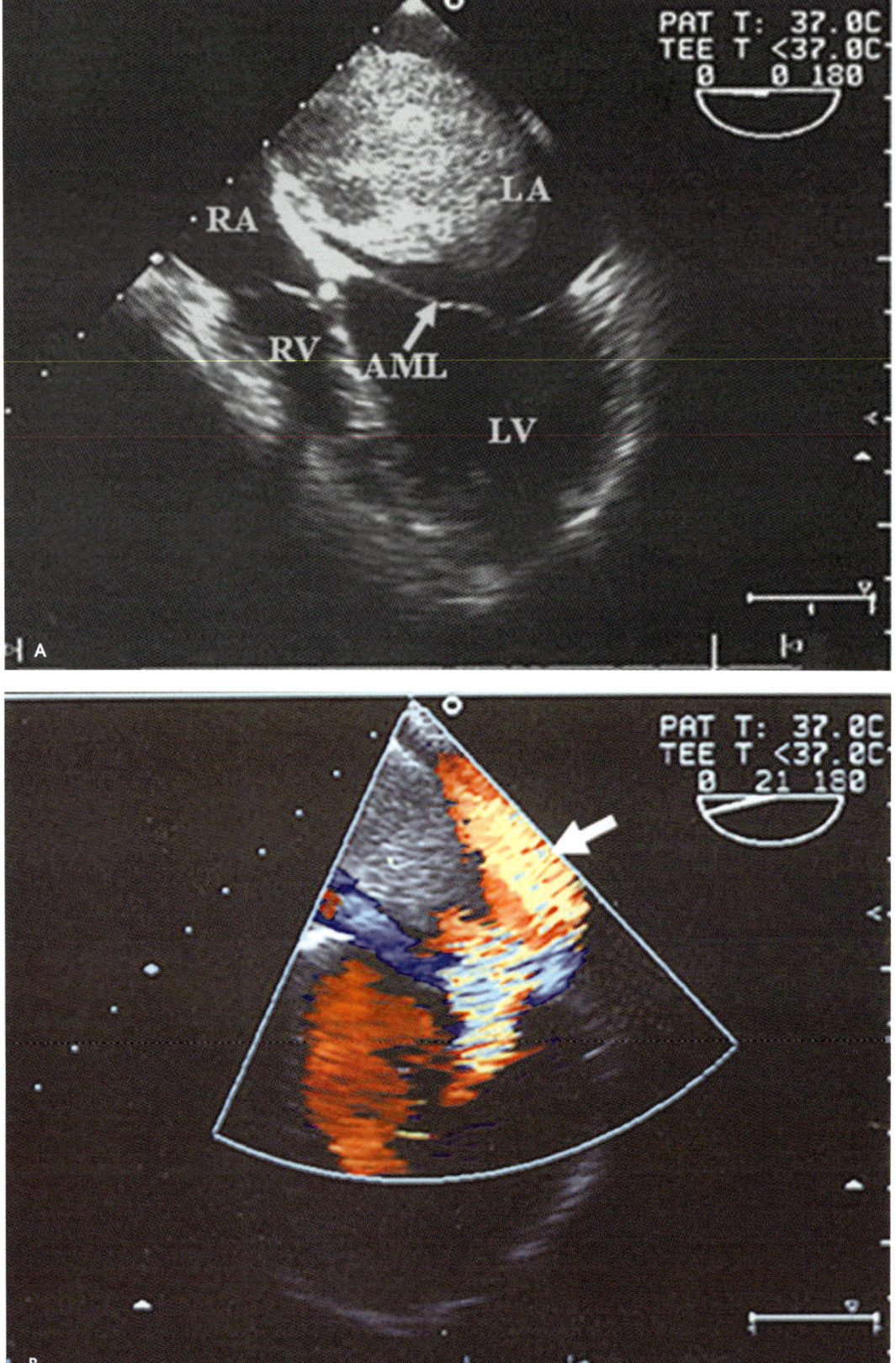

Fig. 10.8: (A) A large left atrial myxoma arising from the inter-atrial septum and projecting over the anterior mitral leaflet (AML). (B) Note the mitral regurgitant jet (arrow) resulting from improper coaptation of the mitral leaflets. (LA: left atrium, RA: right atrium, RV: right ventricle, LV: left ventricle).

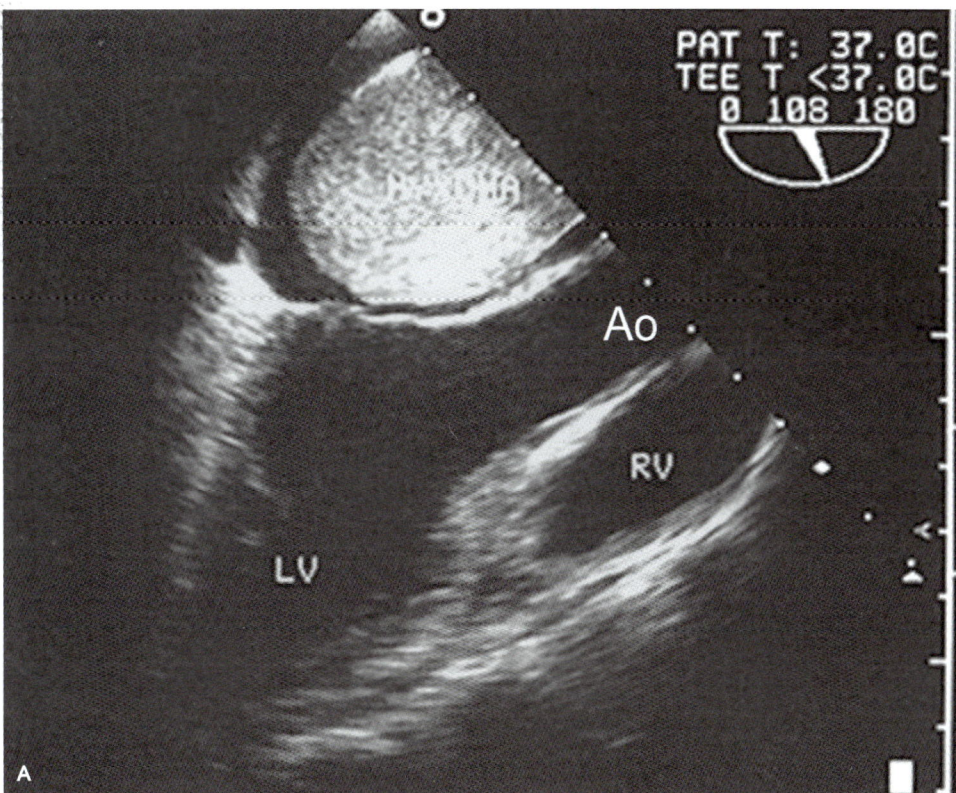

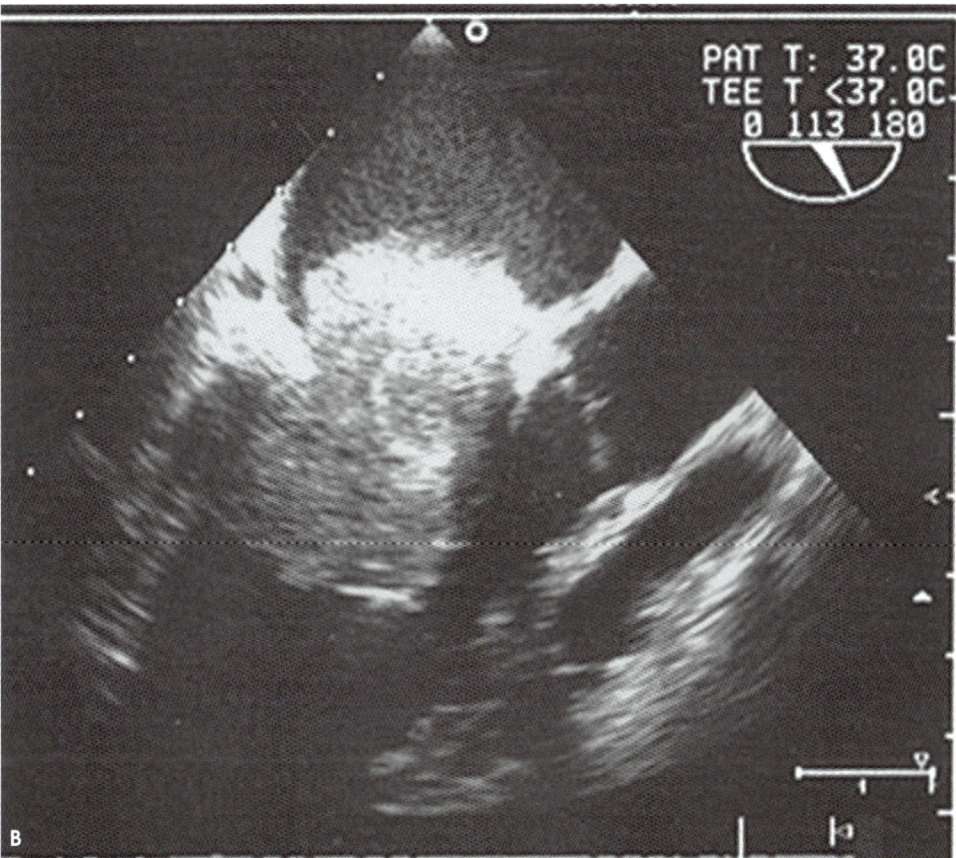

Fig. 10.9: Midesophageal long-axis view of left atrial myxoma in systole (A). The mass is seen to prolapse into the left ventricle in diastole (B). (LV: left ventricle, RV: right ventricle, Ao: aorta).

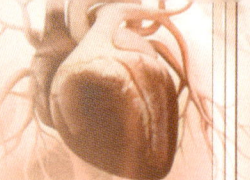

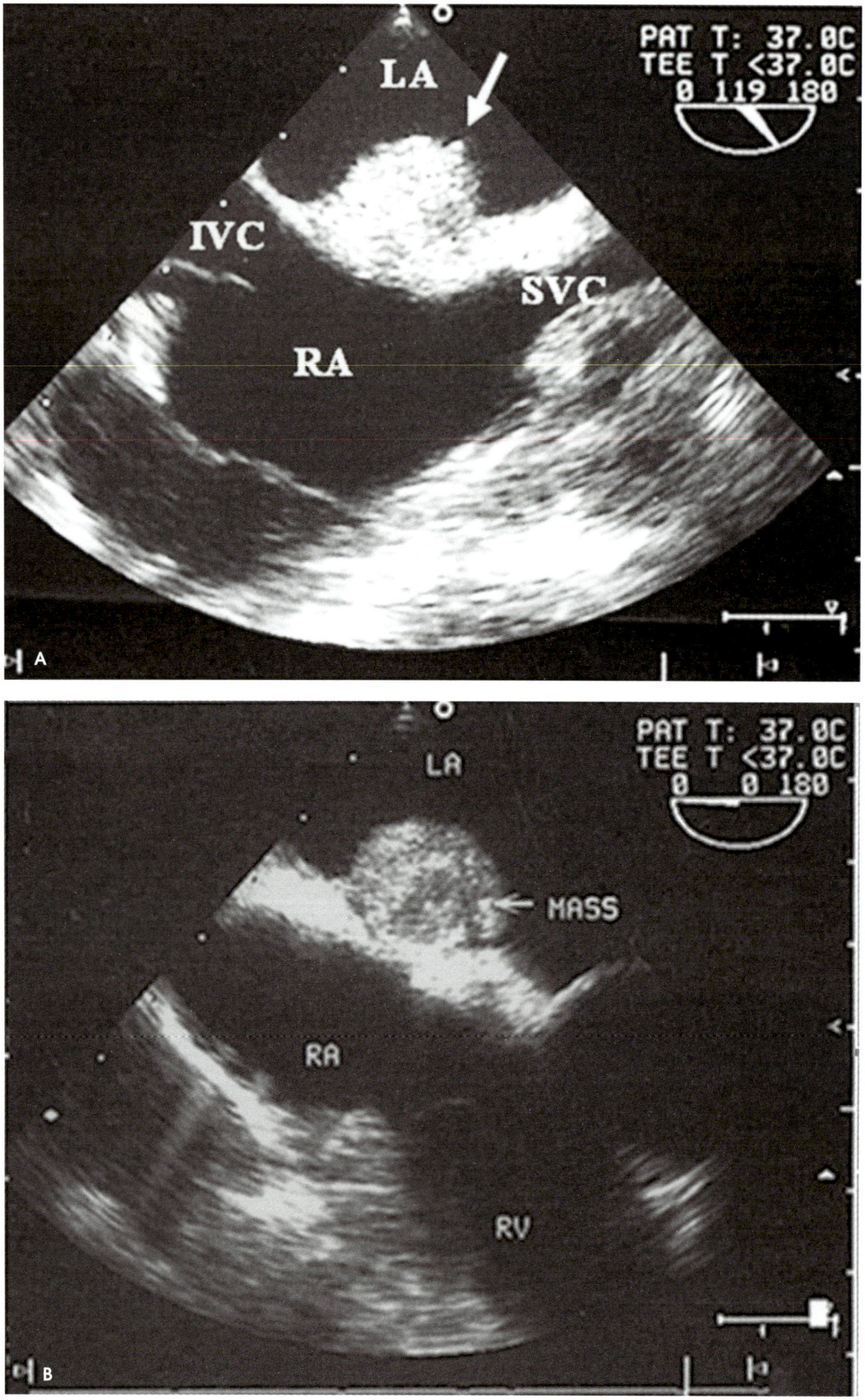

Fig. 10.10: A small left atrial myxoma (arrow) arising from the inter-atrial septum. (A) Bicaval view, (B) Four-chamber view (LA: left atrium, RA: right atrium, RV: right ventricle, SVC: superior vena cava, IVC: inferior vena cava).

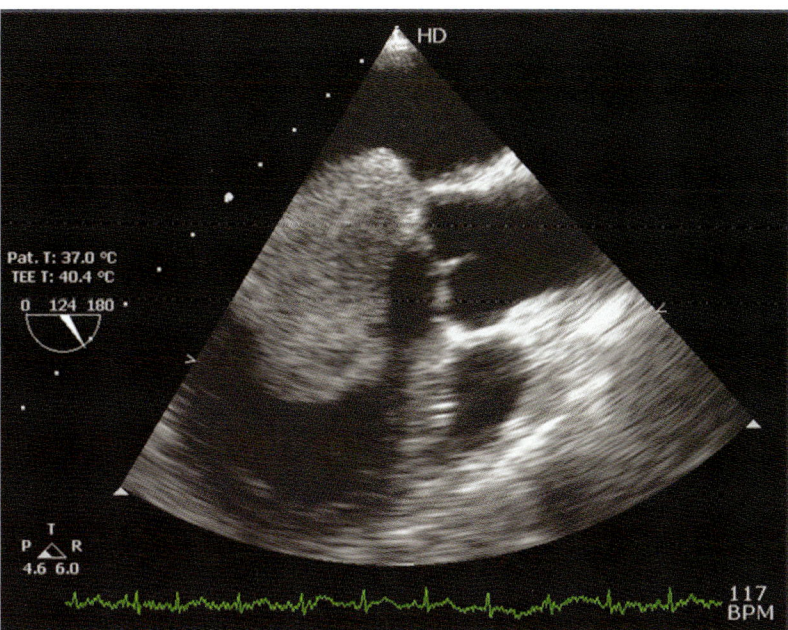

Fig. 10.11: Midesophageal aortic valve long-axis view showing a left atrial myxoma prolapsing into the left ventricle in diastole and obstructing the left ventricular outflow tract.

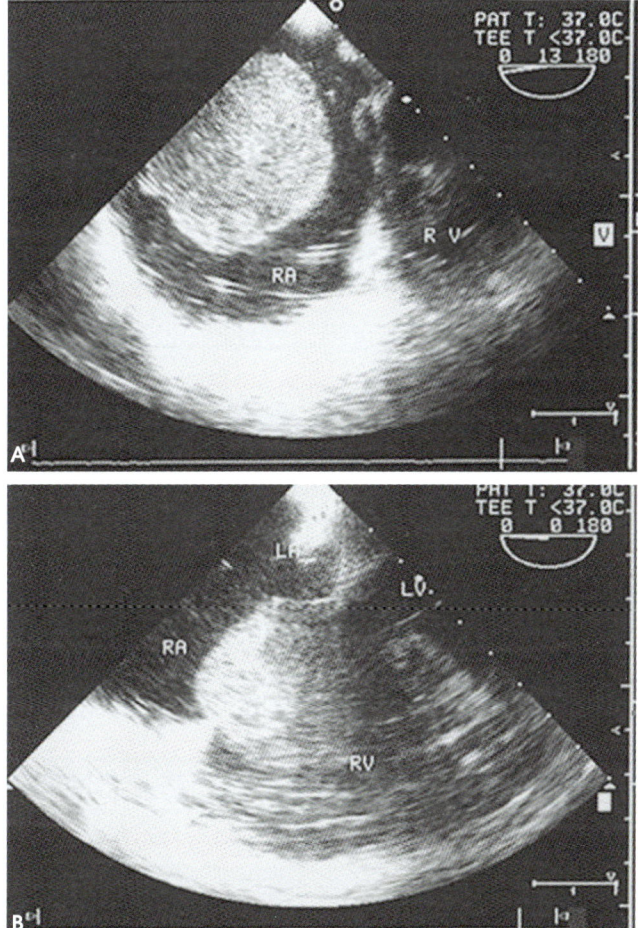

Fig. 10.12A and B: A large right atrial myxoma prolapsing across the tricuspid valve (LA: left atrium, RA: right atrium, RV: right ventricle, LV: left ventricle).

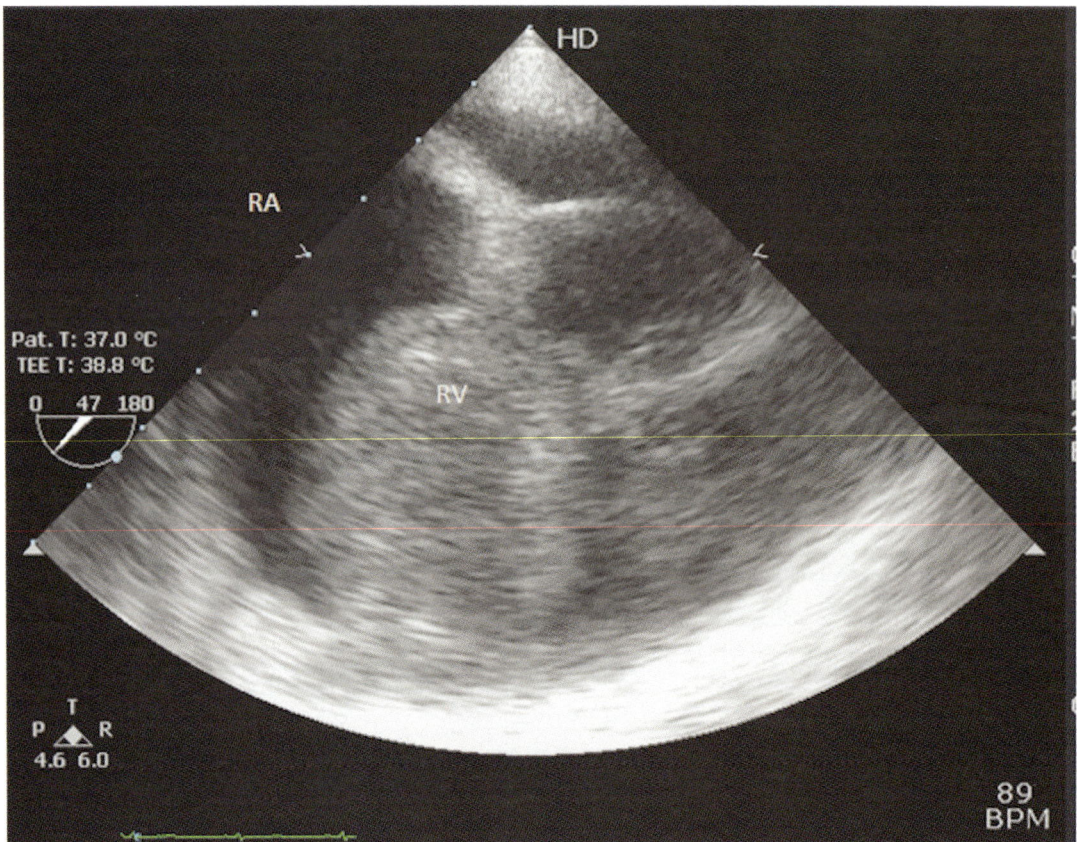

Fig. 10.13: A large right atrial myxoma prolapsing into right ventricle (RA: right atrium, RV: right ventricle).

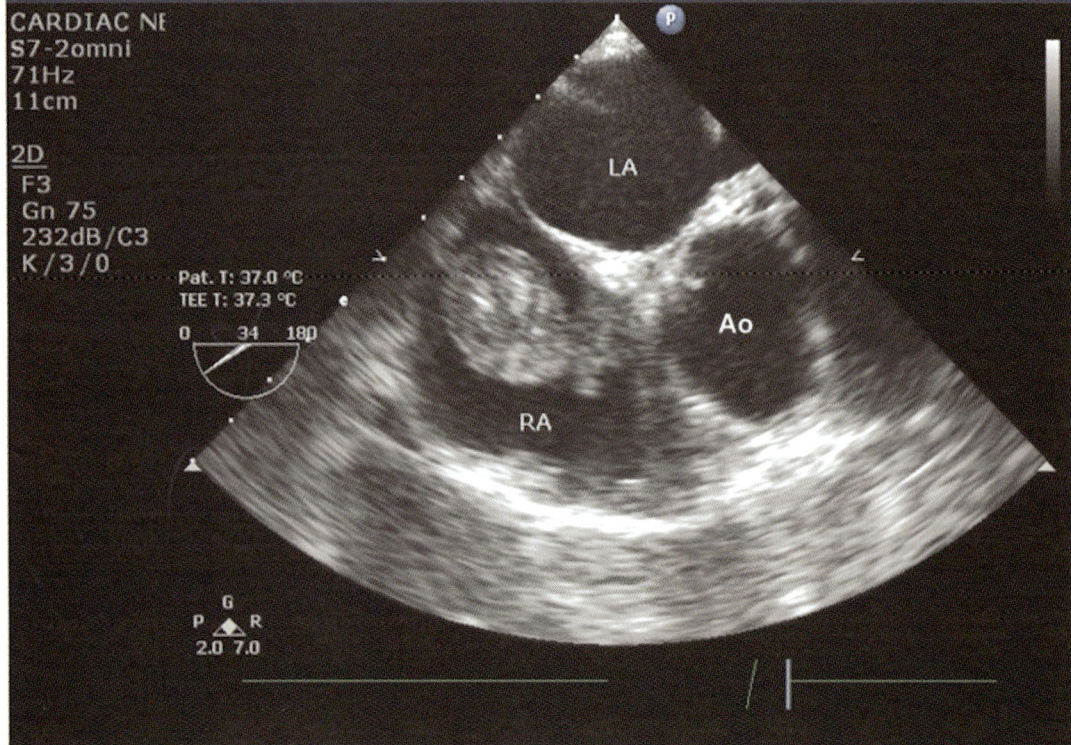

Fig. 10.14: Another patient with a relatively smaller right atrial myxoma (RA: right atrium, LA: left atrium, Ao: aorta).

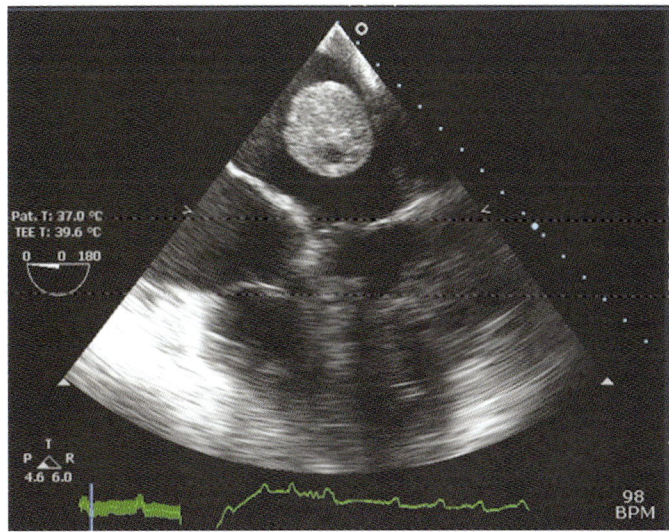

Fig. 10.15: Midesophageal four-chamber view showing a freely mobile mass in the left atrium, turned out to be a thrombus on histopathology (*refer* to the video).

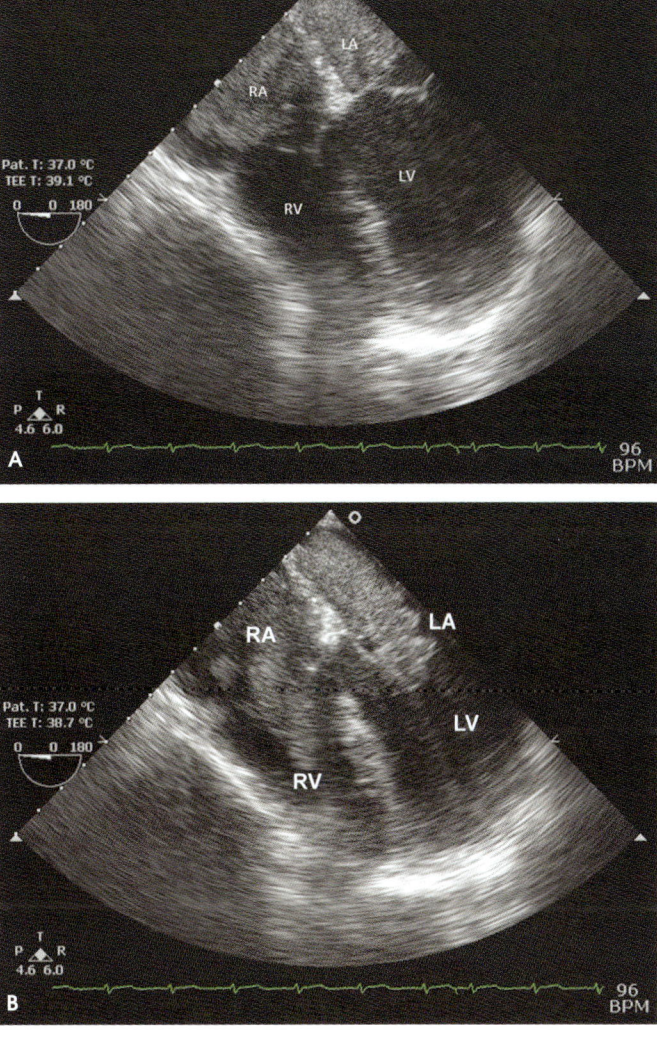

Fig. 10.16: Midesophageal four-chamber view showing biatrial myxoma in systole (A) and prolapsing into their respective ventricles in diastole (B). (RA: right atrium , LA: left atrium, RV: right ventricle, LV: left ventricle).

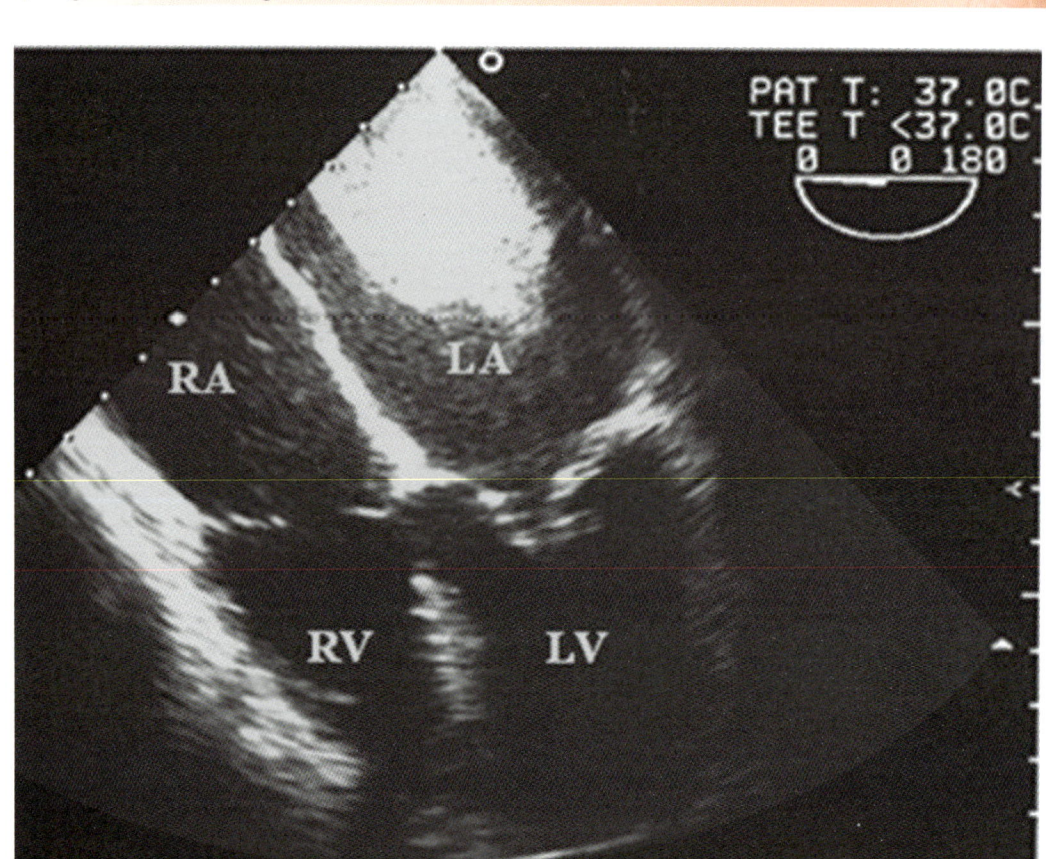

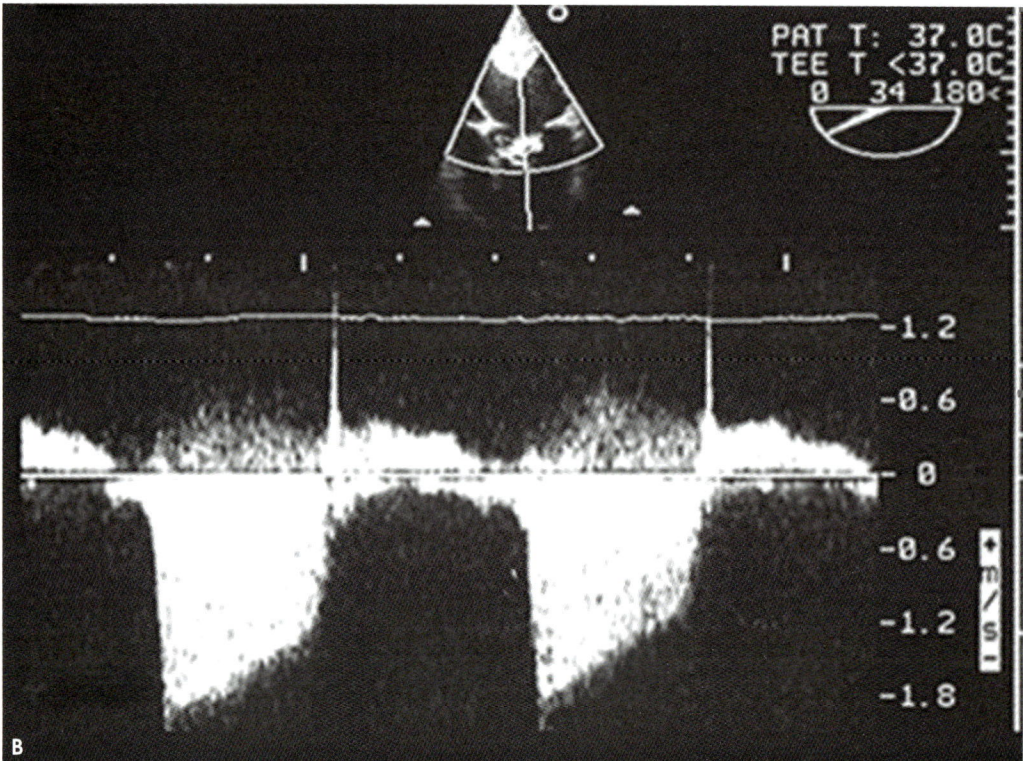

Fig. 10.17: (A) Four-chamber view showing a large left atrial thrombus in a patient with rheumatic mitral stenosis. (B) Transmitral continuous wave Doppler in the same patient showed a peak gradient of 14 mm Hg and mean gradient of 9 mm Hg (RA: right atrium, LA: left atrium, RV: right ventricle, LV: left ventricle).

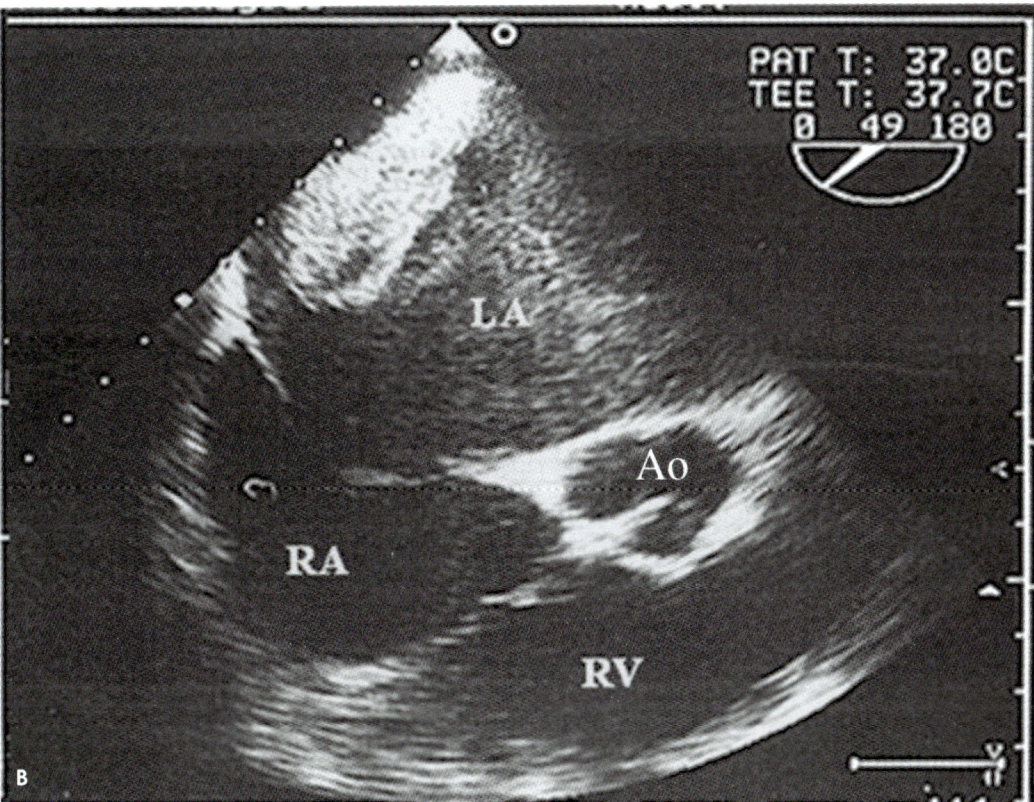

Fig. 10.18A and B: Spontaneous echo contrast and left atrial thrombus (arrow) in a patient with rheumatic mitral stenosis (LA: left atrium, RA: right atrium, RV: right ventricle, LV: left ventricle, Ao: aorta).

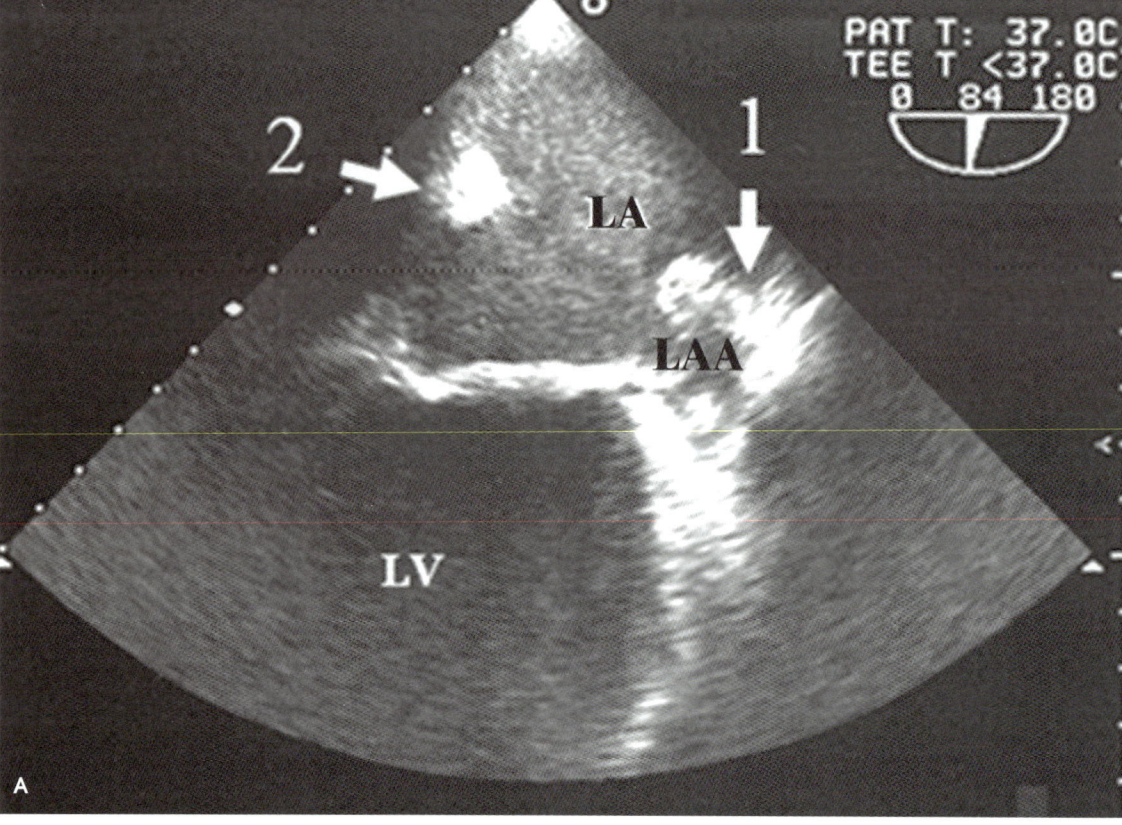

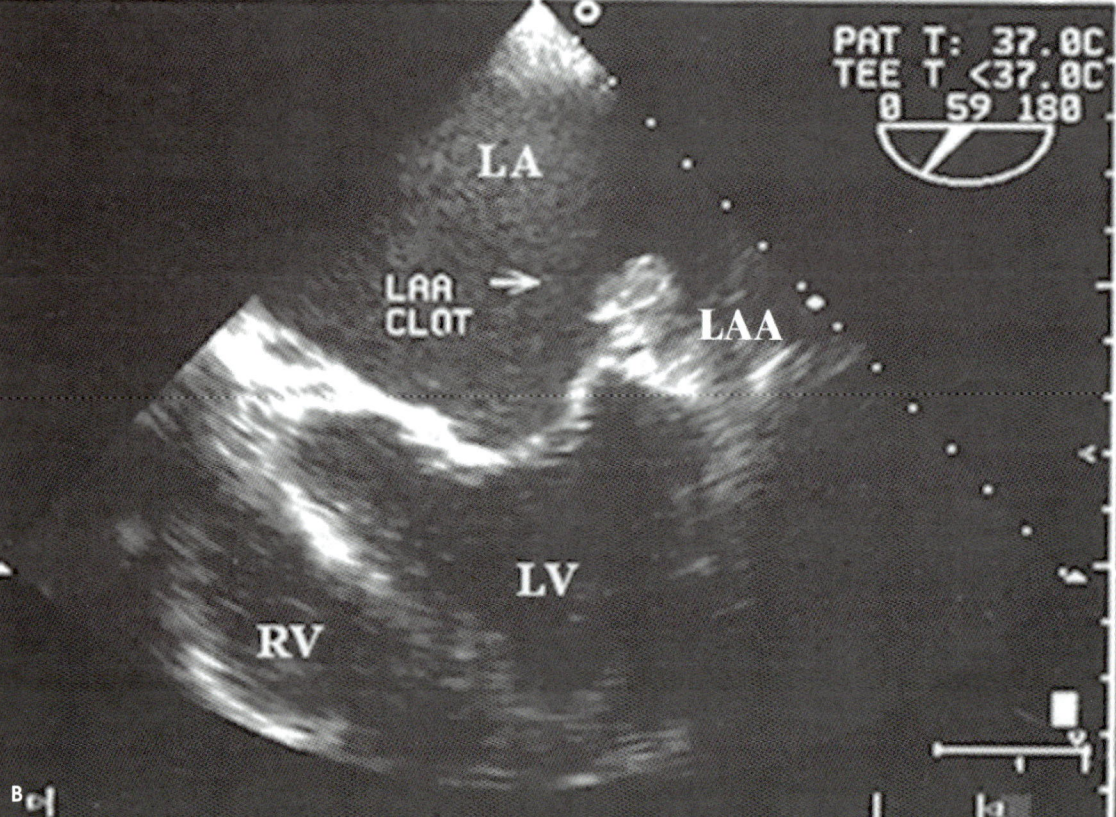

Fig. 10.19: Left atrial appendage thrombus (arrow 1 in panel A and Panel B) and left atrial body thrombus (arrow 2) in a patient with severe mitral stenosis. (LA: left atrium, LV: left ventricle, RV: right ventricle, LAA: left atrial appendage).

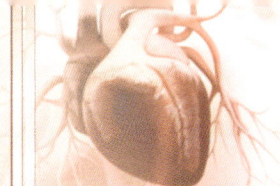

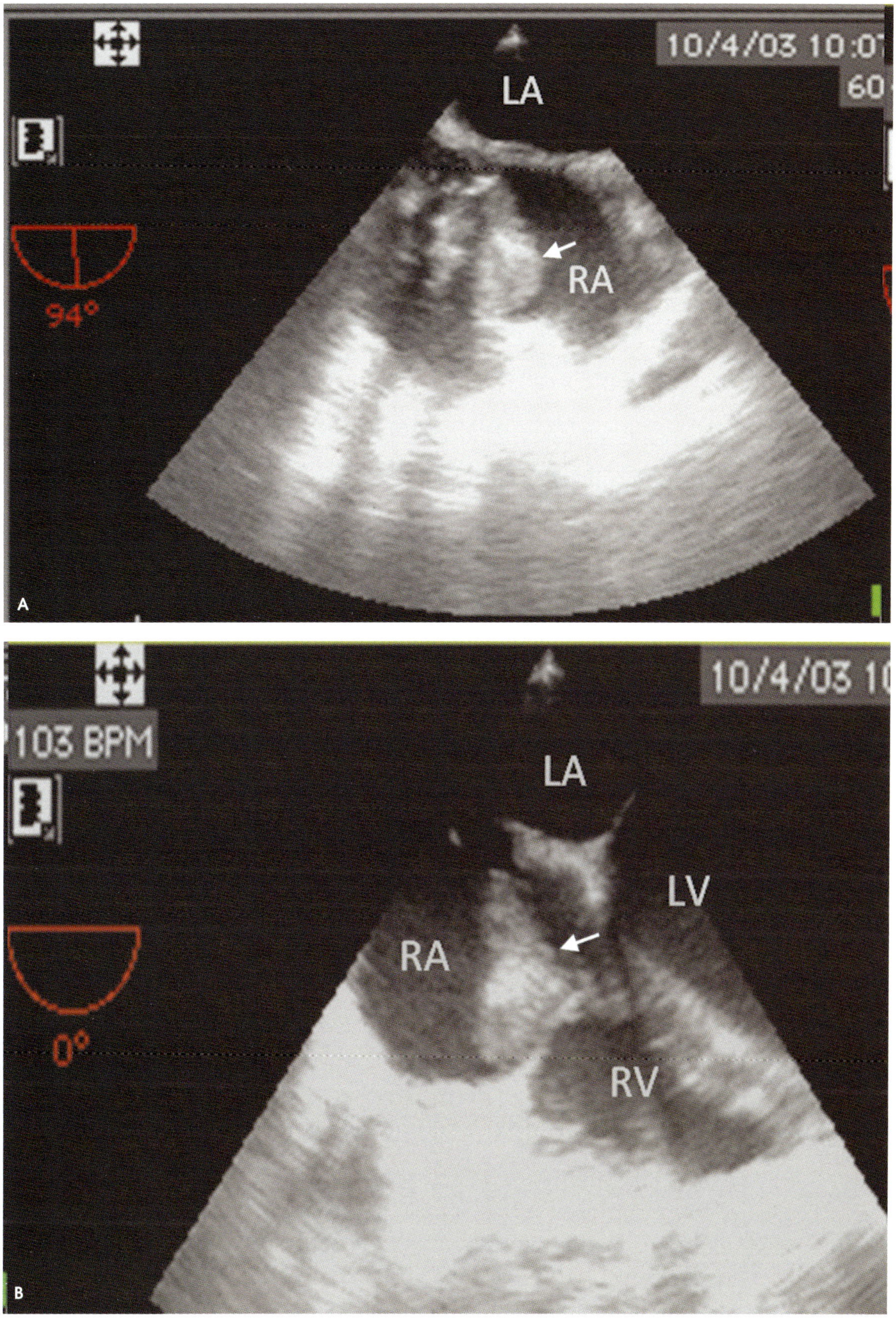

Fig. 10.20: Right atrial thrombus (arrow) in bicaval view (A) and four-chamber view (B) (LA: left atrium, RA: right atrium, LV: left ventricle, RV: right ventricle).

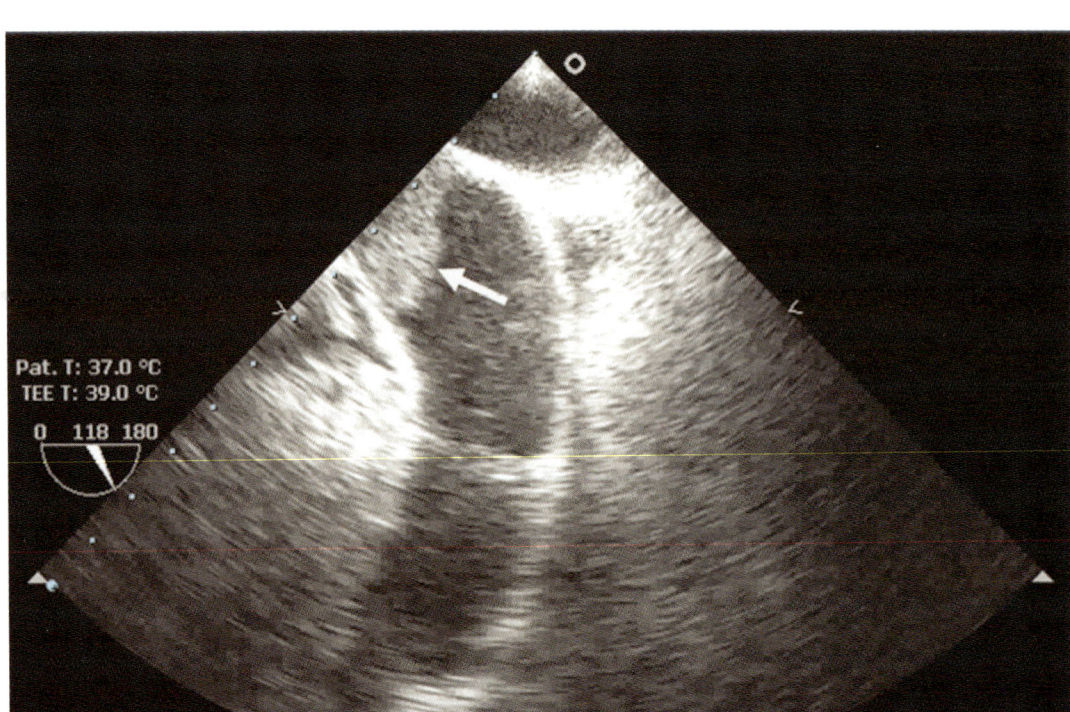

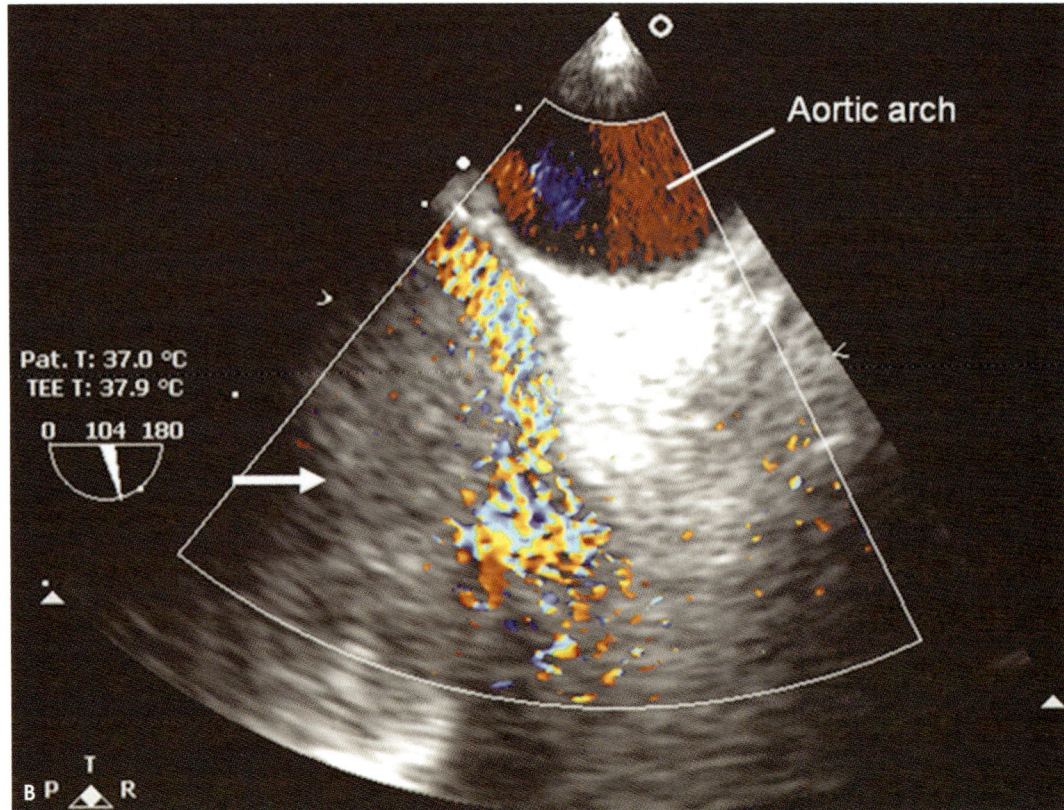

Fig. 10.21: Upper esophageal aortic arch short-axis view showing a mass in the main pulmonary artery (A), (arrow) causing turbulent flow (B). Arrow shows homogenous mass occupying the main pulmonary artery .

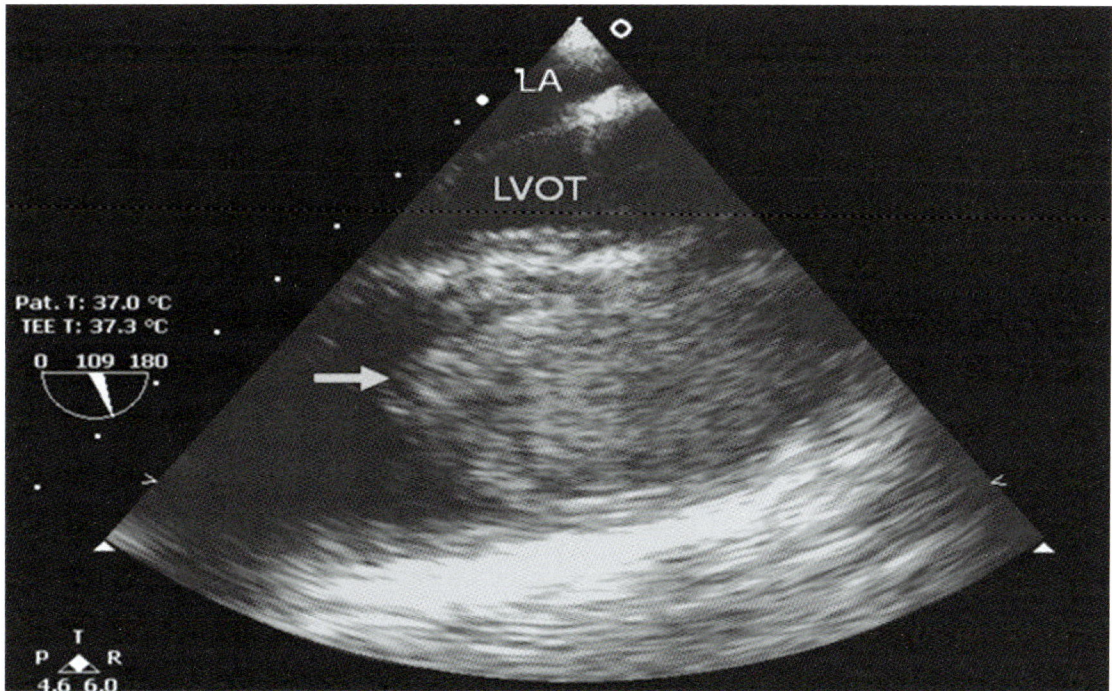

Fig. 10.22: Midesophageal long-axis view showing a homogenous mass (arrow) occupying the right ventricular outflow tract (LA: left atrium, LVOT: left ventricular outflow tract).

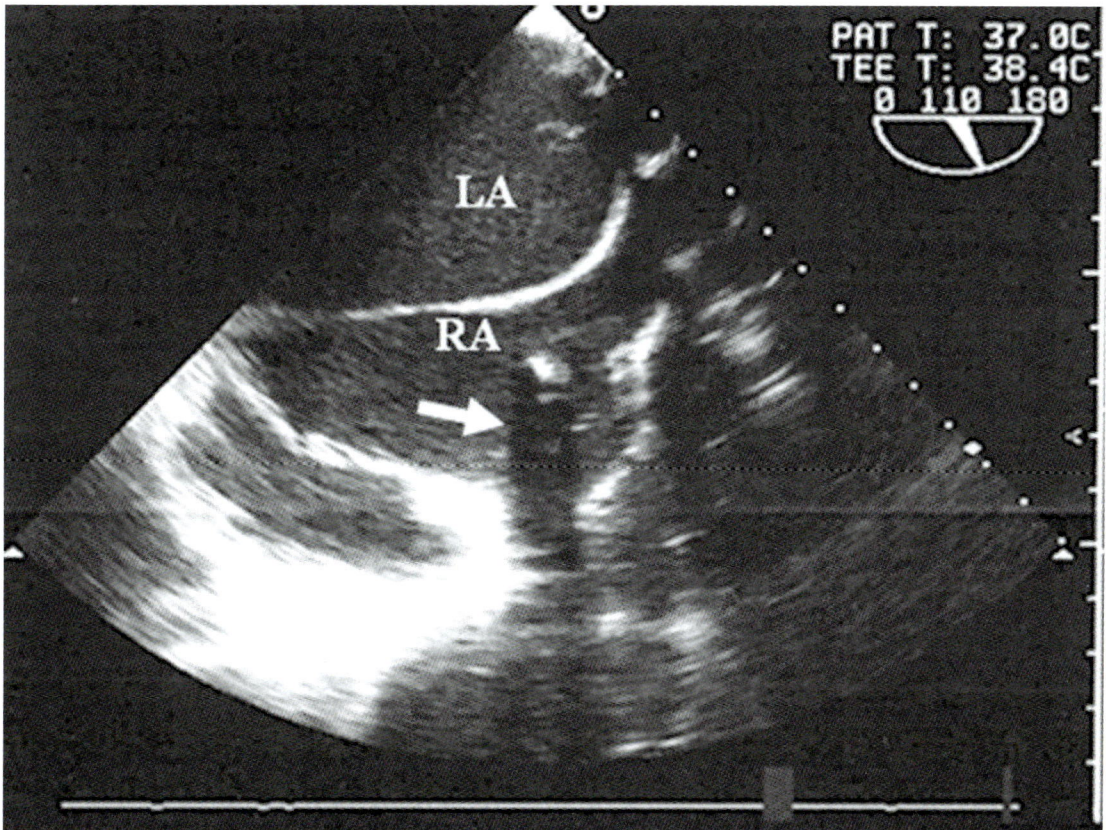

Fig. 10.23: Midesophageal bicaval view showing a venous cannula (arrow) in the right atrium (LA: left atrium, RA: right atrium).

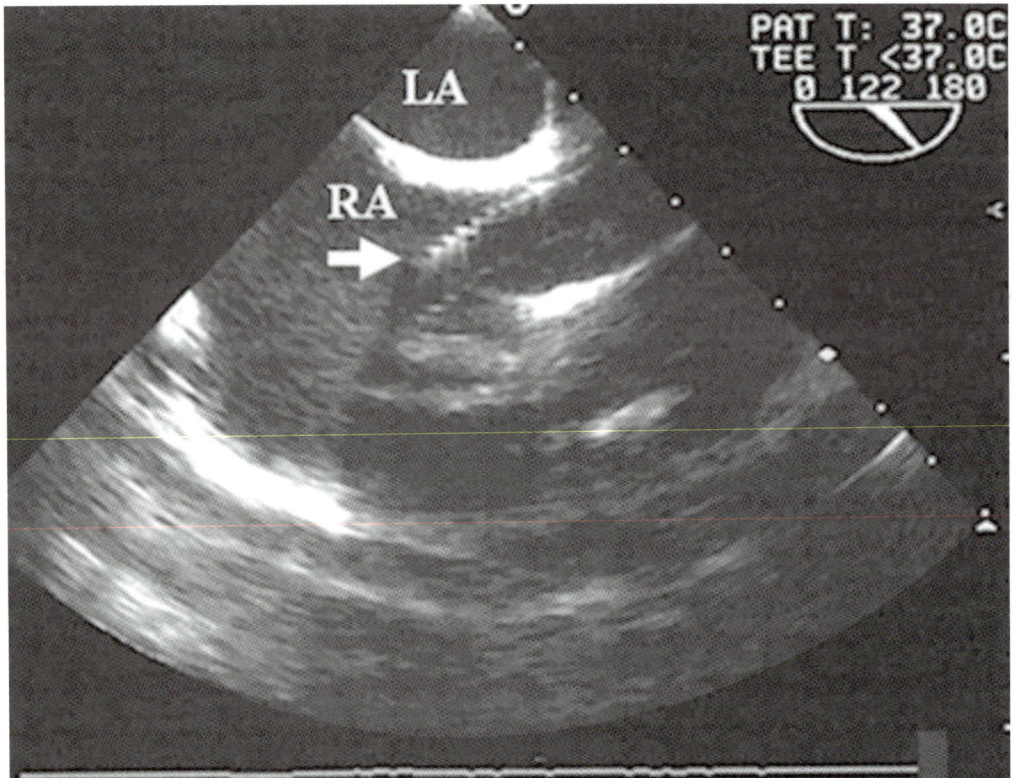

Fig. 10.24: Midesophageal bicaval view showing a venous cannula (arrow) directed in the superior vena cava. (LA: left atrium, RA: right atrium).

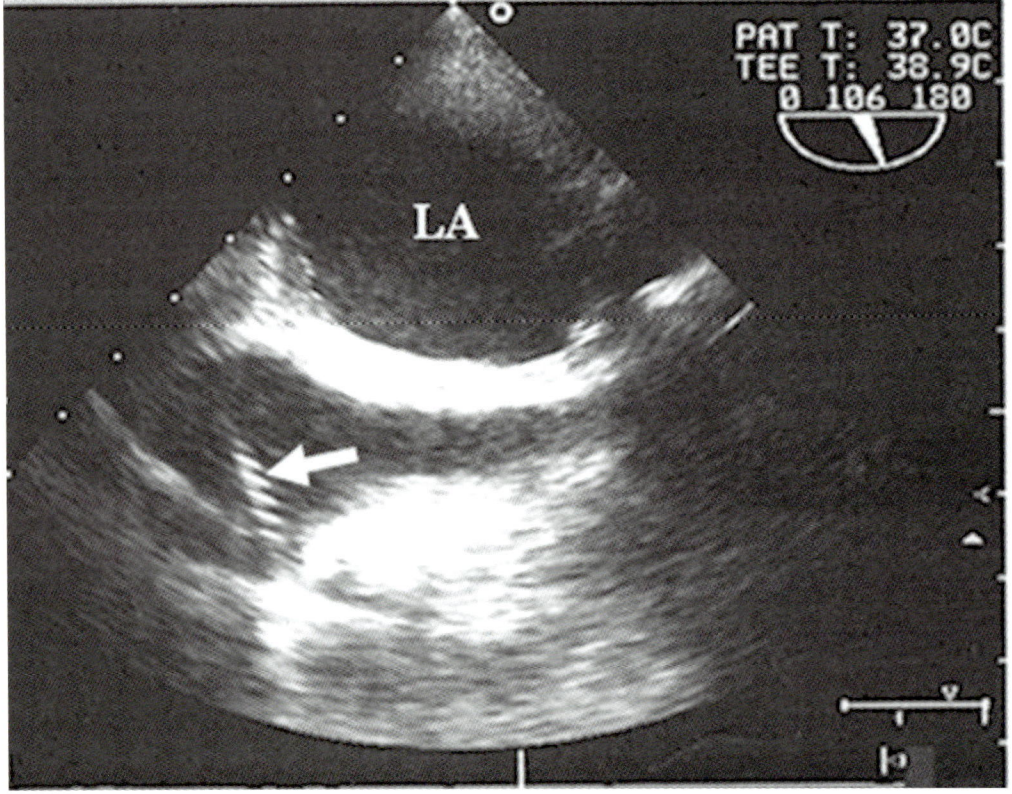

Fig. 10.25: Midesophageal bicaval view showing a venous cannula (arrow) directed in the inferior vena cava. (LA: left atrium).

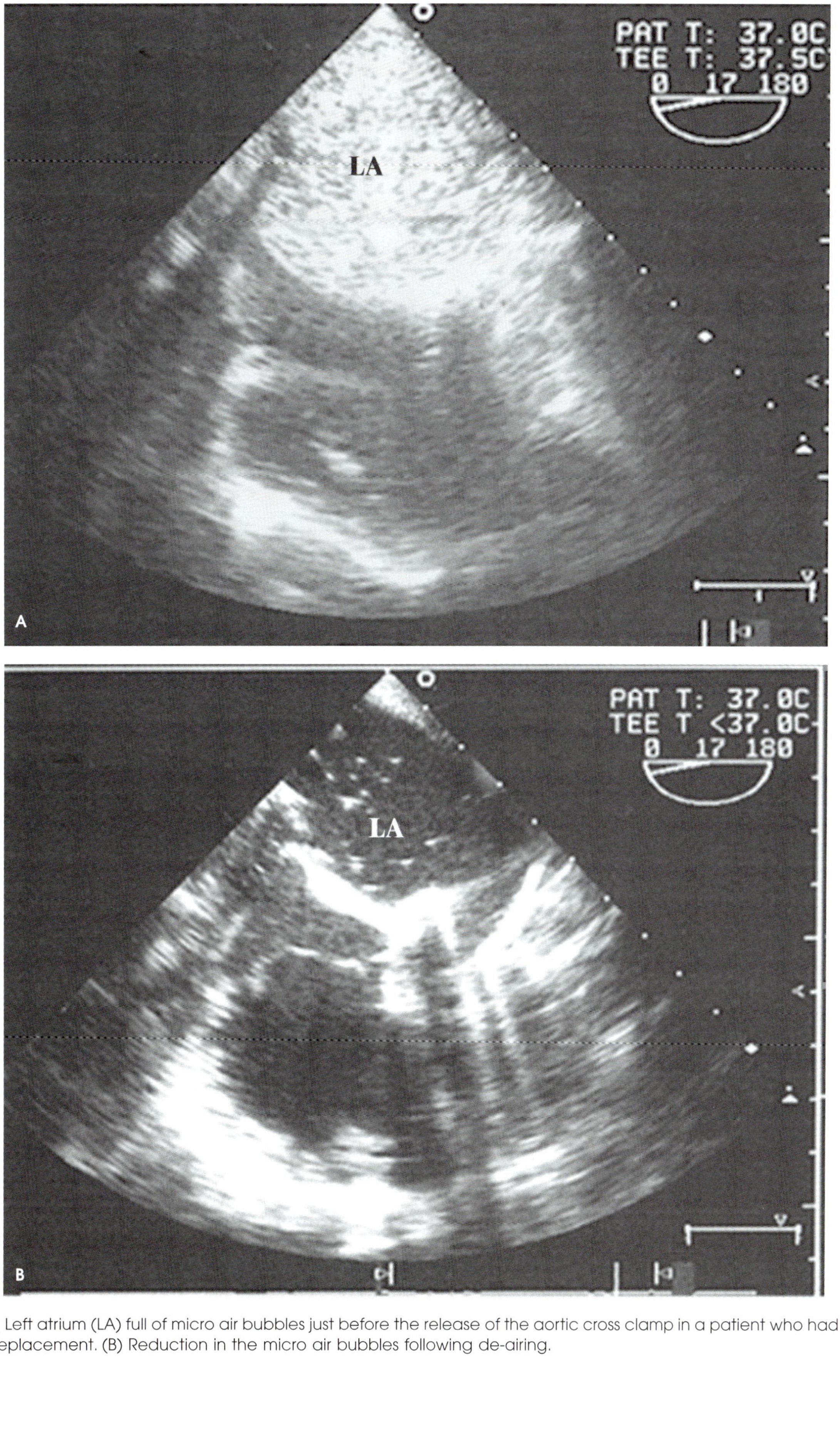

Fig. 10.26: (A) Left atrium (LA) full of micro air bubbles just before the release of the aortic cross clamp in a patient who had undergone mitral valve replacement. (B) Reduction in the micro air bubbles following de-airing.

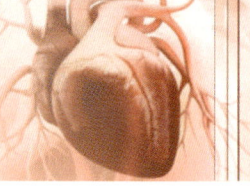

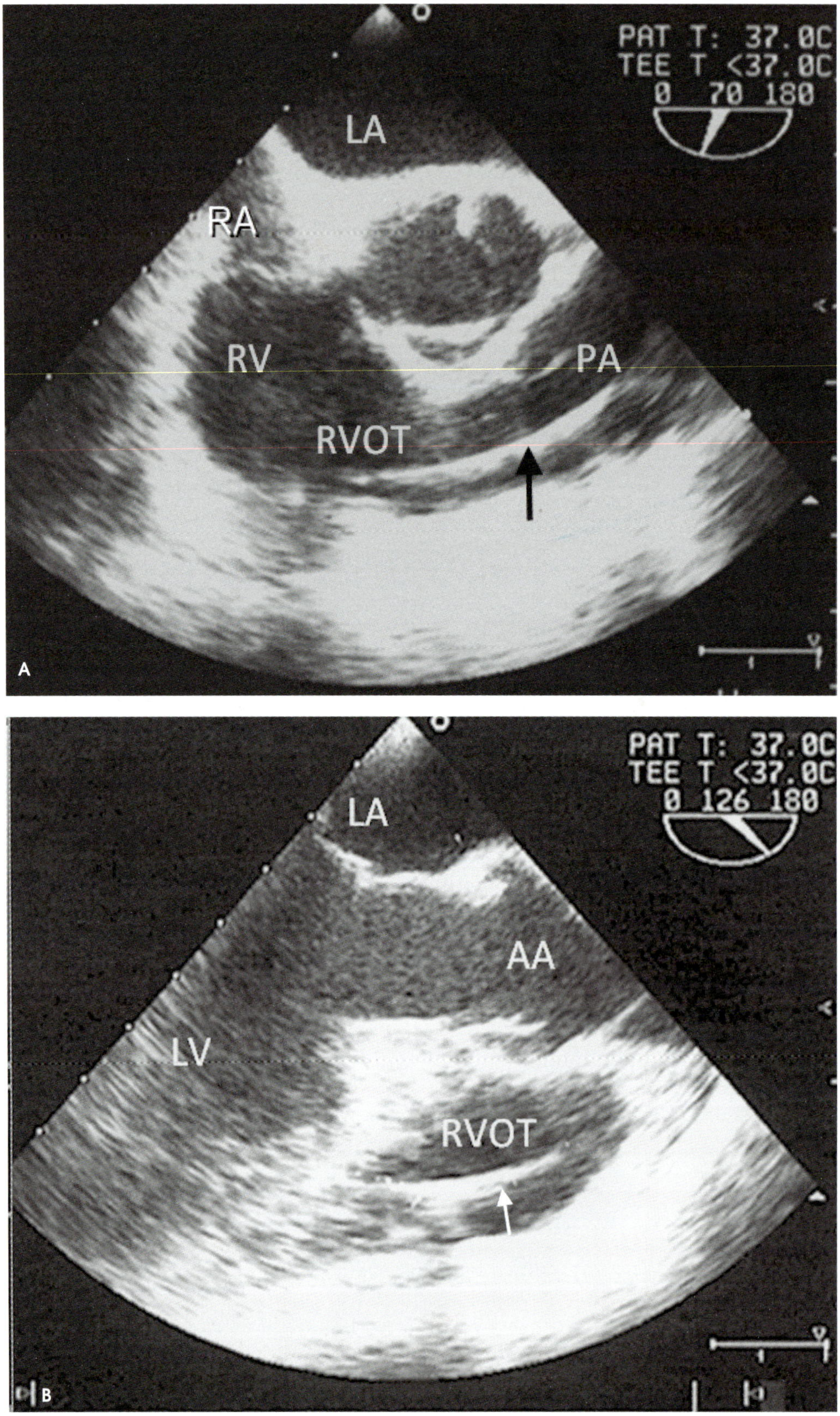

Fig. 10.27: Appearance of the pulmonary artery catheter (arrow) in RV inflow-outflow view (A) and midesophageal long-axis view (B) (LA: left atrium, RA: right atrium, LV: left ventricle, RV: right ventricle, PA: pulmonary artery, AA: ascending aorta, RVOT: right ventricular outflow tract).

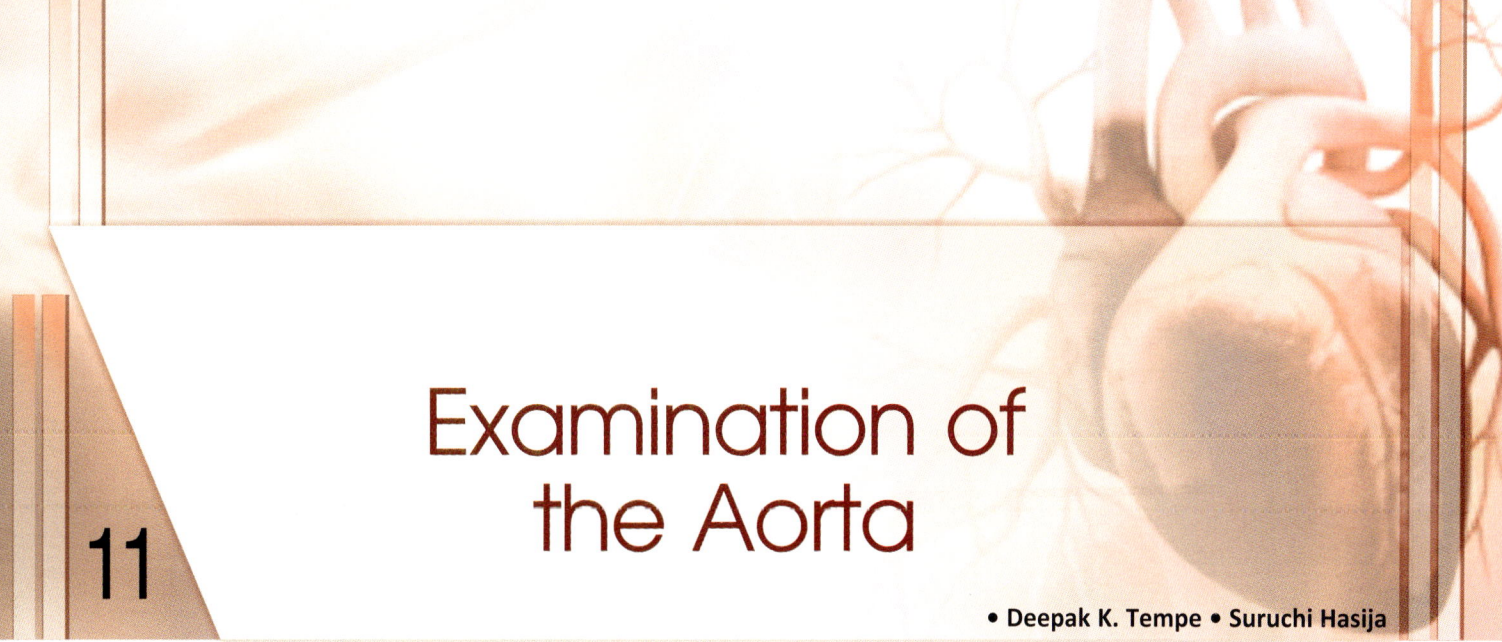

Examination of the Aorta

• Deepak K. Tempe • Suruchi Hasija

11

Examination of the thoracic aorta with transeso-phageal echocardiography (TEE) is an important aspect during the operative period. The examination of the ascending aorta especially with the view to detect atheromas is important in patients undergoing coronary artery bypass grafting. The detection of the atheromas can help to alter the surgical technique so that manipulation of the aorta is avoided. Thereby, the risk of systemic embolization (in particular cerebral) can be prevented. TEE is also an important tool for the diagnosis of dissection of the ascending aorta.

This chapter depicts some images of the aorta.

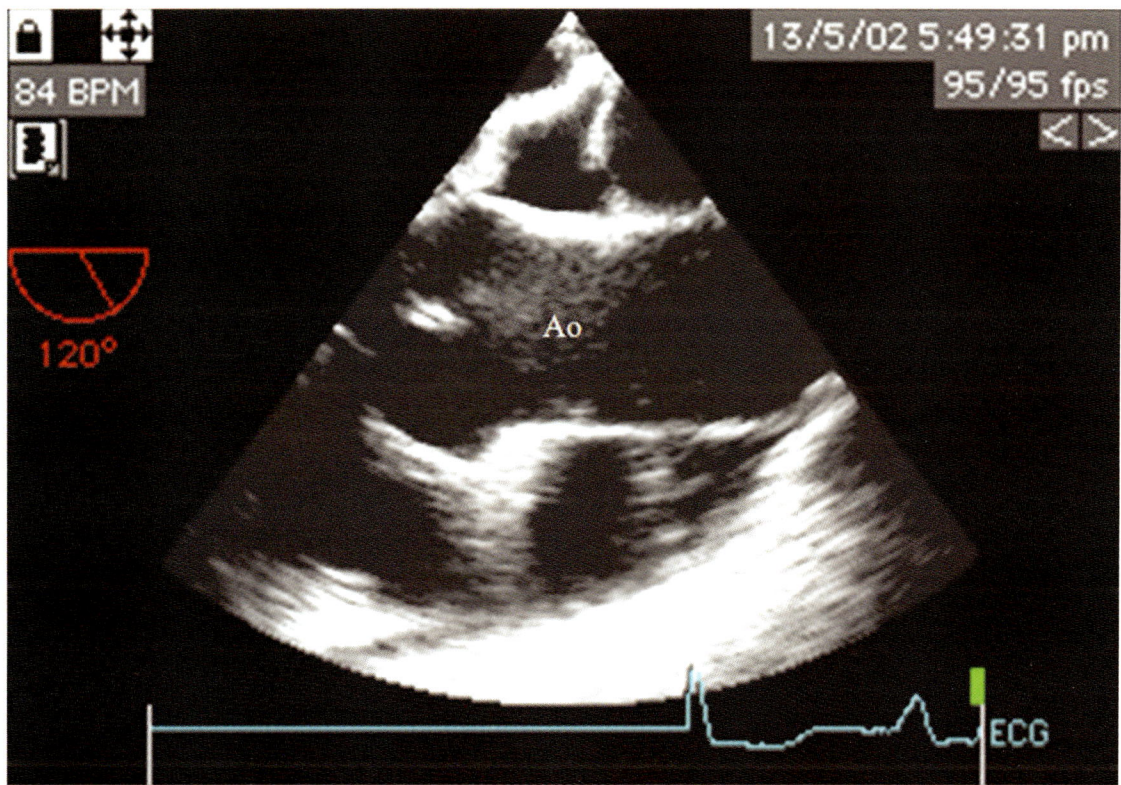

Fig. 11.1: Midesophageal ascending aorta long-axis view showing the ascending thoracic aorta (Ao).

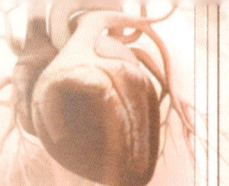

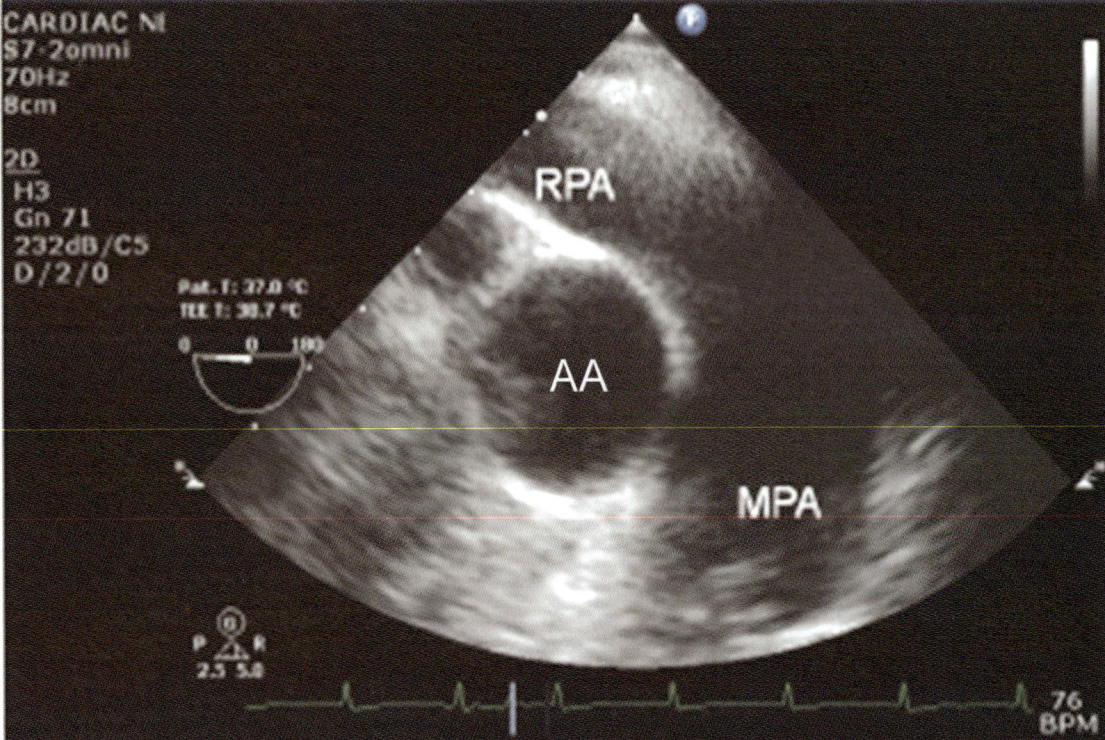

Fig. 11.2: Midesophageal ascending aortic short-axis view showing the ascending aorta in short-axis. By withdrawing or advancing the probe, almost entire length of the ascending aorta can be examined. (AA: ascending aorta, MPA: main pulmonary artery, RPA: right pulmonary artery).

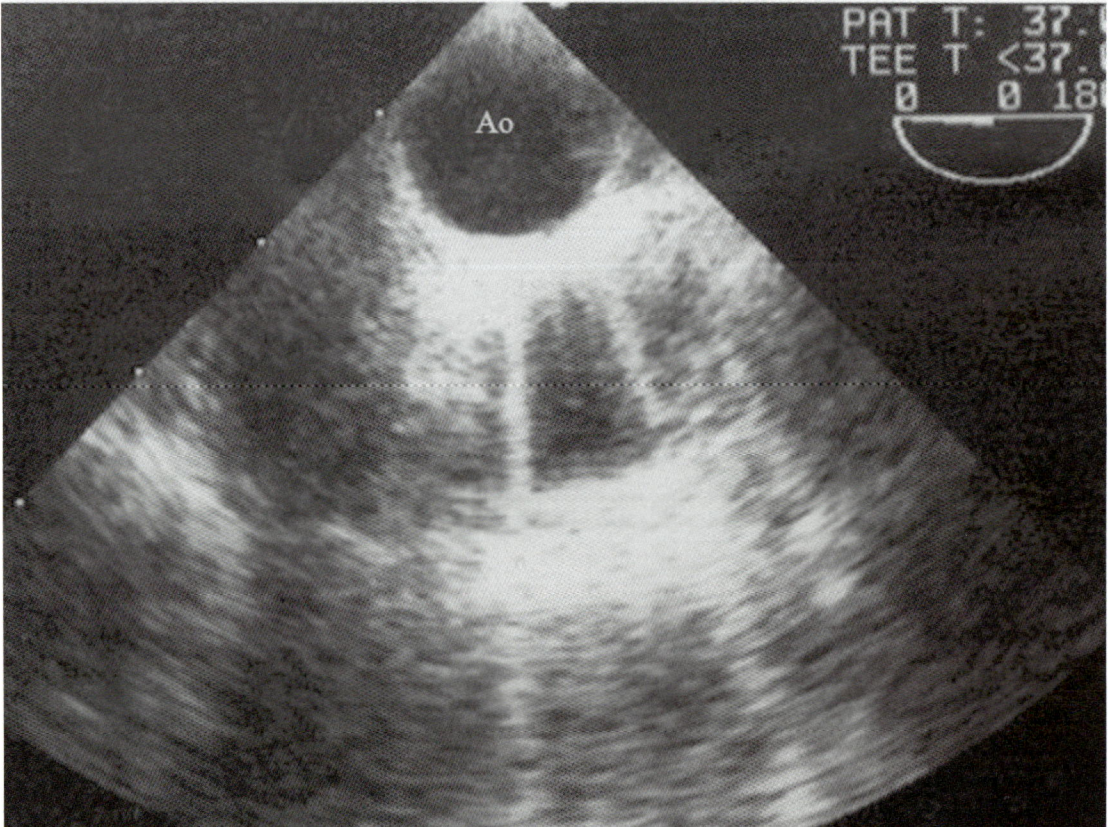

Fig. 11.3: Midesophageal descending aorta short-axis view for examining the descending thoracic aorta (Ao). By advancing the probe, almost the entire length of the descending aorta can be visualized.

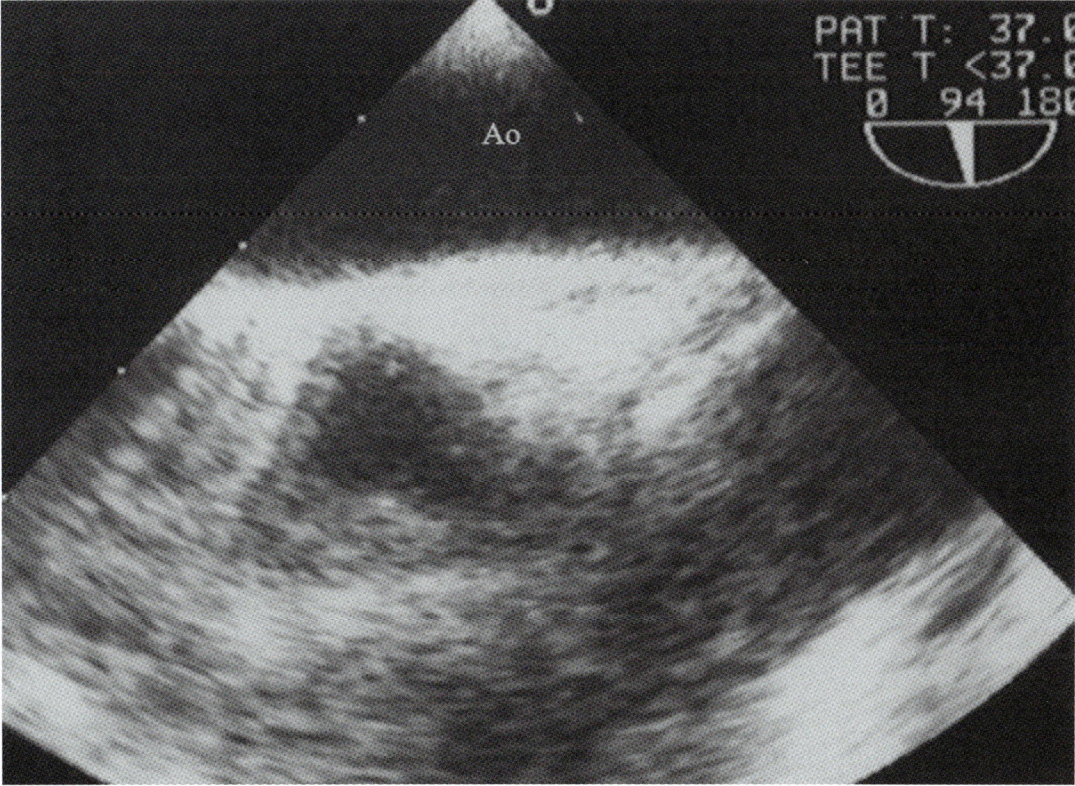

Fig. 11.4: Midesophageal descending aorta long-axis view for assessing descending thoracic aorta in its long-axis. (Ao: aorta). By advancing the probe, almost the entire descending aorta can be visualized.

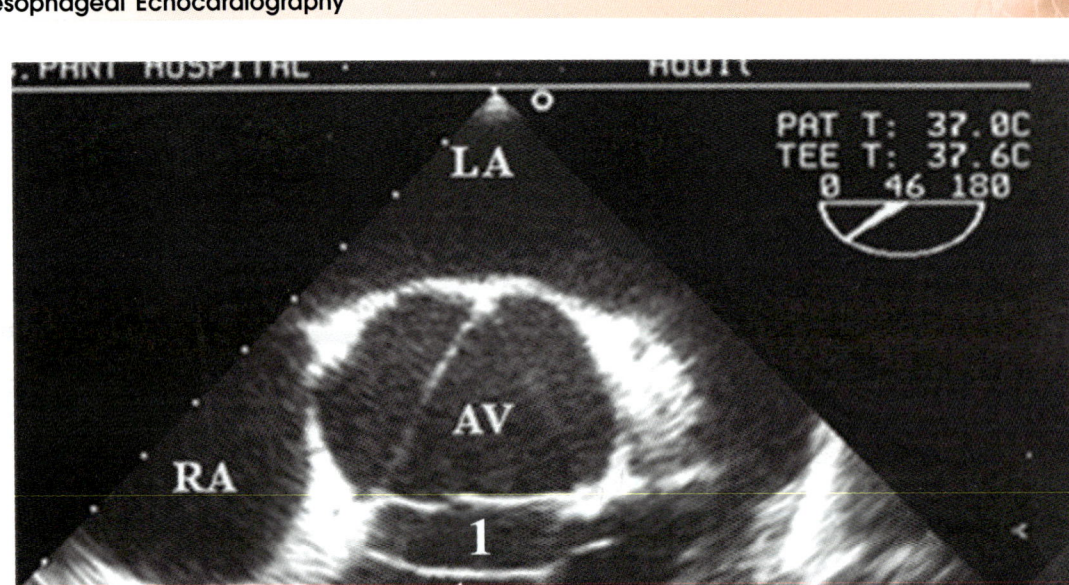

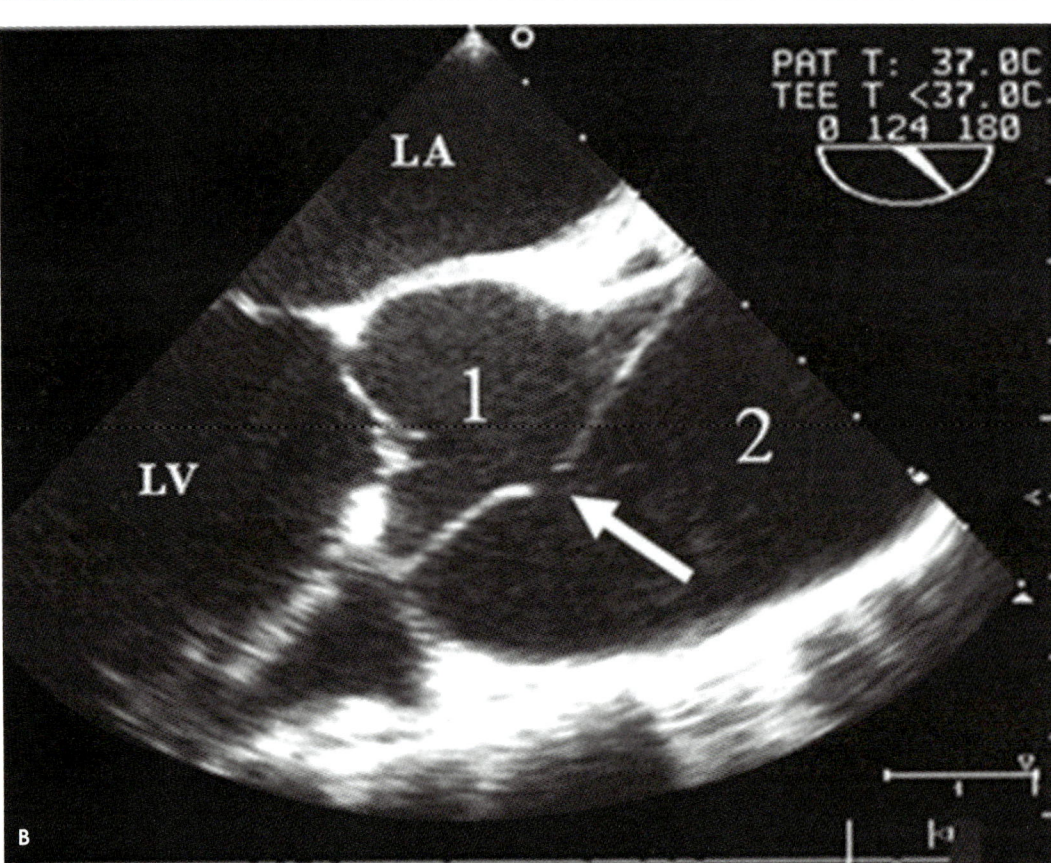

Fig. 11.5A and B: Transesophageal echocardiography in a patient with aortic dissection. Note the dissection flap (arrow) dividing the aortic lumen into true (1) and false lumens (2). (RA: right atrium, LA: left atrium, LV: left ventricle, AV: aortic valve).

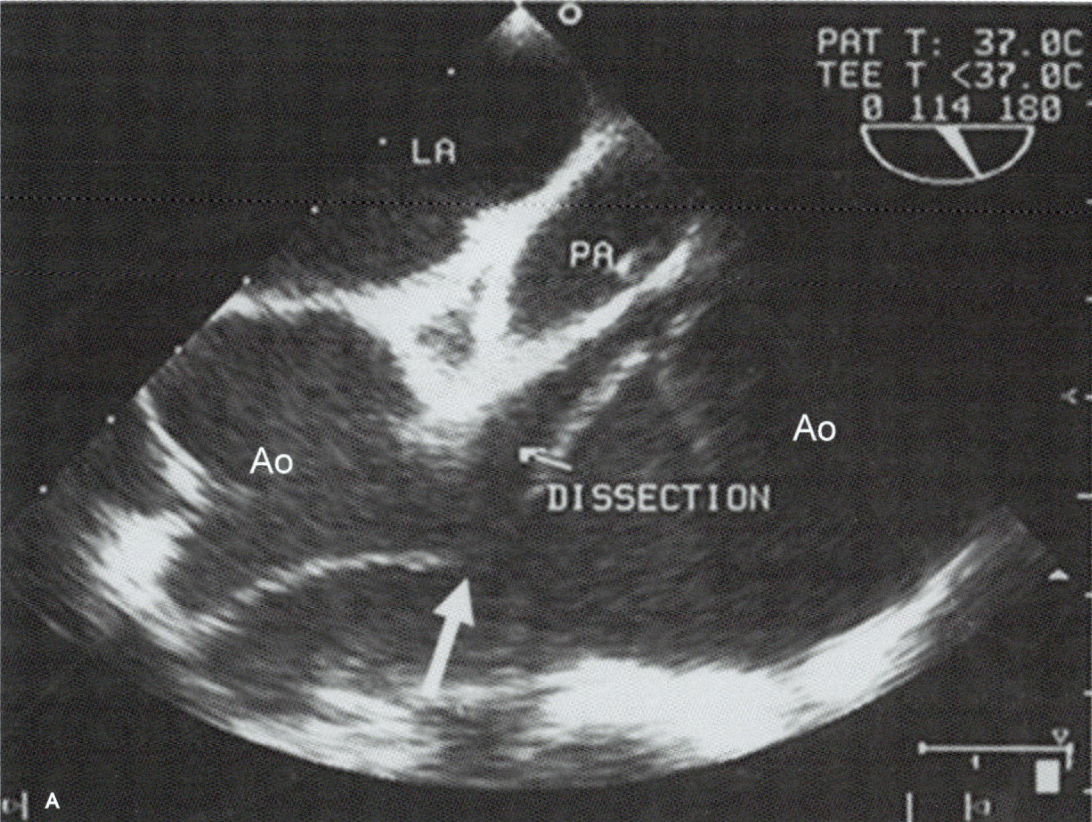

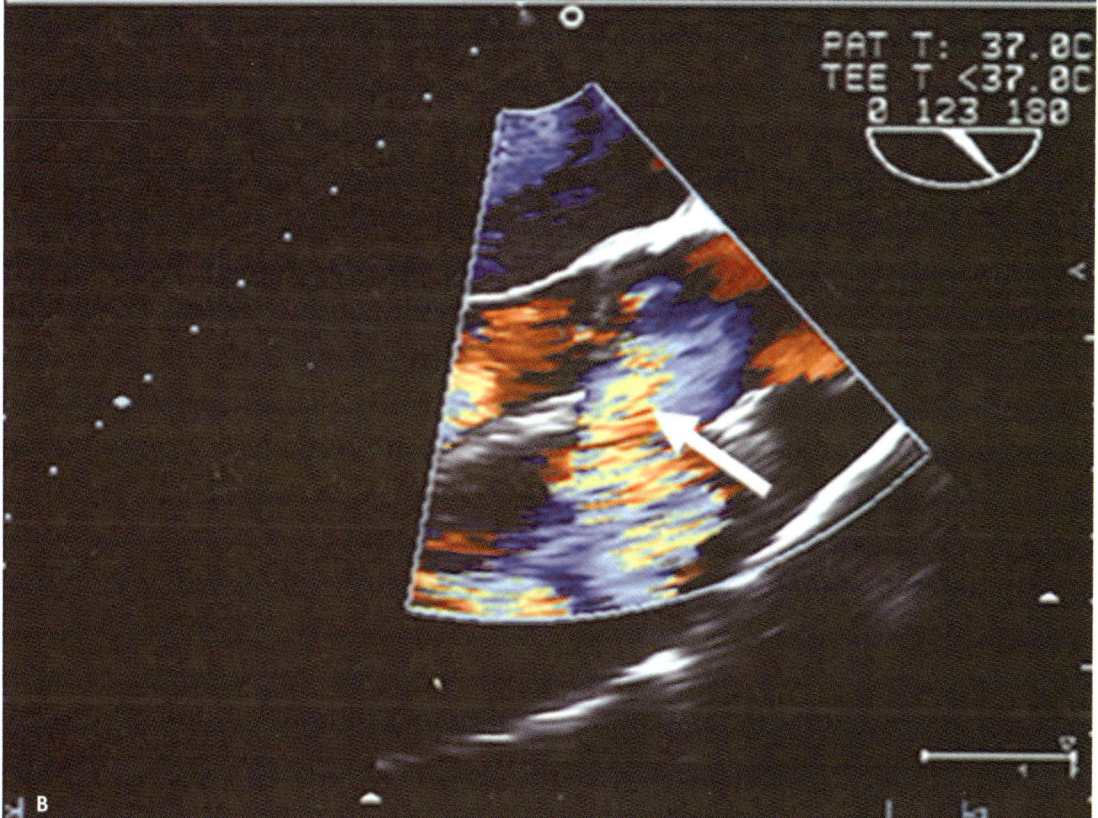

Fig. 11.6A and B: Midesophageal ascending aorta long-axis view in a patient with aortic dissection. Note the entry point (arrow). Color flow showing flow of blood from true lumen to false lumen. (LA: left atrium, Ao: aorta, PA: pulmonary artery).

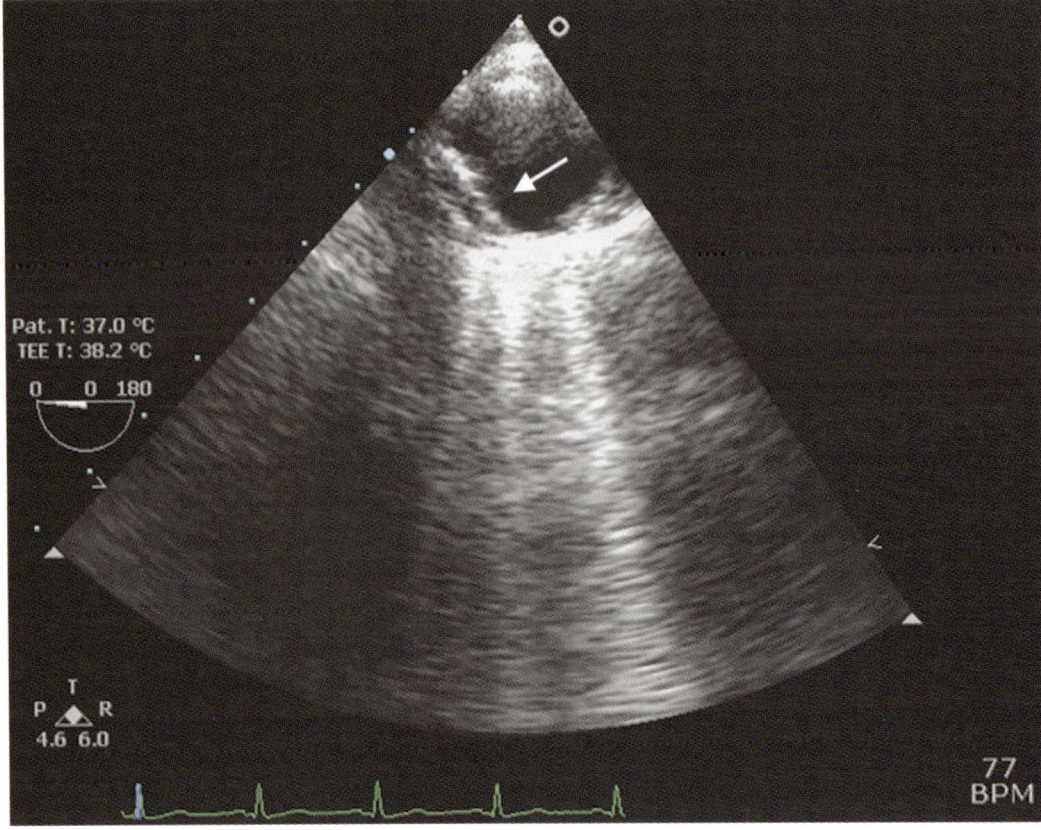

Fig. 11.7: Midesophageal descending aorta short-axis view showing intimal atheromatous plaque at 6 to 9 o' clock position (arrow).

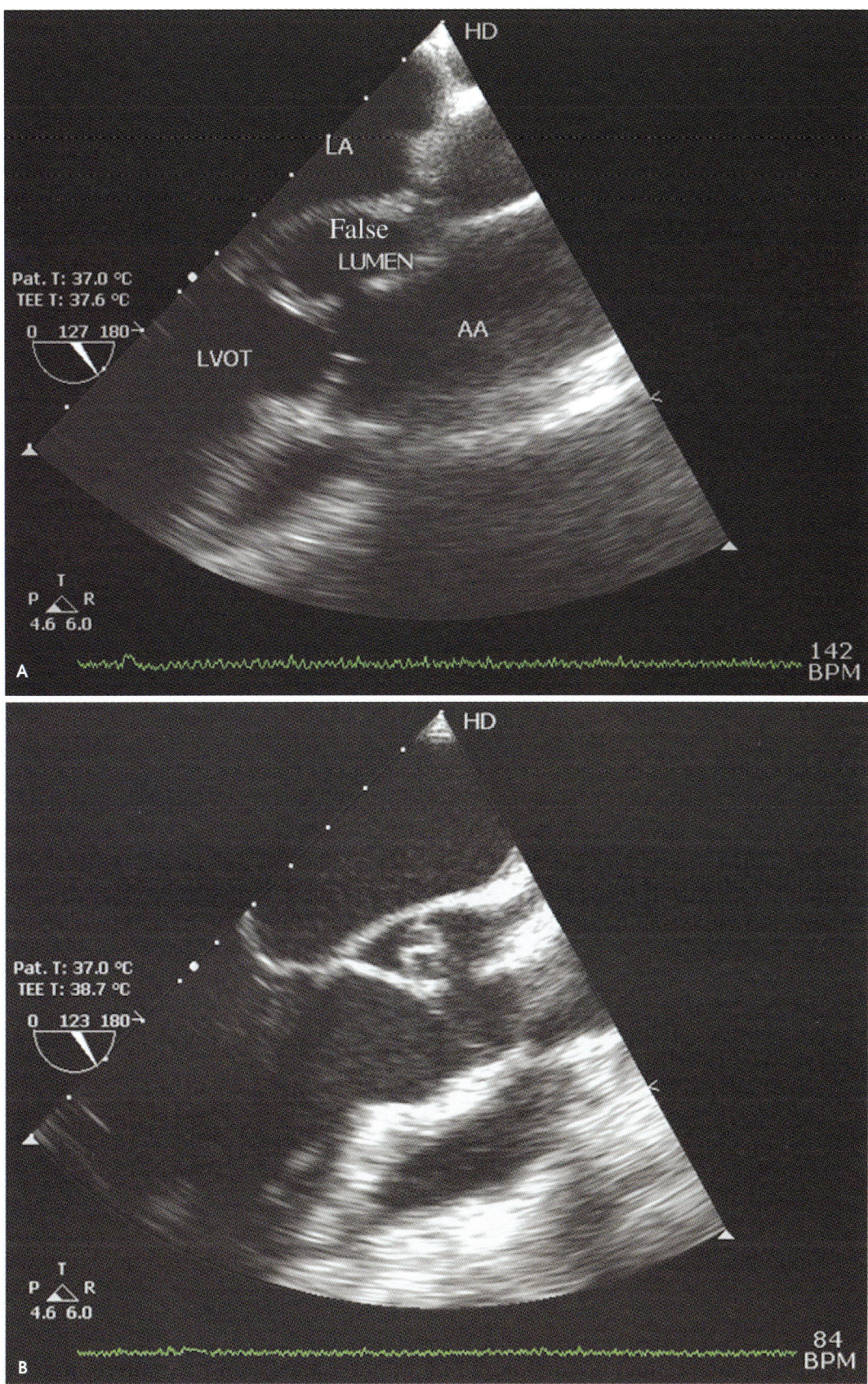

Fig. 11.8: Midesophageal long-axis view showing an ascending aorta pseudoaneurysm in diastole (A) and systole (B) (LA: left atrium, LVOT: left ventricular outflow tract, AA: ascending aorta).

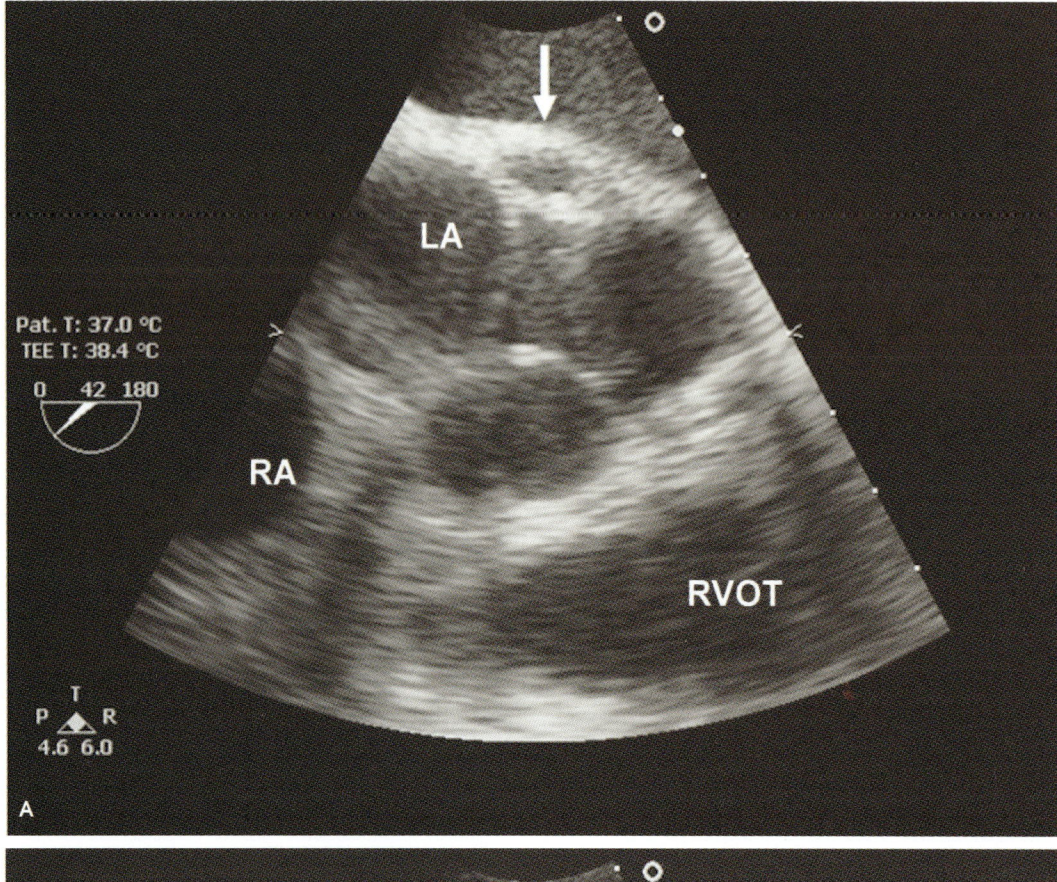

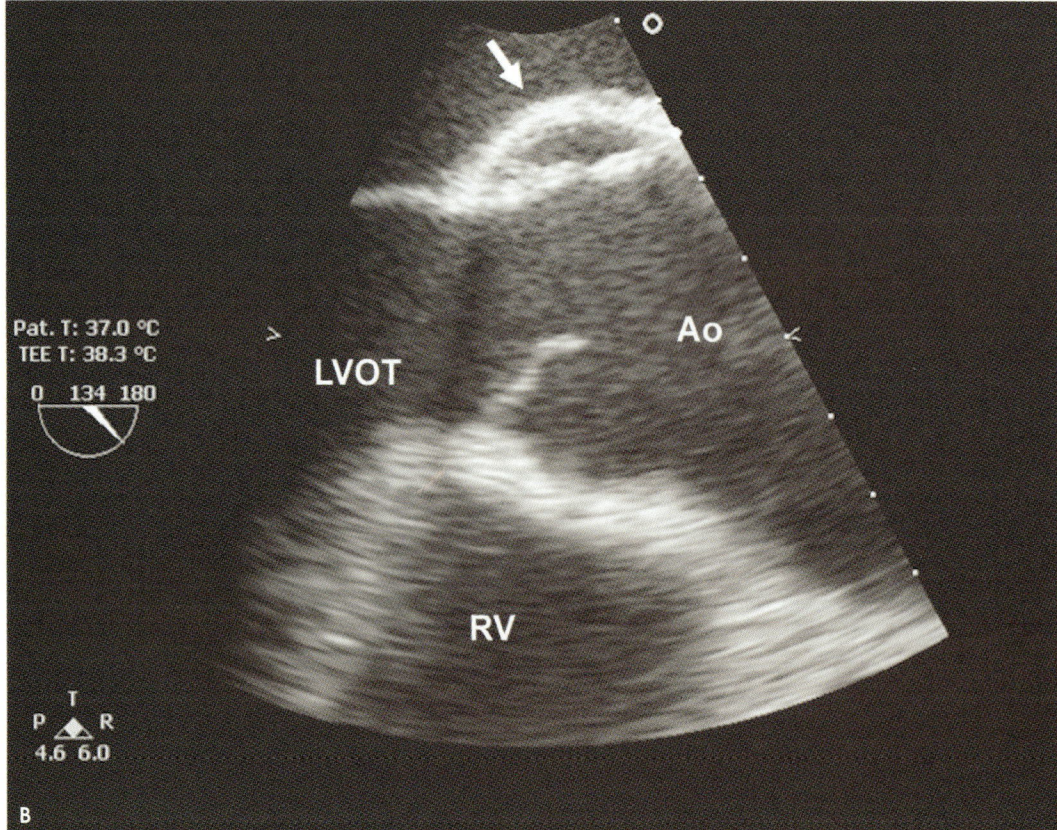

Fig. 11.9: Midesophageal aortic valve short-axis (A) and long-axis view (B) showing aortic root abscess (arrow) (RA: right atrium, LA: left atrium, RVOT: right ventricular outflow tract, LVOT: left ventricular outflow tract, Ao: aorta, RV: right ventricle).

Evaluation of Prosthetic Valve Function

12

• Deepak K. Tempe • Suruchi Hasija

Assessment of the prosthetic valve function is one of the most important applications of the transesophageal echocardiography (TEE). However, evaluation of the prosthetic valves can be complex, especially due to the fact that a large variety and different sizes of valves are available, each one of which has unique flow characteristics. Nevertheless, functional assessment of a newly implanted prosthetic valve during surgery can be effectively performed in most patients. The metallic echodense components of mechanical prosthetic valves and the sewing ring and stents of bioprosthetic valves generate acoustic artifacts that may interfere with the visualization of the prosthetic valve structure. In addition, these structures cast acoustic shadows, which interfere with the visualization of structures on the side of the prosthesis facing away from the ultrasound transducer. For the same reason the blood flow on the side of the prosthesis that is facing away from the ultrasound transducer is masked, thereby interfering with the Doppler interrogation. As the TEE probe lies directly posterior to the left atrium, the left atrial aspect of the prosthetic mitral valve is clearly visualised. Such an unobstructed view is not readily achieved with the transthoracic probe. The TEE examination of the prosthetic valve should be targeted to ensure the stability and seating of the prosthetic valve, leaflet mobility, and absence of paravalvular leak and left ventricular outflow tract obstruction. The transvalvular pressure gradient and effective orifice area must be within acceptable limits. Prosthesis-patient mismatch is suspected if the indexed effective orifice area (EOA) (EOAi = EOA/body surface area) is ≤ 1.2 cm^2/m^2 after mitral valve replacement or ≤ 0.85 cm^2/m^2 after aortic valve replacement. The presence of any of these findings necessitates reinstitution of the cardiopulmonary bypass to carry-out the necessary repair. Assessment during the postoperative period can detect pathological conditions such as dehiscence, thrombosis, pannus formation, calcification, degeneration, vegetations, regurgitation and stenosis. In this chapter, normal appearance of some of the commonly implanted prosthetic valves is shown. In addition, some pathological conditions have also been depicted.

MITRAL VALVE PROSTHESIS

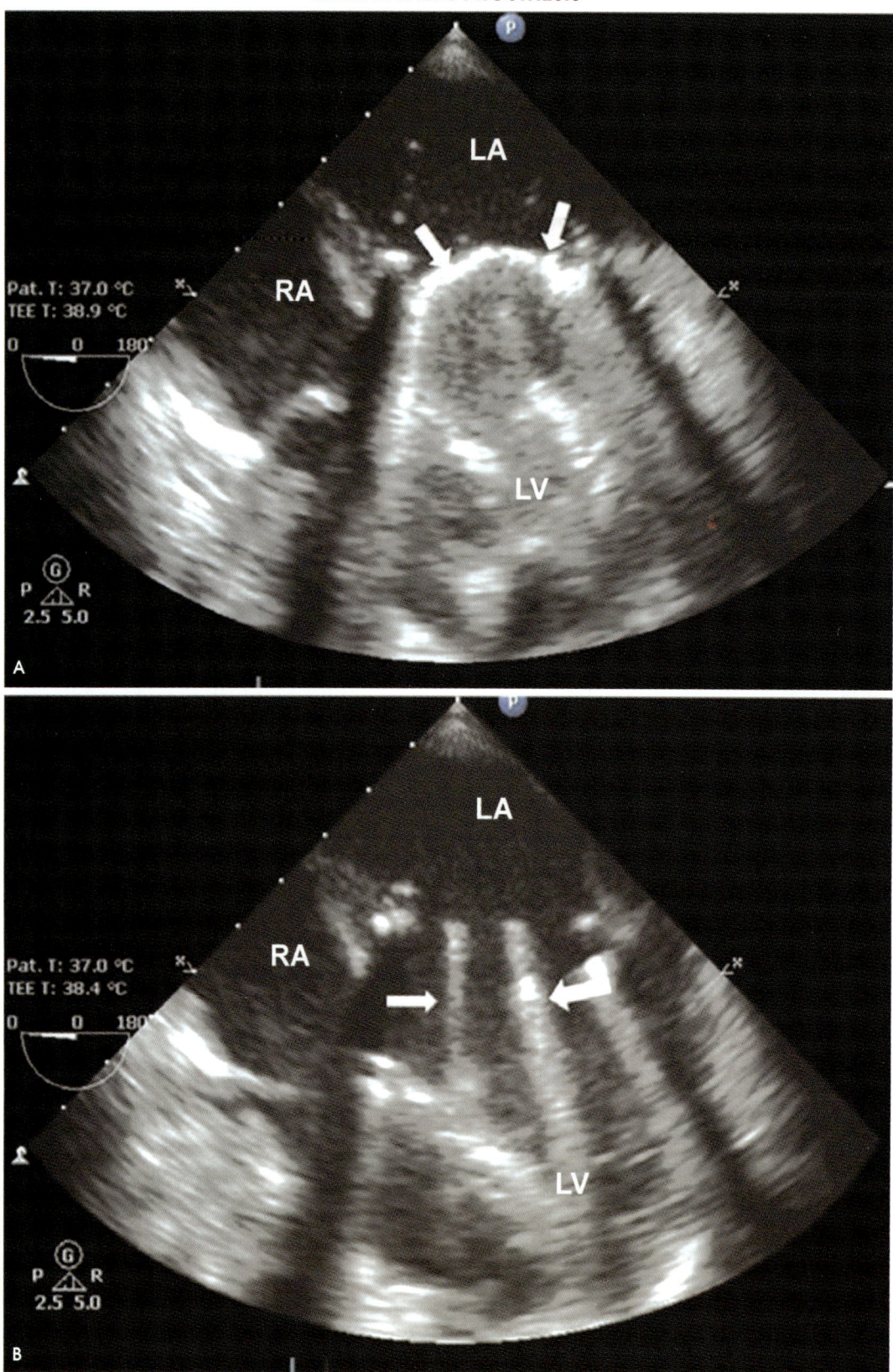

Fig. 12.1: Midesophageal 4-chamber view showing bileaflet mitral valve prosthesis (Medtronic) in closed (A) and open (B) positions. Arrows indicate the leaflets. In case of bileaflet valves, it is important to know that the two leaflets open symmetrically to an angle of 85° to 90° and close at an angle of 30° with the plane of the annulus (LA: left atrium, RA: right atrium, LV: left ventricle).

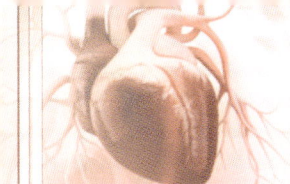

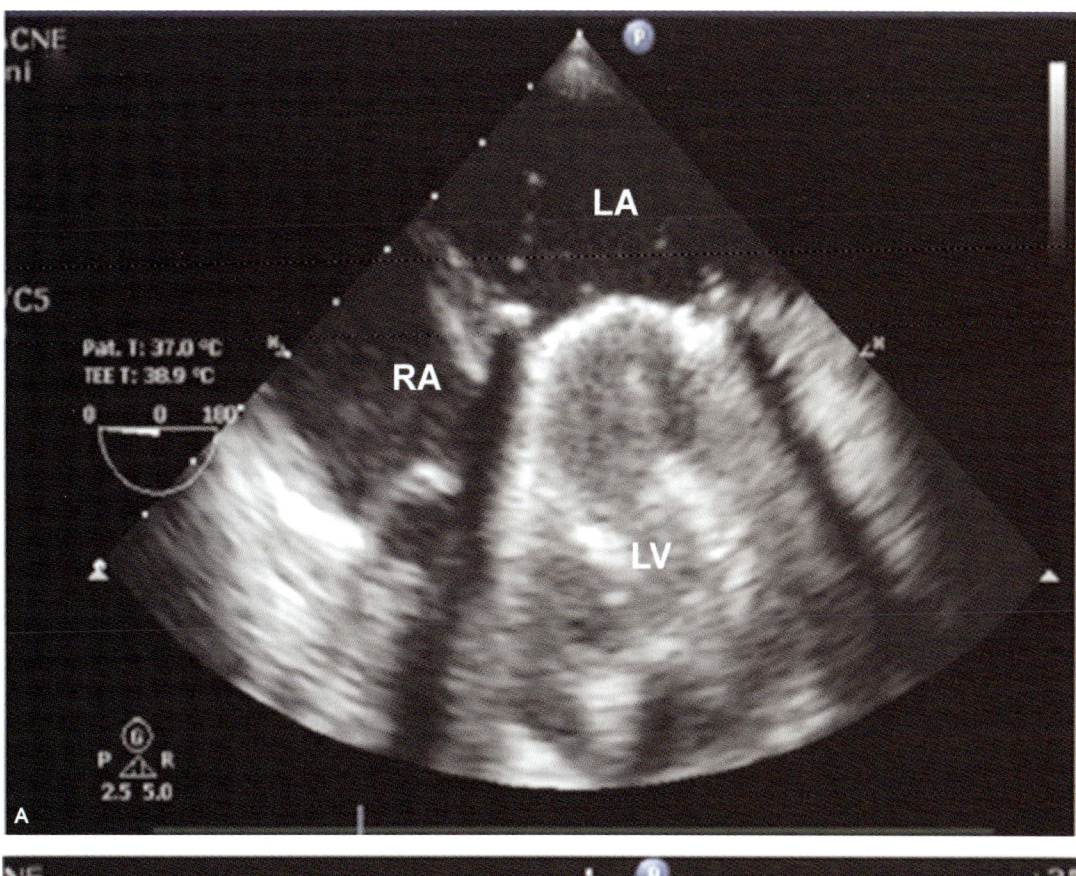

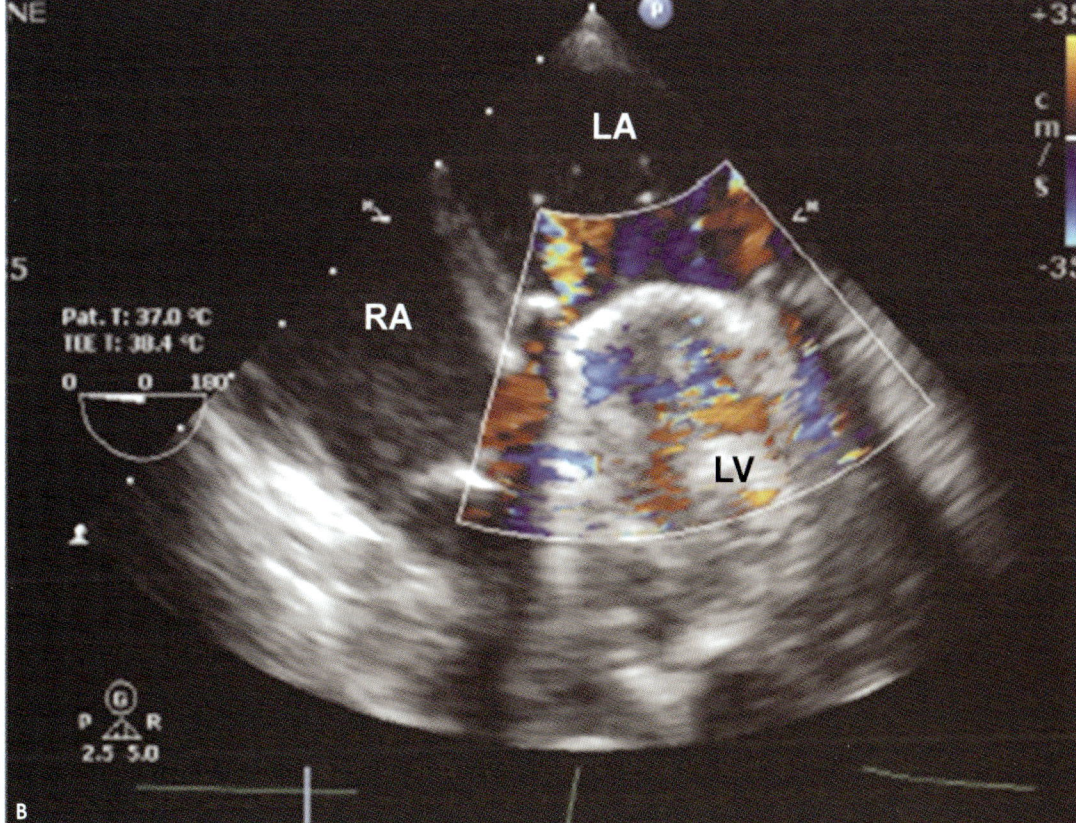

Fig. 12.2: Midesophageal 4-chamber view showing bileaflet mitral valve prosthesis in closed position (A) and color flow showing normal washing jets (B) (LA: left atrium, RA: right atrium, LV: left ventricle).

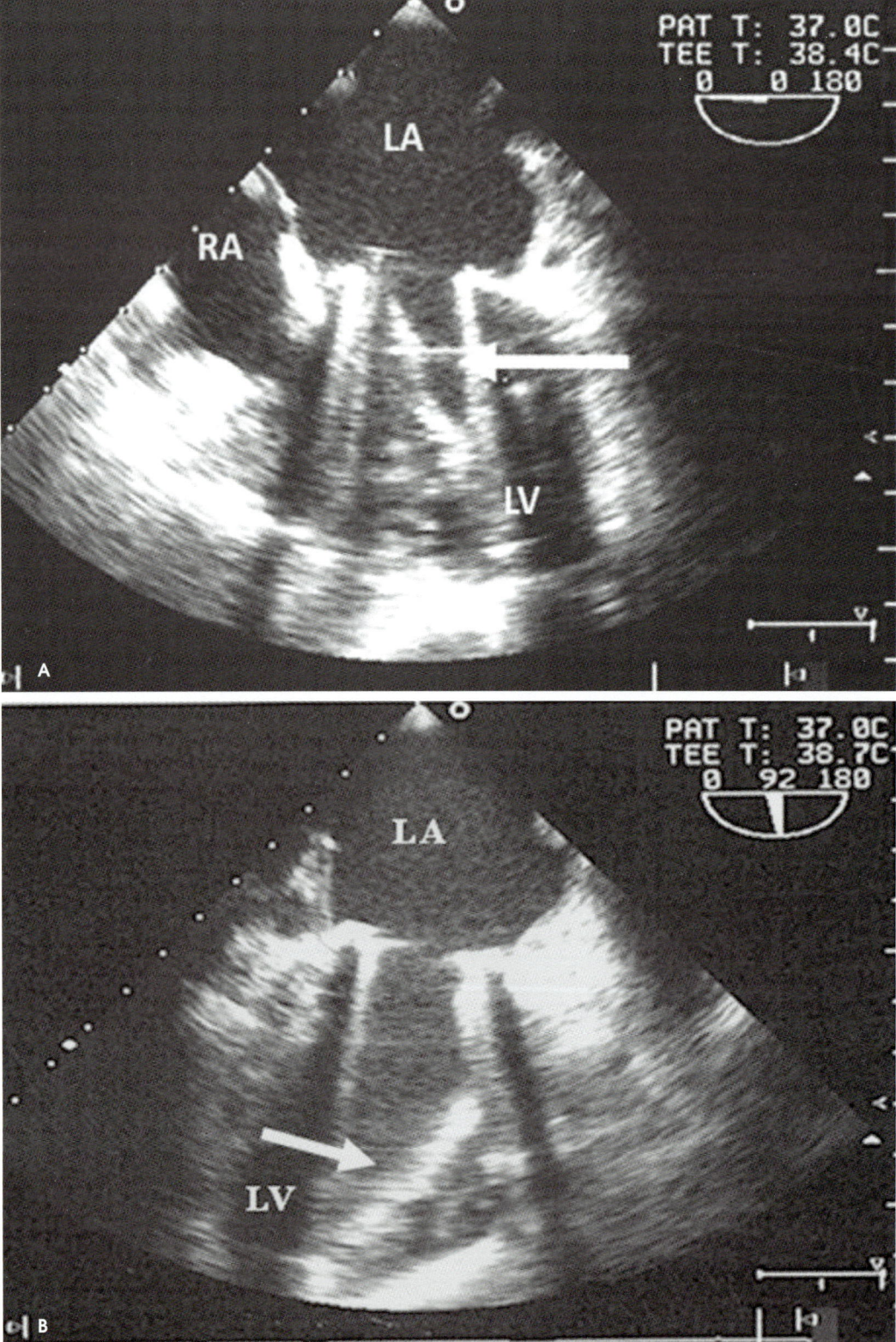

Fig. 12.3: Appearance of the Bjork-Shiley tilting disc valve in the mitral position in the midesophageal four-chamber view (A) and two-chamber view (B). In tilting disc valves, the single disc opens 60 to 80° to form two orifices of different size and shape. The gradient is measured across the major orifice in such valves. Note the acoustic shadowing caused by the metallic disc (arrow). To overcome acoustic shadowing, the valve should be examined in multiple views for leaflet/disc motion and sewing ring stability. Imaging in the transgastric, deep transgastric or other non-standard planes provides details that are not discernible in the midesophageal views. (LA: left atrium, RA: right atrium, LV: left ventricle).

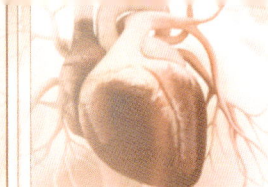

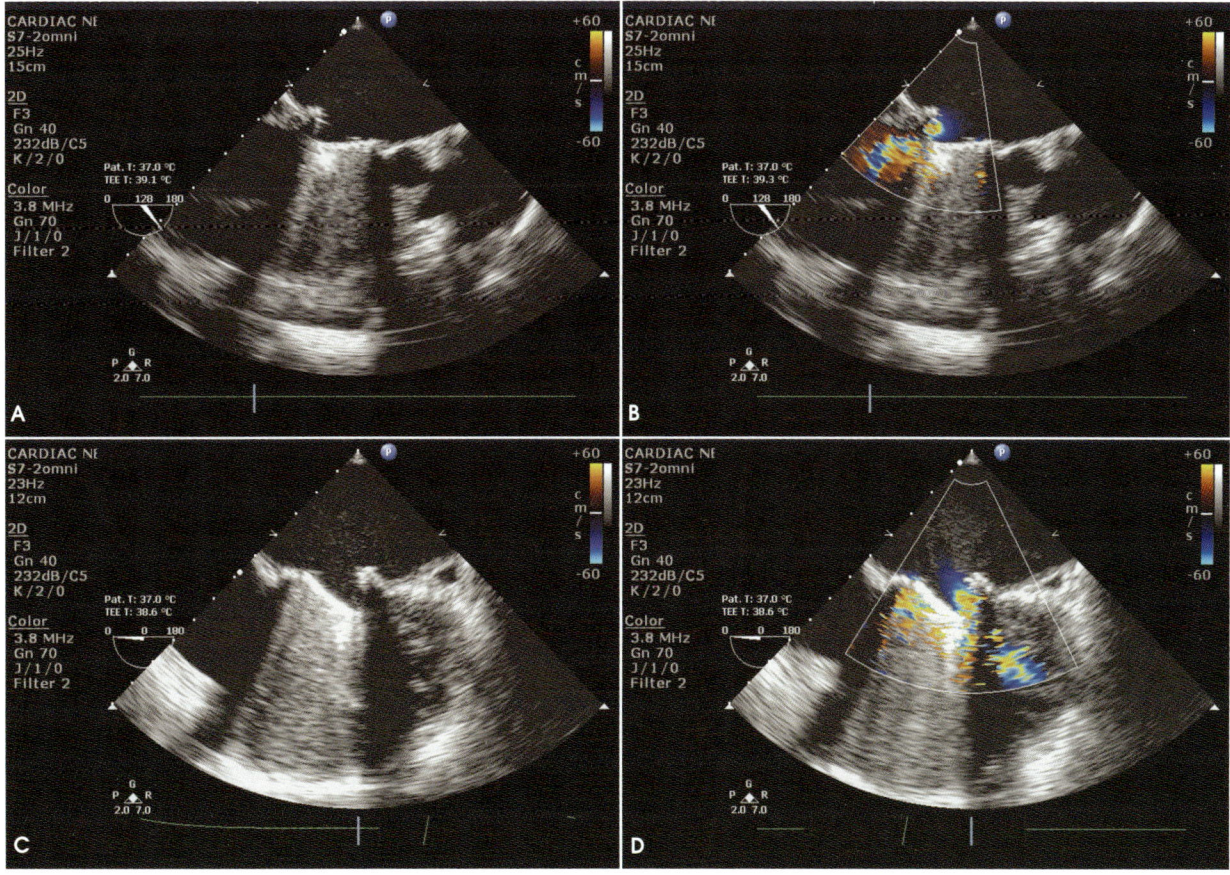

Fig. 12.4: Midesophageal aortic valve long-axis view (A, B) and four-chamber view (C,D) showing a tilting disc mitral valve prosthesis with restricted mobility and color flow showing turbulent flow.

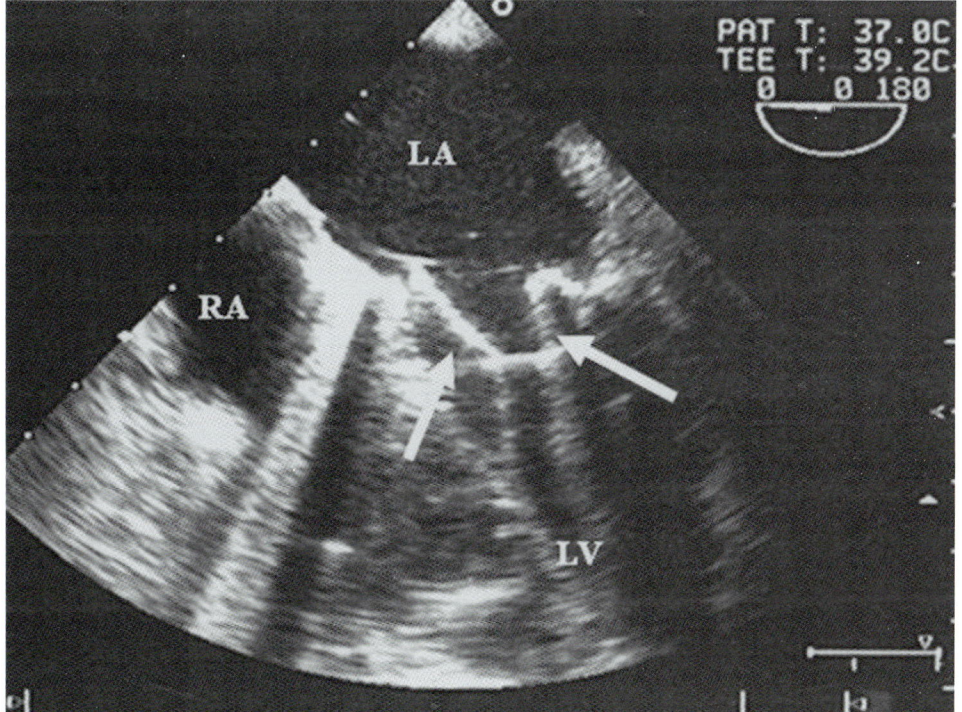

Fig. 12.5: Midesophageal 4-chamber view showing St. Jude prosthesis in the mitral position. Note the two discs (arrows). (LA: left atrium, RA: right atrium, LV: left ventricle).

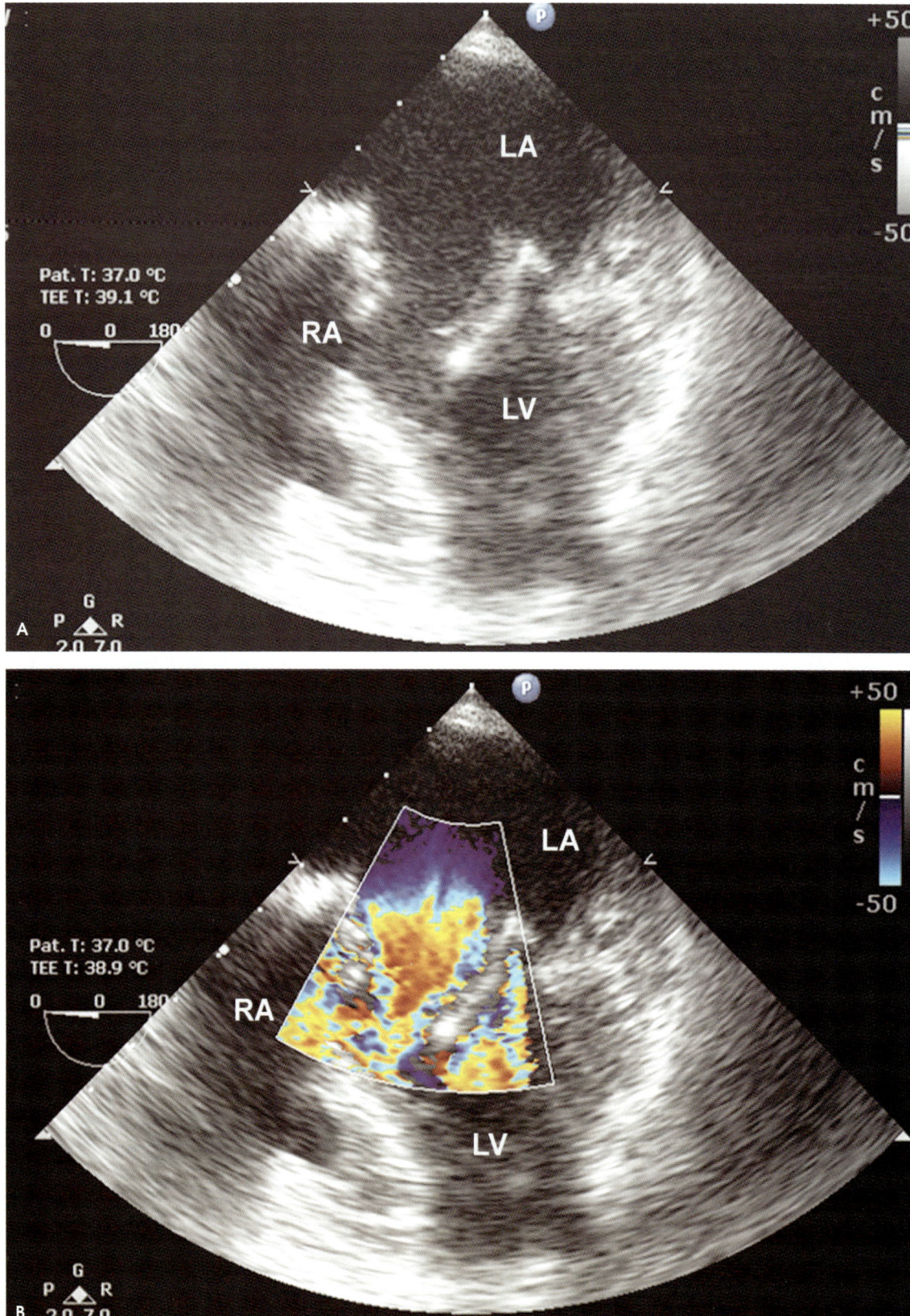

Fig. 12.6: Midesophageal 4-chamber view showing a bioprosthetic valve in situ in mitral position showing thickening and calcification of the leaflets caused by chronic degenerative changes (A), leading to turbulent flow across it suggestive of stenosis (B) (LA: left atrium, RA: right atrium, LV: left ventricle).

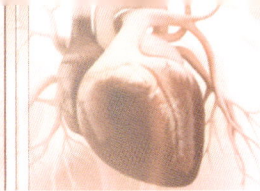

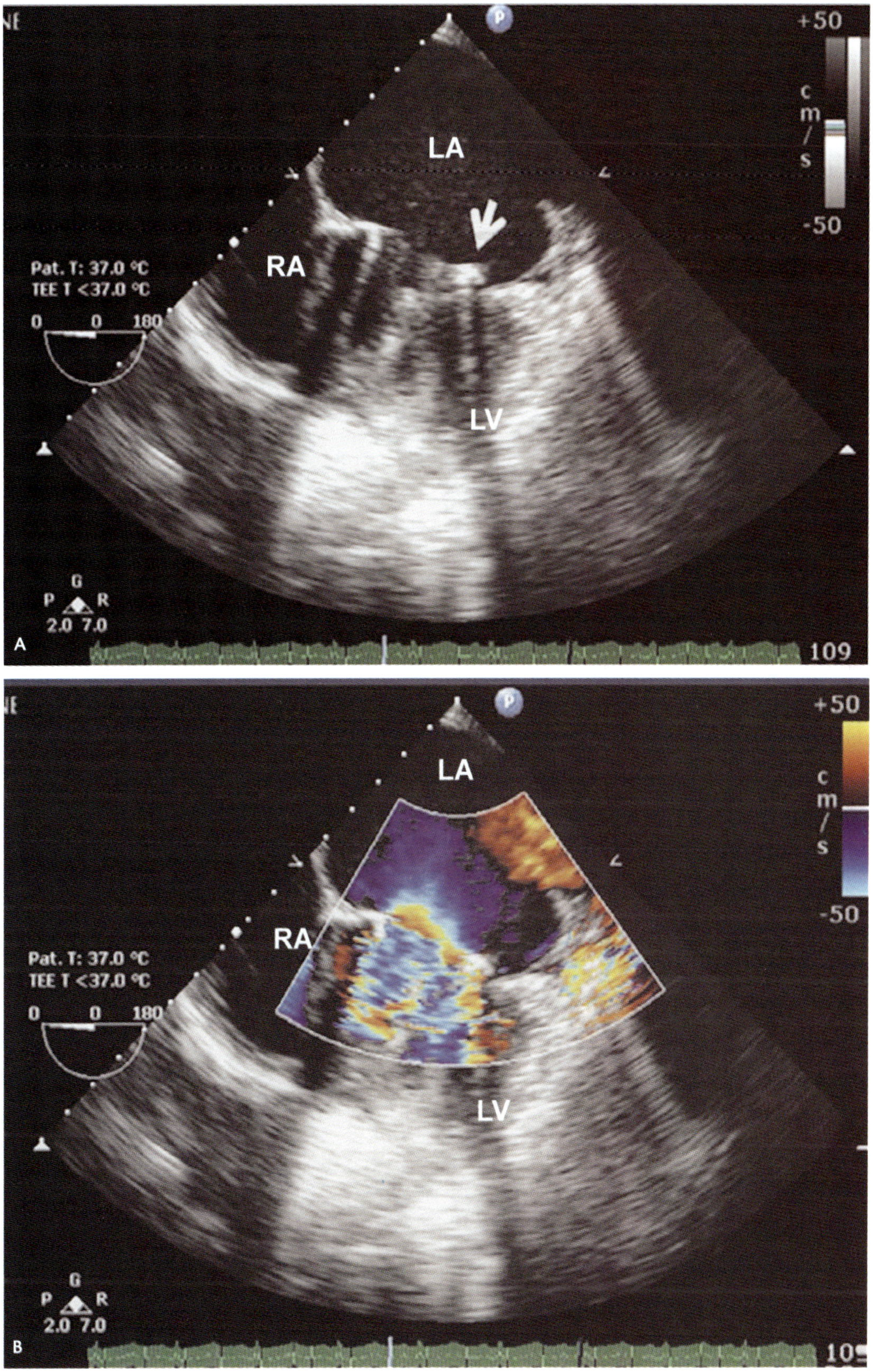

Fig. 12.7: Midesophageal 4-chamber view showing mitral valve prosthesis in situ with a pannus (arrow) (A) leading to turbulent flow across the prosthesis (B). Thrombosis and pannus formation (fibroconnective tissue ingrowth) are the etiological causes of mechanical valve stenosis (LA: left atrium, RA: right atrium, LV: left ventricle).

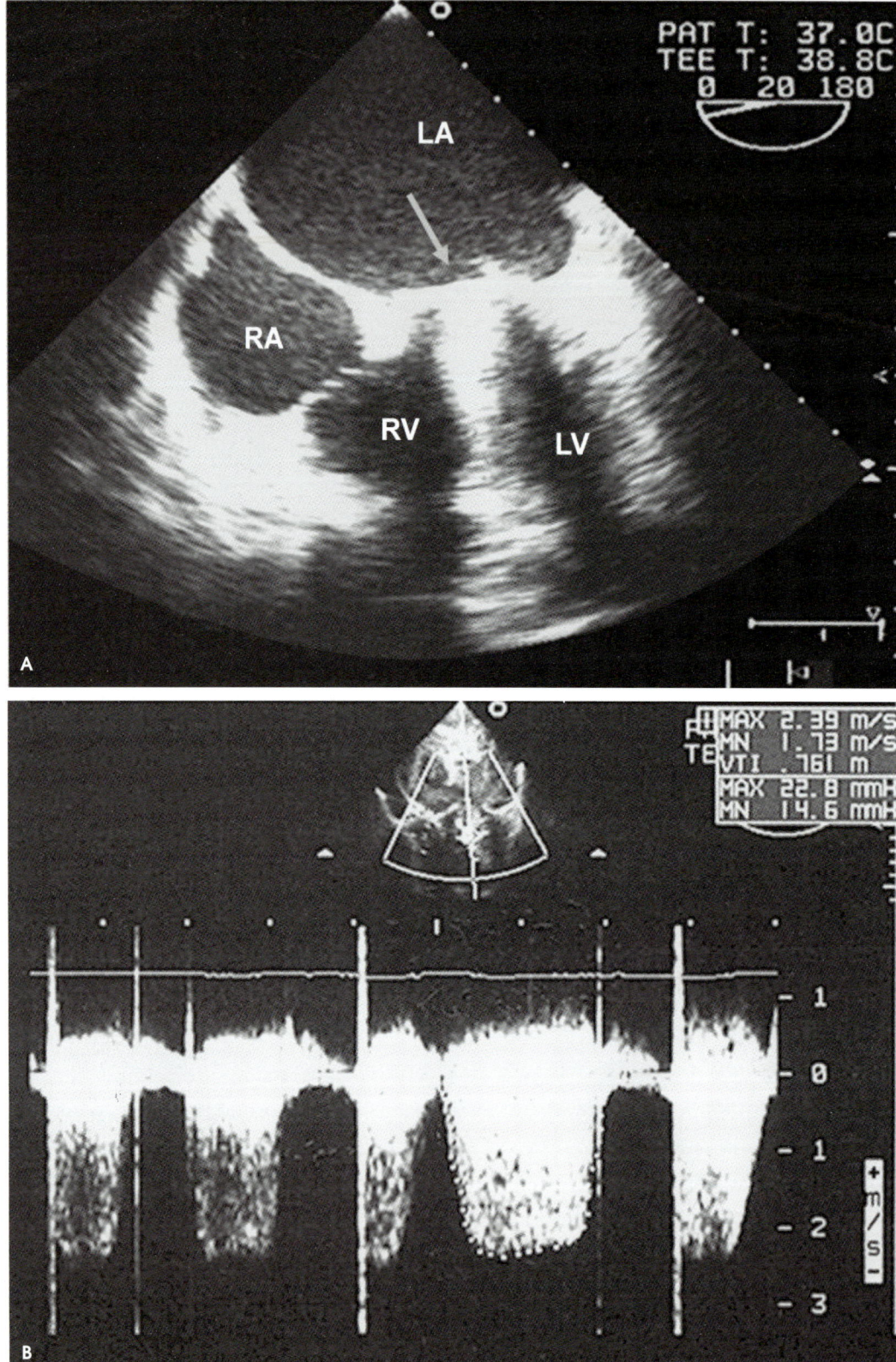

Fig. 12.8: Panel A: Midesophageal 4-chamber view showing pannus formation (fibrous tissue overgrowth) on the St. Jude valve in the mitral position (arrow) causing prosthetic valve stenosis. Panel B: Note the continuous wave Doppler tracing across the mitral valve showing a large transmitral gradient and a prolonged pressure half time. The peak and mean gradients across the valve decrease with increasing prosthesis size. In general, the peak transvalvular gradient for mitral bioprostheses ranges from 3 to 4 mm Hg. (LA: left atrium, RA: right atrium, LV: left ventricle, RV: right ventricle).

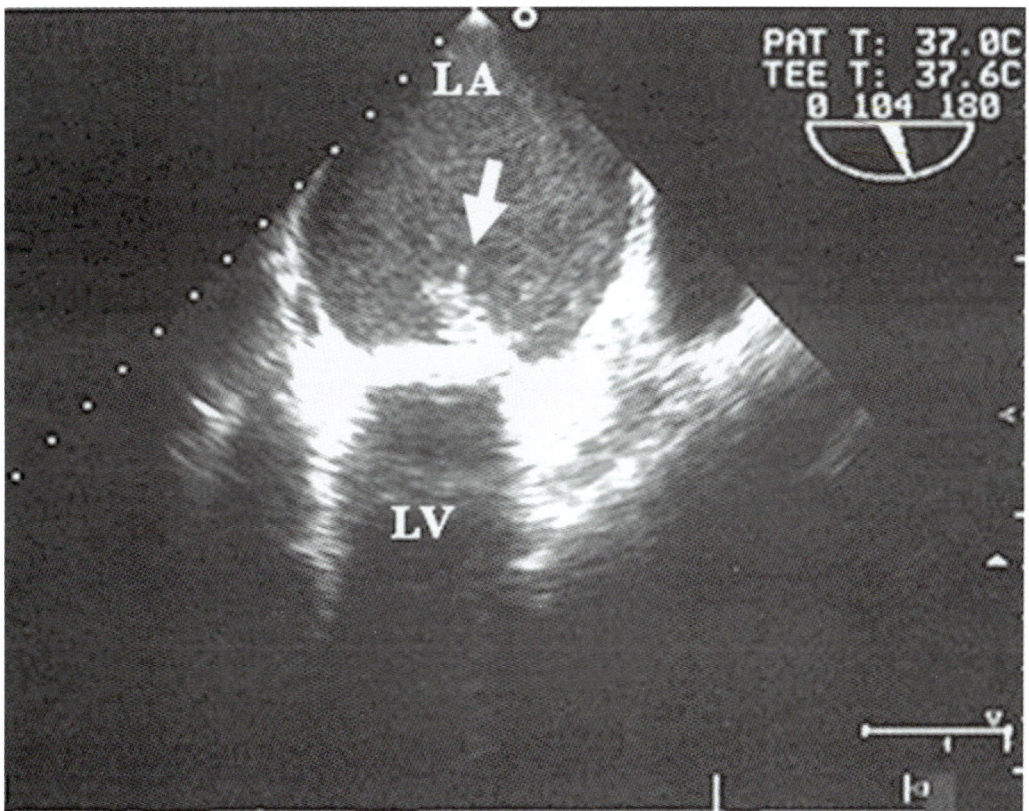

Fig. 12.9: Continuous wave spectral Doppler across the stuck mitral valve prosthesis showing high velocity (3.6 m/sec) indicating high gradient.

Fig. 12.10: Prosthetic valve dysfunction due to formation of a large thrombus (arrow) in a patient with Bjork-Shiley tilting disc valve prosthesis in mitral position. A thrombus is usually large in size and generally fixed, however, if mobile, it moves along with the underlying structure to which it is attached. (LA: left atrium, LV: left ventricle).

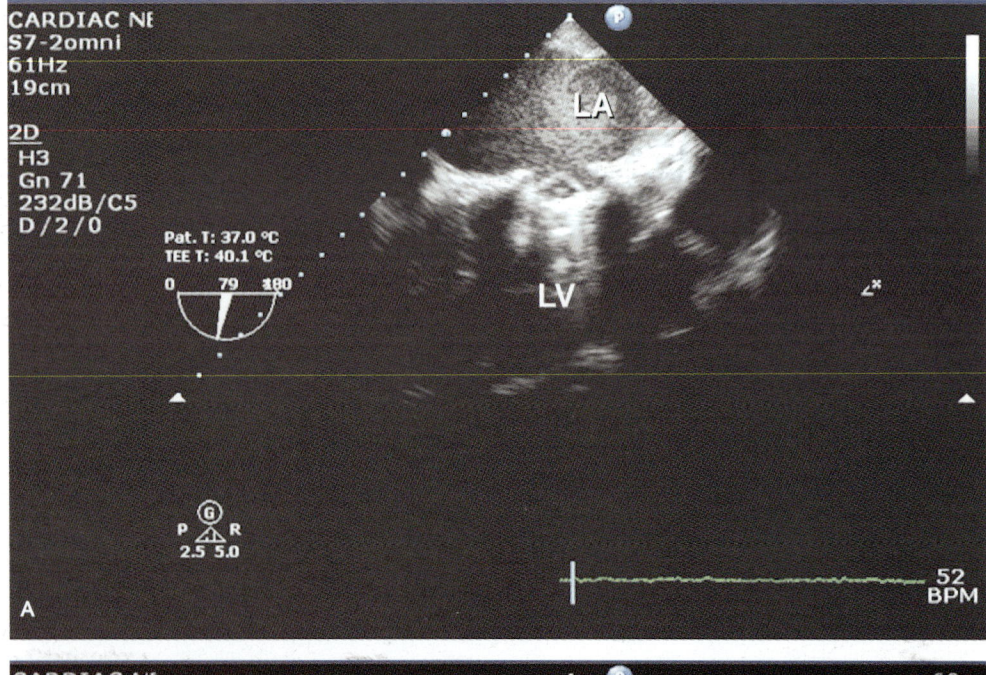

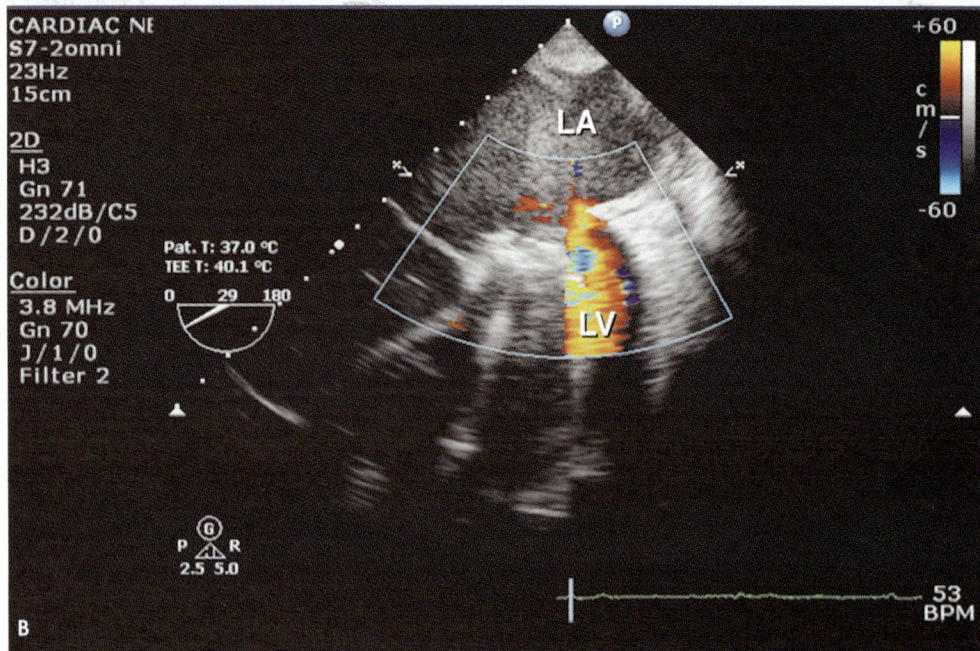

Fig. 12.11: Stuck leaflet of the bileaflet prosthesis (A) and color flow showing turbulent flow across the other leaflet that is mobile (B). Also note the spontaneous echo contrast and thrombus in the left atrium (LA: left atrium, LV: left ventricle).

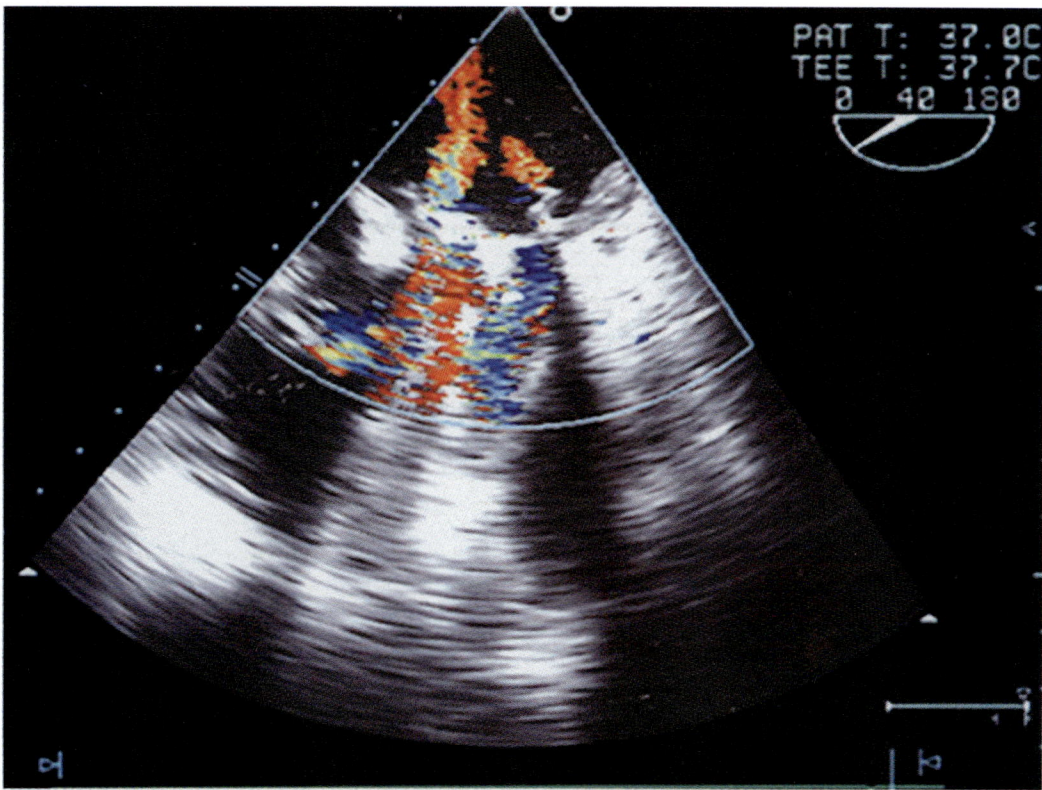

Fig. 12.12: Prosthetic valve thrombosis causing mitral regurgitation.

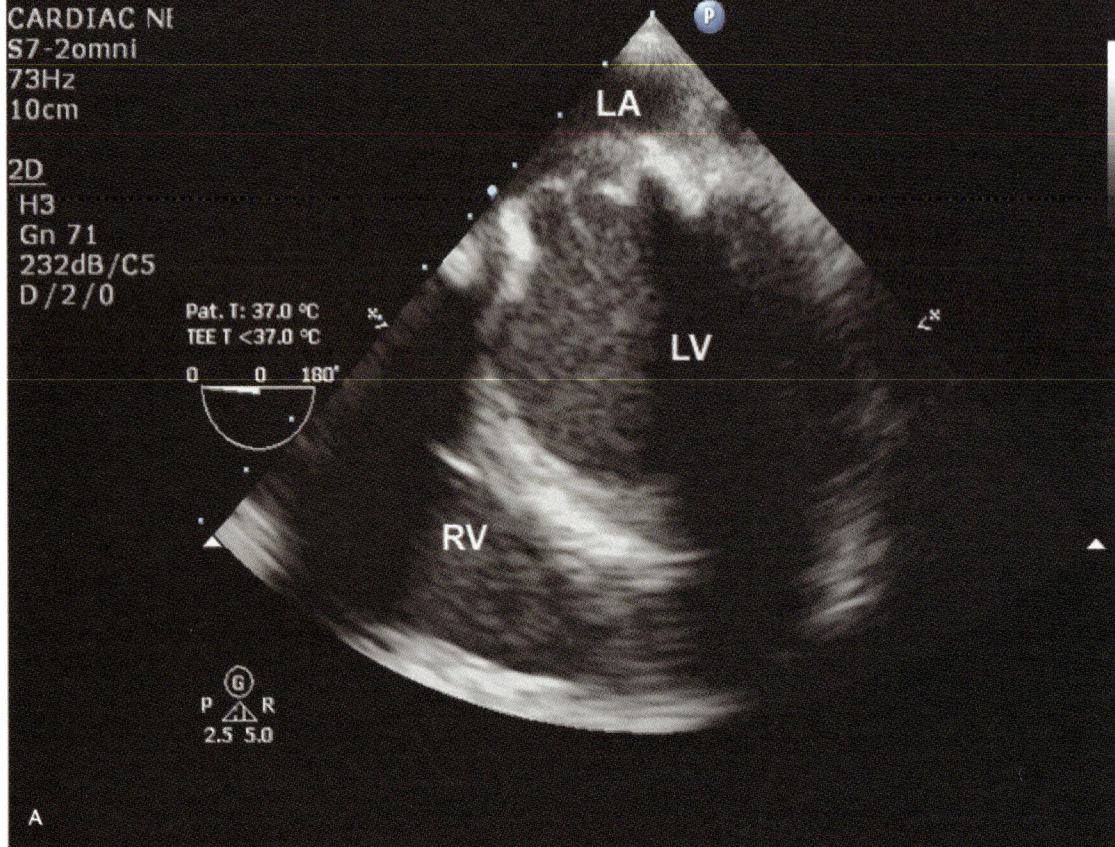

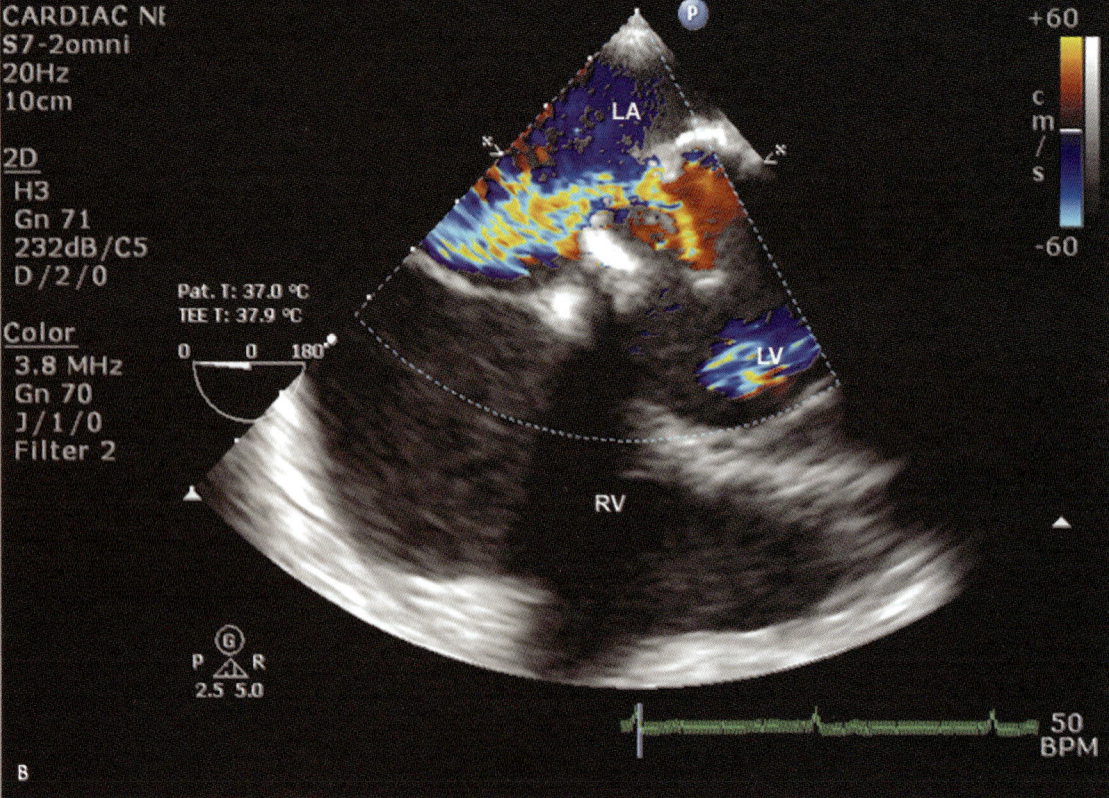

Fig. 12.13: Midesophageal four-chamber view showing a tissue valve in mitral position (A) and severe regurgitation caused by degeneration (B) (LA: left atrium, LV: left ventricle, RV: right ventricle).

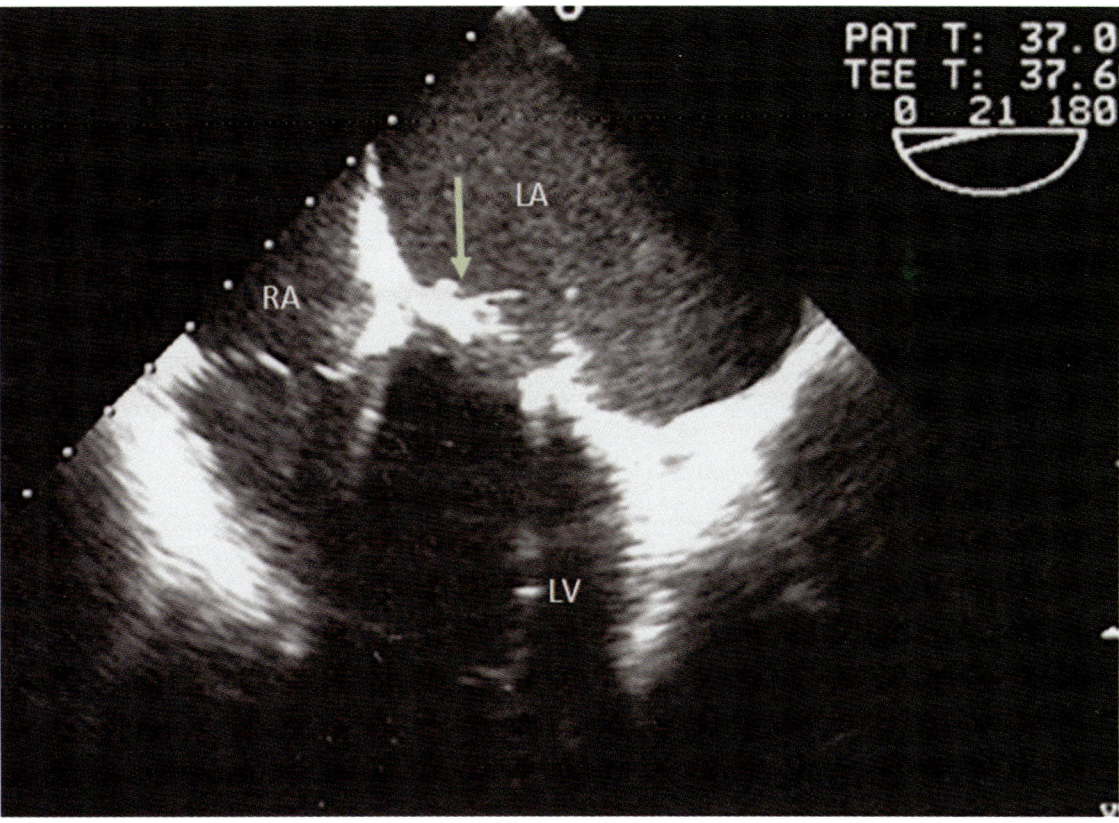

Fig. 12.14: Formation of a large vegetation (arrow) in a patient with a tilting disc prosthesis in the mitral position. (LA: left atrium, RA: right atrium, LV: left ventricle).

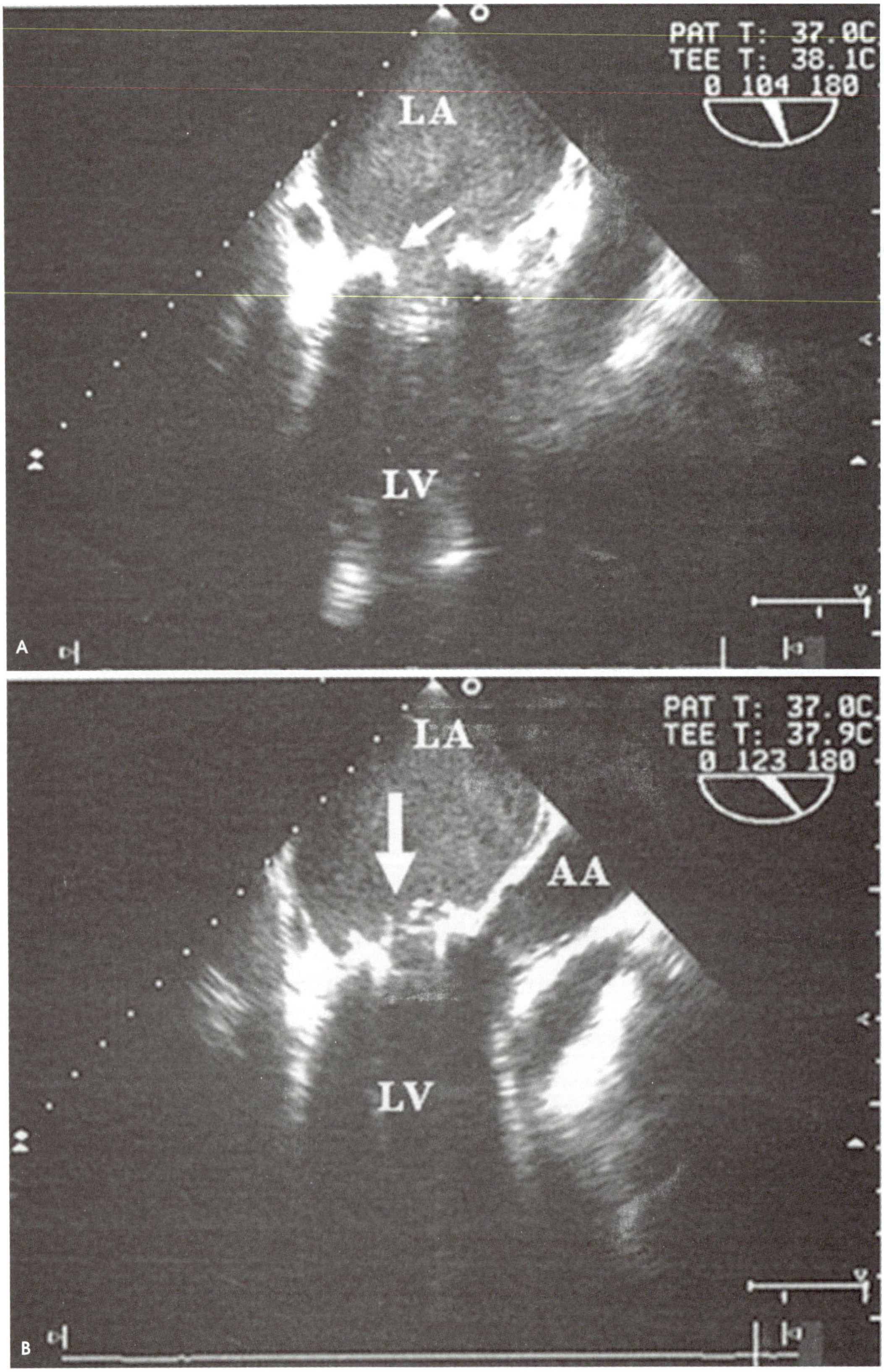

Fig. 12.15A and B: Vegetations (arrows) in a patient with the Starr-Edwards prosthesis in mitral position. Vegetations, suture material and fibrous strands growing from valves resemble each other and are differentiated based upon their location, appearance and movement. Vegetations have a characteristic off-axis motion, which is independent of and lags from the underlying tissue. (LA: left atrium, LV: left ventricle, AA: ascending aorta).

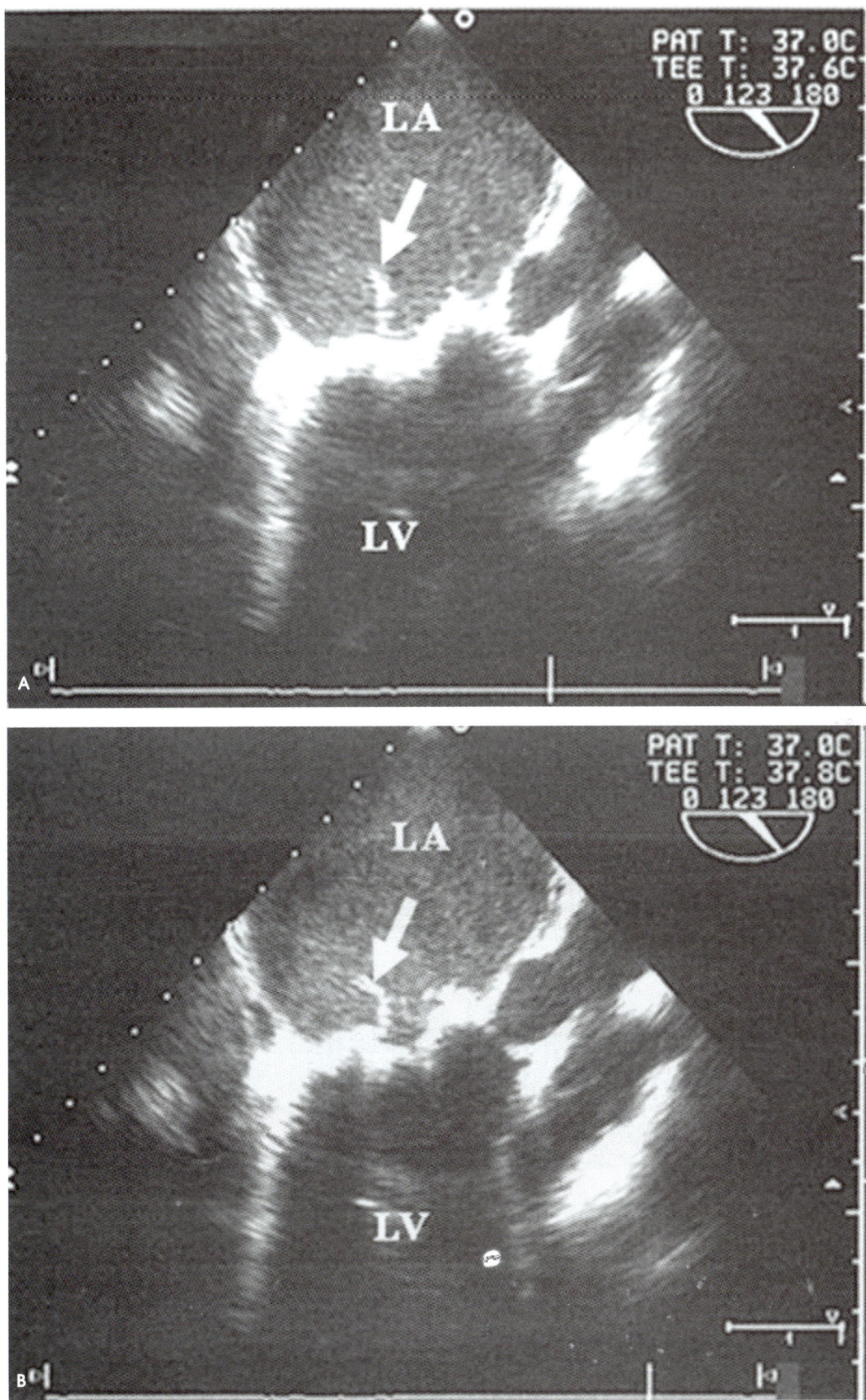

Fig. 12.16A and B: Mobile vegetations (arrow) over the mitral prosthesis (LA: left atrium, LV: left ventricle).

AORTIC VALVE PROSTHESIS

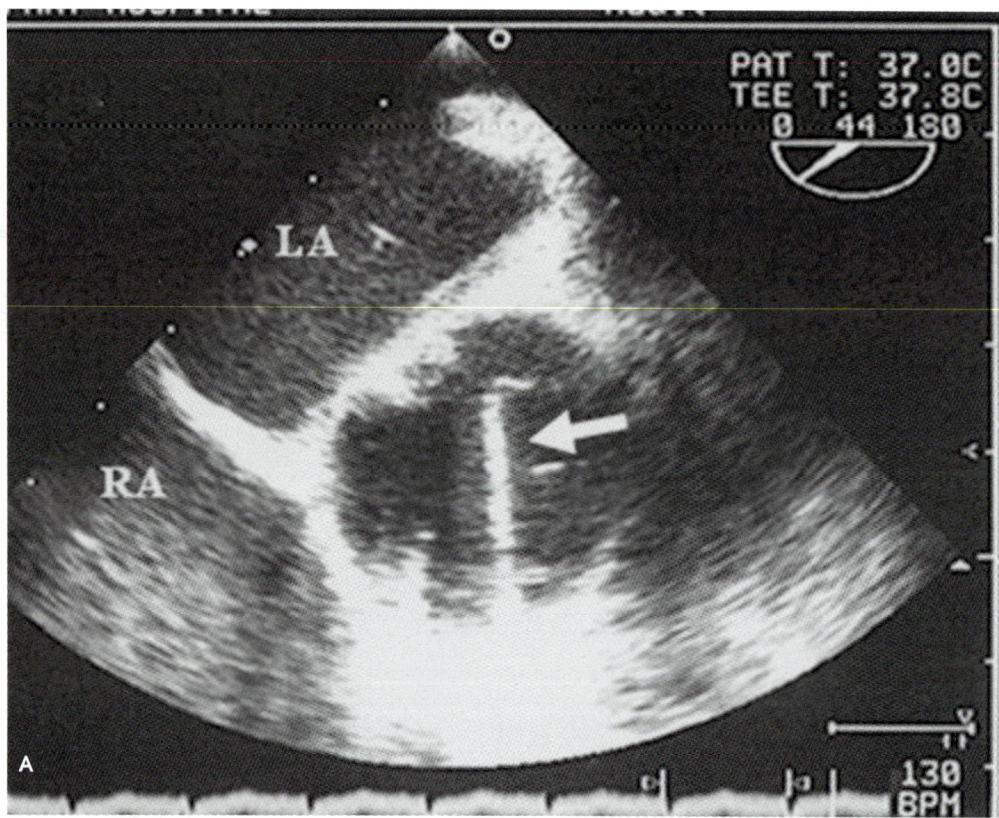

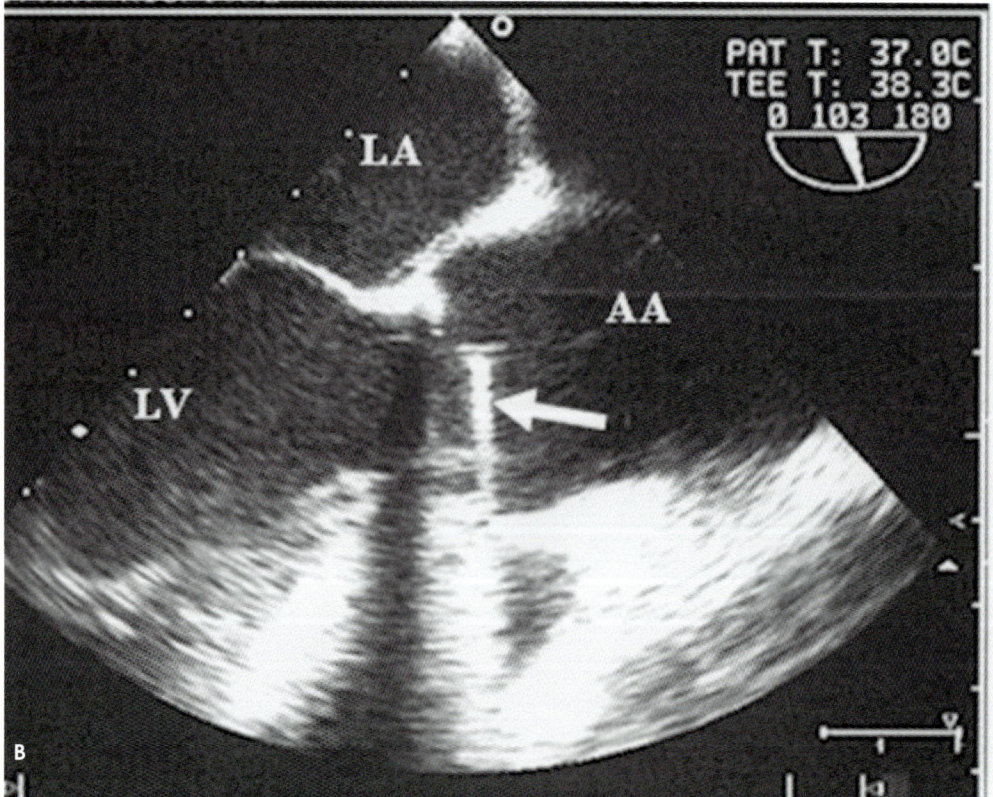

Fig. 12.17: Bjork-Shiley tilting disc valve in the aortic position. Note the appearance of disc (arrow) in midesophageal aortic valve short-axis view (A) and long-axis view (B). (LA: left atrium, RA: right atrium, LV: left ventricle, AA: ascending aorta).

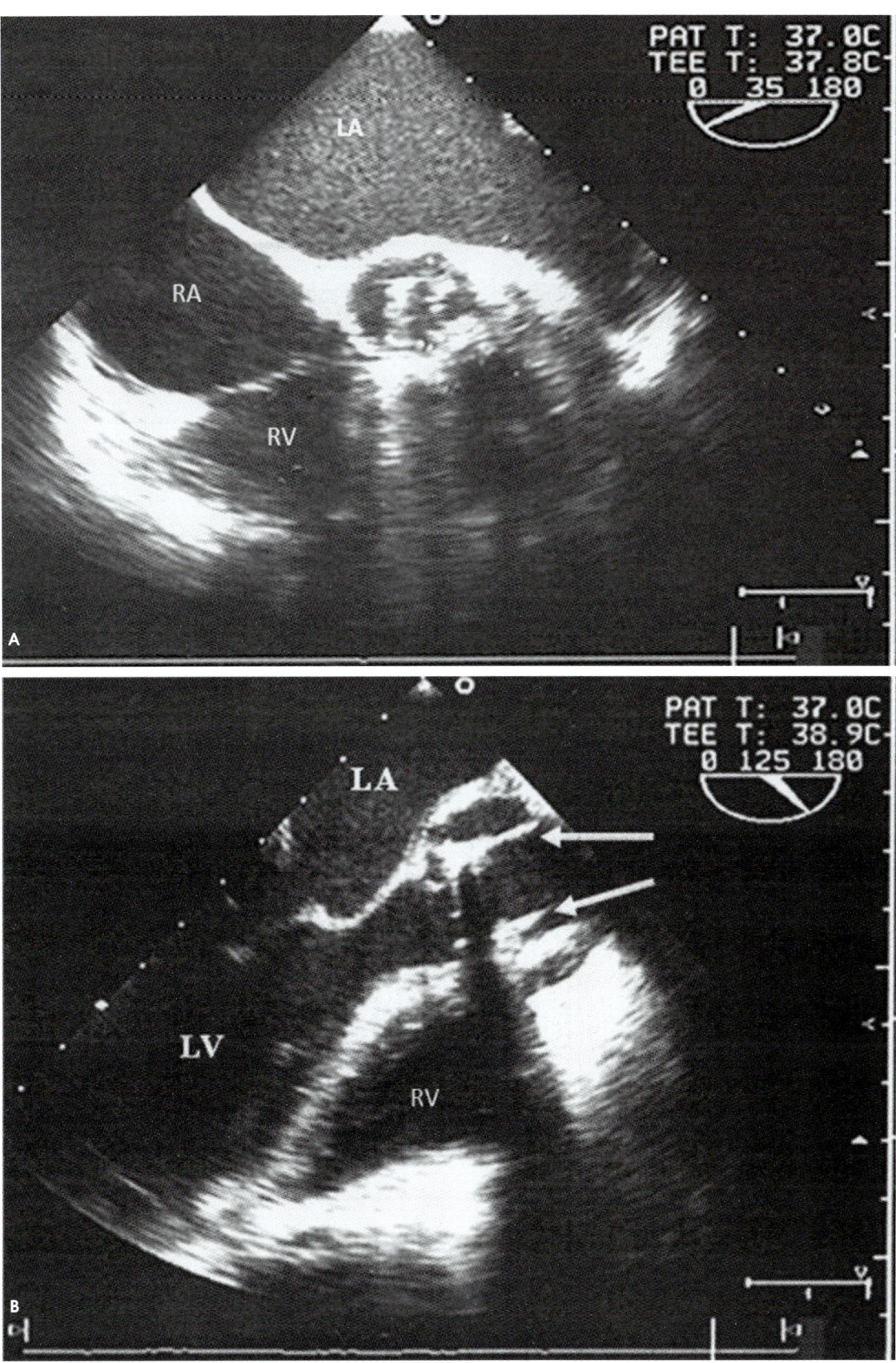

Fig. 12.18: Appearance of the St. Jude bileaflet prosthesis in the aortic position in short-axis view (A) and long-axis view (B). Note the two leaflets (arrows). (RA: right atrium, RV: right ventricle, LA: left atrium, LV: left ventricle).

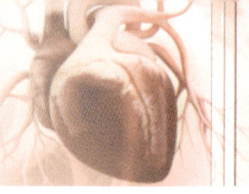

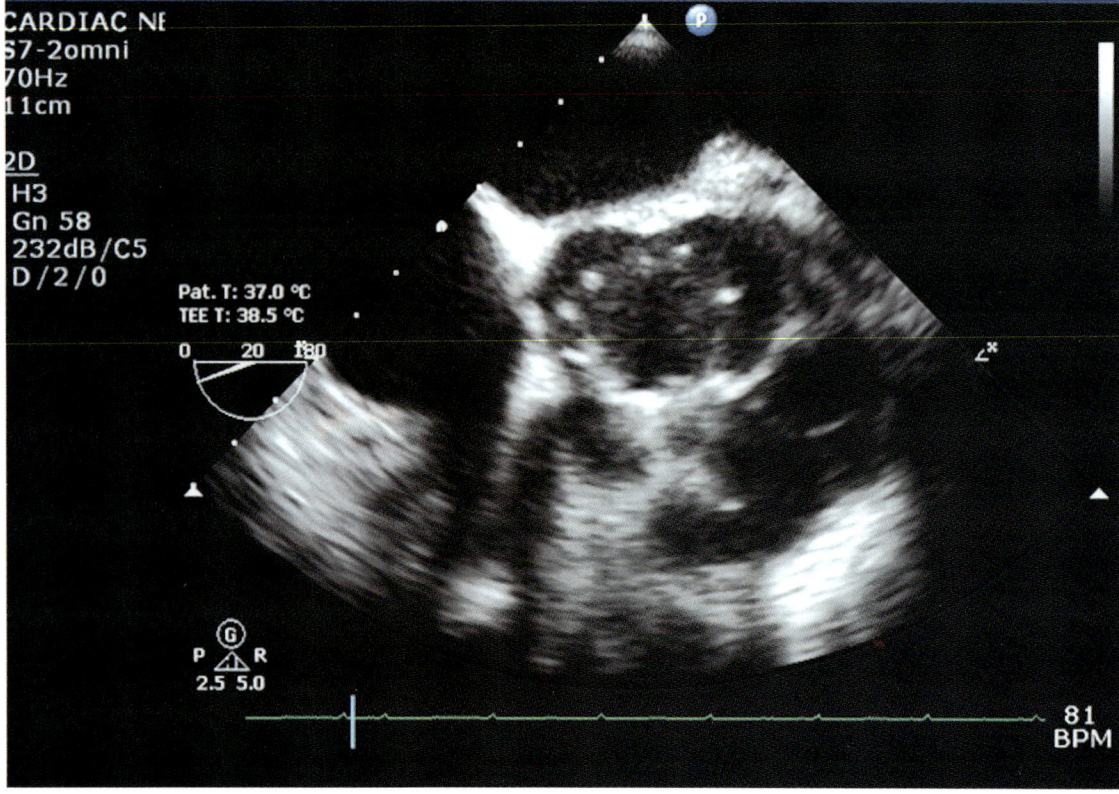

Fig. 12.19: Midesophageal aortic valve short-axis view showing the circumferential suture line in a patient with aortic valve replacement.

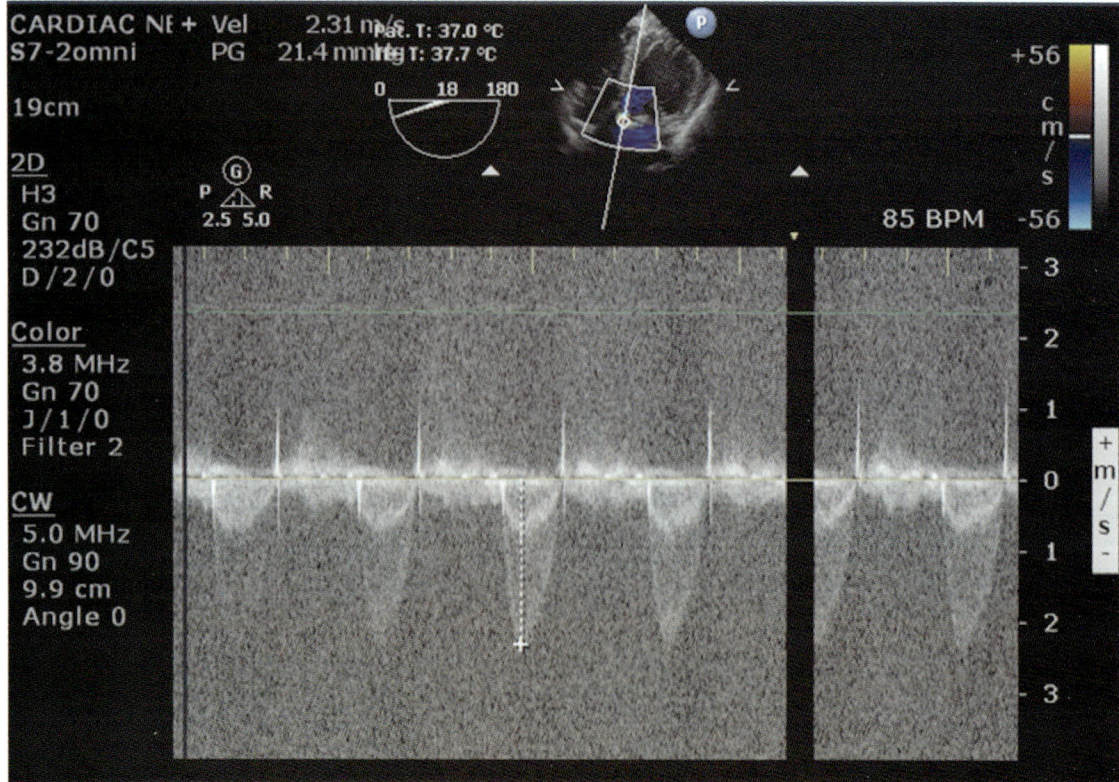

Fig. 12.20: Pulsed wave Doppler across the prosthetic aortic valve showing two envelops, the smaller at the level of the left ventricular outflow tract and the larger at the aortic valve due to the inherent gradient offered by the prosthetic valve.

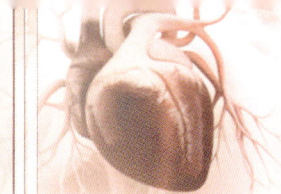

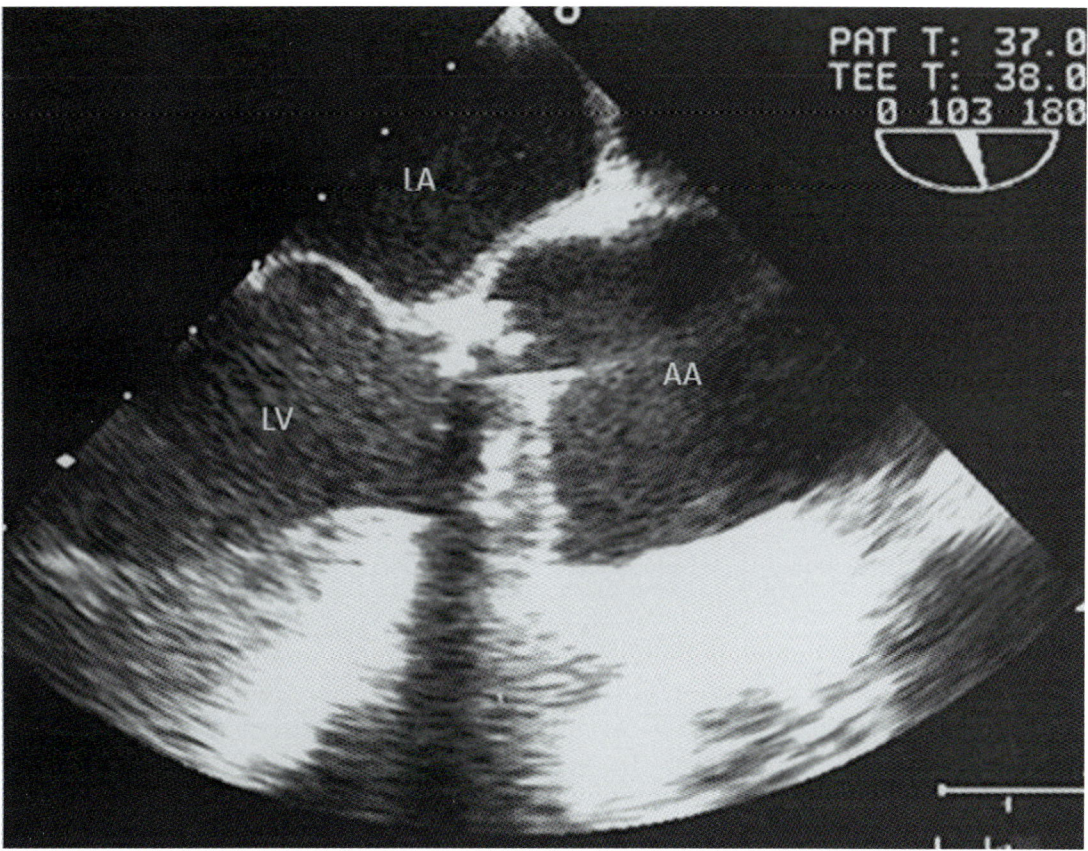

Fig. 12.21: Midesophageal aortic valve long-axis view showing vegetations over a tilting disc aortic valve prosthesis. (LA: left atrium, LV: left ventricle, AA: ascending aorta)

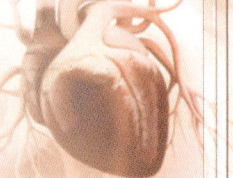

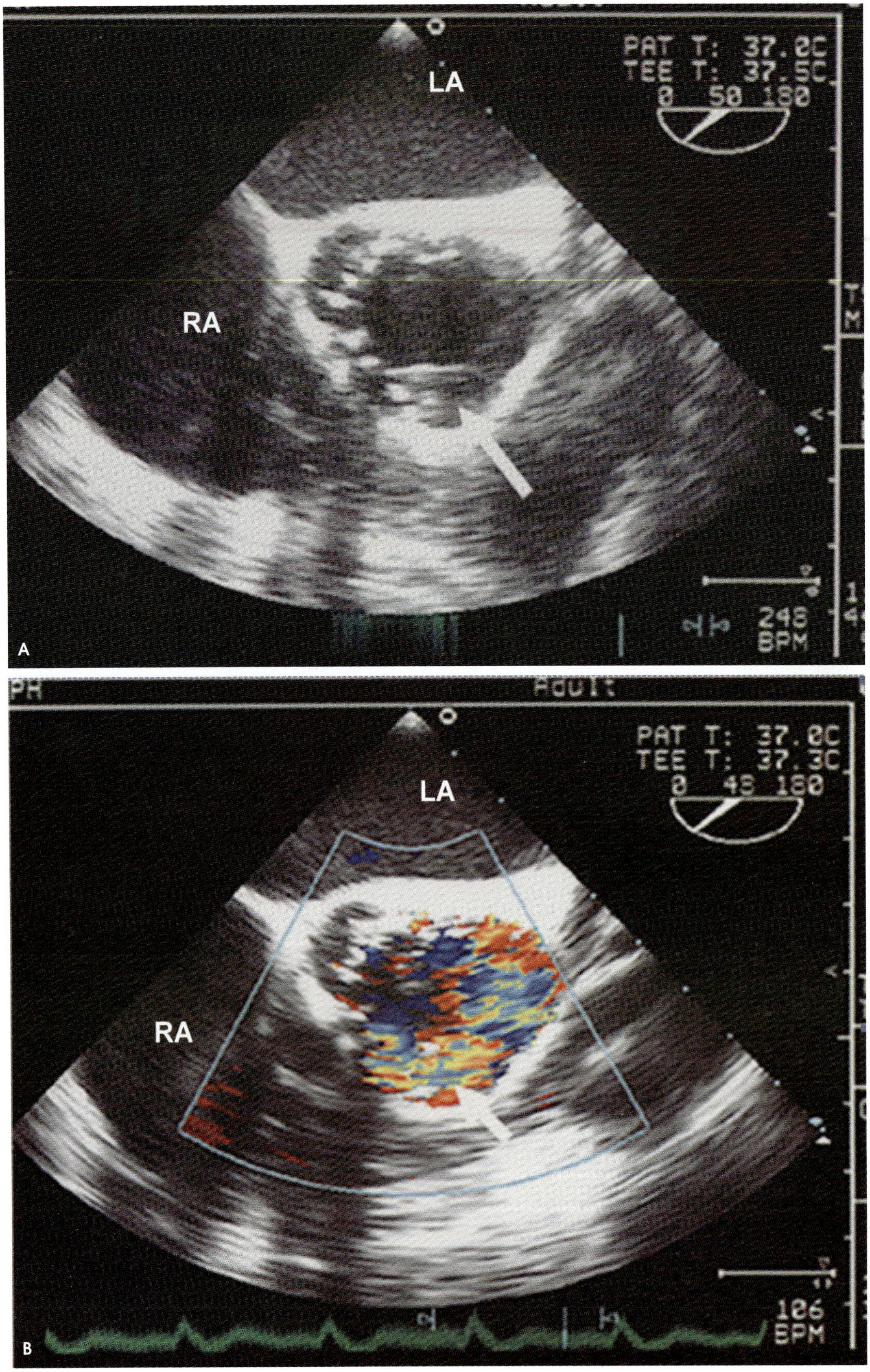

Fig. 12.22: Midesophageal aortic valve short-axis view showing paravalvular leak in a patient with aortic homograft. Note the paravalvular space (arrow in A) and the regurgitant jet through that area (arrow in B) (LA: left atrium, RA: right atrium).

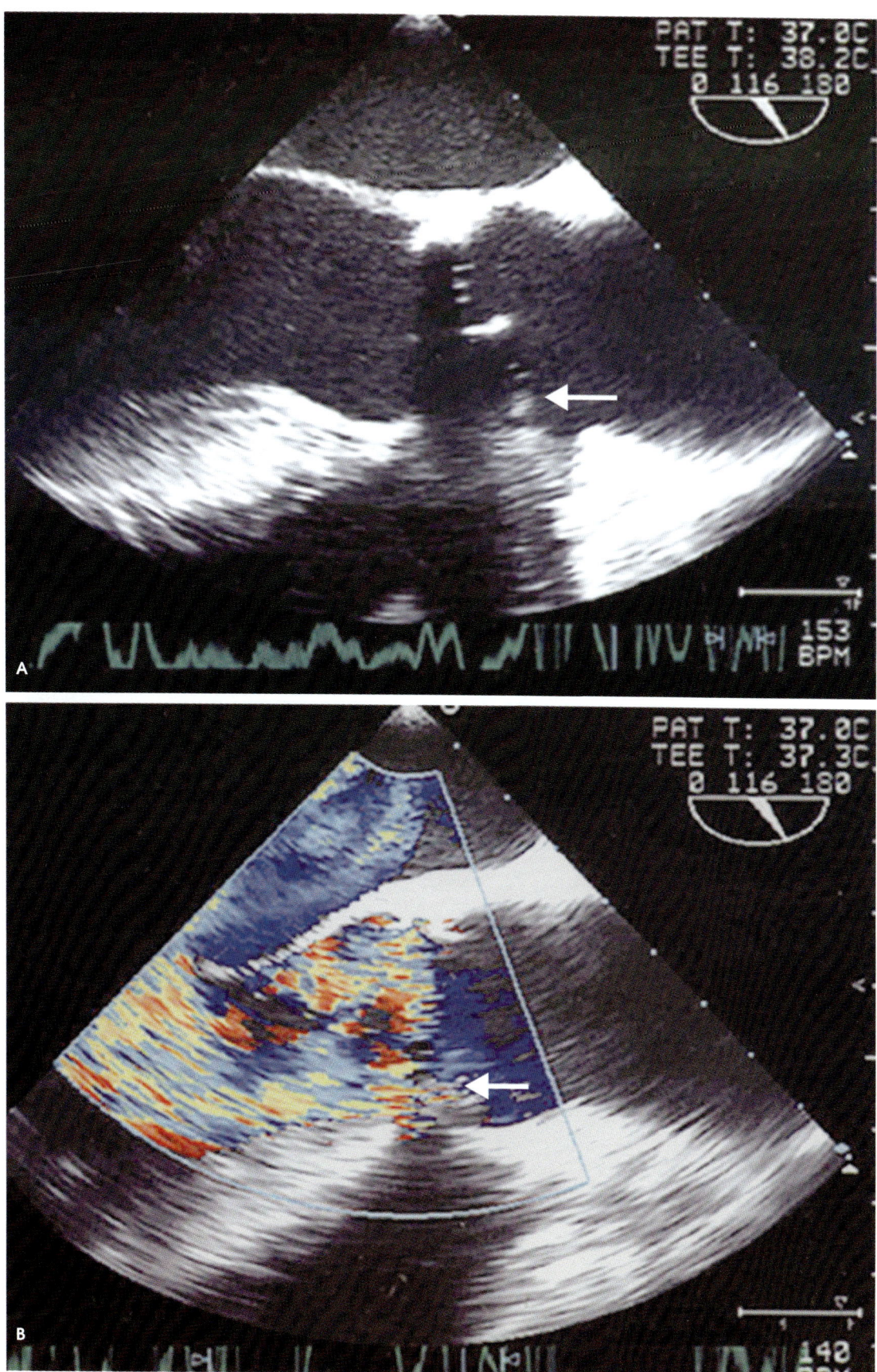

Fig. 12.23: Appearance of the paraprosthetic space (arrow, A) and aortic regurgitation (arrow, B) in aortic valve long-axis view.

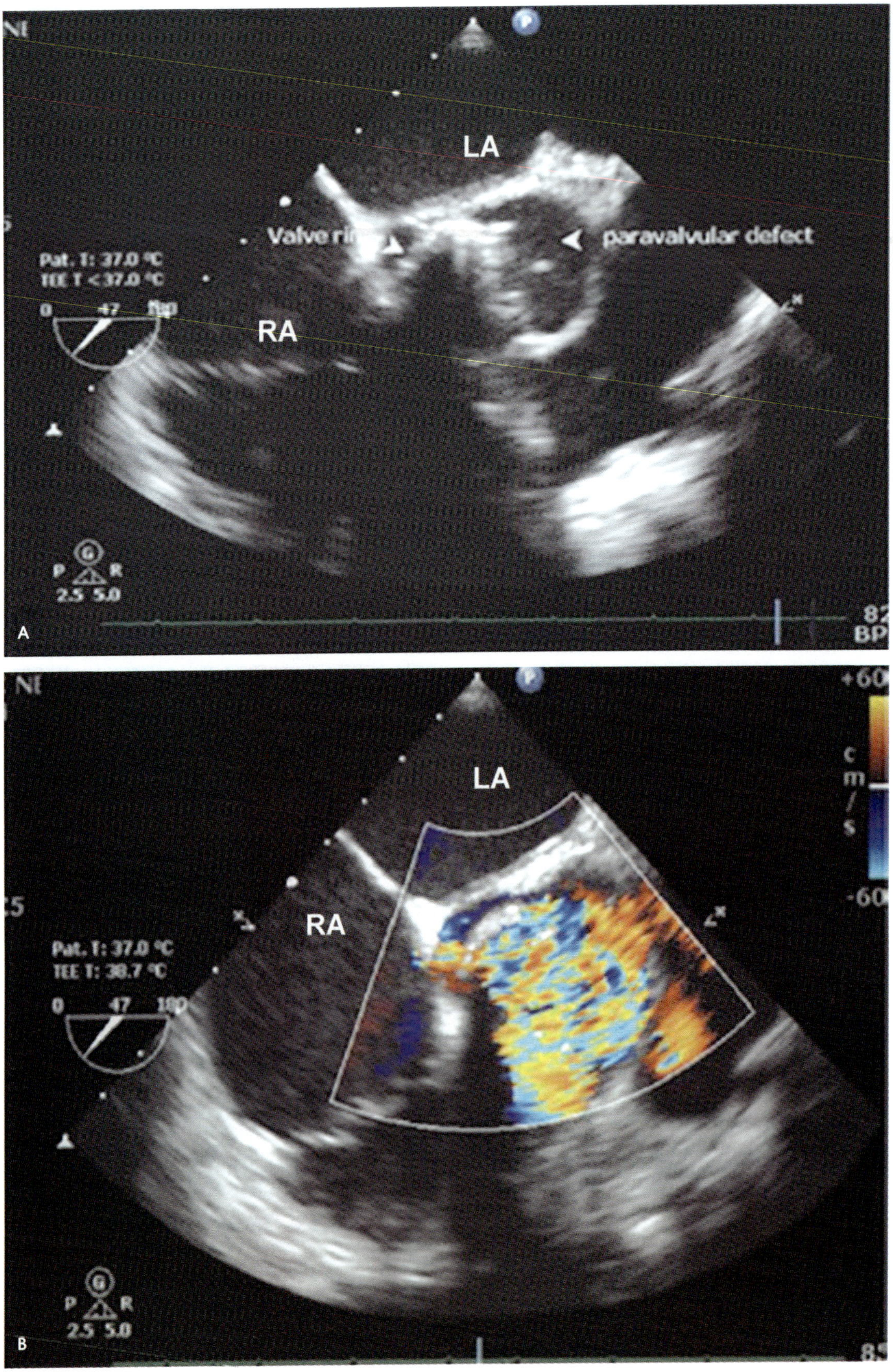

Fig. 12.24: Midesophageal aortic valve short-axis view showing a paravalvular defect around the aortic valve prosthesis (A) and color flow showing severe regurgitation (B) (LA: left atrium, RA: right atrium).

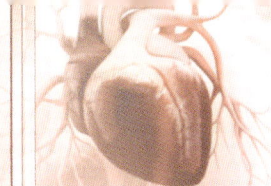

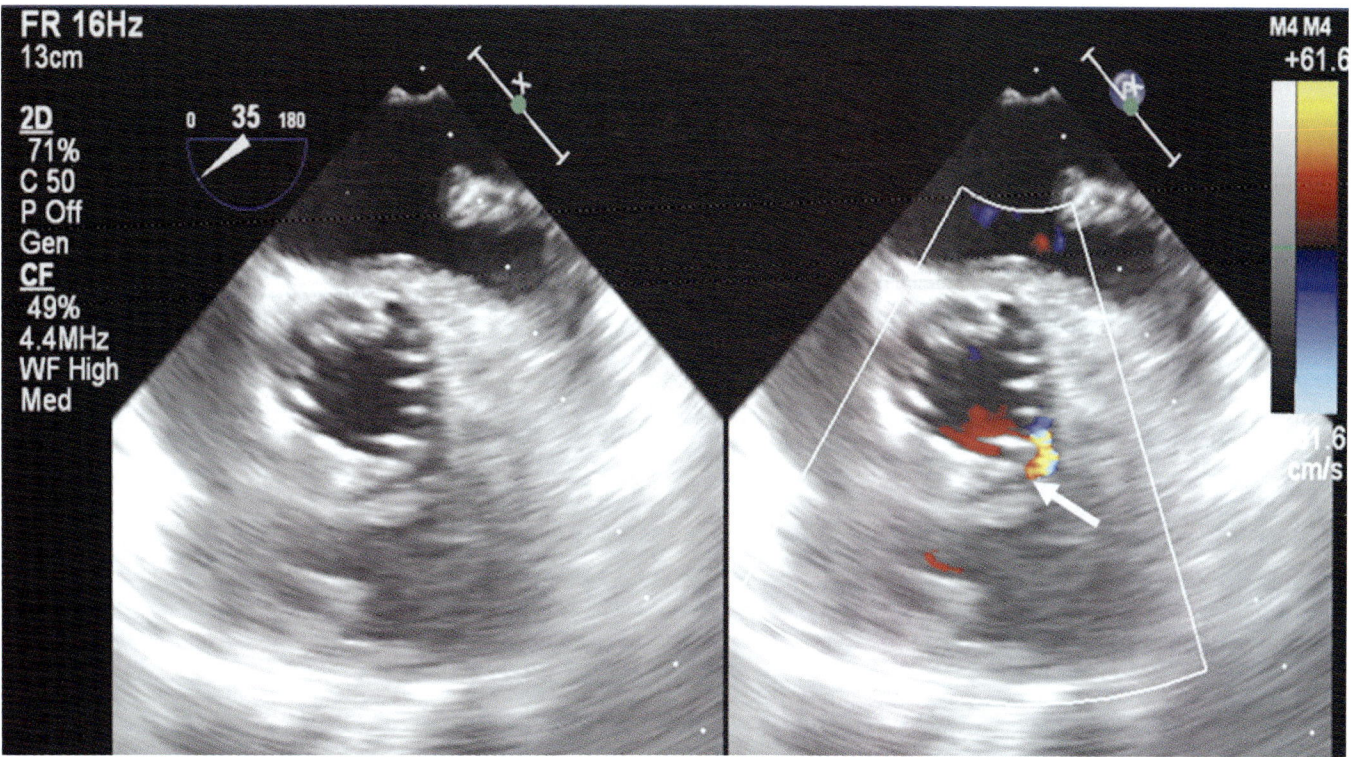

Fig. 12.25: Midesophageal aortic valve short-axis view with color showing an aortic prosthesis in situ and the presence of paravalvular leak at the junction of right and left coronary sinuses (arrow).

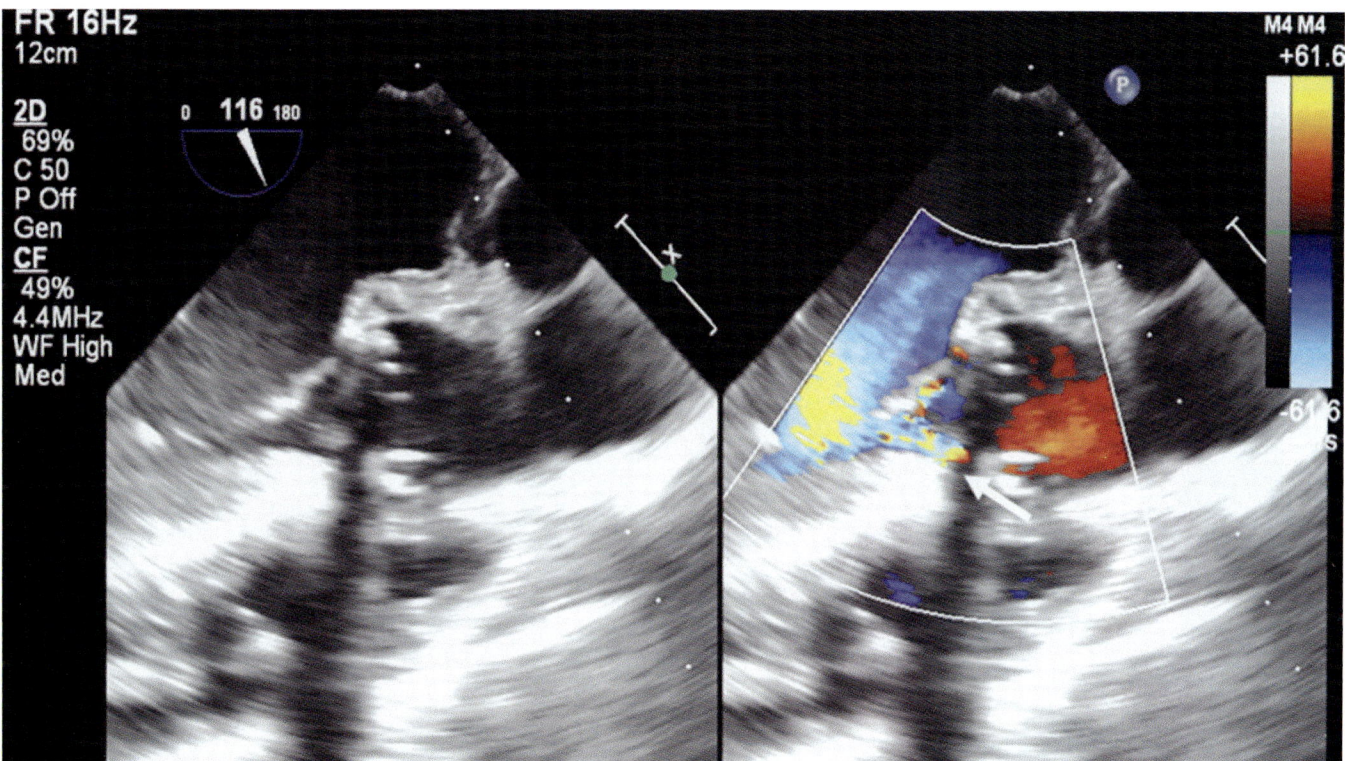

Fig. 12.26: Midesophageal aortic valve long-axis view with color showing a mechanical aortic prosthesis in situ and the presence of paravalvular leak at the junction of right and left coronary sinuses (arrow).

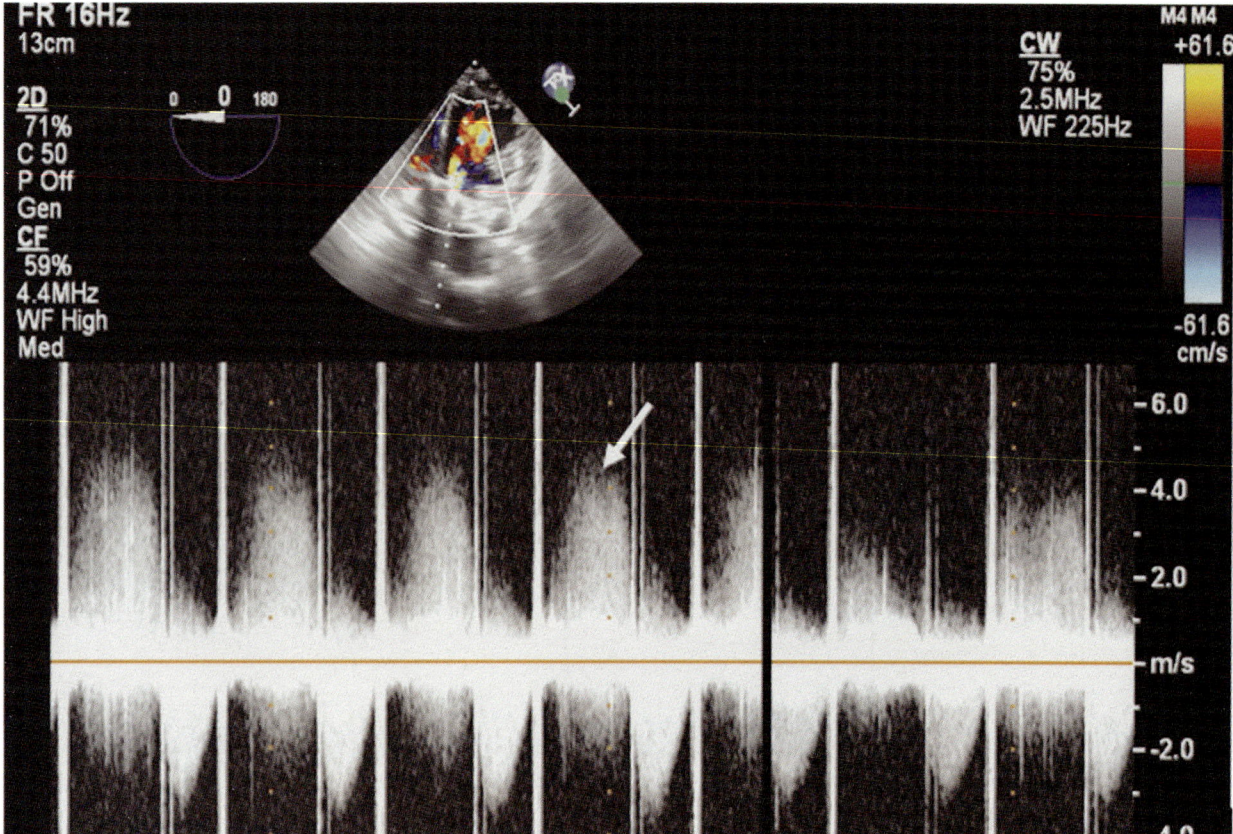

Fig. 12.27: Deep transgastric long-axis view with continuous wave Doppler showing regurgitant flow due to paravalvular leak (arrow) in addition to the inherent gradient of a mechanical aortic prosthesis.

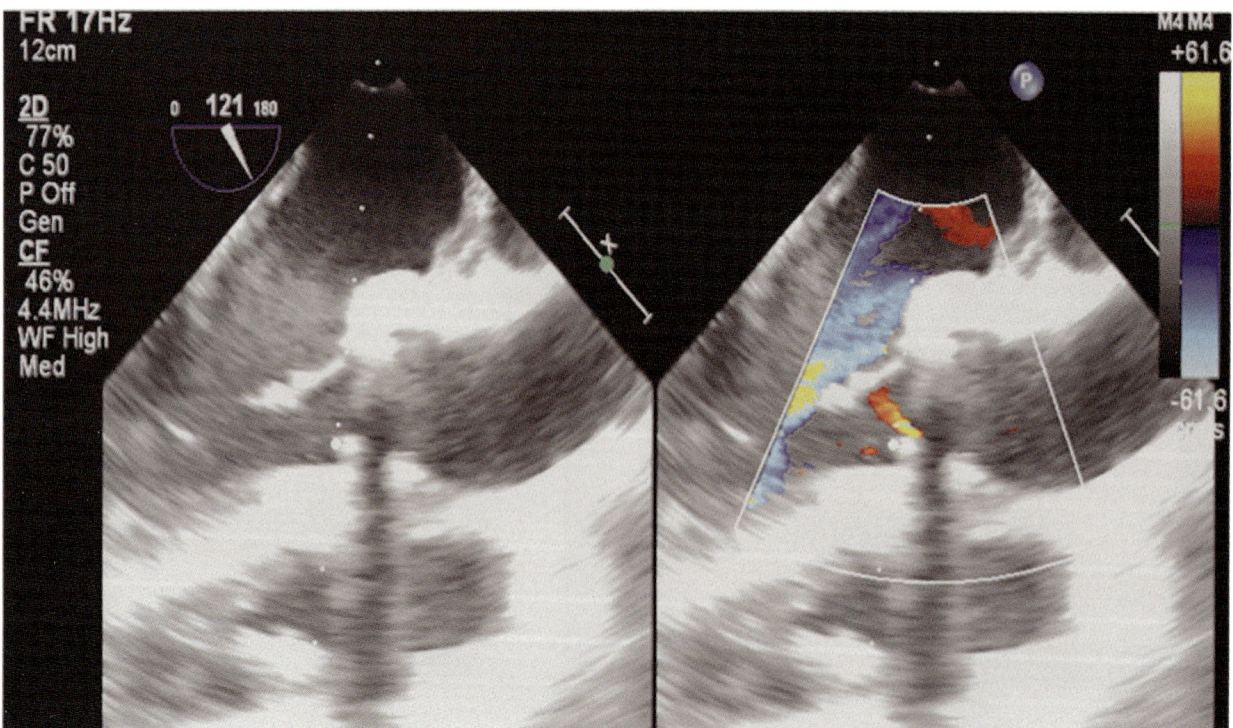

Fig. 12.28: Midesophageal aortic valve long-axis view after correction of the paravalvular leak shows disappearance of the regurgitant jet outside the sewing ring.

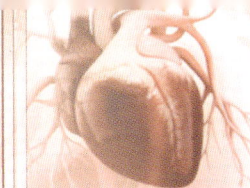

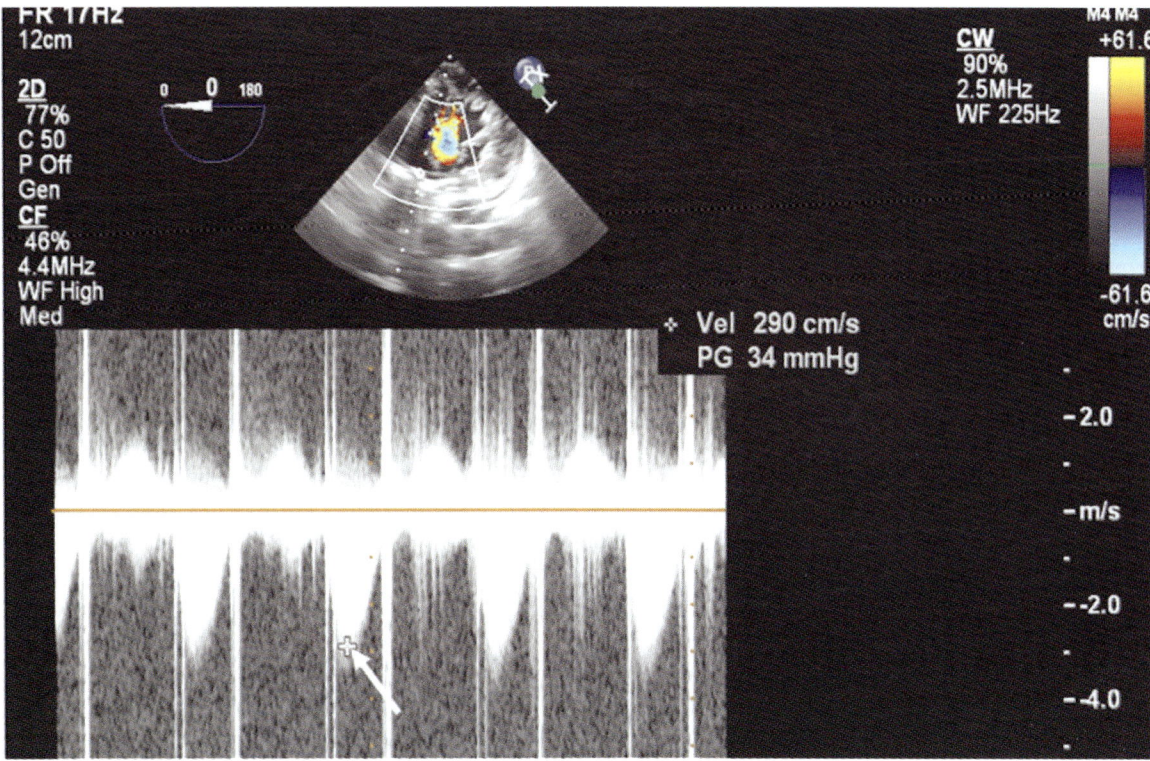

Fig. 12.29: Deep transgastric long-axis view with continuous wave Doppler after correction of the paravalvular leak shows the disappearance of the regurgitant jet. The native aortic valve was replaced with a size 19 mechanical prosthesis which had an inherent gradient (arrow).

Congenital Heart Disease

• Deepak K. Tempe • Suruchi Hasija

13

Transthoracic echocardiography currently is considered as a gold standard for diagnosing structural defects in patients with congenital heart disease (CHD). Transesophageal echocardiography (TEE) aids in confirming the diagnosis, judging the adequacy of the repair, deairing, detection and

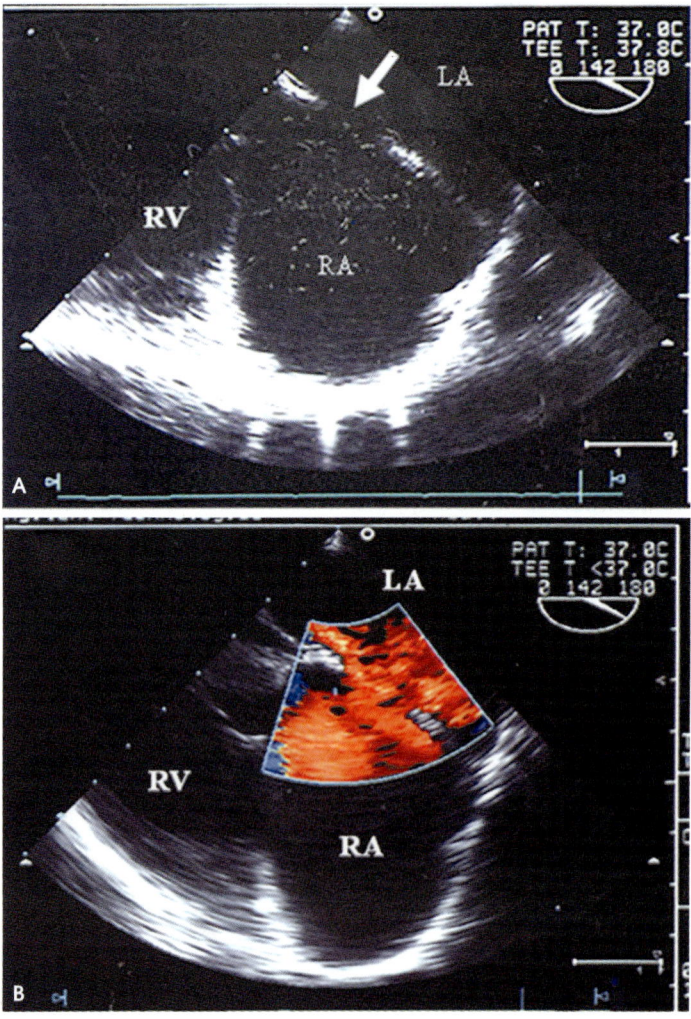

Fig. 13.1: Midesophageal modified bicaval view showing an ostium secundum atrial septal defect (ASD) (arrow). Note the margins of the defect (A) and right to left atrial shunt on color flow (B) (RA: right atrium, LA: left atrium, RV: right ventricle). In patients with isolated ASD having right to left shunt, pulmonary hypertension is likely to be present.

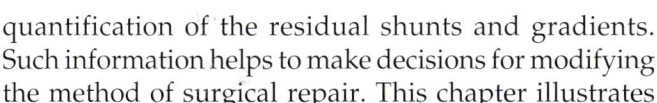

quantification of the residual shunts and gradients. Such information helps to make decisions for modifying the method of surgical repair. This chapter illustrates the TEE appearance of some commonly encountered congenital heart defects.

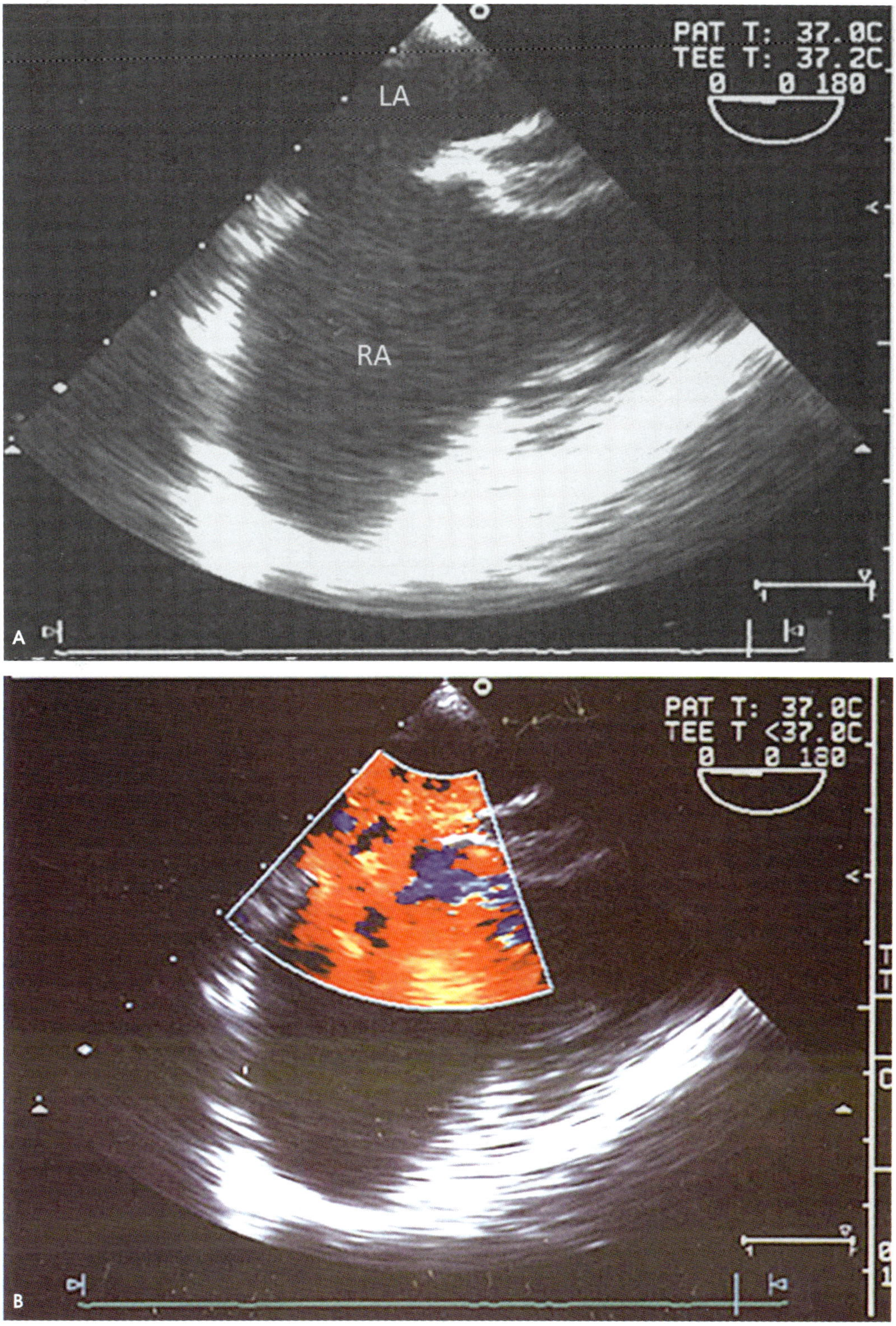

Fig. 13.2: Midesophageal view at zero degree, (A) A large ostium secundum atrial septal defect. Note the margins of atrial septal defect which are relatively deficient. The patient had a bidirectional shunt due to significant pulmonary arterial hypertension (subsystemic). Panel B shows the right to left component of the bidirectional flow in this patient. (RA: right atrium, LA: left atrium).

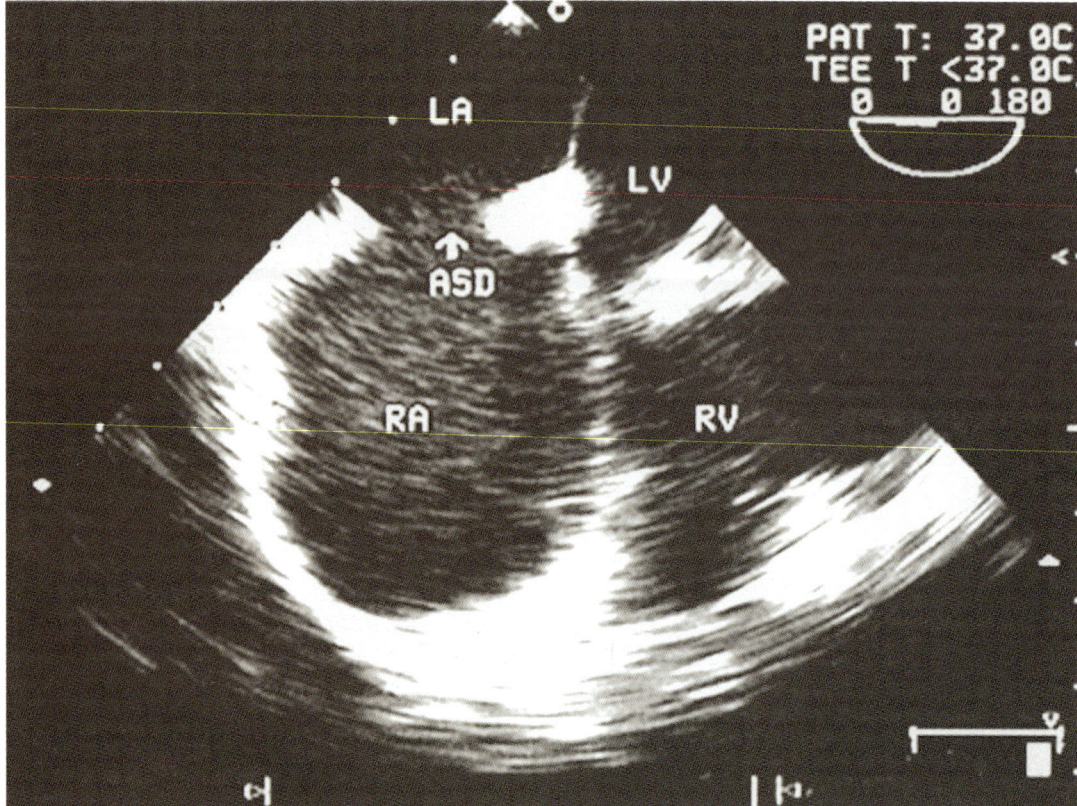

Fig. 13.3: Modified midesophageal four-chamber view showing a large secundum atrial septal defect (ASD). (LA: left atrium, RA: right atrium, LV: left ventricle, RV: right ventricle).

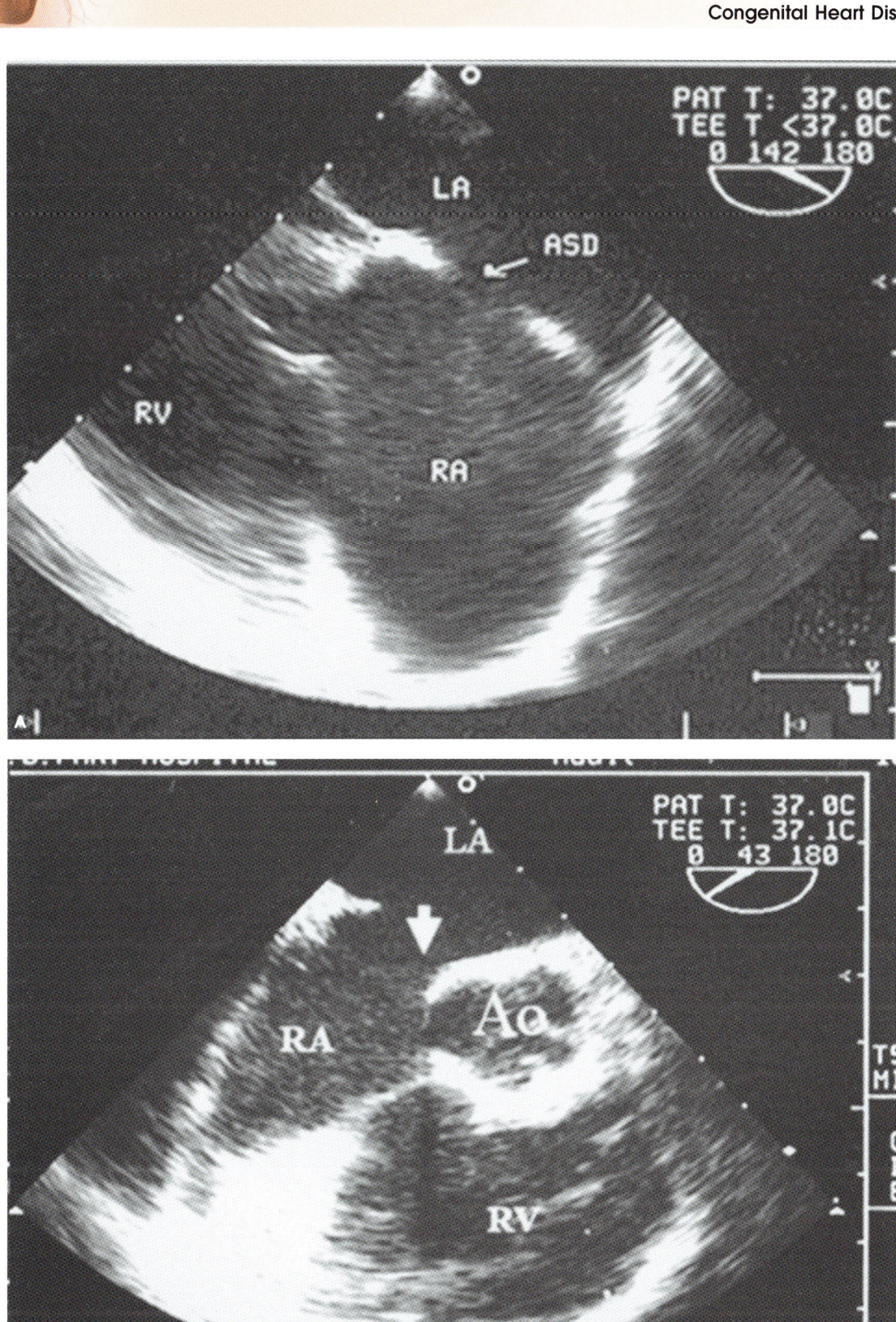

Fig. 13.4: Appearance of the atrial septal defect (ASD) in different views. Note the well formed superior and inferior margins (A) and deficient aortic margin (arrow, B) (LA: left atrium, RA: right atrium, Ao: aorta, RV: right ventricle).

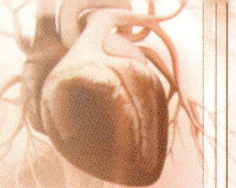

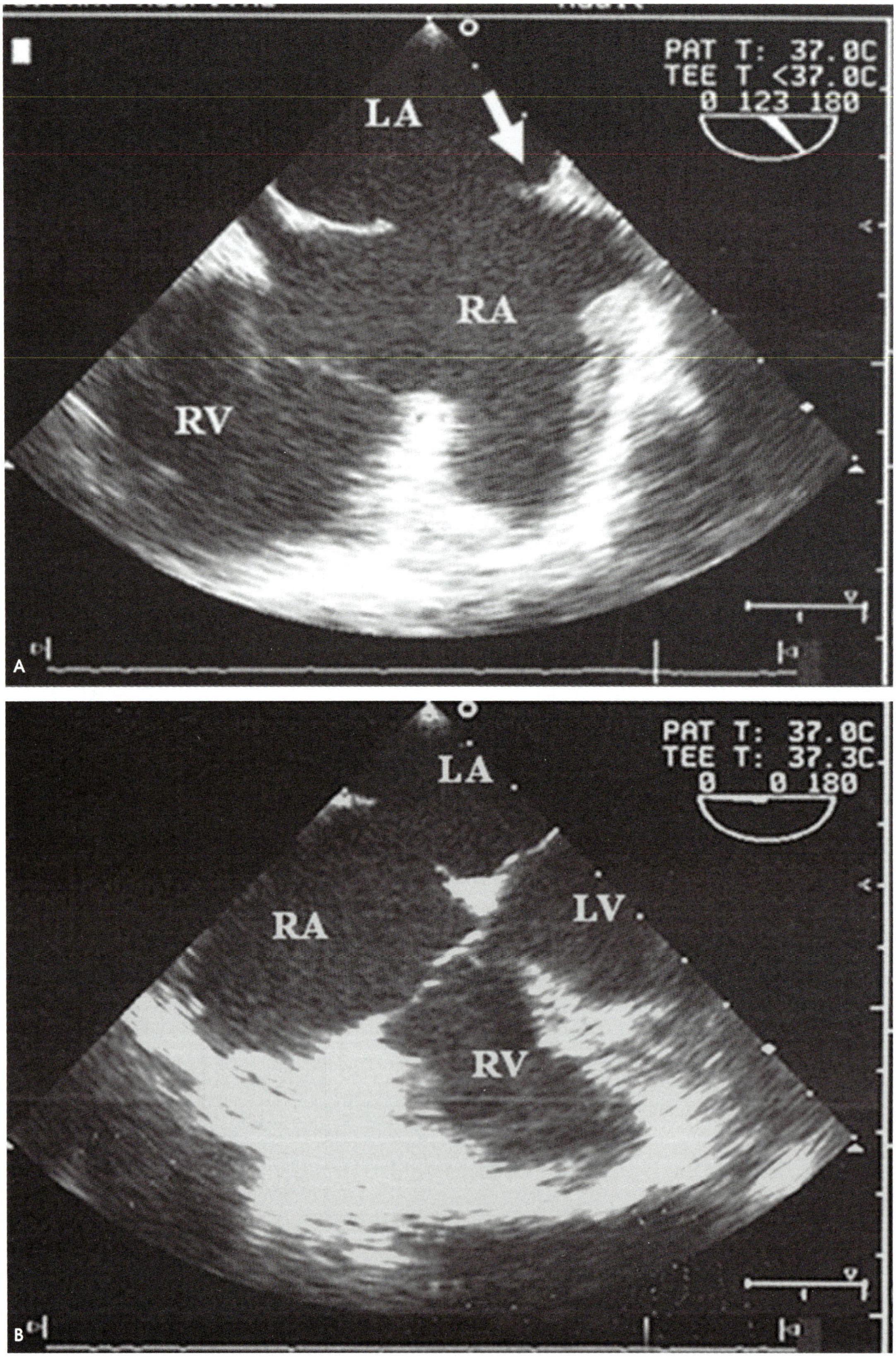

Fig. 13.5: Modified bicaval view showing a large secundum atrial septal defect with inadequate superior margin (arrow, A), although it appears adequate in the four chamber view (B). Adequate margins are a prerequisite for percutaneous device closure of atrial septal defect, and its absence necessitates surgical closure as in this case (LA: left atrium, RA: right atrium, RV: right ventricle, LV: left ventricle).

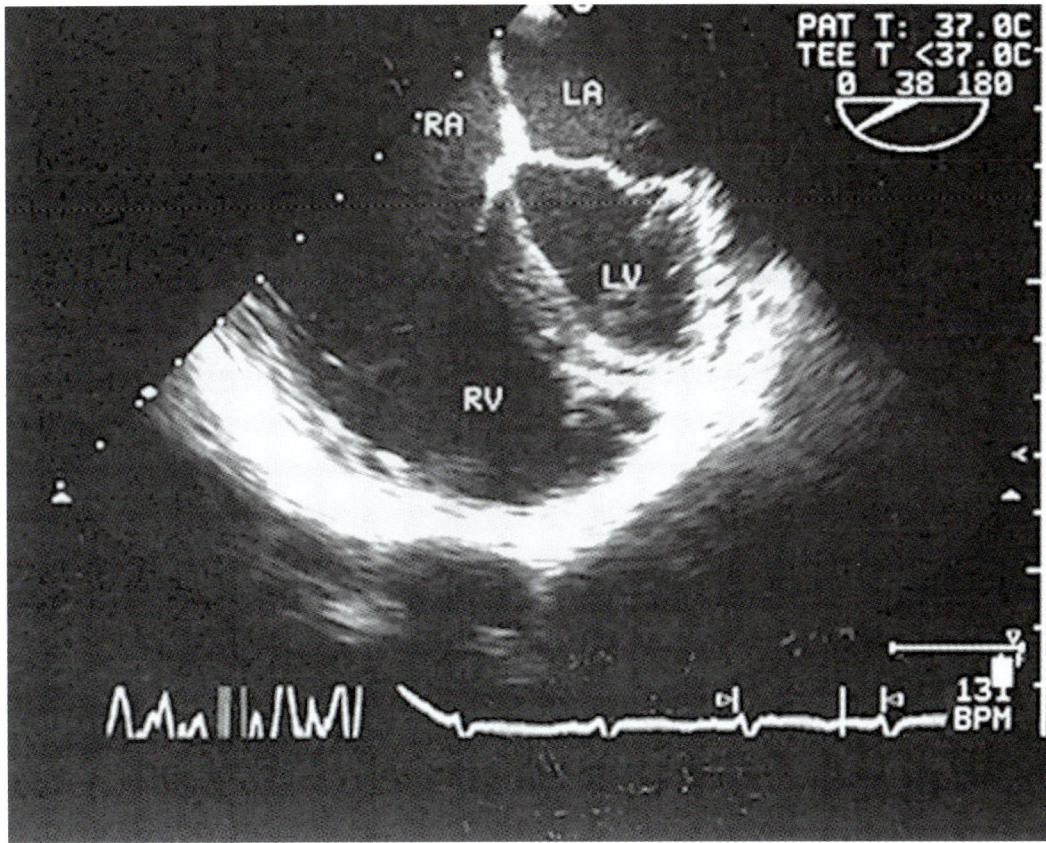

Fig. 13.6: Dilated right side due to massive Left-to-right shunt in a patient with an atrial septal defect. Normal size of the right ventricle is less than 60% of that of the left ventricle. (RA: right atrium, LA; left atrium, RV: right ventricle, LV; left ventricle).

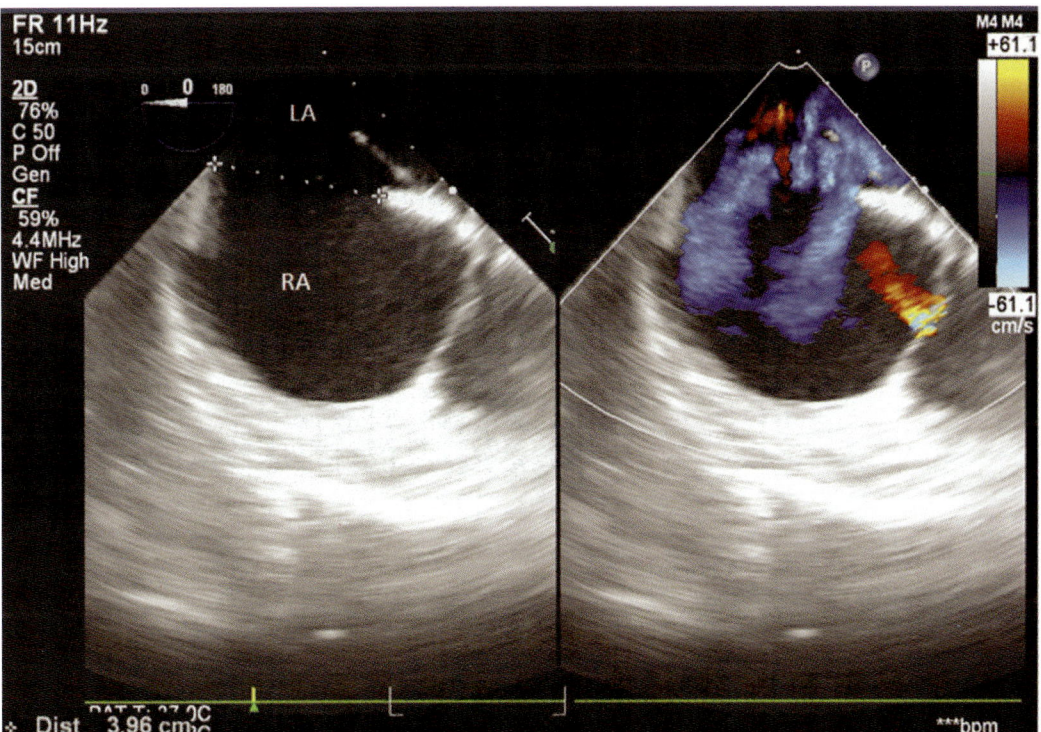

Fig. 13.7: Midesophageal four-chamber view with rightward rotation showing a large ostium secundum atrial septal defect with left to right shunt (LA: left atrium, RA: right atrium).

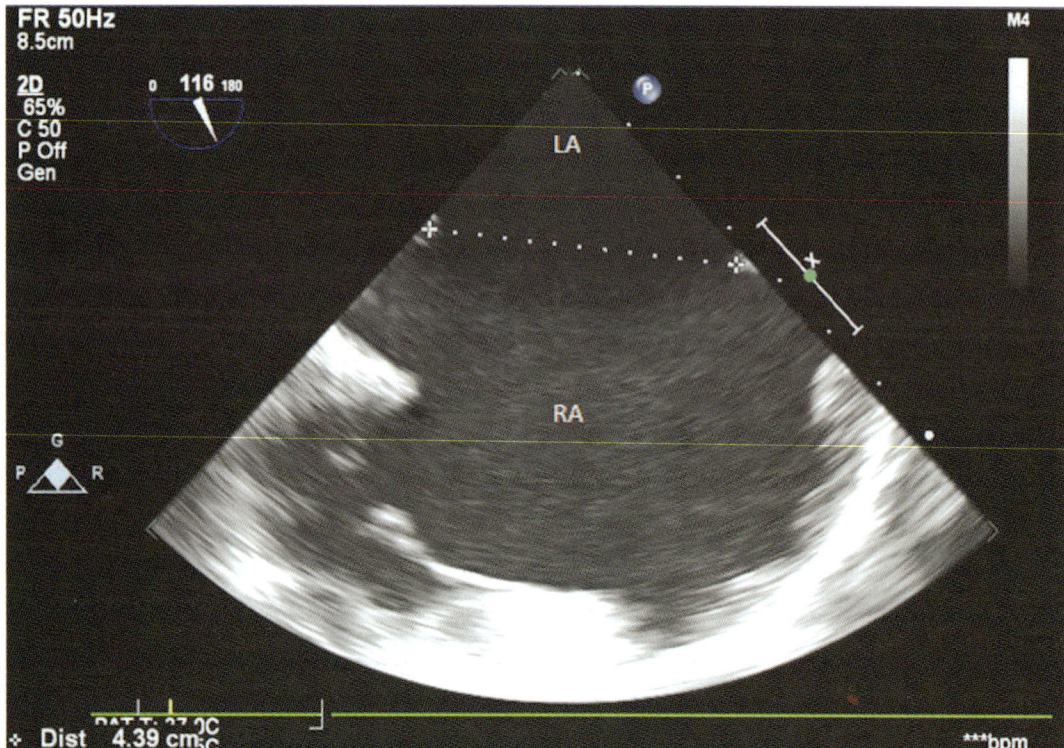

Fig. 13.8: Midesophageal modified bicaval view showing a large ostium secundum atrial septal defect (LA: left atrium, RA: right atrium).

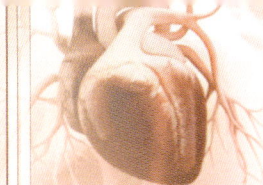

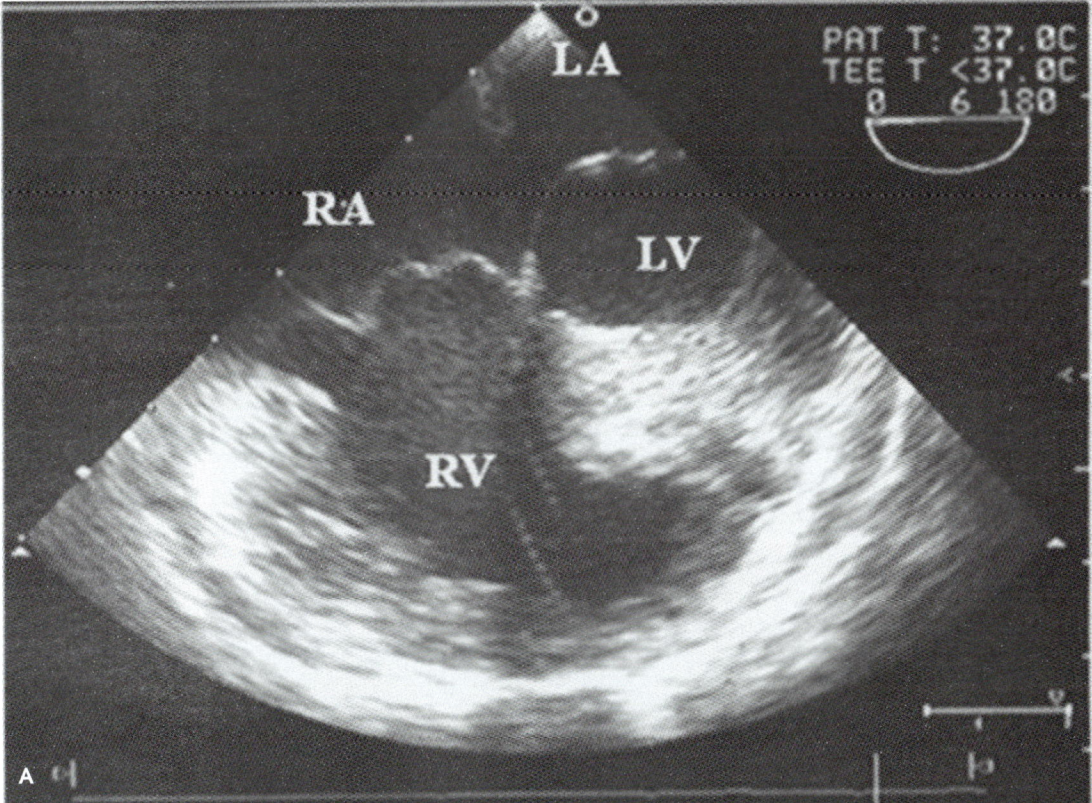

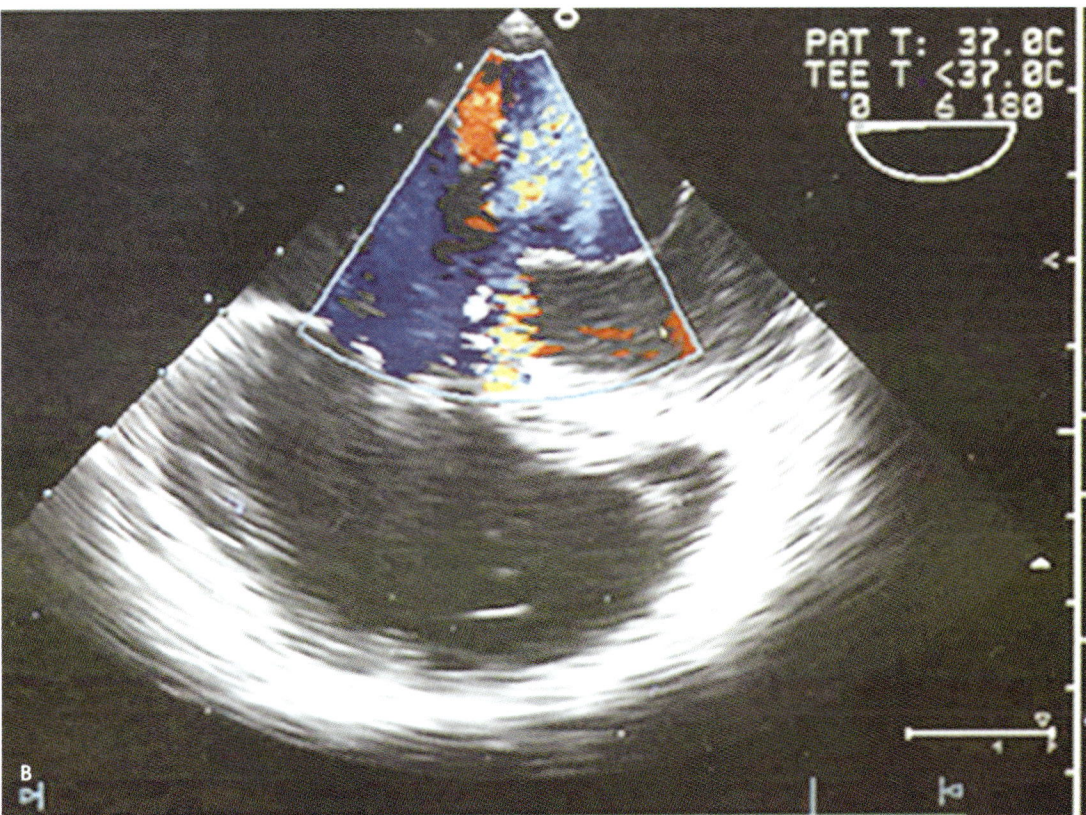

Fig. 13.9: Midesophageal four-chamber view. Panel A: Appearance of the ostium primum atrial septal defect. Note the volume overloaded right ventricle. Panel B: Color flow across the defect shows a large left to right shunt across the defect (LA: left atrium, RA: right atrium, LV: left ventricle, RV: right ventricle).

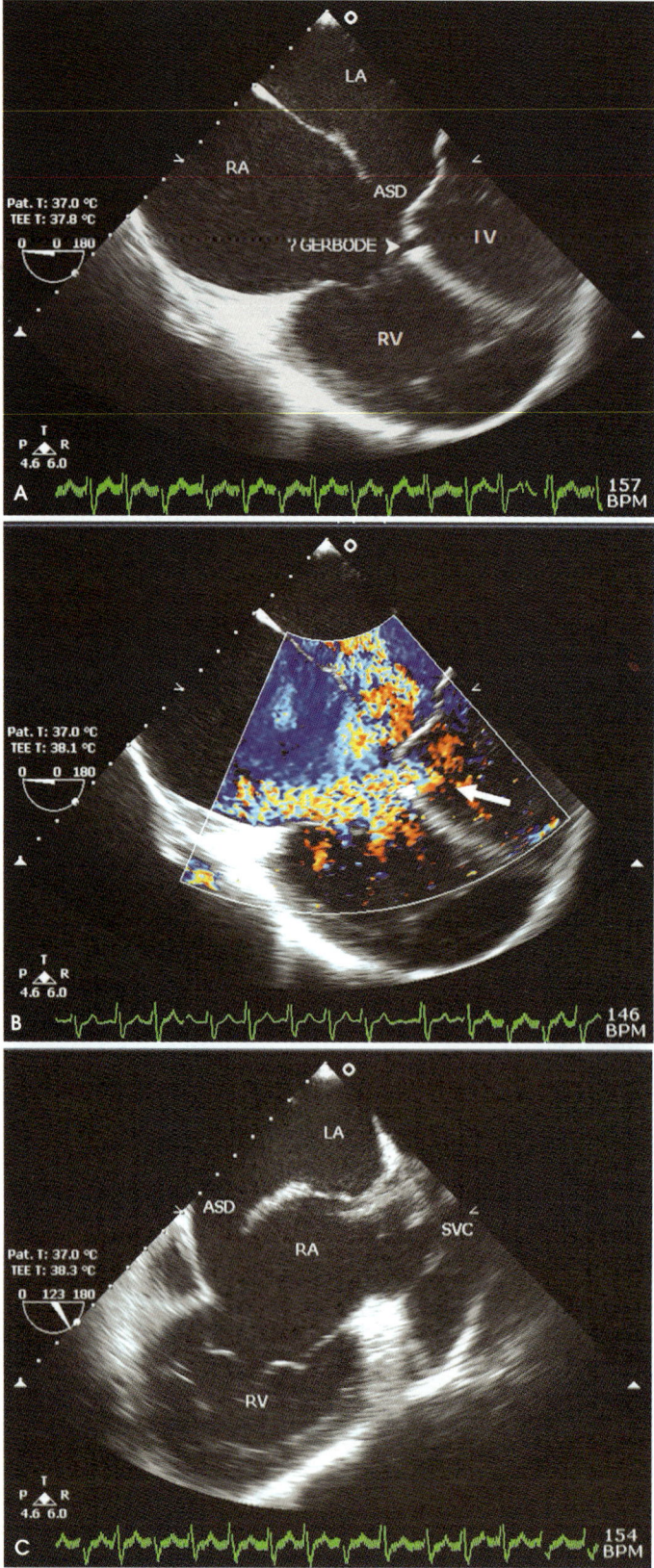

Fig. 13.10: Midesophageal four-chamber view (A) with color flow Doppler (B) and midesophageal modified bicaval view (C) showing an ostium primum atrial septal defect. Note the shunt across the atrial septal defect as well as at Gerbode defect. The Gerbode defect is a communication between the left ventricle and the right atrium (B, arrow). (RA: right atrium, LA: left atrium, RV: right ventricle, LV: left ventricle, ASD: atrial septal defect, SVC: superior vena cava).

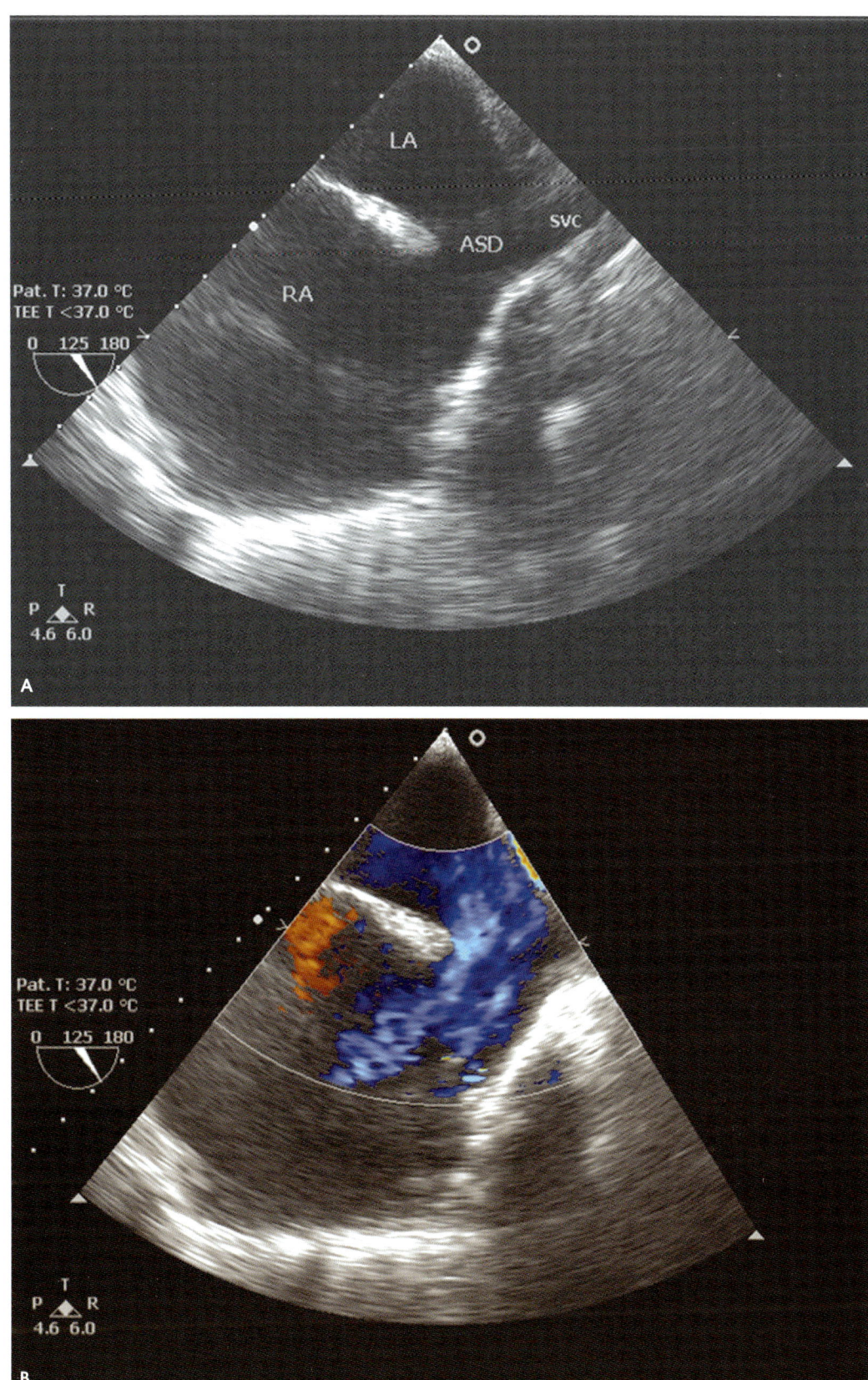

Fig. 13.11: Midesophageal bicaval view (A) with color flow Doppler (B) showing a sinus venosus (SVC type) atrial septal defect (ASD) with left to right shunt. The superior margin of the defect cannot be seen in the sinus venous type of defect (LA: left atrium, RA: right atrium, SVC: superior vena cava).

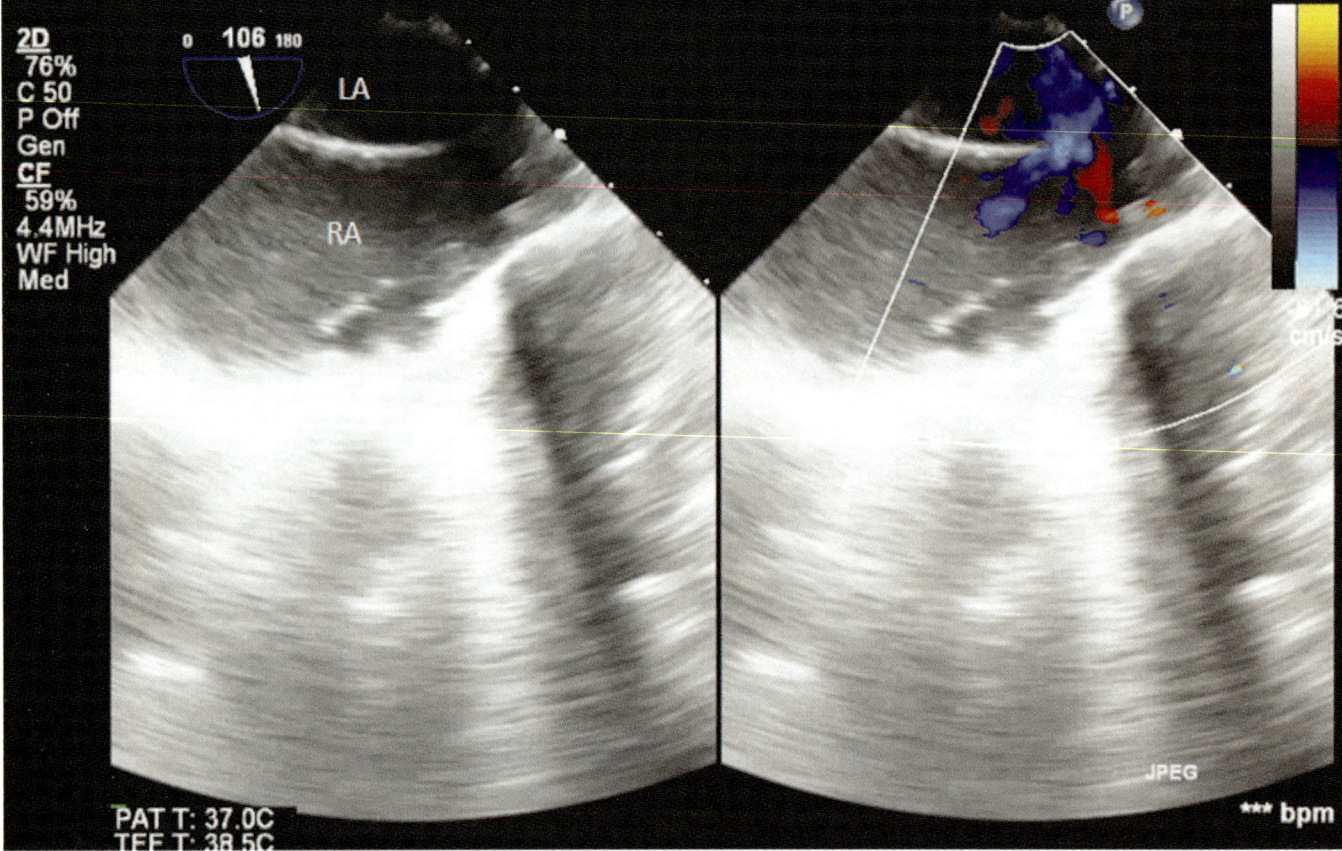

Fig. 13.12: Midesophageal bicaval view with color flow Doppler in another patient showing a sinus venosus (superior vena cava type) atrial septal defect with left to right shunt (LA: left atrium, RA: right atrium).

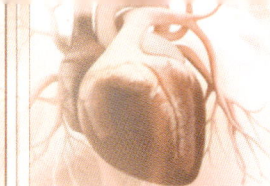

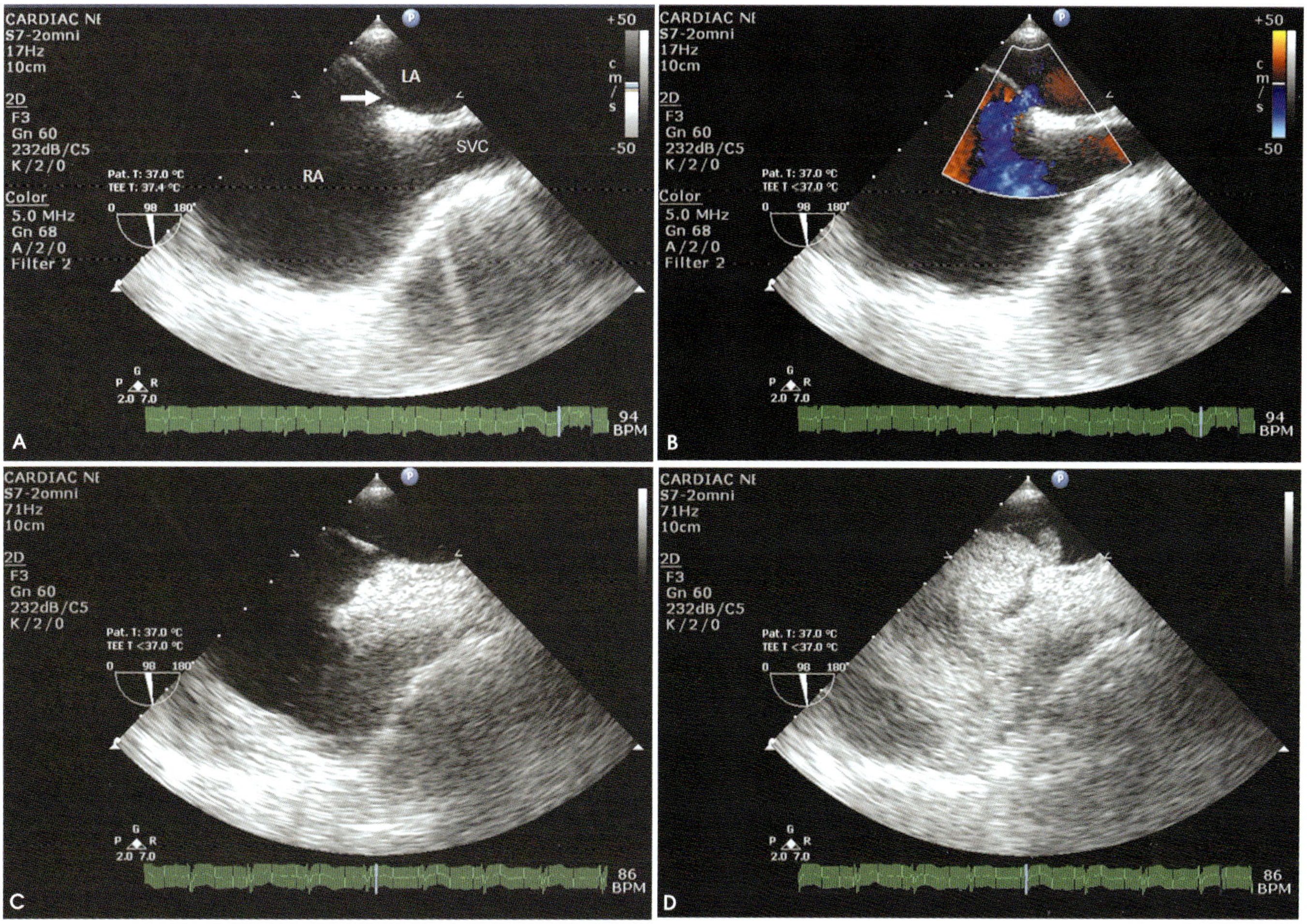

Fig. 13.13: Midesophageal bicaval view showing a patent foramen ovale (A, arrow) shunting from left atrium to right atrium (B). Injection of agitated saline into a peripheral upper limb vein opacifies the superior vena cava, right atrium (C) and sequentially the left atrium (D). (LA: left atrium, RA: right atrium, SVC: superior vena cava).

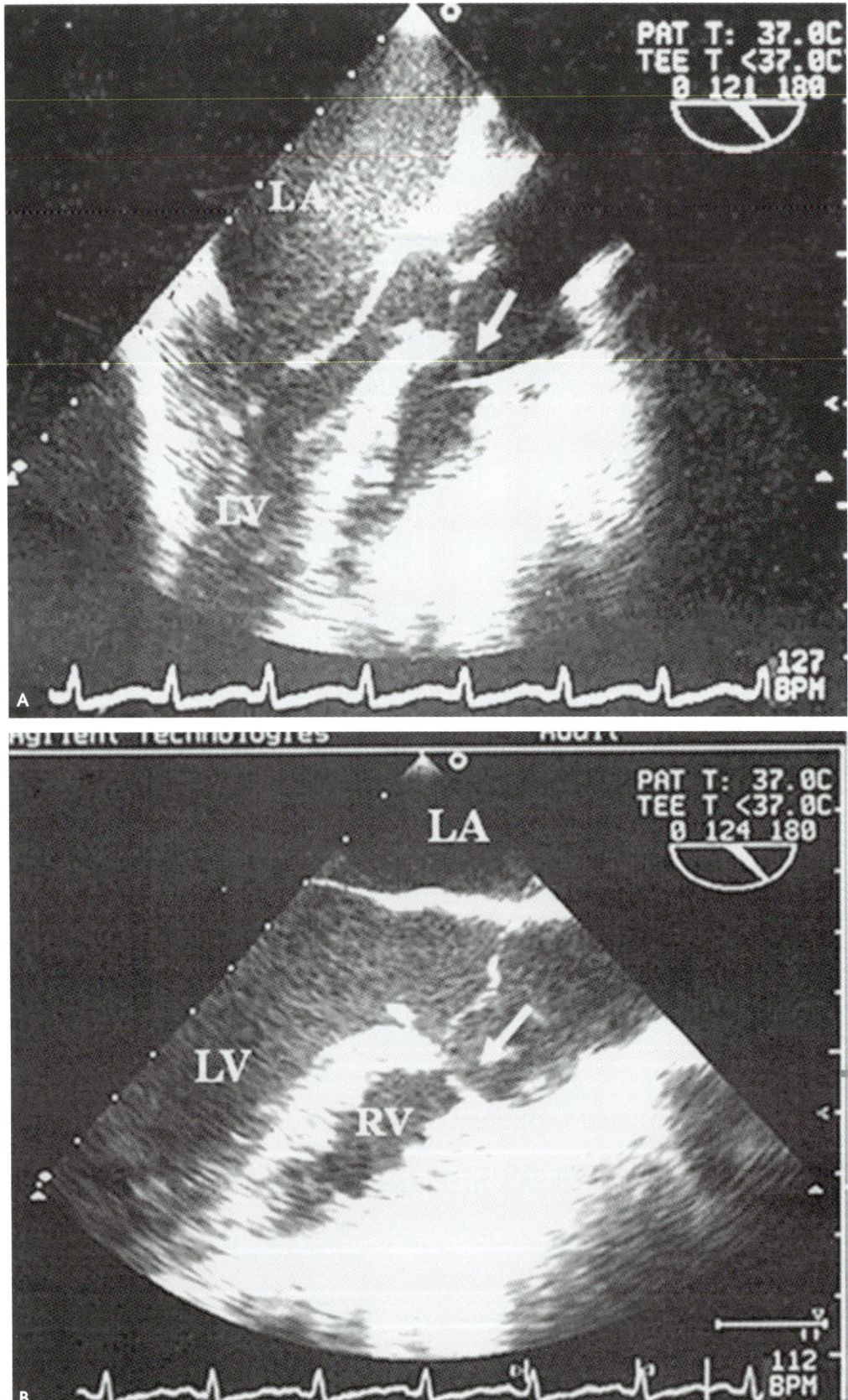

Fig. 13.14A and B: Midesophageal aortic valve long-axis view showing perimembranous ventricular septal defect. Note the prolapsing aortic cusp (arrows) (LA: left atrium, LV: left ventricle, RV: right ventricle).

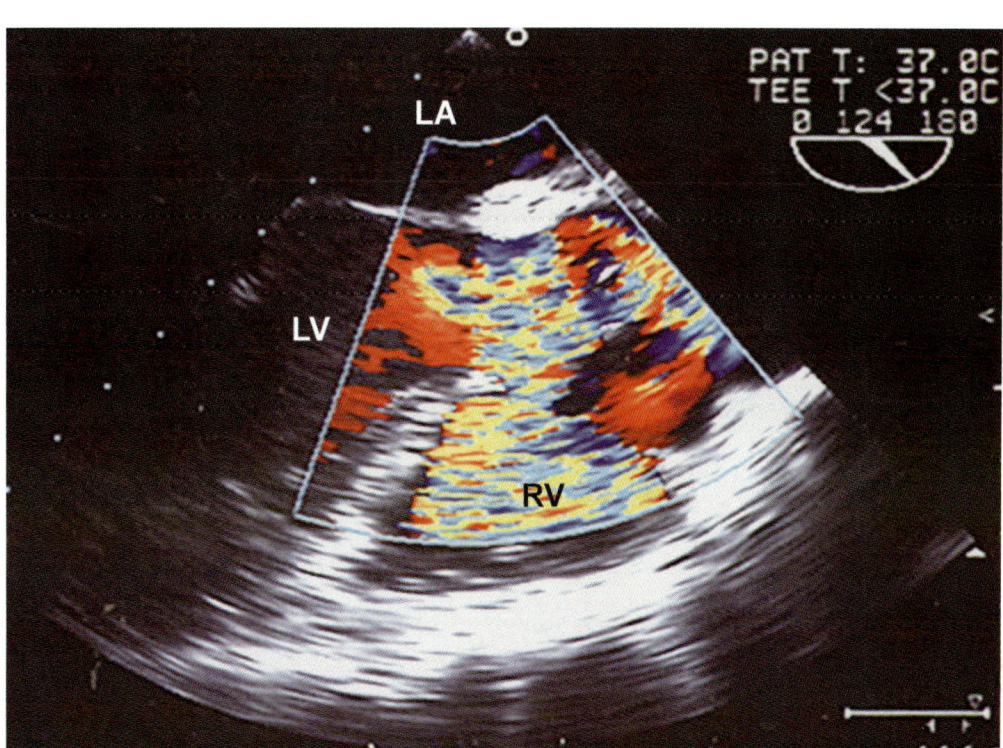

Fig. 13.15: Color flow across the perimembranous ventricular septal defect revealing a large left to right shunt across the defect (LA: left atrium, LV: left ventricle, RV: right ventricle).

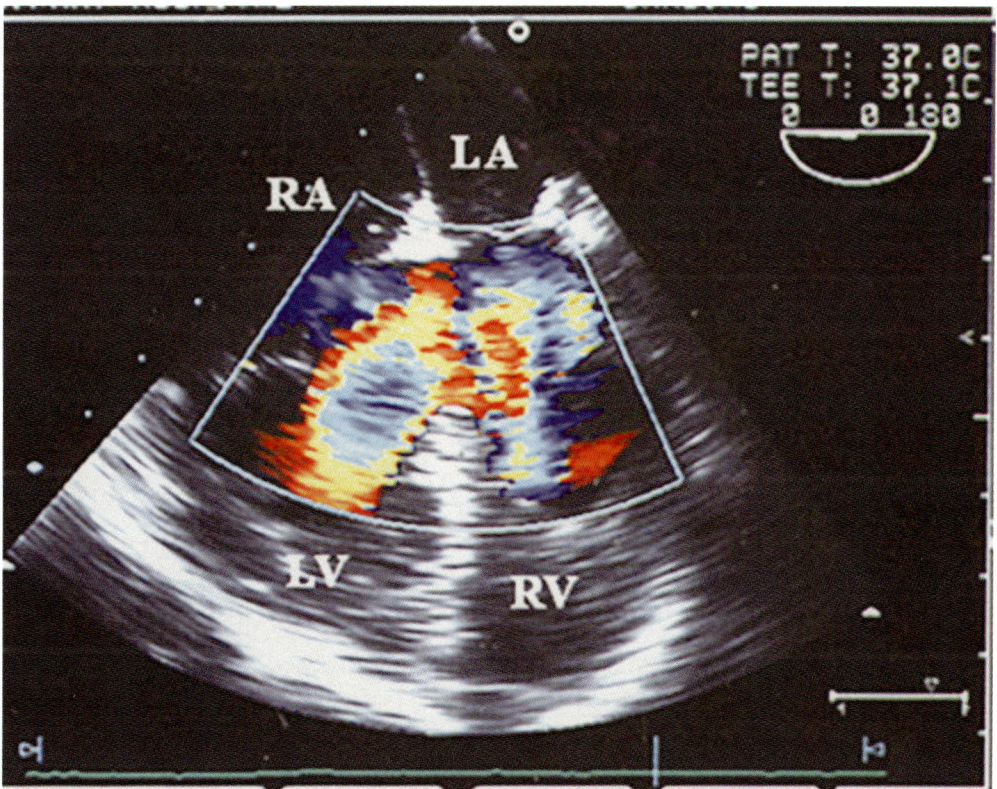

Fig. 13.16: Midesophageal four-chamber view showing the color flow across a muscular ventricular septal defect. Note the left to right ventricular shunt (LA: left atrium, LV: left ventricle, RA: right atrium, RV: right ventricle).

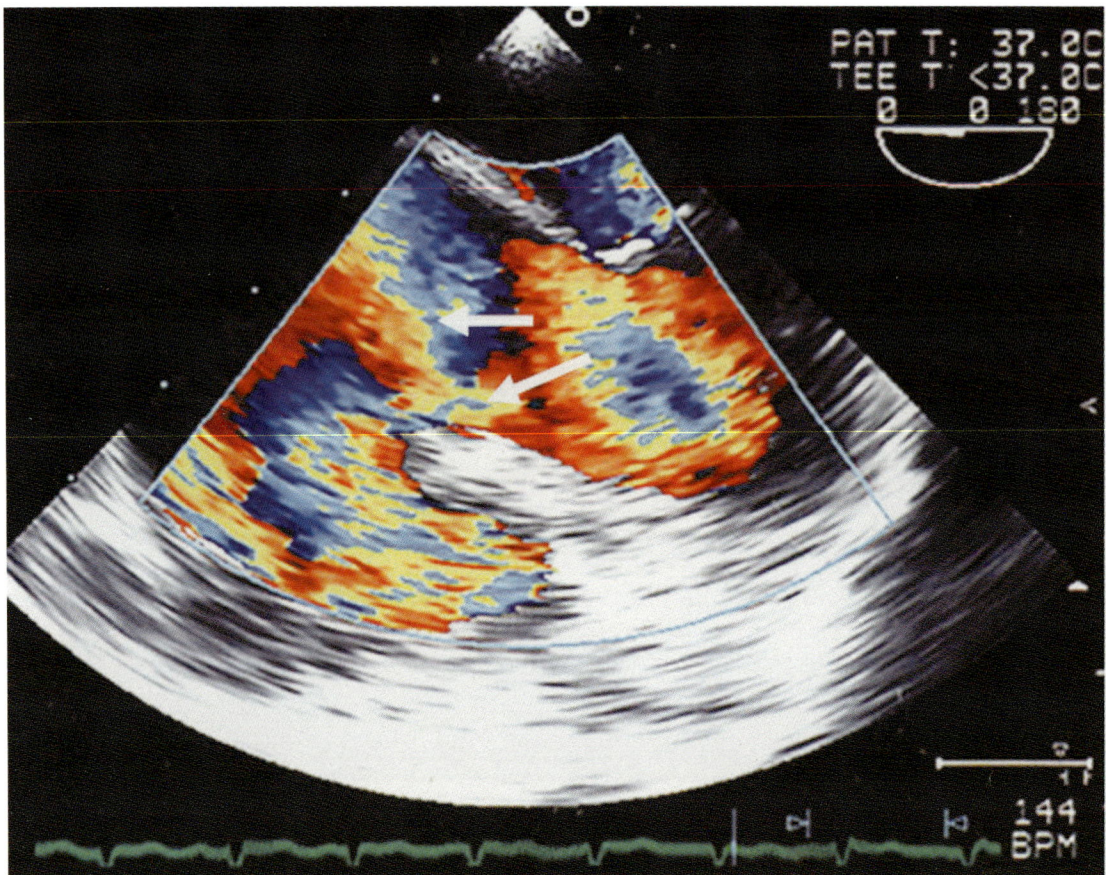

Fig. 13.17: Midesophageal four-chamber view showing the perimembranous ventricular septal defect. Color flow across the defect shows two jets (arrows); an upper left ventricular to right atrial shunt and a lower left to right ventricular shunt.

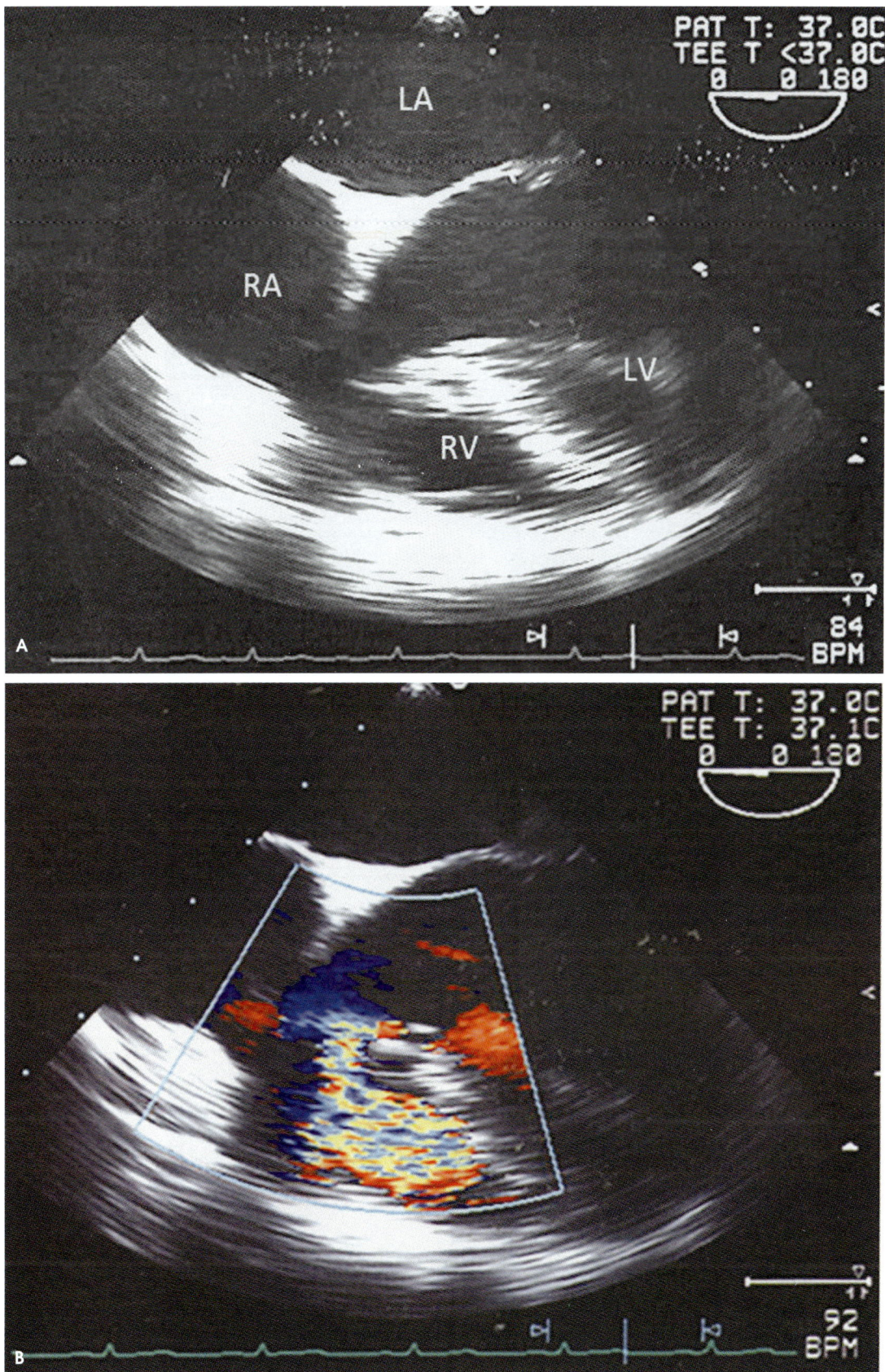

Fig. 13.18: Midesophageal four-chamber view showing inlet ventricular septal defect (A) and color flow across it (B). (LA: left atrium, RA: right atrium, LV: left ventricle, RV: right ventricle).

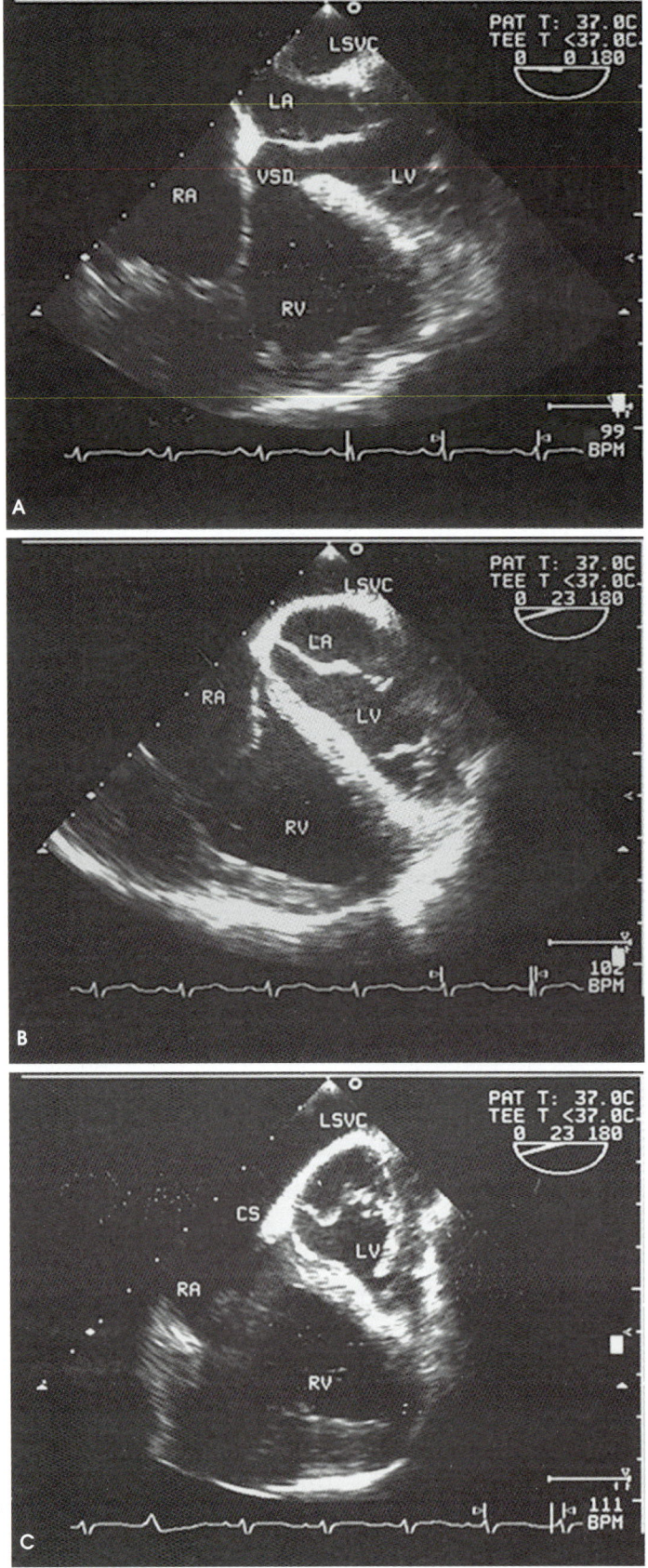

Fig. 13.19: Serial images from a patient with a ventricular septal defect (VSD) and left superior vena cava (LSVC) opening into the coronary sinus (CS). (LA: left atrium, RA: right atrium, LV: left ventricle, RV: right ventricle).

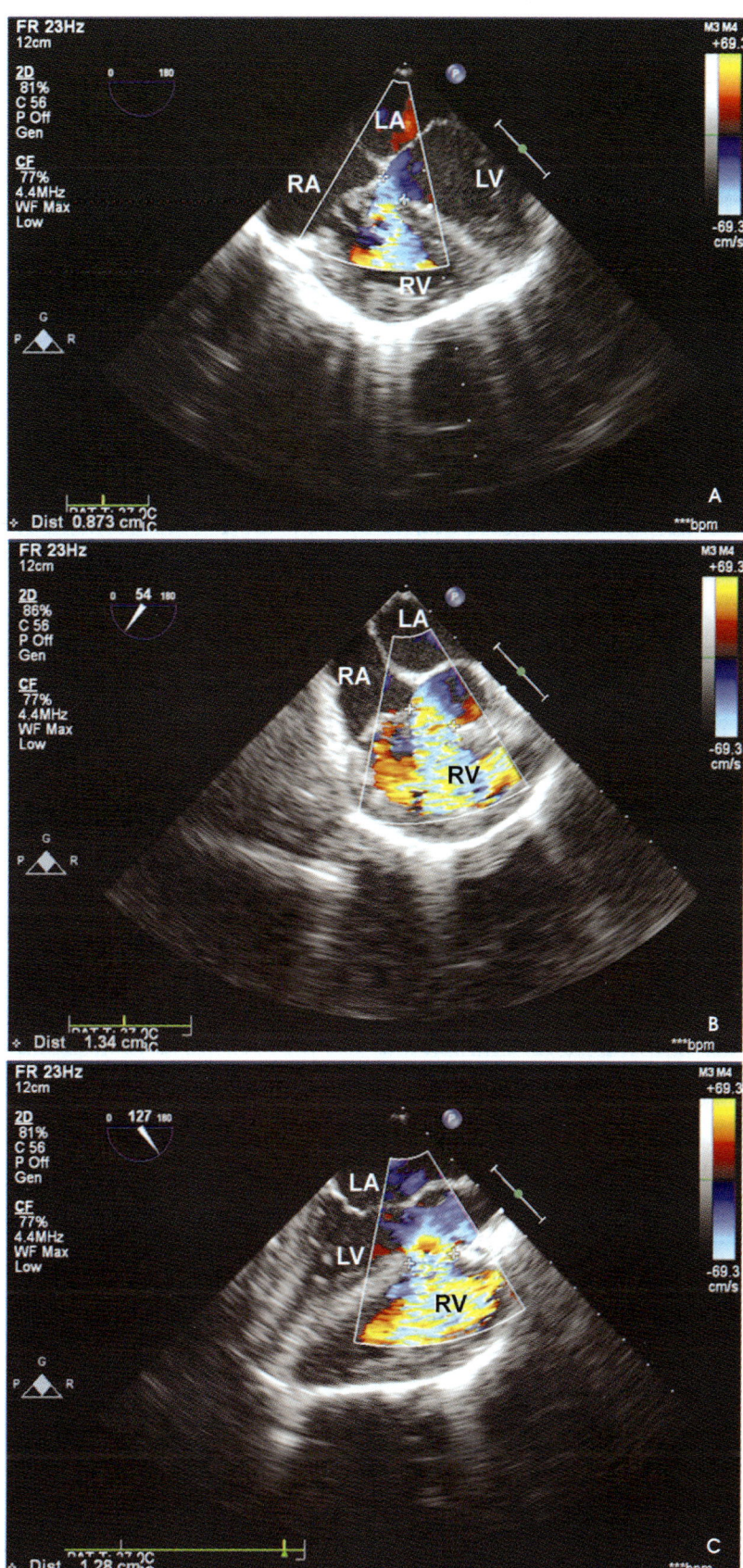

Fig. 13.20: Perimembranous ventricular septal defect with left to right shunt in midesophageal four-chamber view (A), right ventricle inflow-outflow view (B) and aortic valve long-axis view (C) (LA: left atrium, RA: right atrium, RV: right ventricle, LV: left ventricle).

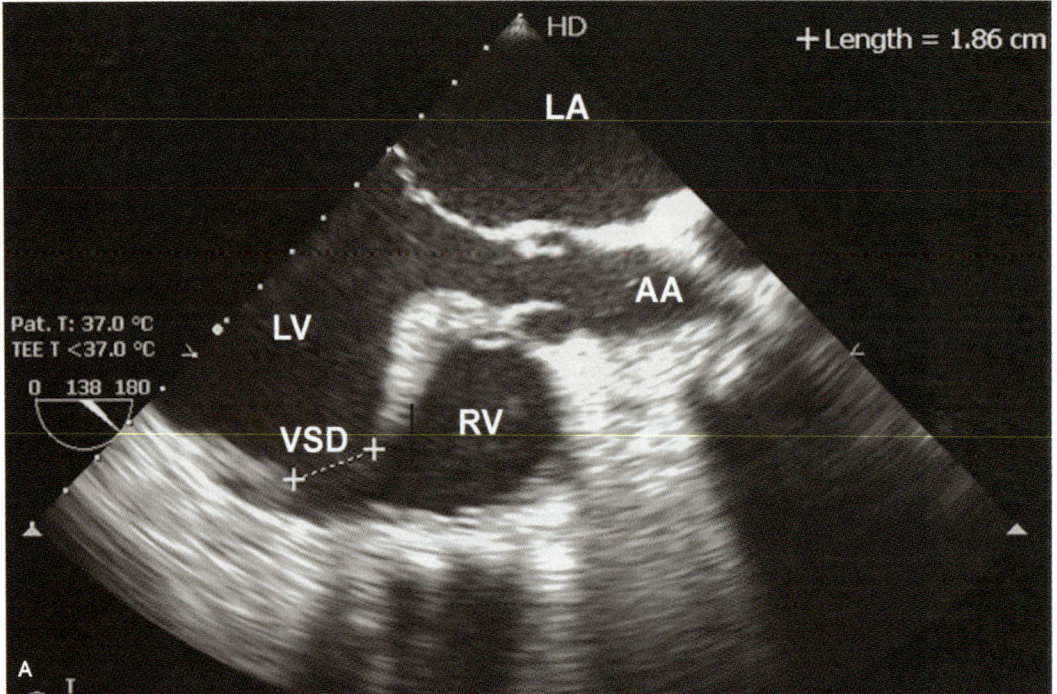

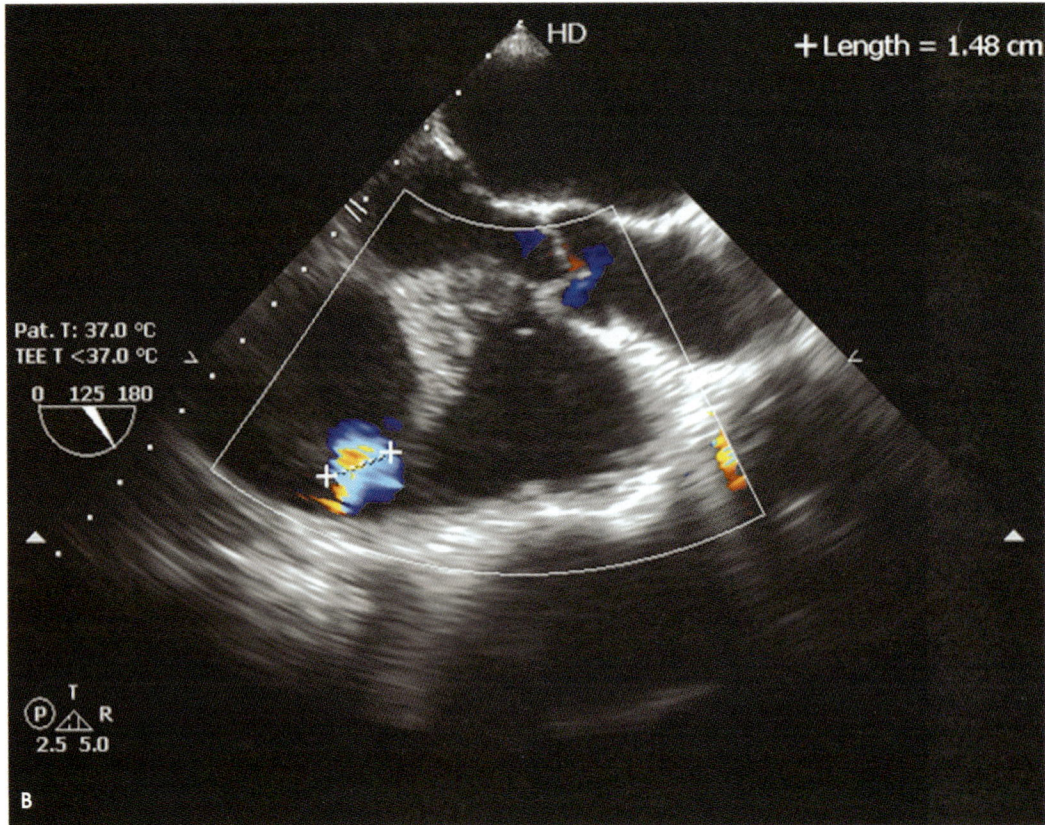

Fig. 13.21: (A) Midesophageal aortic valve long-axis view in a patient with muscular ventricular septal defect (VSD). (B) Color flow Doppler showing left to right shunt through the defect. (LA: left atrium, LV: left ventricle, RV: right ventricle, AA: ascending aorta).

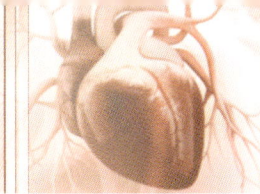

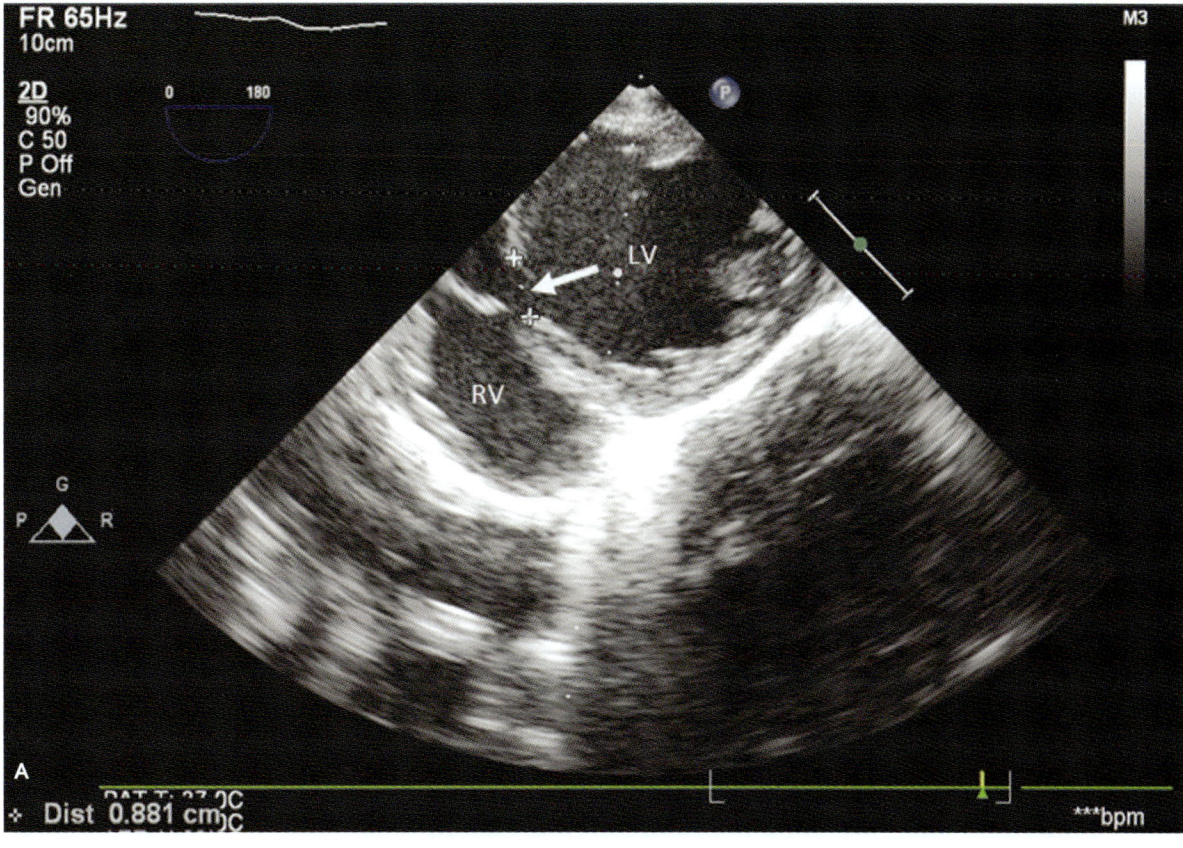

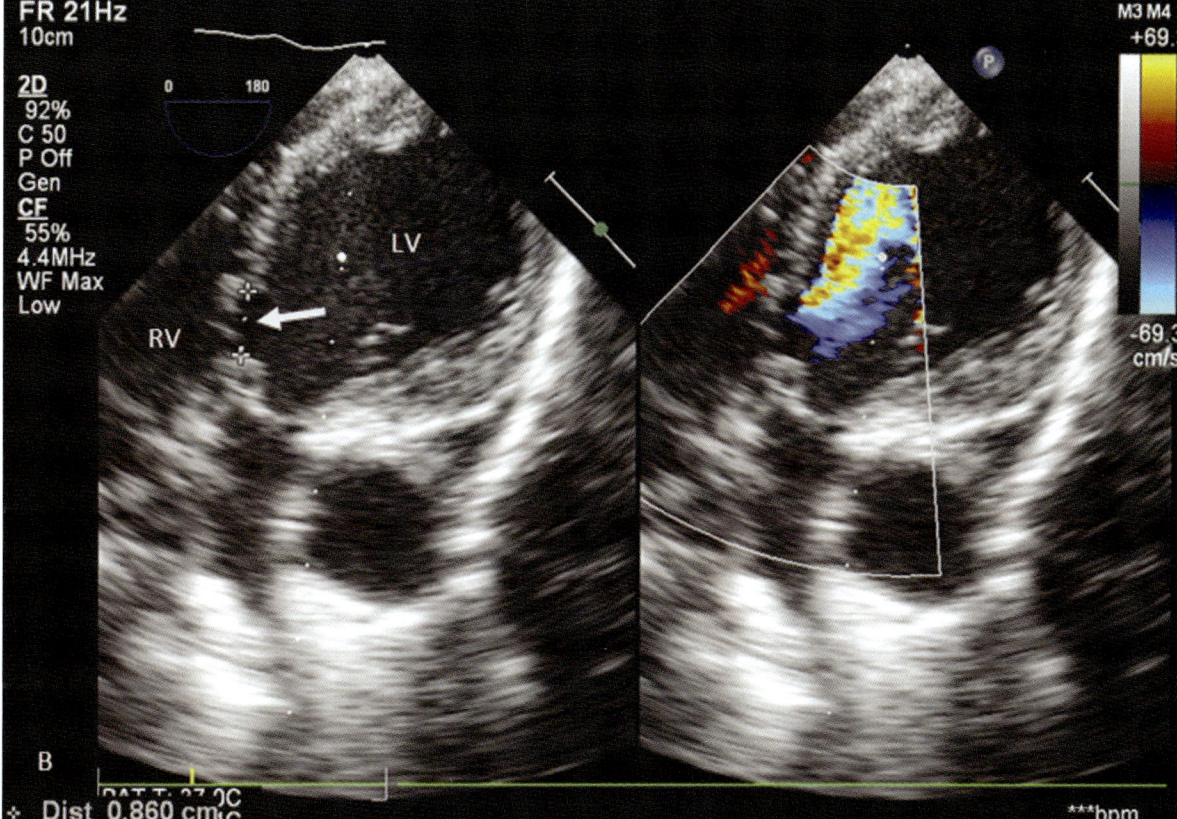

Fig. 13.22: Muscular ventricular septal defect (arrow) with left to right shunt in transgastric mid-papillary view (A) and deep transgastric long-axis view (B). (LV: left ventricle, RV: right ventricle).

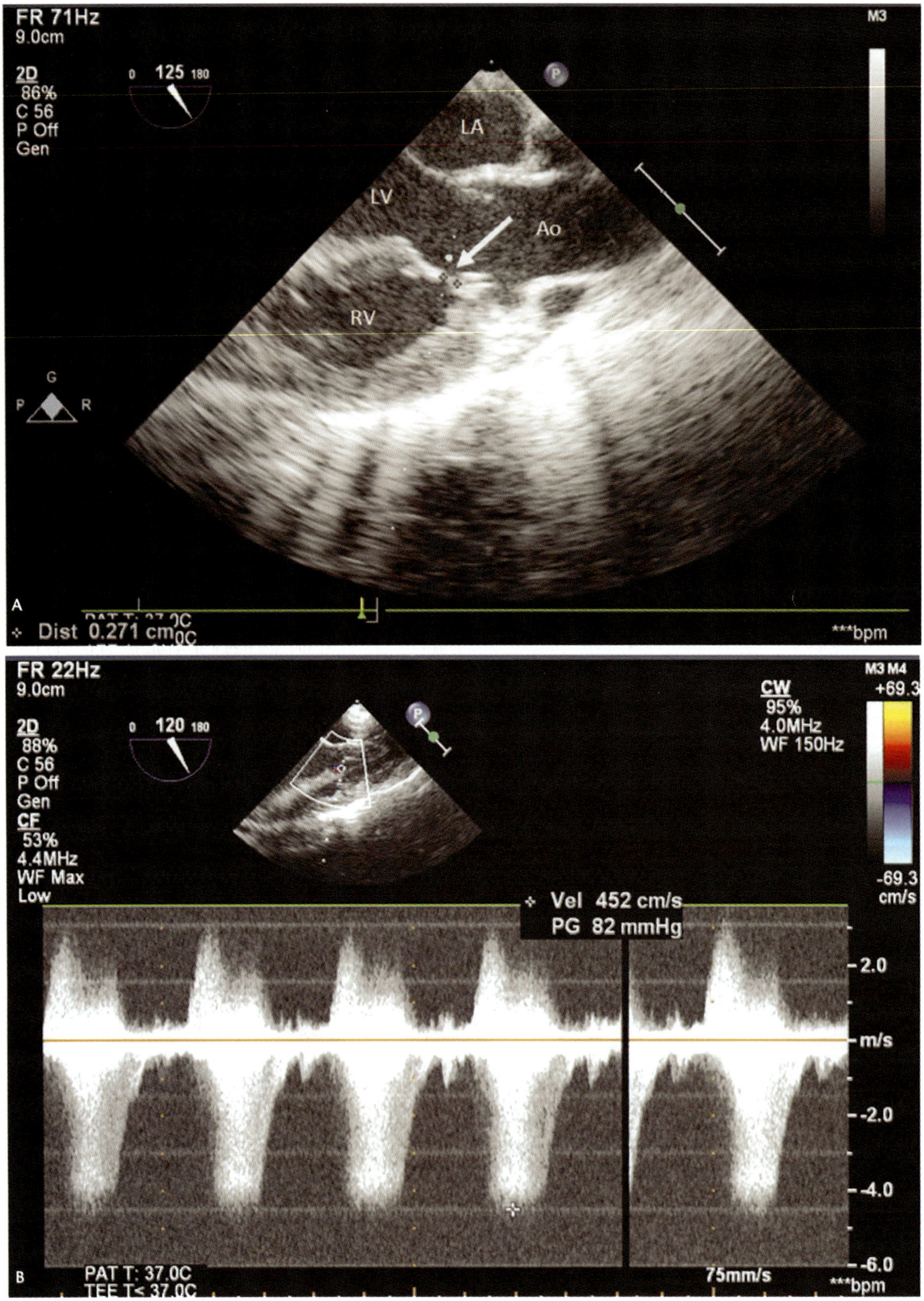

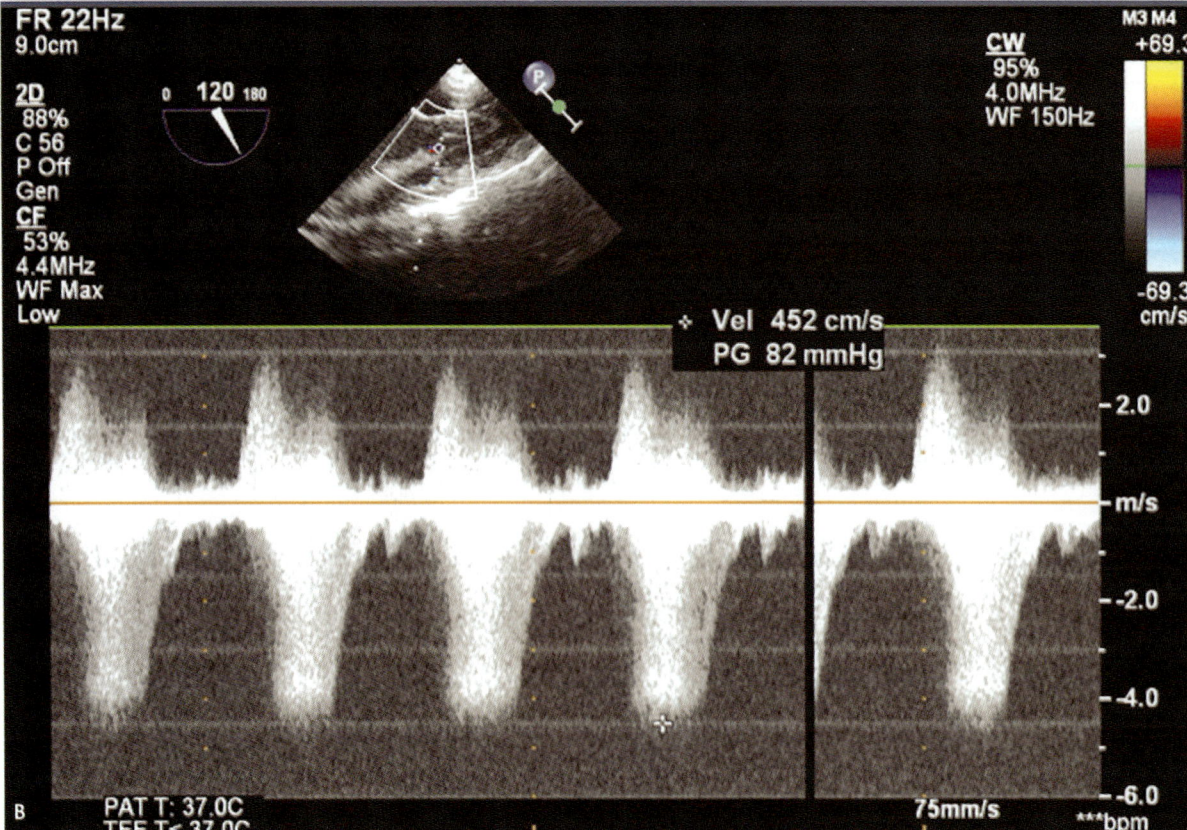

Fig. 13.23: Outlet ventricular septal defect in midesophageal long-axis view (A, arrow) with continuous wave Doppler showing high flow velocity (around 4 m/s) indicating a restrictive left to right flow (B). (LA: left atrium, LV: left ventricle, RV: right ventricle, Ao: aorta).

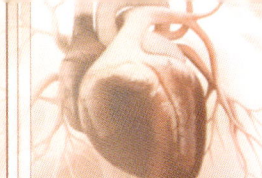

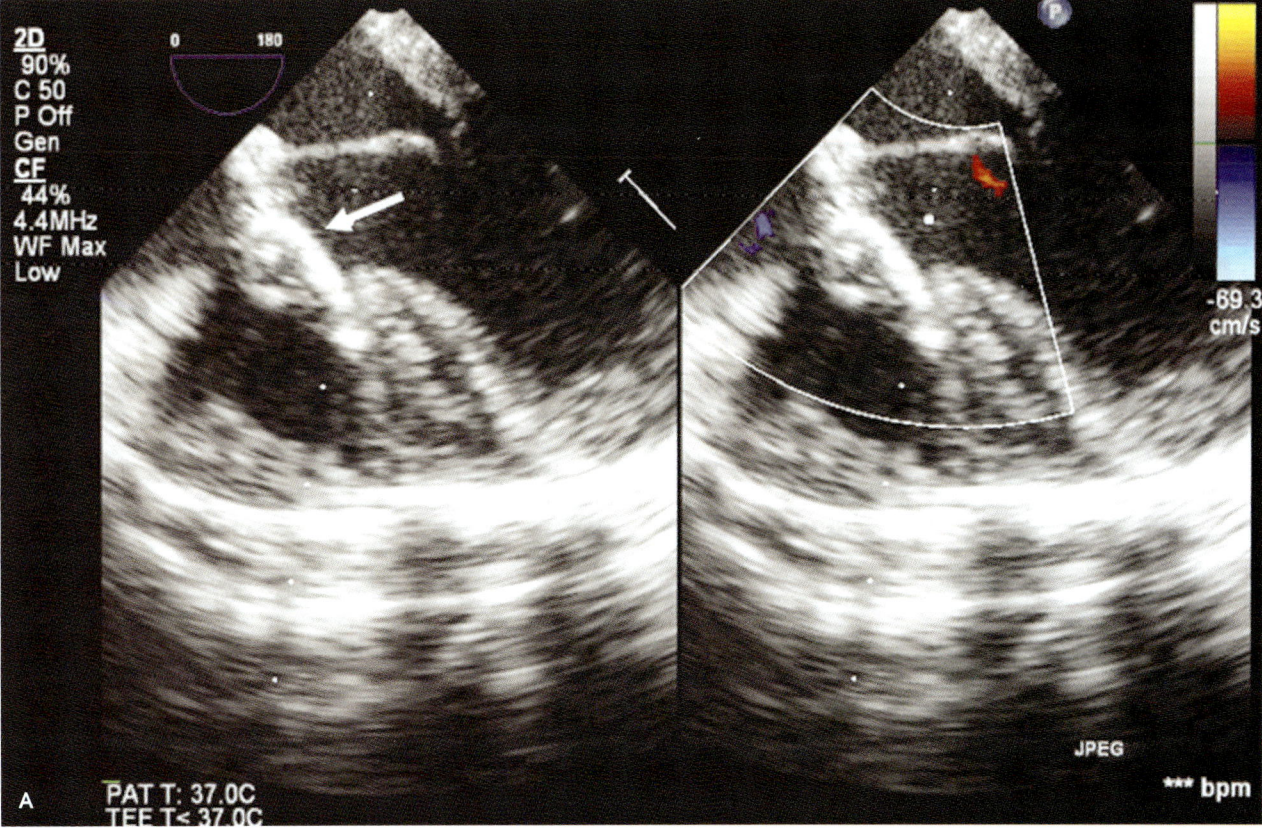

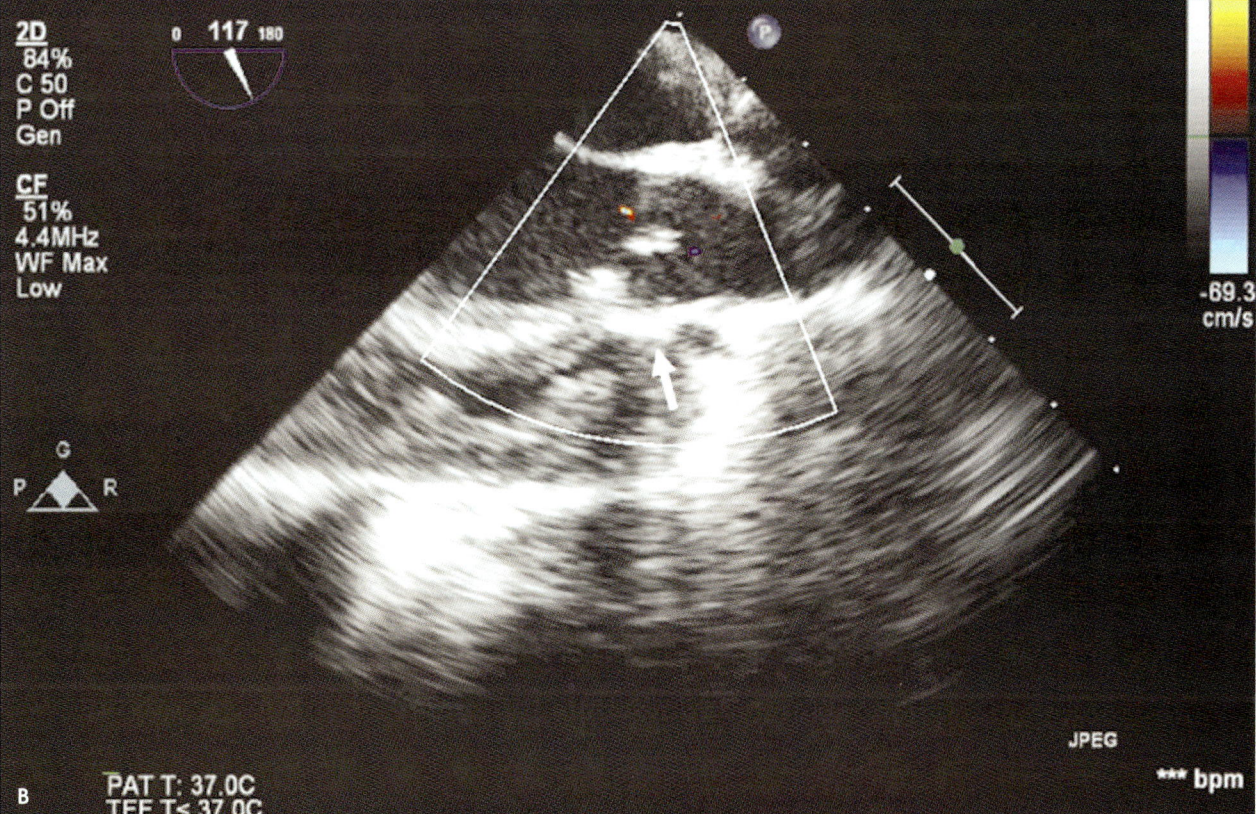

Fig. 13.24: Postoperative midesophageal four-chamber view (A) and long-axis view (B) after VSD patch closure (arrow) showing abolition of left to right shunt. The patch is seen as a dense echogenic shadow.

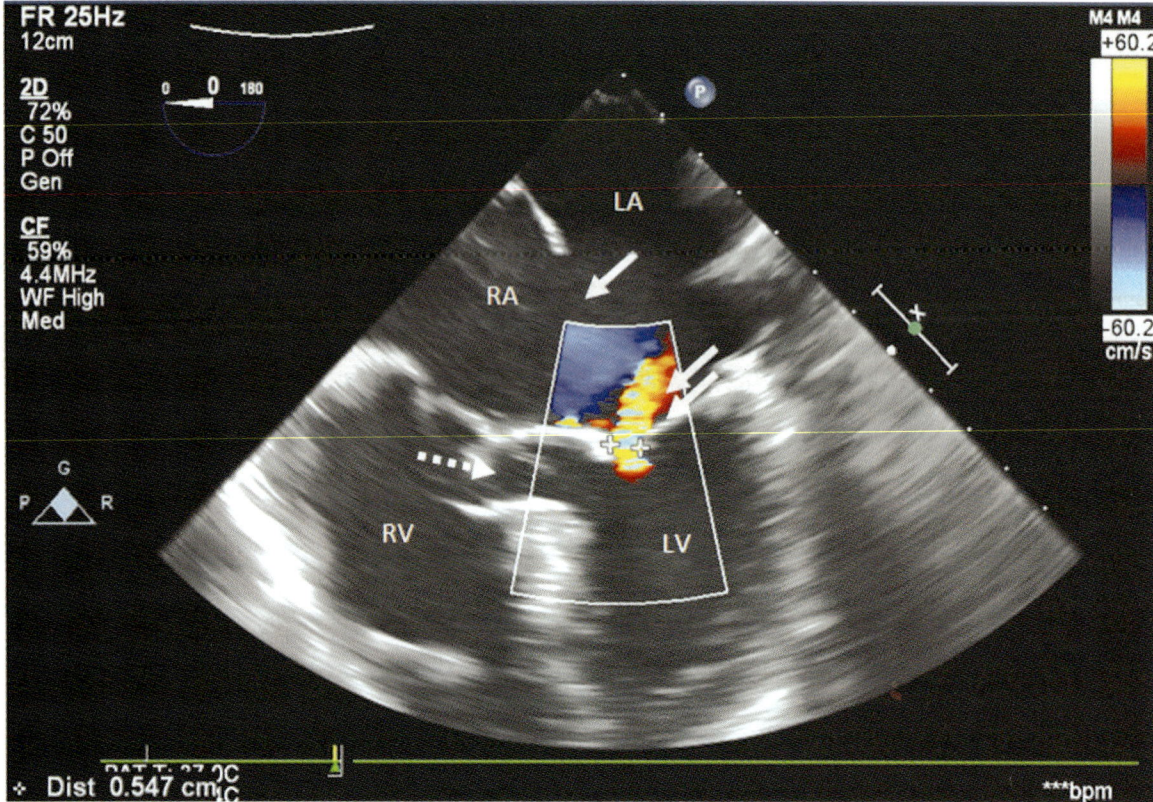

Fig. 13.25: Atrioventricular septal defect: Midesophageal four-chamber view with color flow Doppler showing a large ostium primum atrial septal defect (arrow), inlet ventricular septal defect (dashed arrow) and left atrioventricular valve regugtitation (double arrow) (RA: right atrium, LA: left atrium, RV: right ventricle, LV: left ventricle).

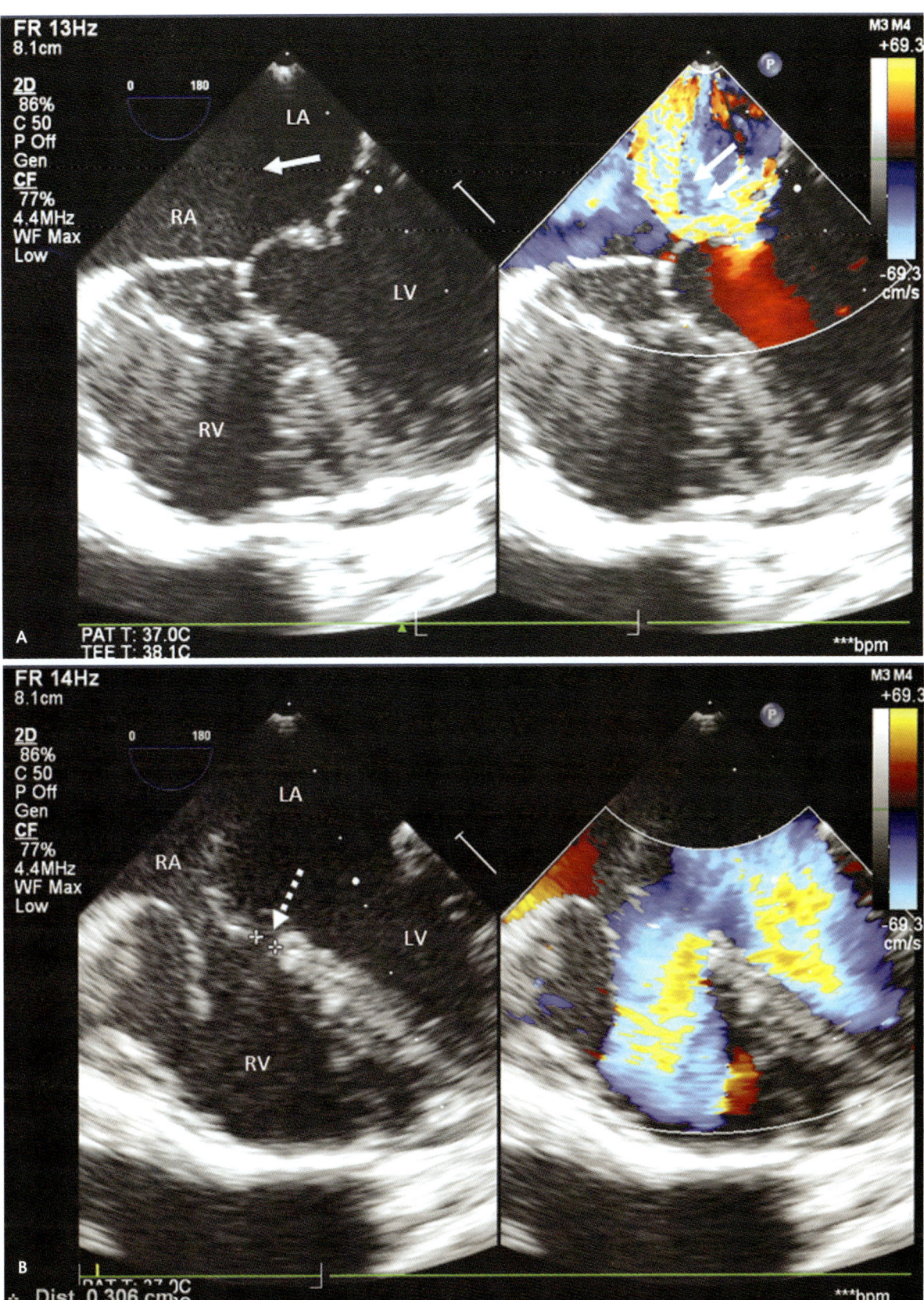

Fig. 13.26: Midesophageal four-chamber view with color flow Doppler showing a large ostium primum atrial septal defect (arrow) and severe left atrioventricular valve regugtitation (double arrow, A) and inlet ventricular septal defect (B, dashed arrow) (RA: right atrium, LA: left atrium, RV: right ventricle, LV: left ventricle).

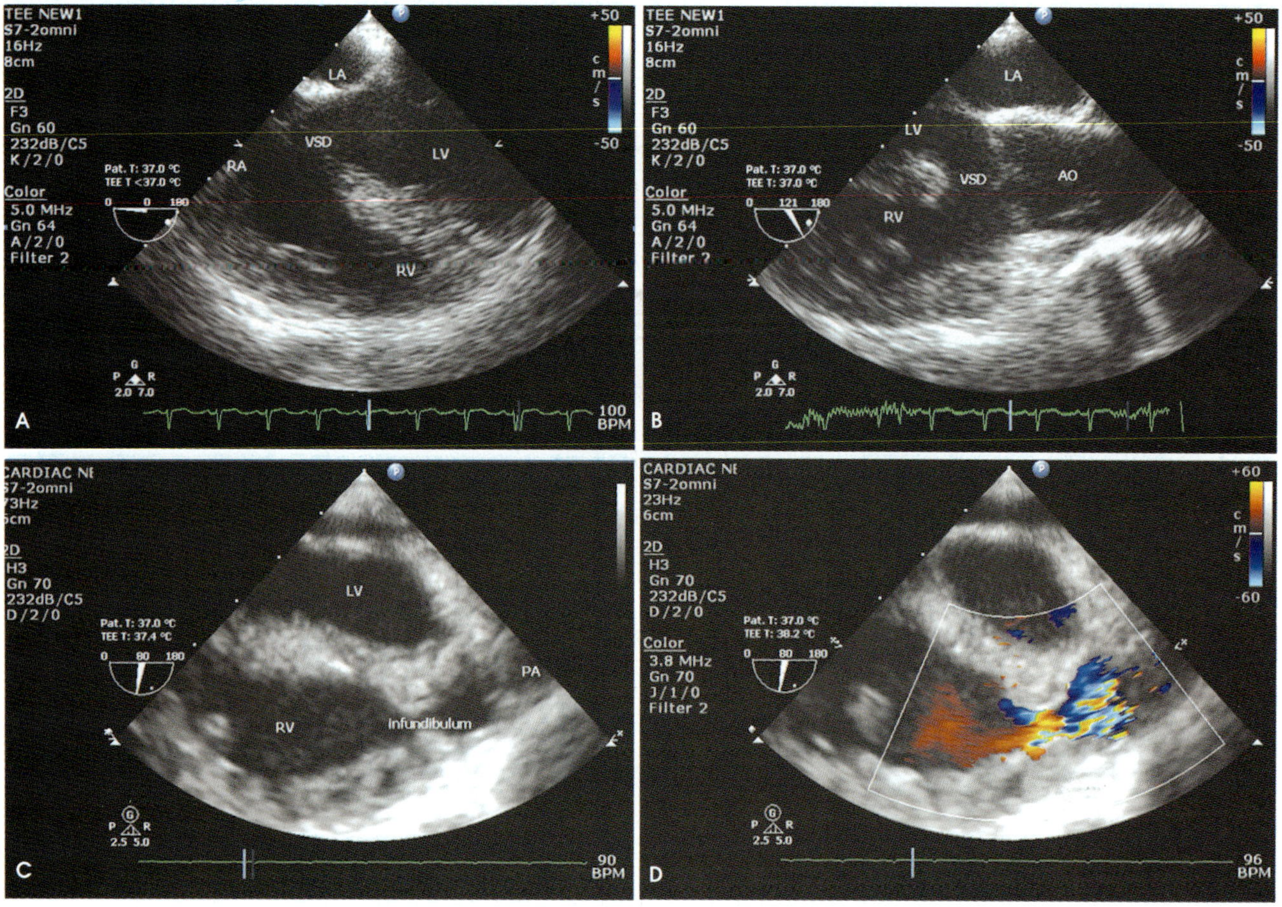

Fig. 13.27: Tetralogy of Fallot: Midesophageal views showing a large subaortic ventricular septal defect (A), overriding of aorta (B), infundibular and valvular pulmonary stenosis (C, D) and right ventricular hypertrophy (C, D). (RA: left atrium, LA: left atrium, RV: right ventricle, LV: left ventricle, PA: pulmonary artery, Ao: aorta, VSD: ventricular septal defect).

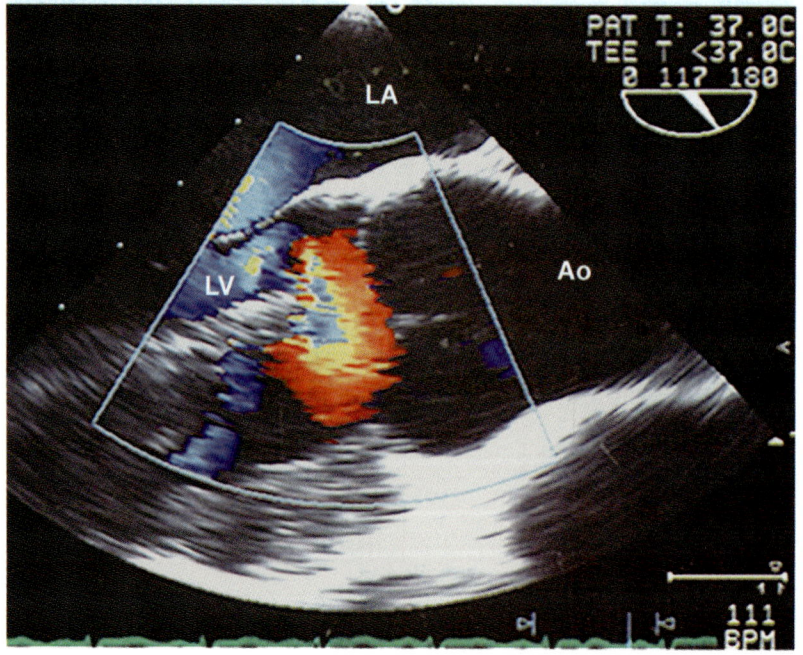

Fig. 13.28: Midesophageal aortic valve long-axis view showing aortic override and malaligned ventricular septal defect in a patient with tetralogy of Fallot (LA: left atrium, LV: left ventricle, Ao: aorta).

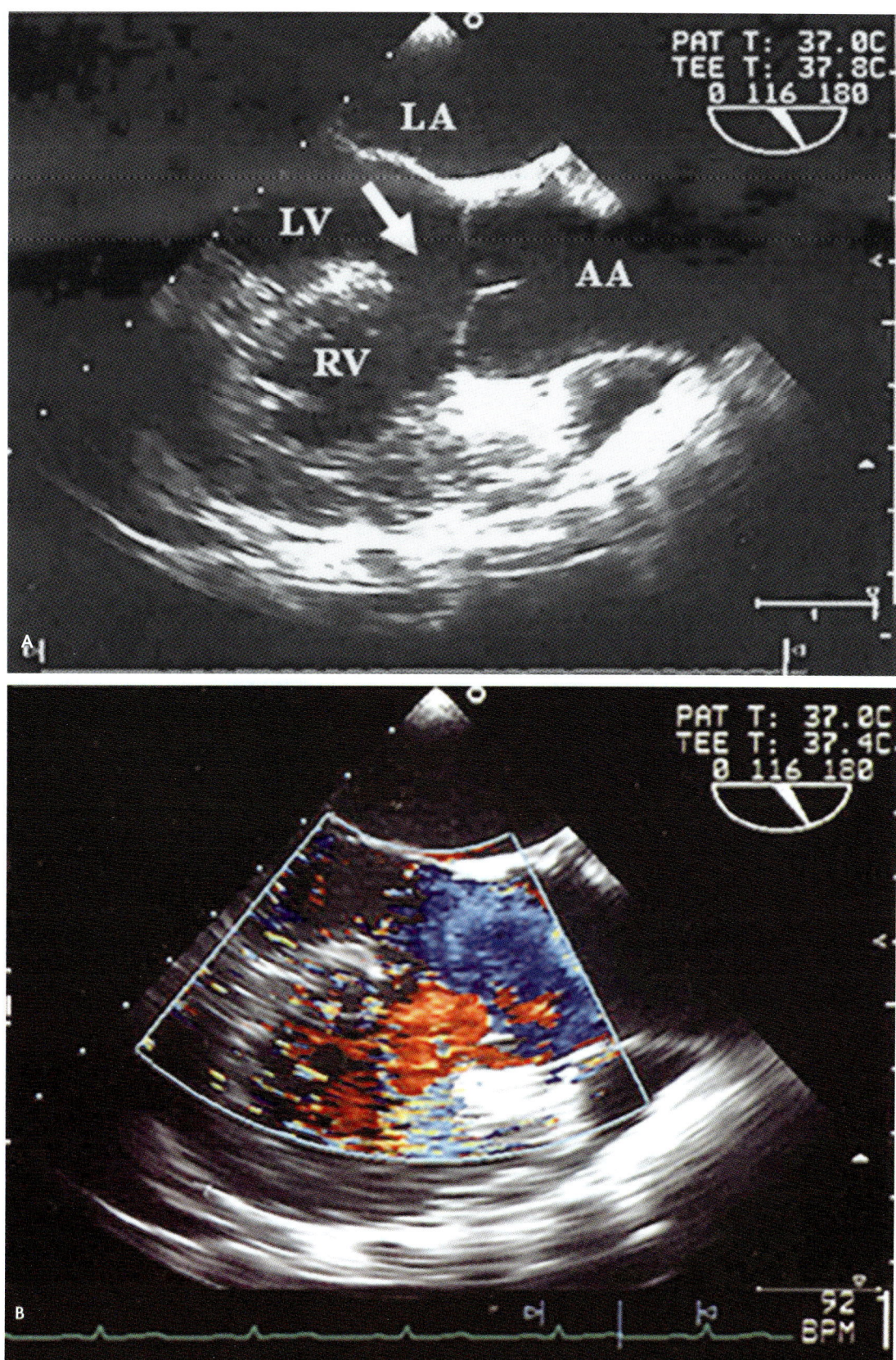

Fig. 13.29: Panel A: Midesophageal aortic valve long-axis view showing a large sub-aortic ventricular septal defect (arrow) in a patient with tetralogy of Fallot with 50% aortic over-ride. Panel B: Color flow across the defect and over-riding aorta shows streaming of blood from both right and left ventricles into the aorta (LA: left atrium, LV: left ventricle, RV: right ventricle, AA: ascending aorta).

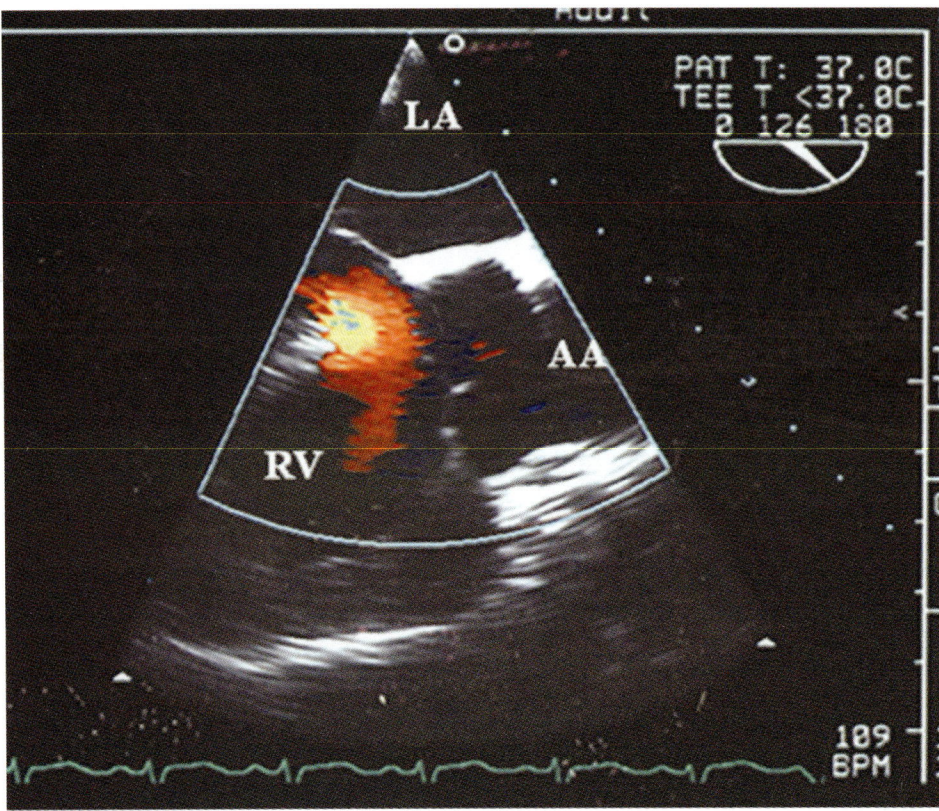

Fig. 13.30: Midesophageal aortic valve long-axis view showing ventricular septal defect caused by mal-alignment of the aorta. Note the absence of turbulence due to a relatively large defect size causing equalization of pressure in both the chambers and a low velocity left to right shunt across the defect (LA: left atrium, RV: right ventricle, AA: ascending aorta).

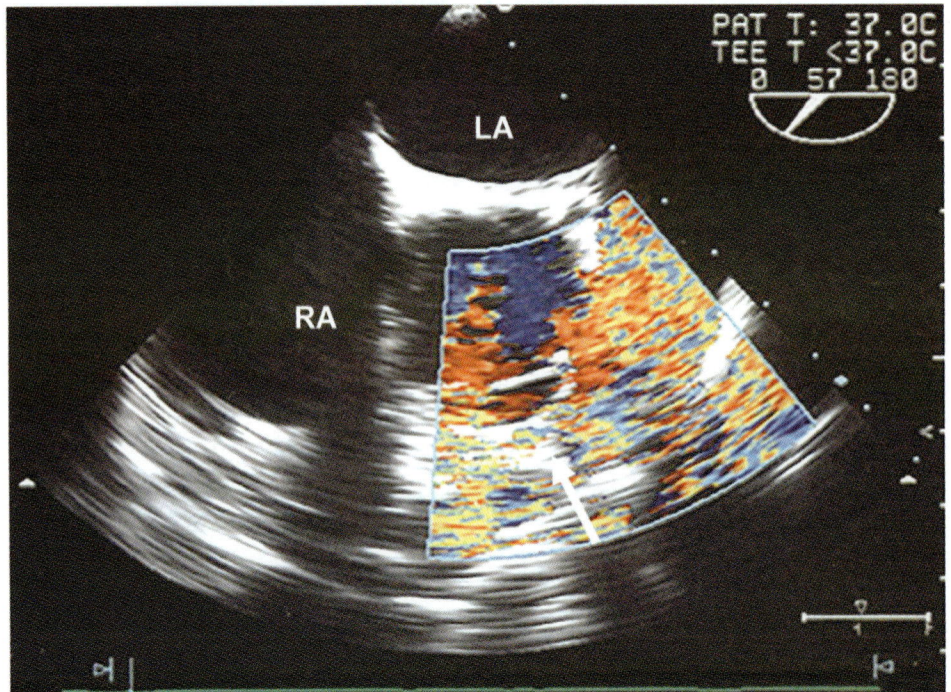

Fig. 13.31: Midesophageal right ventricle inflow-outflow view with color flow Doppler across the right ventricular outflow tract in a patient with tetralogy of Fallot showing turbulence (arrow) caused by the stenosed right ventricular infundibulum (LA: left artrium, RA: right atrium).

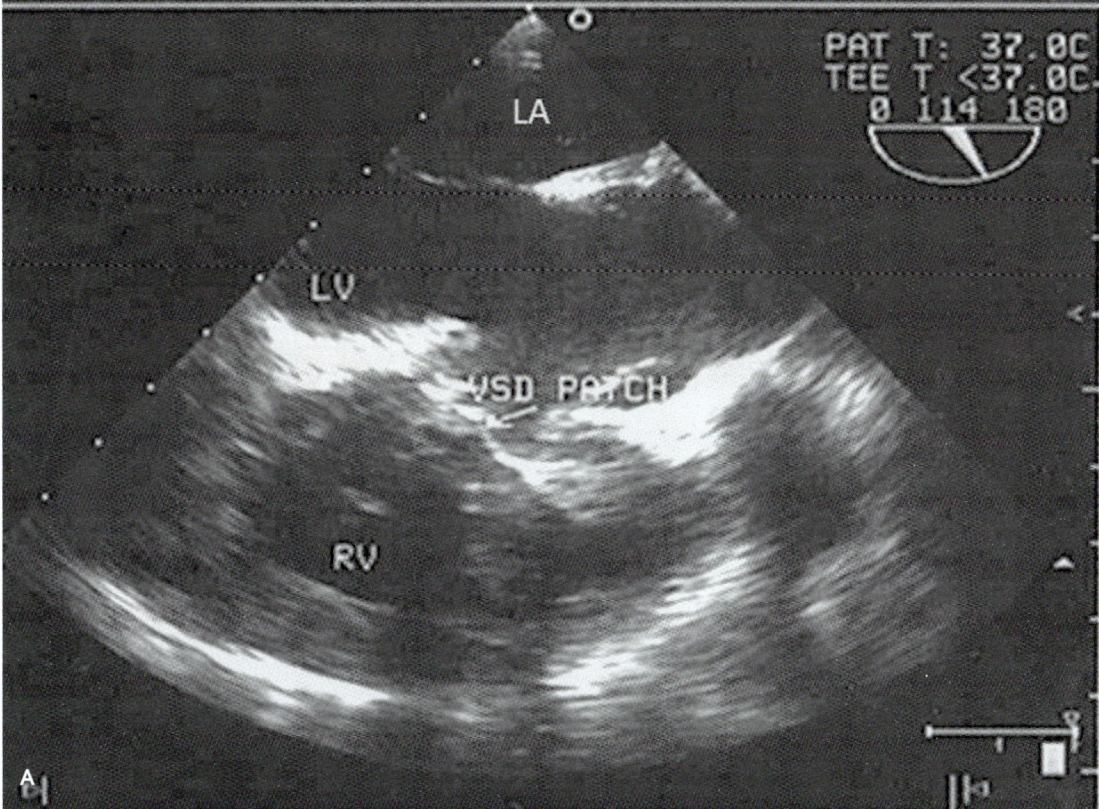

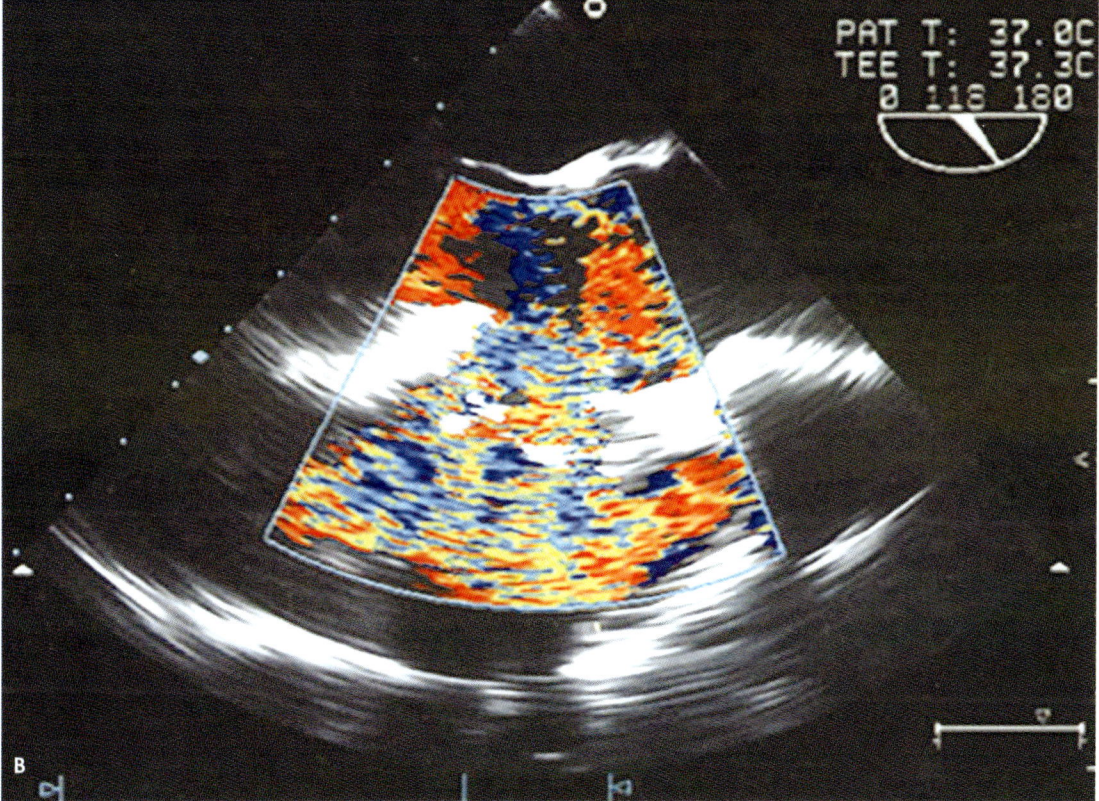

Fig. 13.32: Images from a patient with tetrology of Fallot who underwent intracardiac repair. Note the Dacron patch across the ventricular septal defect (VSD) (A, arrow). Color flow (B) shows a large residual shunt across the VSD. (LA: left atrium, LV: left ventricle, RV: right ventricle).

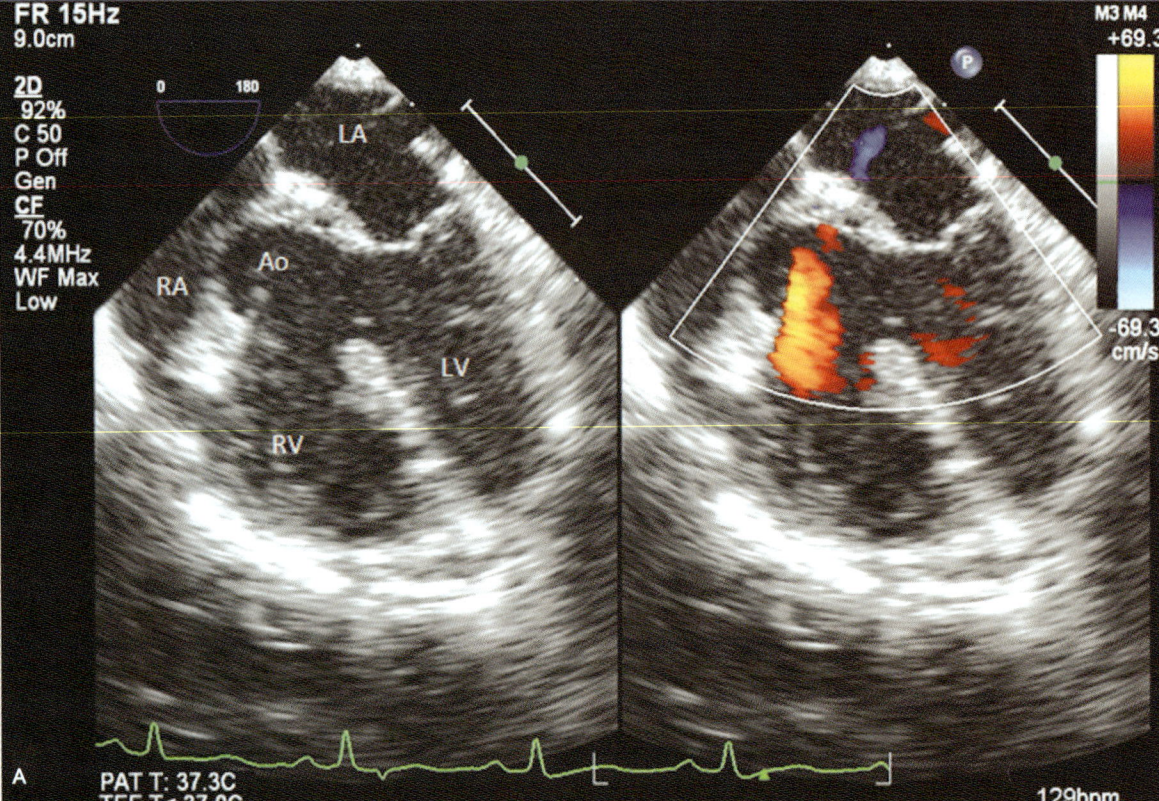

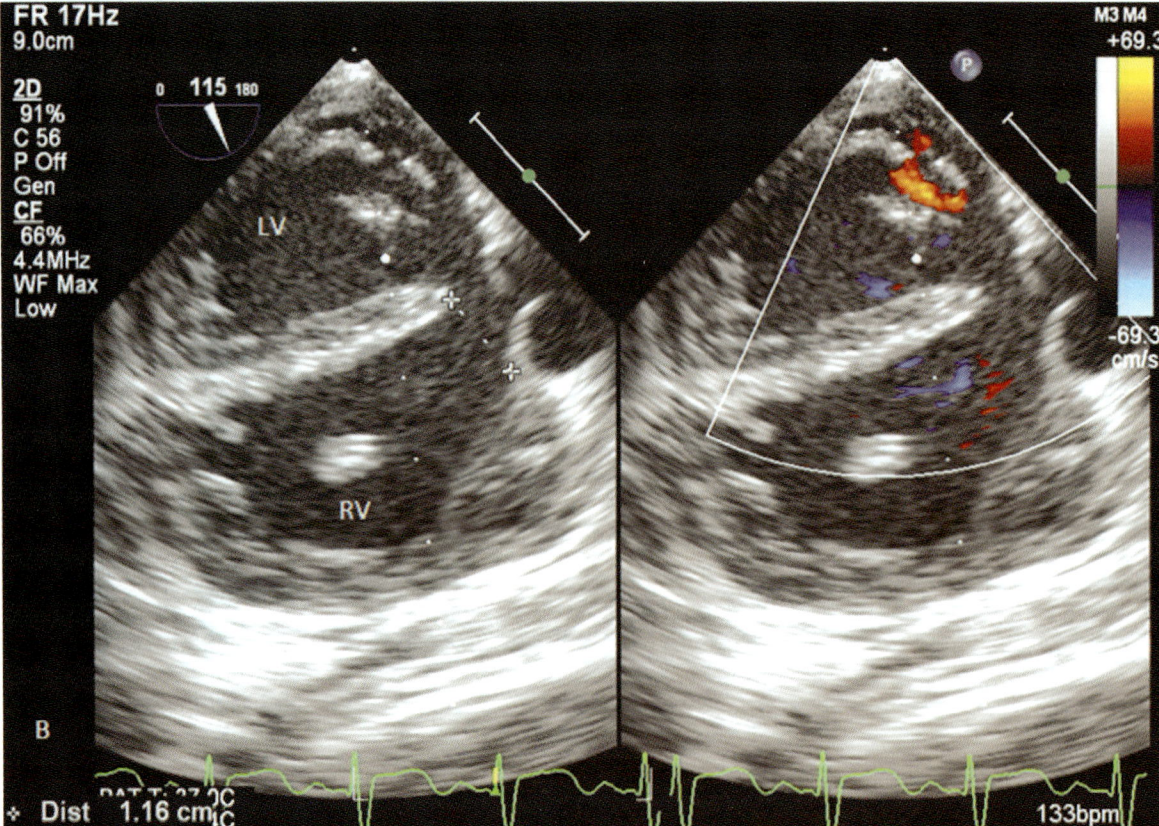

Fig. 13.33: Tetralogy of Fallot: Midesophageal five-chamber view (A) and long-axis view (B) showing overriding of the aorta and a large sub-aortic ventricular septal defect with right-to-left shunt. (RA: right atrium, RV: right ventricle, LA: left atrium, LV: left ventricle, Ao: aorta).

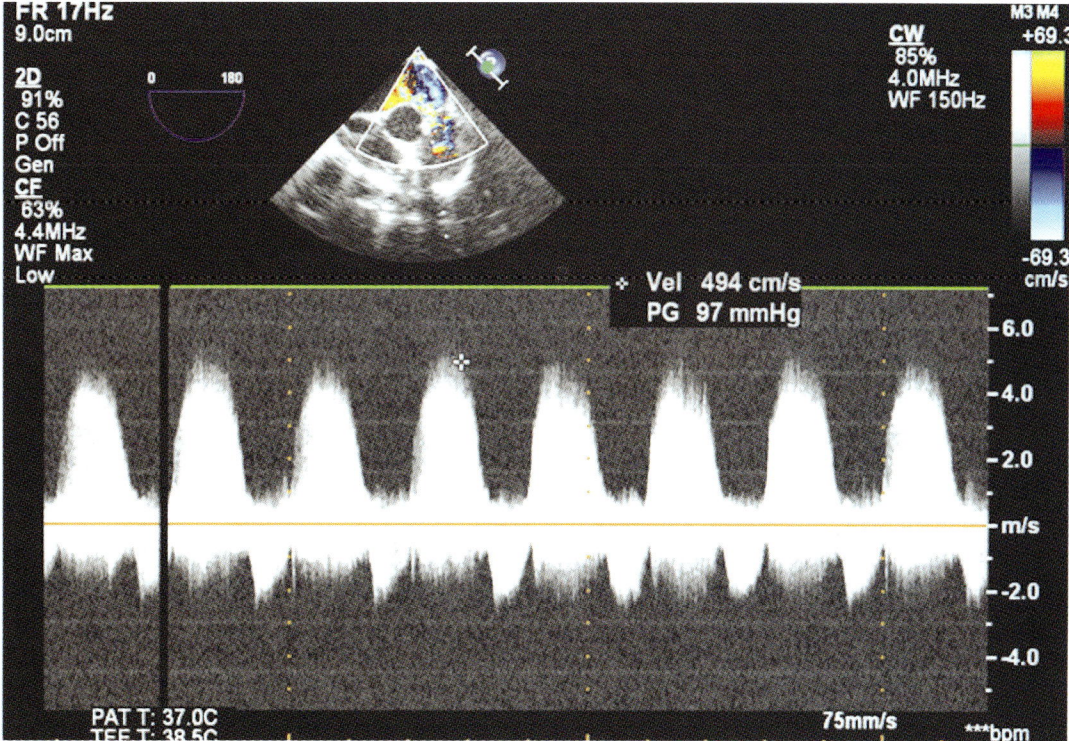

Fig. 13.34: Midesophageal ascending aorta short-axis view with continuous wave Doppler across the pulmonary valve in a patient with tetralogy of Fallot. Note the tight pulmonary stenosis (gradient~100 mm Hg), pulmonary regurgitation (gradient $4 \times 2^2 = 16$ mm Hg) and dilated main pulmonary artery.

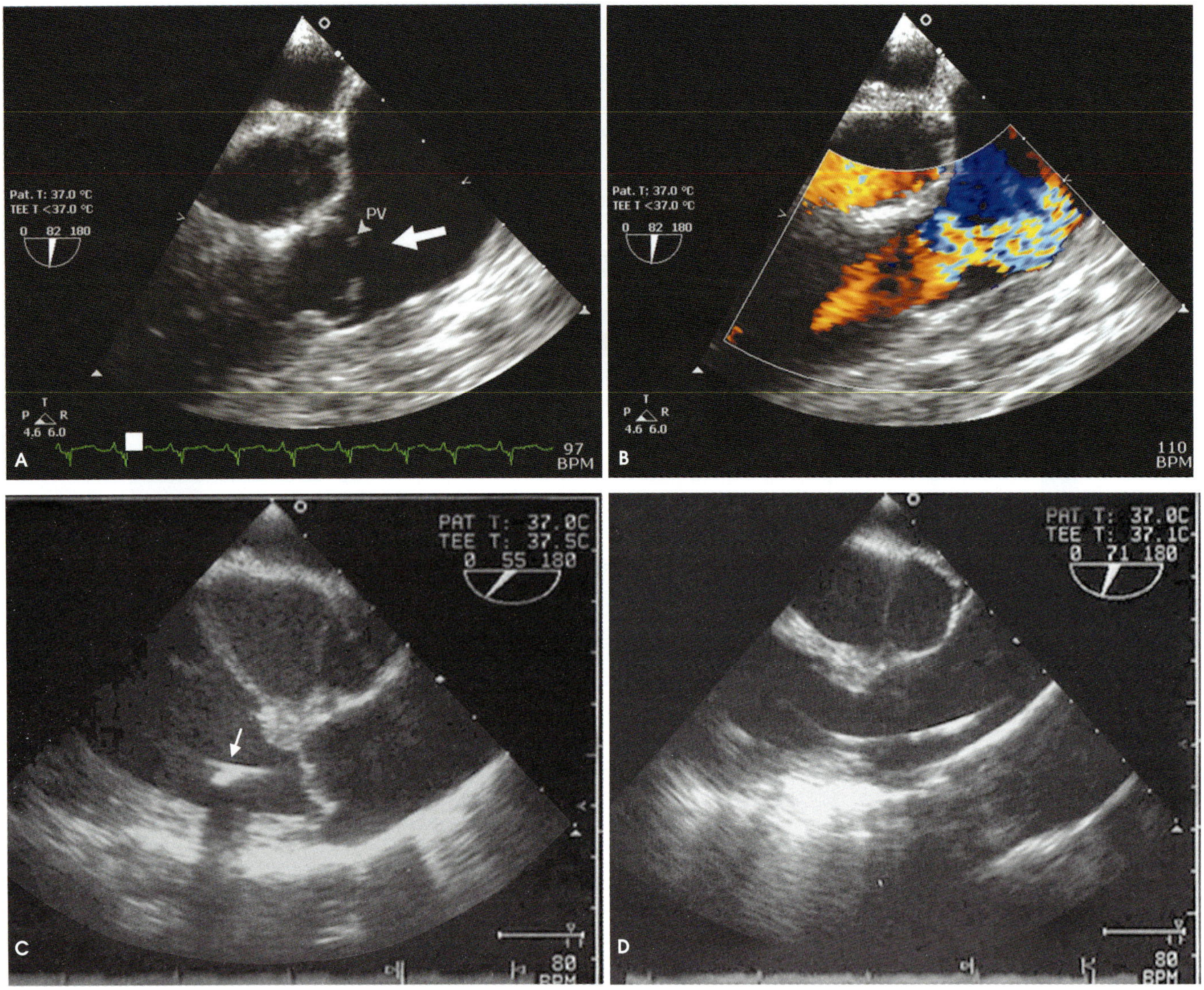

Fig. 13.35: A patient with pulmonary valvular stenosis. Note the doming pulmonary valve (A, arrow) with turbulent flow across the valve on color flow (B). Panels C and D show a Swan-Ganz pulmonary artery catheter (C, arrow) being passed across the stenosed pulmonary valve (D). (The pulmonary artery catheter was inserted as a part of a research project in this patient).

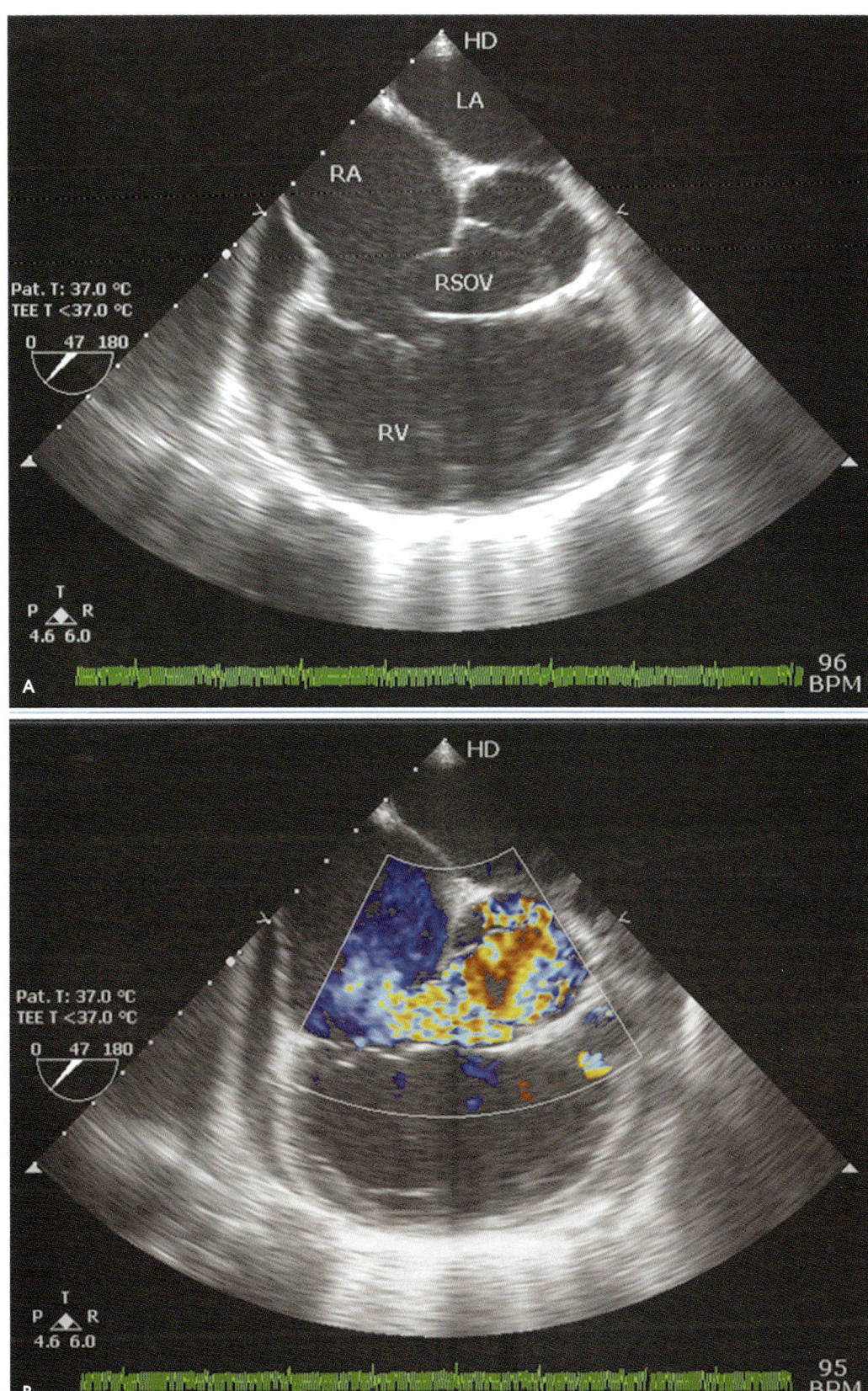

Fig. 13.36: Panel A: Appearance of the ruptured sinus of valsalva (RSOV). Note the tract arising from the right aortic sinus and opening into the right atrium. Panel B: Color flow across the fistulous tract showing a continuous shunt from the aorta to the right atrium (LA: left atrium, RA: right atrium, RV: right ventricle).

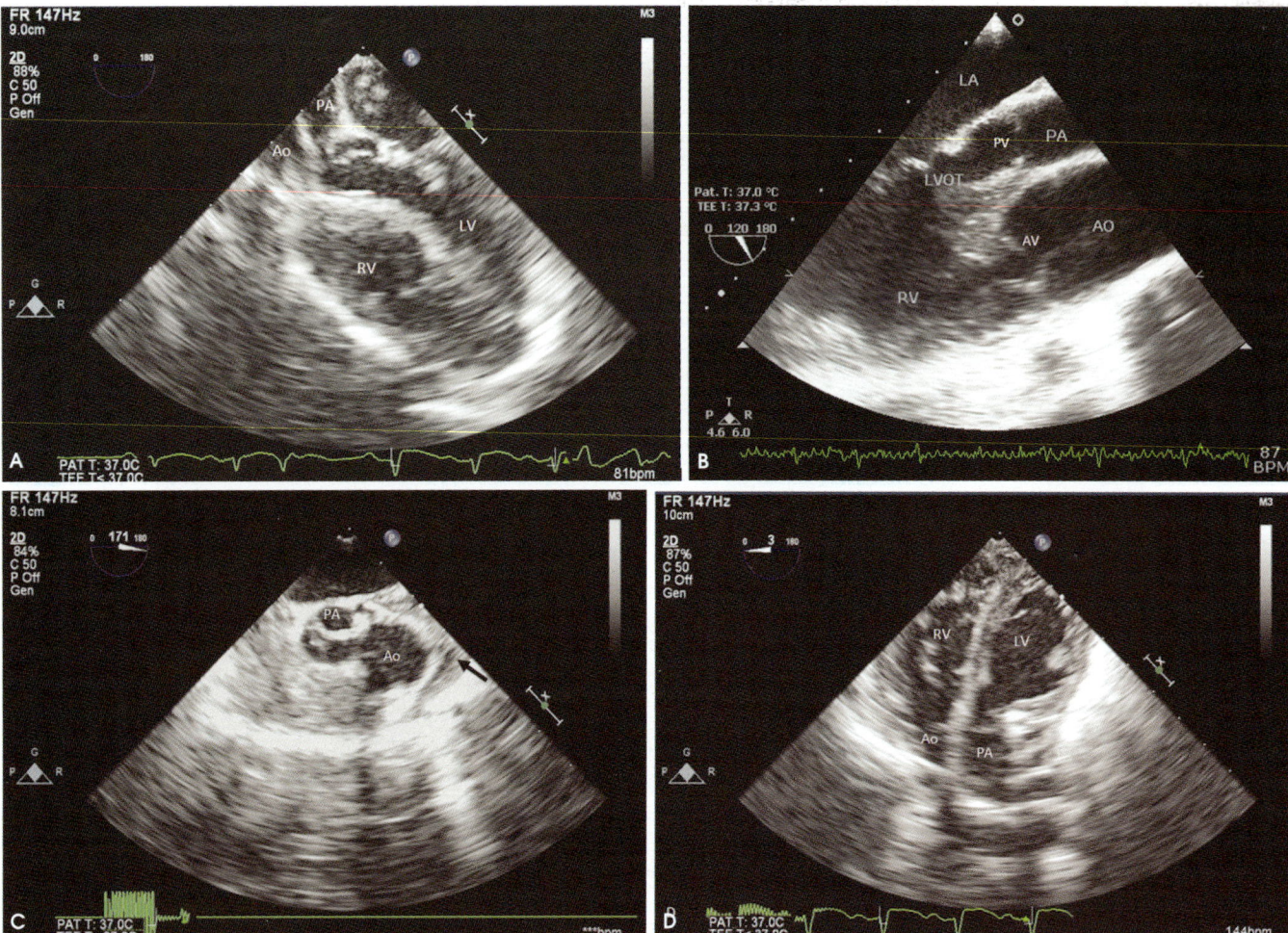

Fig. 13.37: Transposition of great arteries: Midesophageal five chamber view (A), midesophageal long-axis view (B), modified midesophageal view with extreme angulation (C) and deep transgastric long-axis view (D) showing the parallel orientation of the great vessels. The aorta arises from the right ventricle and the pulmonary artery arises from the left ventricle. The aorta can be identified by the origin of the coronary arteries (arrow, C). Note the regressed (D-shaped) left ventricle. (RV: right ventricle, LV: left ventricle, Ao: aorta, PA: pulmonary artery, LA; left atrium, LVOT: left ventricular outflow tract, PV: pulmonary valve, AV: aortic valve).

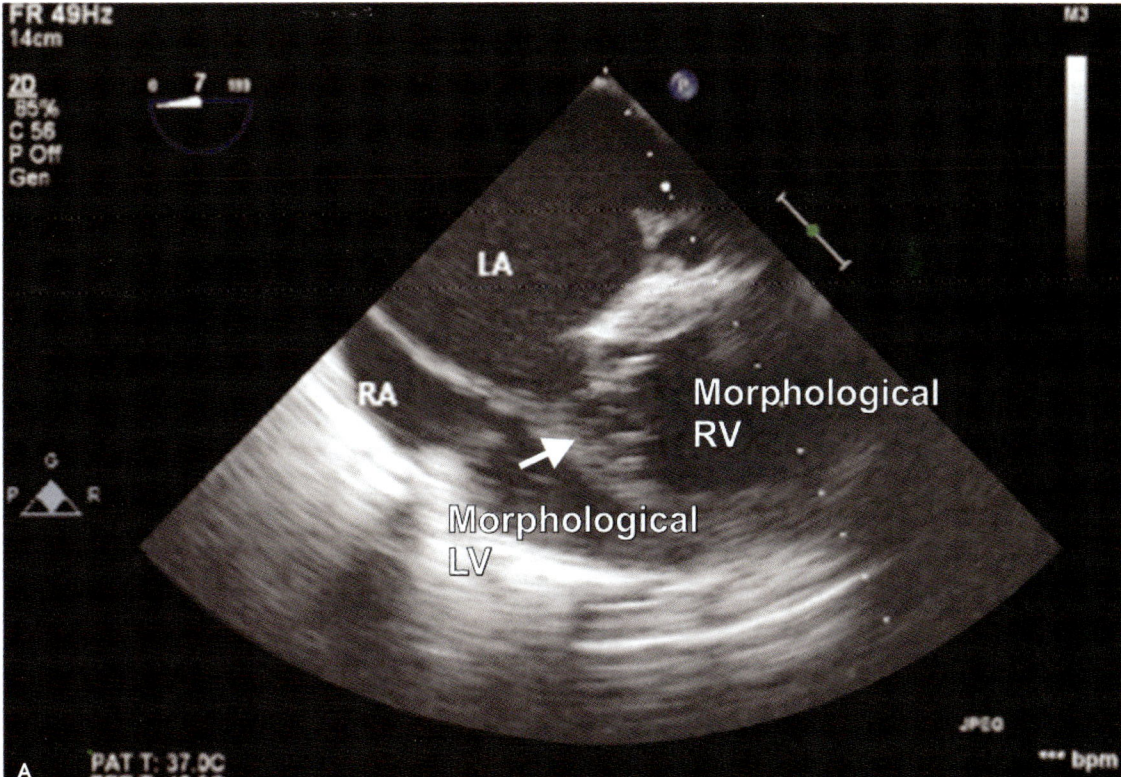

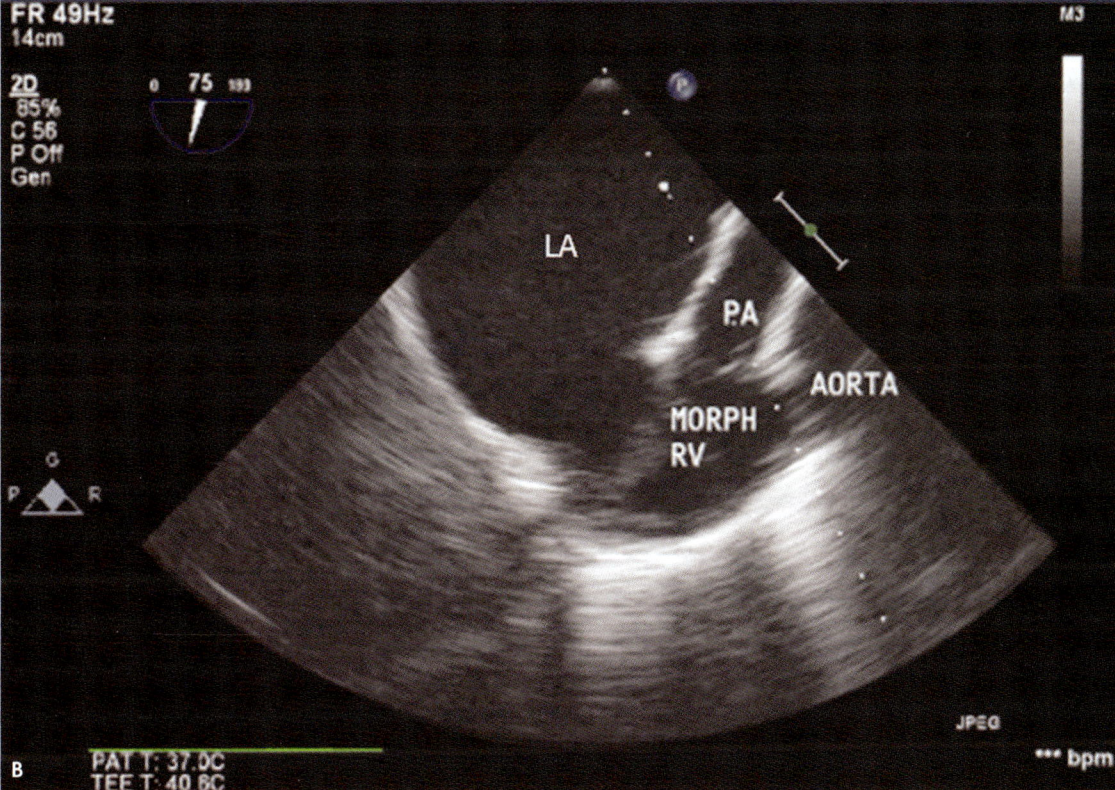

Fig. 13.38: Congenitally corrected transposition of great arteries or ventricular inversion: Midesophageal four-chamber view (A) and midesophageal long-axis view (B) showing the right atrium connected to the morphological left ventricle and the left atrium connected to the morphological right ventricle (identified in Panel A by the more apical attachment of the tricuspid valve leaflets compared to the mitral valve leaflets, arrow). The aorta arises from the right ventricle and the pulmonary artery arises from the left ventricle. Note the regressed (D-shaped) left ventricle (RA: right atrium, LA: left atrium, RV: right ventricle, LV: left ventricle, PA: pulmonary artery).

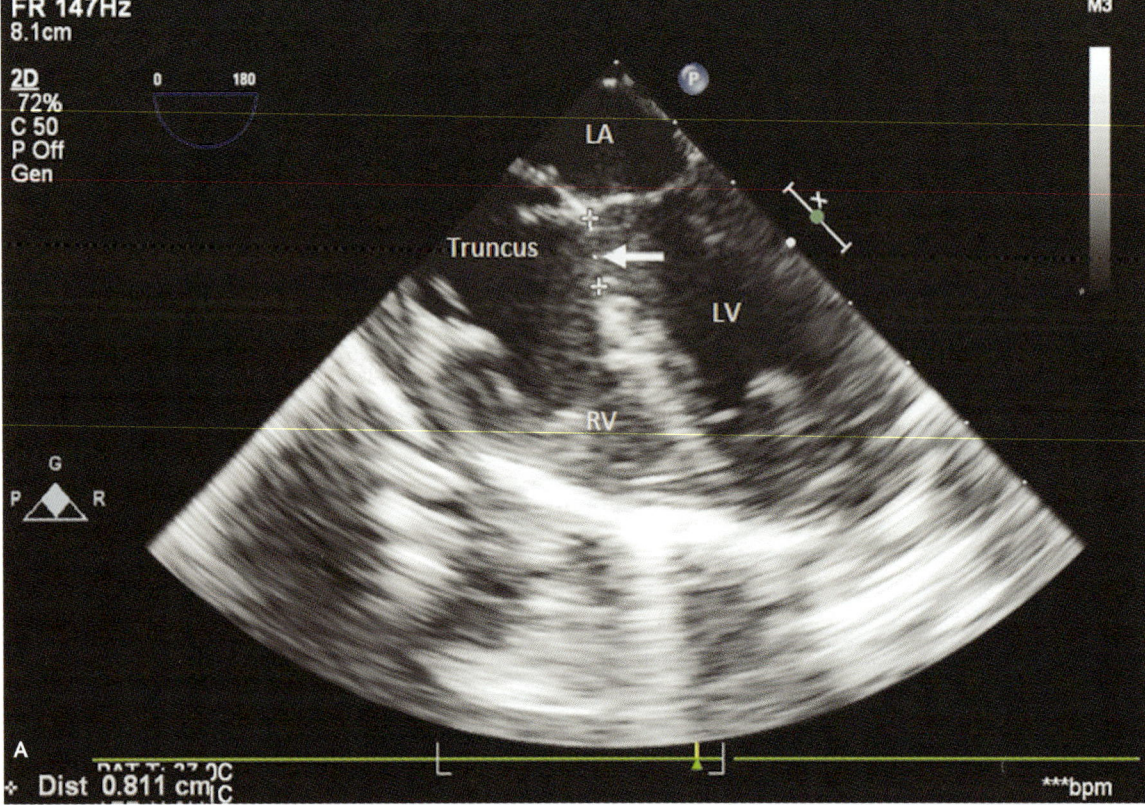

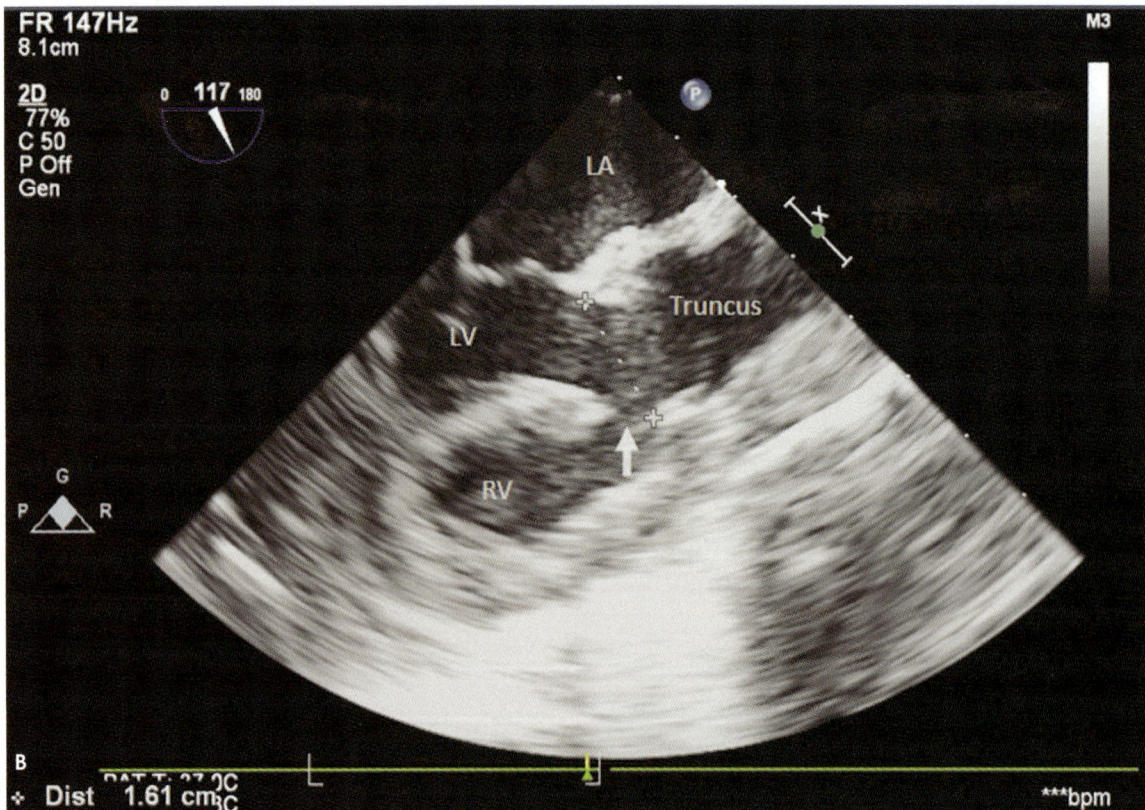

Fig. 13.39: Truncus arteriosus: Midesophageal four-chamber view (A) and long-axis view (B) showing truncus overriding of the ventricular septal defect (arrow). The pulmonary artery could not be seen arising from the right ventricle, instead from the posterior aspect of the truncus. (LA: left atrium, LV: left ventricle, RV: right ventricle).

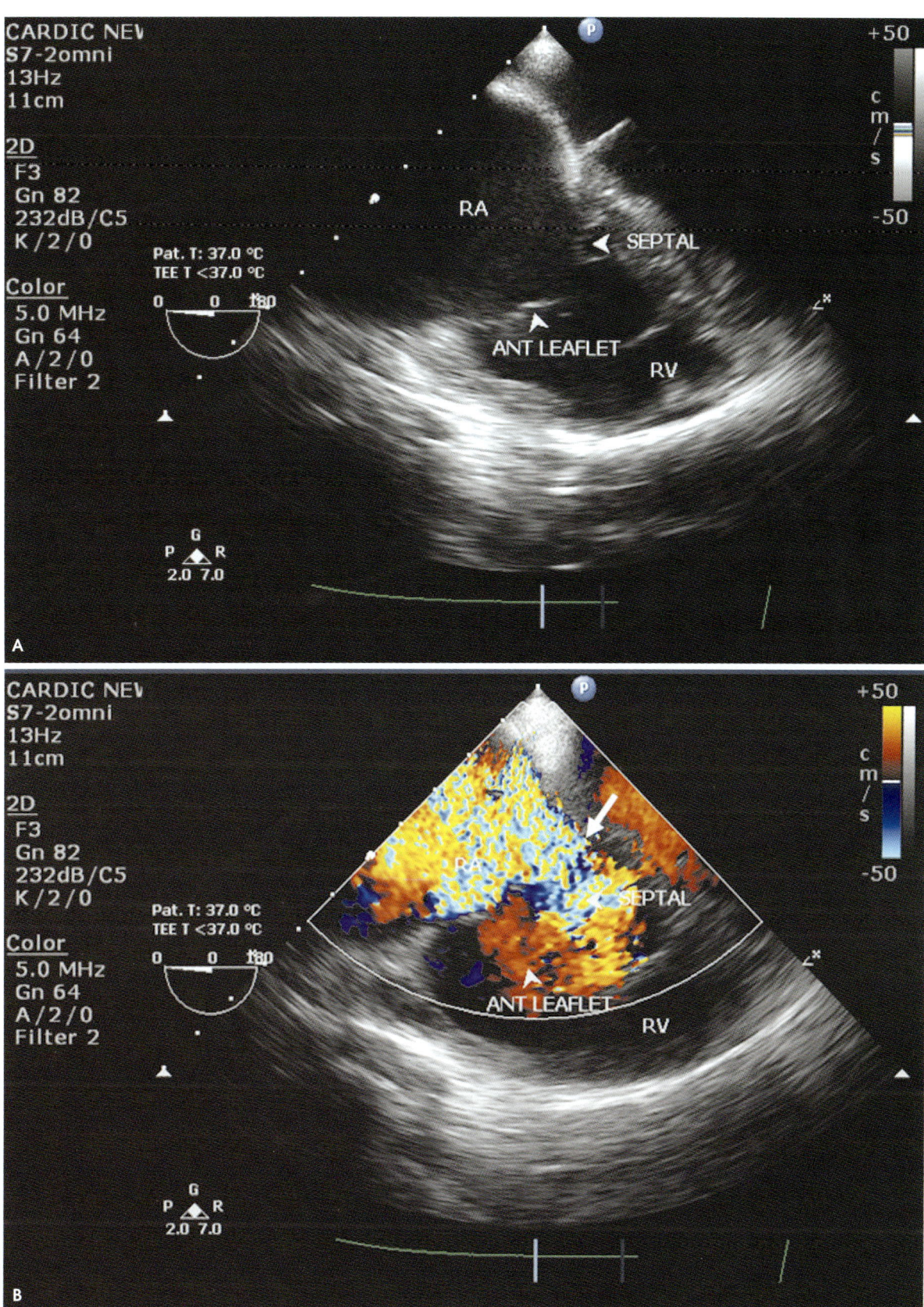

Fig. 13.40: Ebstein's anomaly: Midesophageal four-chamber view showing an apically displaced septal tricuspid leaflet leading to reduced size of the functional right ventricle (A). Color flow Doppler showing severe tricuspid regurgitation (B, arrow) (RA: right atrium, RV: right ventricle).

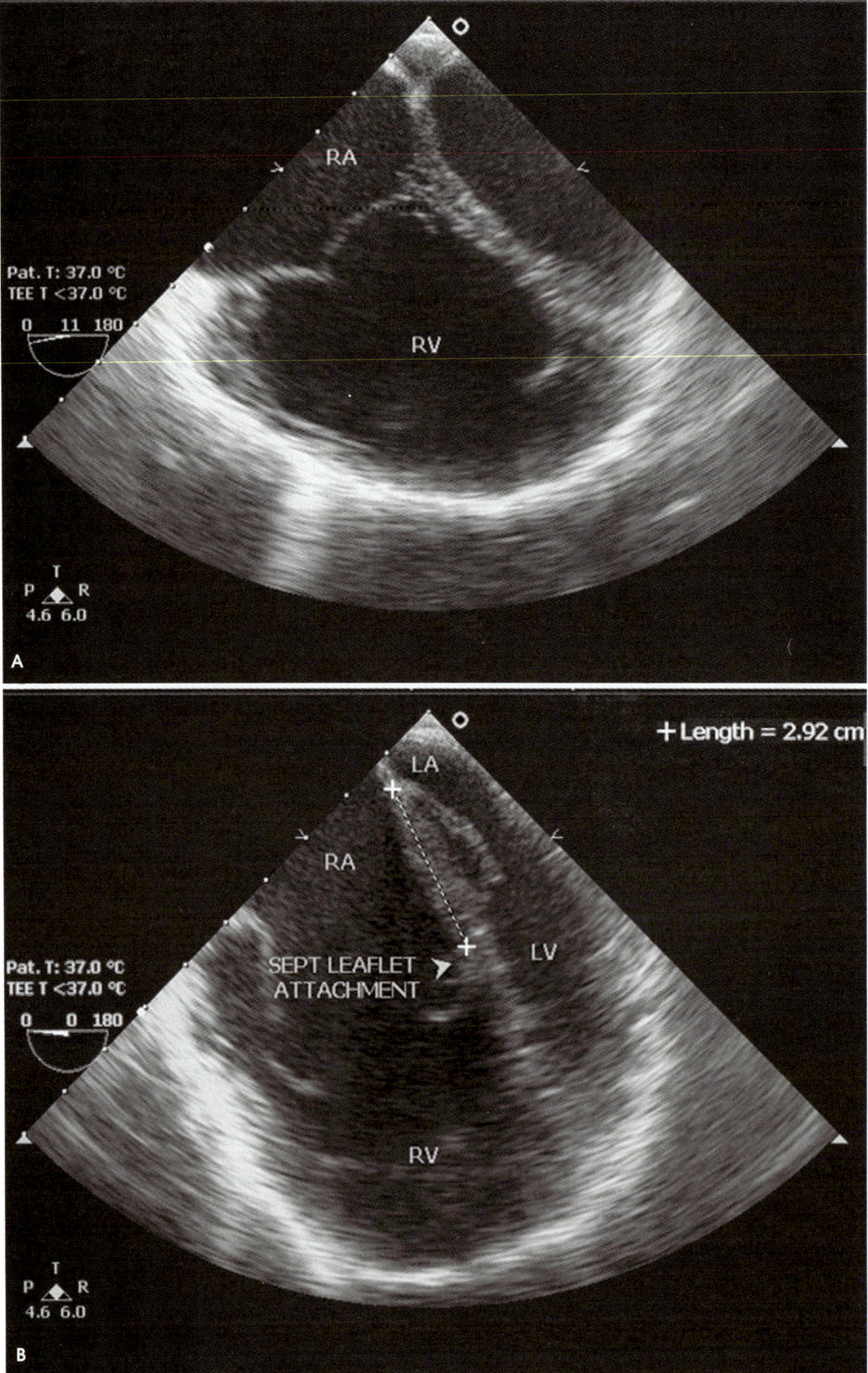

Fig. 13.41: Midesophageal four-chamber view in systole (A) and diastole (B) in a patient with Ebstein's anomaly showing apical displacement of the septal tricuspid leaflet in comparison to the anterior mitral leaflet (RA: right atrium, LA: left atrium, RV: right ventricle, LV: left ventricle).

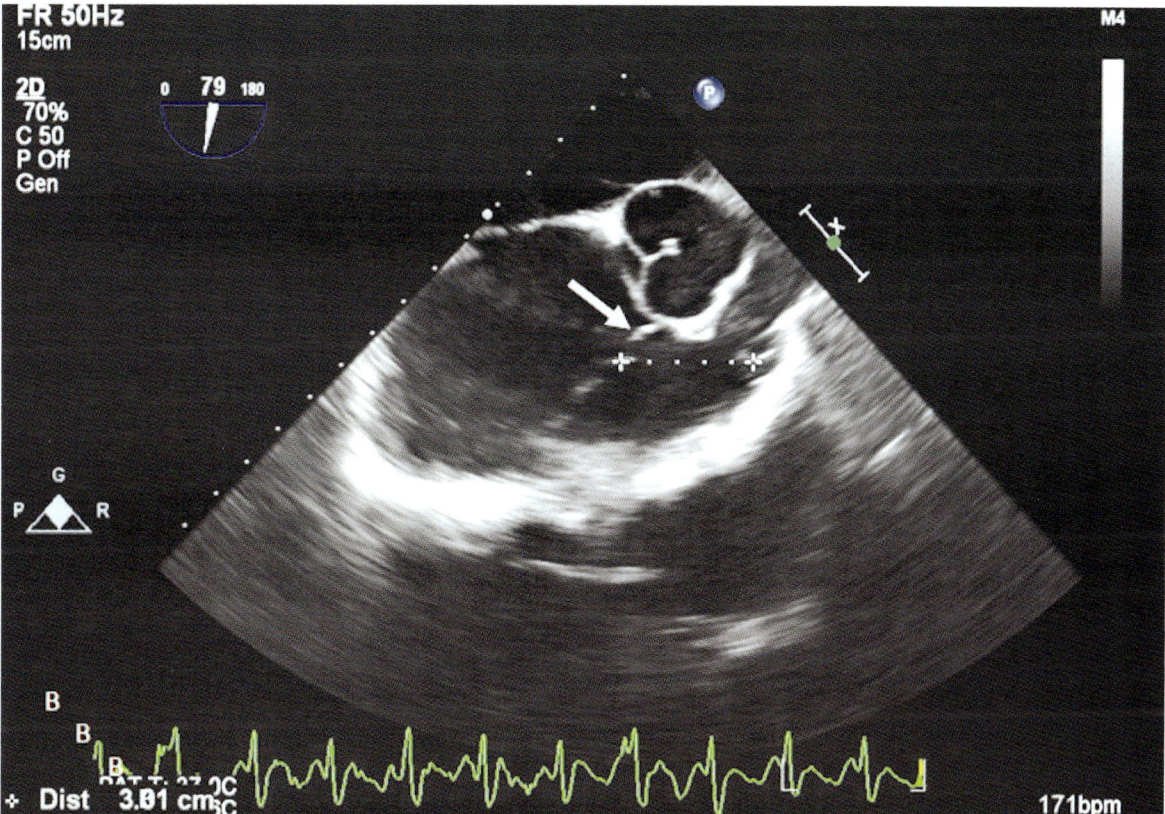

Fig. 13.42: Ebstein's anomaly: Midesophageal four-chamber view (A) and right ventricle inflow-outflow view (B) showing an apically displaced septal tricuspid leaflet (arrow), leading to atrialization of the right ventricle. The functional right ventricle is reduced in size. An atrial septal defect can also be appreciated (dashed arrow). (RA: right atrium, LA: left atrium, RV: right ventricle).

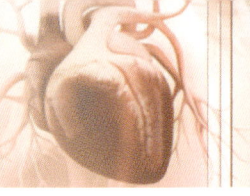

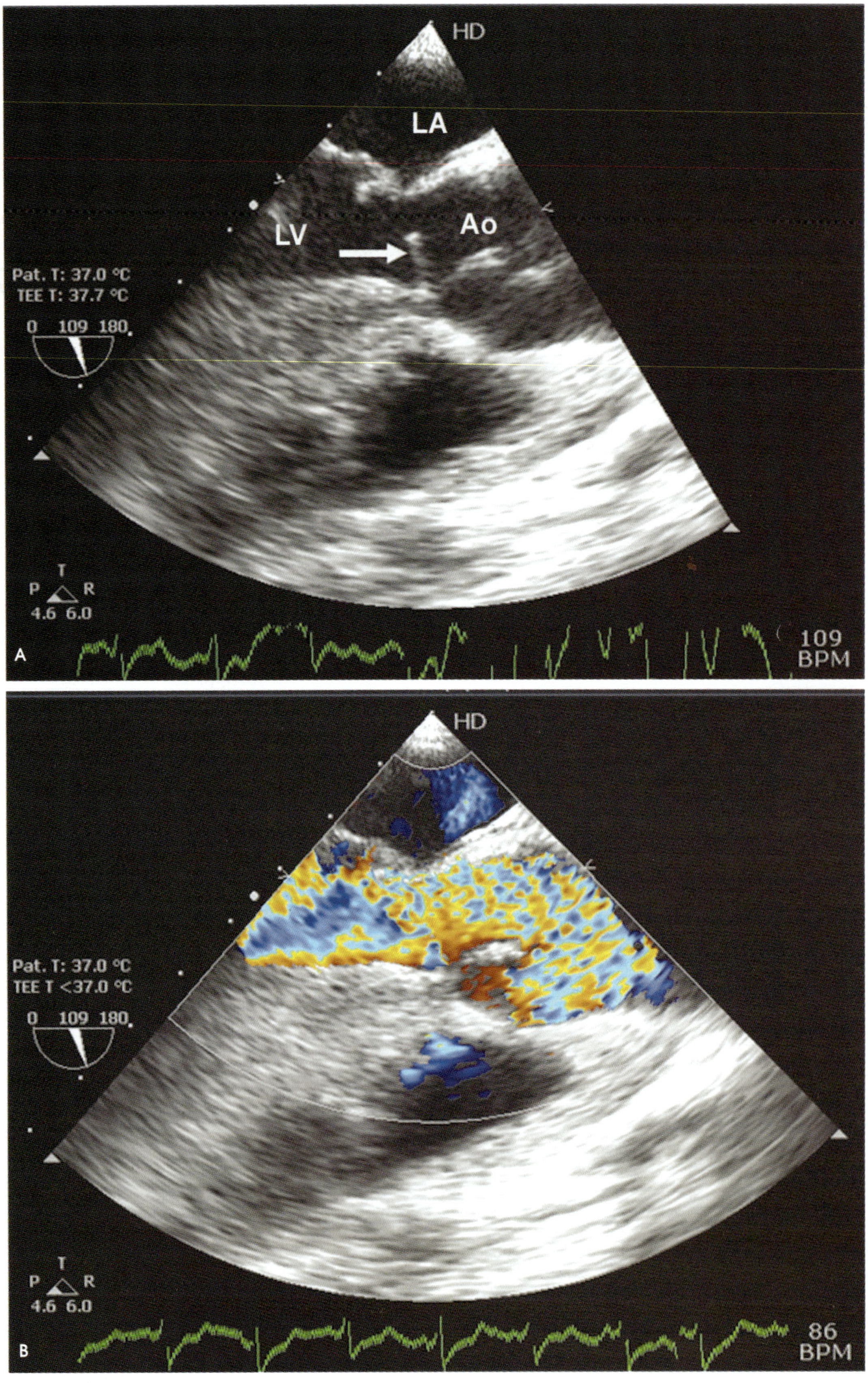

Fig. 13.43: Midesophageal long-axis view showing a subaortic membrane (A, arrow) causing turbulence in forward flow (B) (LA: left atrium, LV: left ventricle, Ao: aorta).

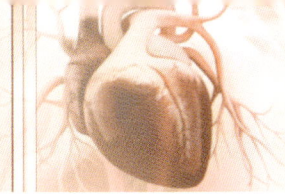

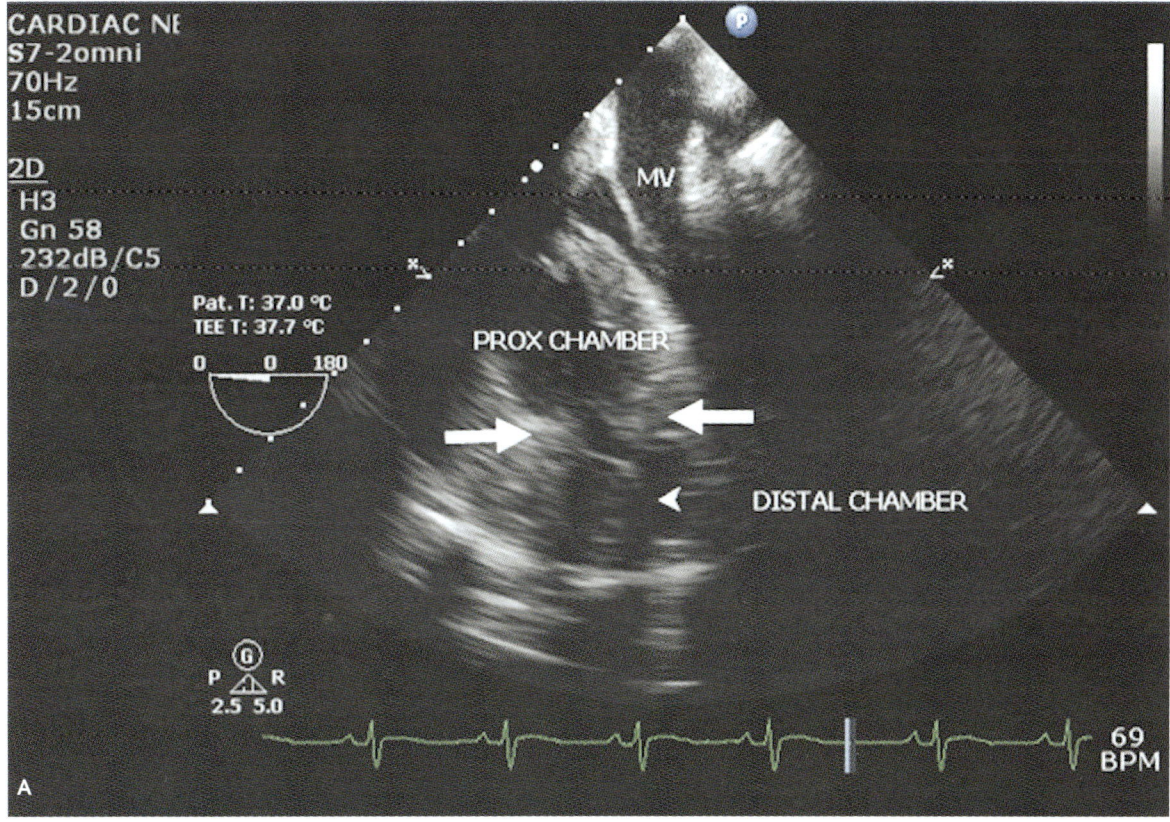

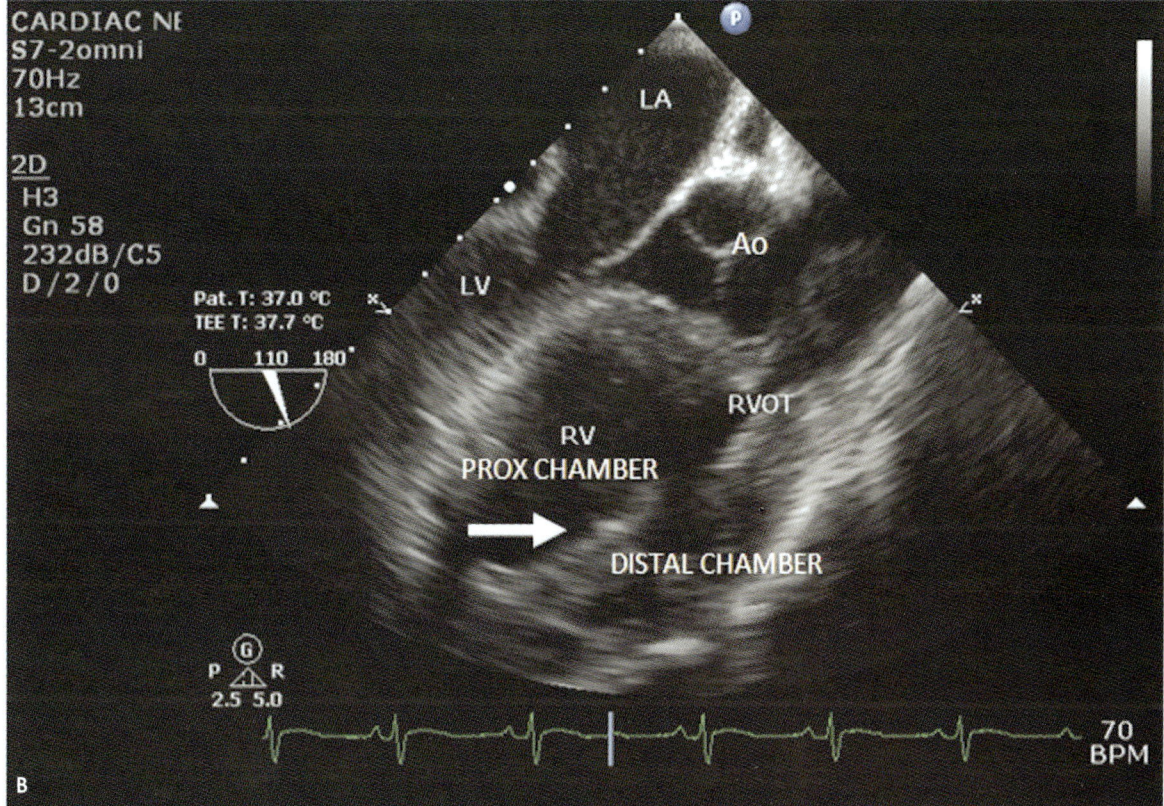

Fig. 13.44: Double chamber right ventricle: Midesophageal four-chamber view (A) and long-axis view (B) showing a dense muscle band (arrow) dividing the right ventricle into a proximal and distal chamber (LA: left atrium, LV: left ventricle, MV: mitral valve, RV: right ventricle, RVOT: right ventricular outflow tract, Ao: aorta).

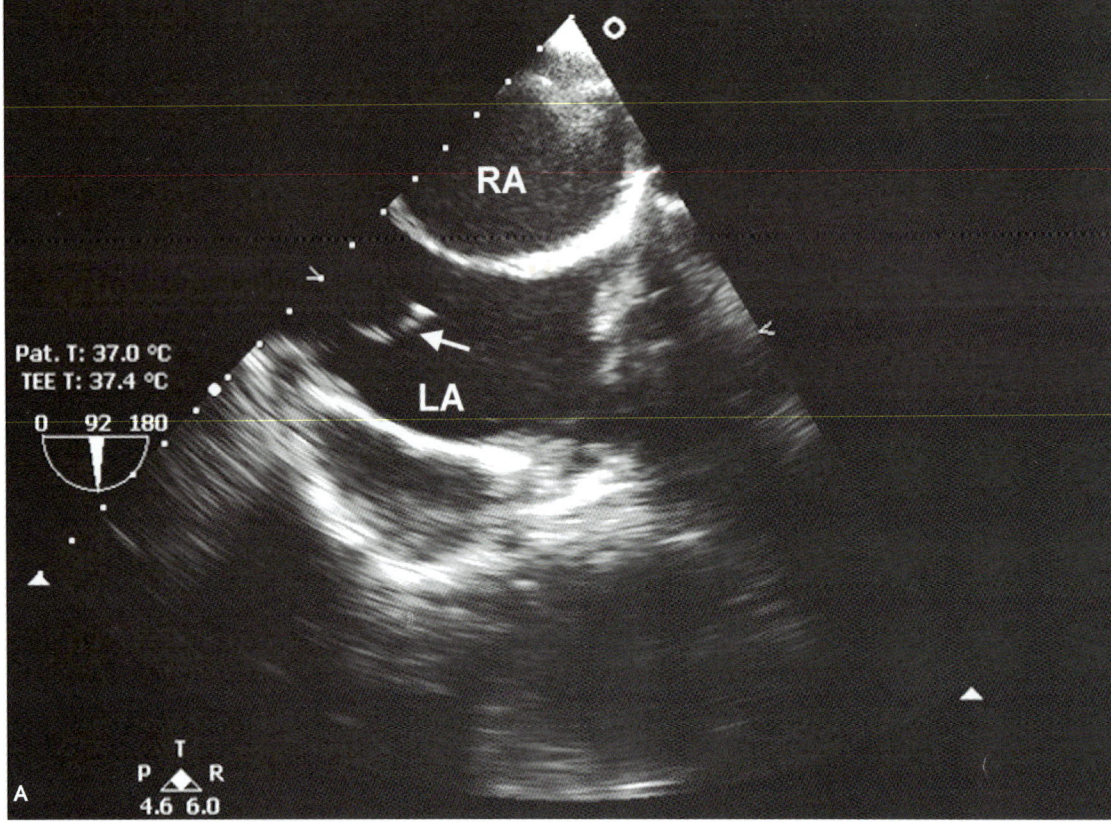

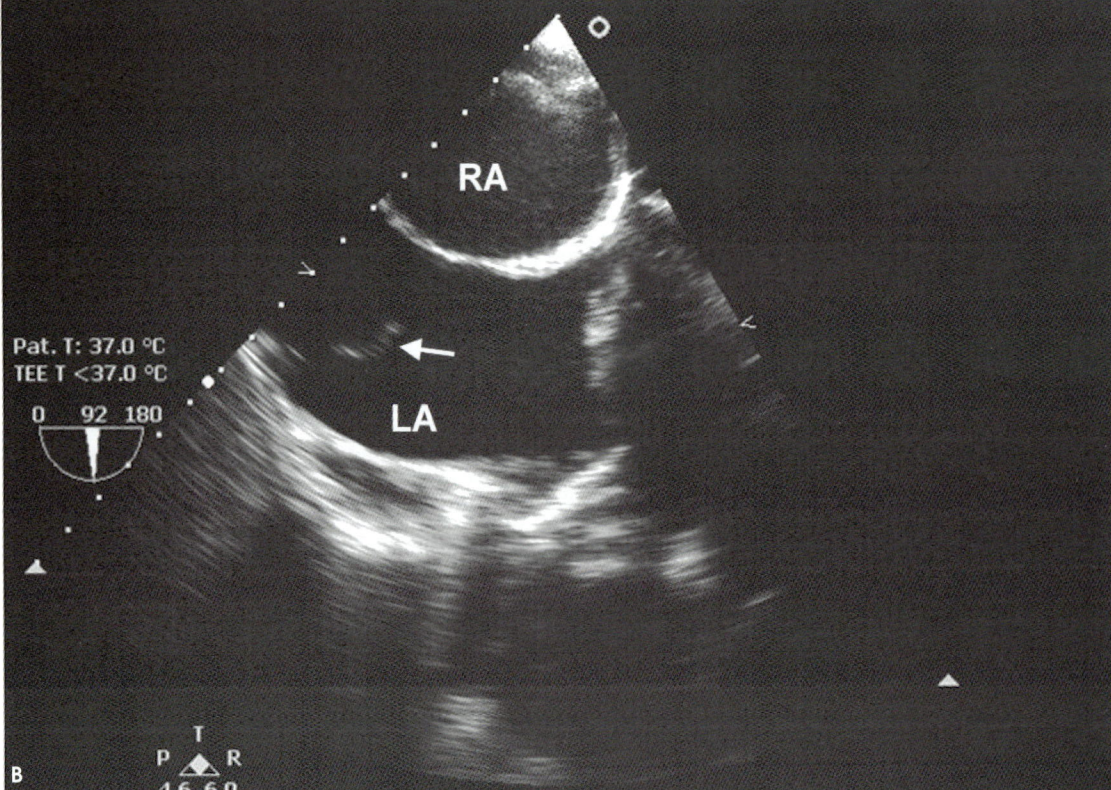

Fig. 13.45 A and B: Chiari network, modified bicaval view showing a Chiari network which is seen as a thread like structure in the right atrium (arrow). It is a mobile whip like structure located near the inferior vena cava and coronary sinus. It is an embryonic remnant of valves of sinus venosus. (refer to video) (RA: right atrium, LA: left atrium).

Three-Dimensional Transesophageal Echocardiography

14

• **Deepak K. Tempe** • **Suruchi Hasija** • **Pawan Jain***

The advent of 3-dimensional (3-D) echocardiography has revolutionized the way of conducting transesophageal echocardiography (TEE) examination. Three-dimensional echocardiography is complimentary to two-dimensional (2-D) echocardiography, but provides enhanced visualization of intracardiac structures from different perspectives. Three-dimensional imaging is based on acquisition of volume datasets. Analytical software allows off-line reconstruction of 3-D datasets for assessment of mitral valve structure and left ventricular function. The echocardiographer can manipulate the 3-D datasets to orient the 3-D images. Three-dimensional systems perform image acquisition in different modes: live 3-D, live 3-D zoom mode, full volume mode and full volume color mode. Real-time 3-D echocardiography is performed using the matrix array transducer which houses 2500 piezoelectric crystals. A matrix probe is a miniaturized beam forming

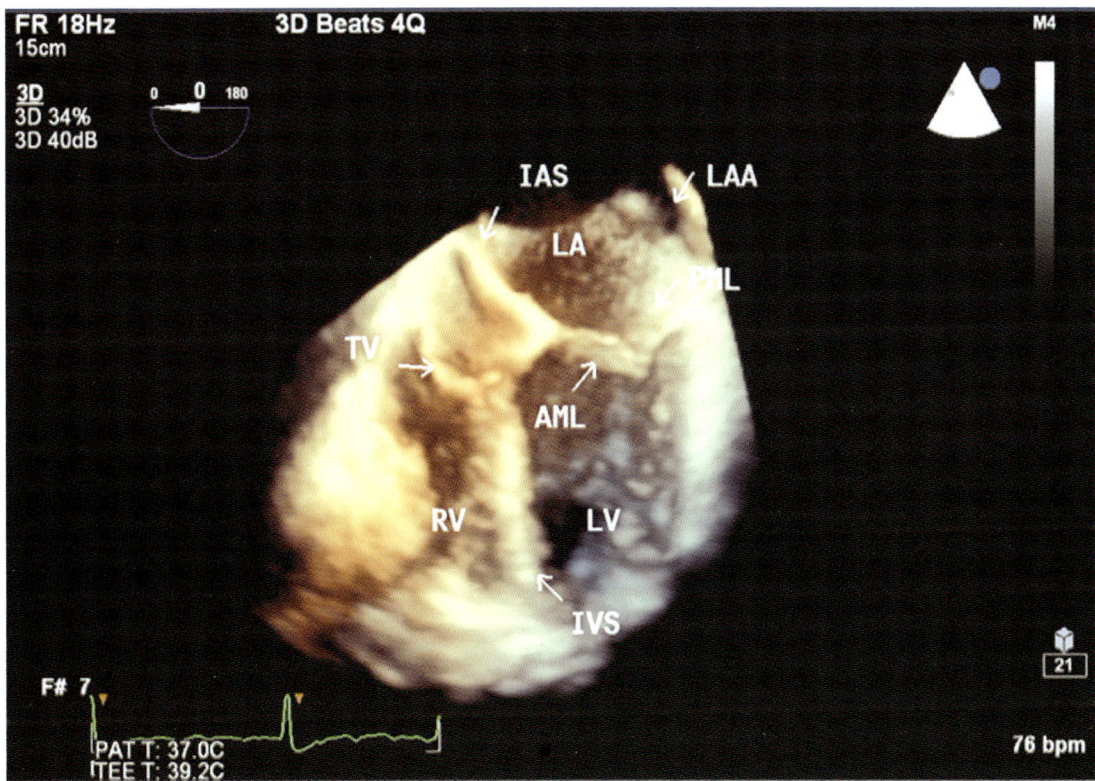

Fig. 14.1: Three-dimensional midesophageal 4-chamber view. (LA: left atrium, RV: right ventricle, LV: left ventricle, LAA: left atrial appendage, IAS: interatrial septum, IVS: interventricular septum, TV: tricuspid valve, AML: anterior mitral leaflet, PML: posterior mitral leaflet).

***Pawan Jain,** Senior resident, Department of Cardiac Anaesthesia, All India Institute of Medical Sciences, New Delhi

technology in the TEE probe. It helps to form a volumetric data set (3D) of an interrogated anatomical structure. 3D echocardiography is an invaluable aid in the echocardiographer's armamentarium that provides accurate information regarding cardiac anatomy and function.

All the views described for 2-D echocardiography can be obtained in 3-D echocardiography. In addition, numerous modified views can be obtained that allow the examination of all the structures of the heart from any angle or plane. The acquired pyramidal volume of information can be visualized from different angles and cropped on any desired plane to focus on any region of interest contained in the volume.

It is essential that the operator is well conversant with the 2-D imaging in order to understand and interpret the 3-D imaging.

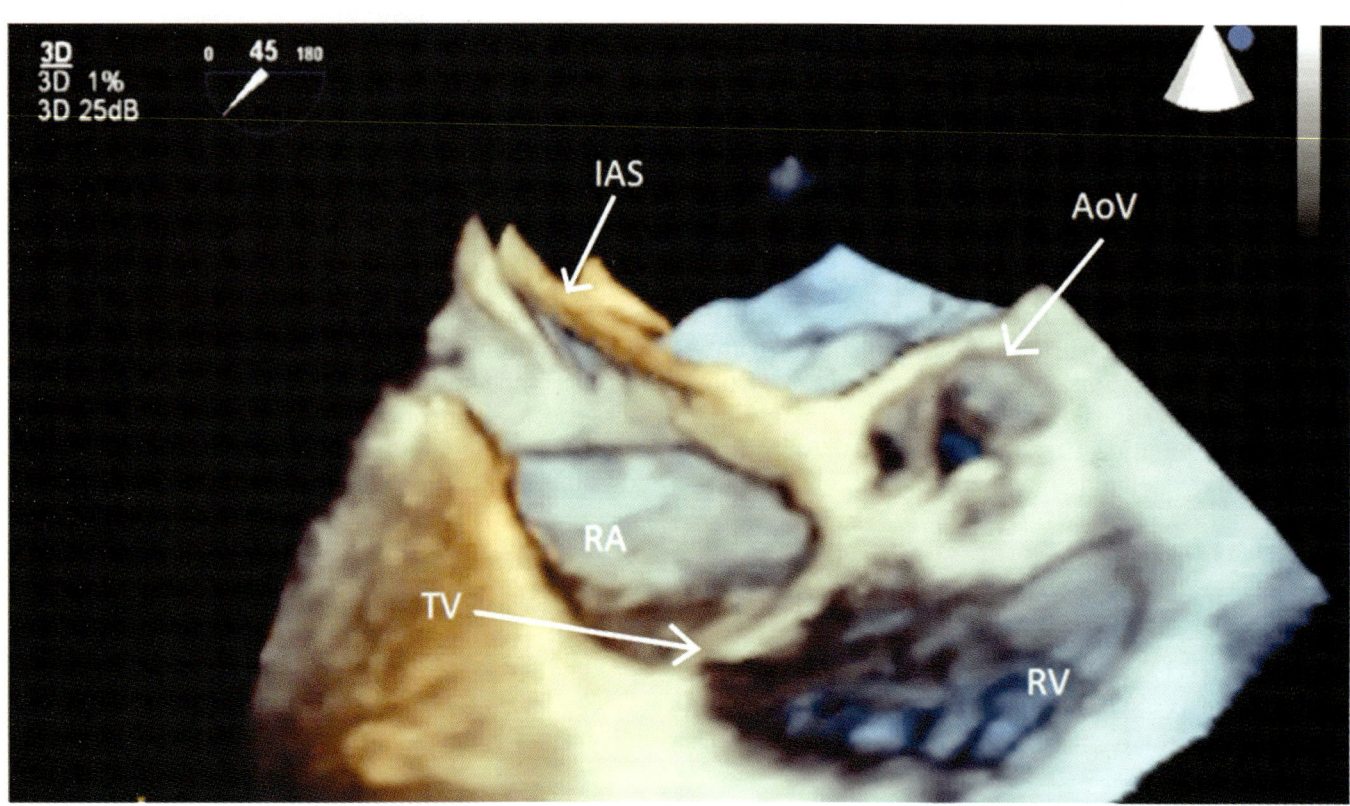

Fig. 14.2: Three-dimensional midesophageal right ventricular inflow-outflow view. (RA: right atrium, TV: tricuspid valve, RV: right ventricle, AoV: aortic valve, IAS: interatrial septum).

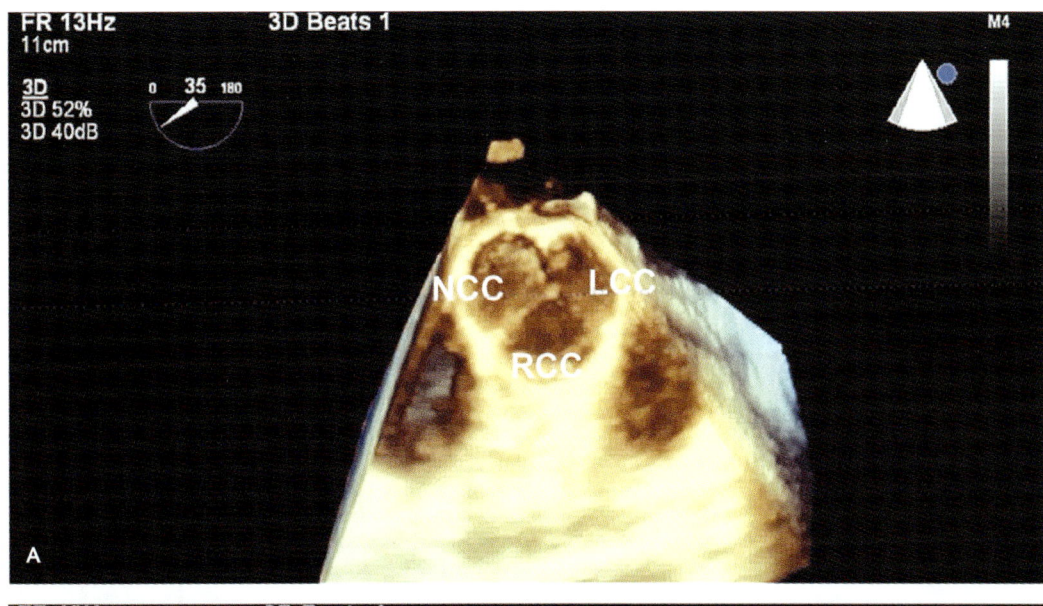

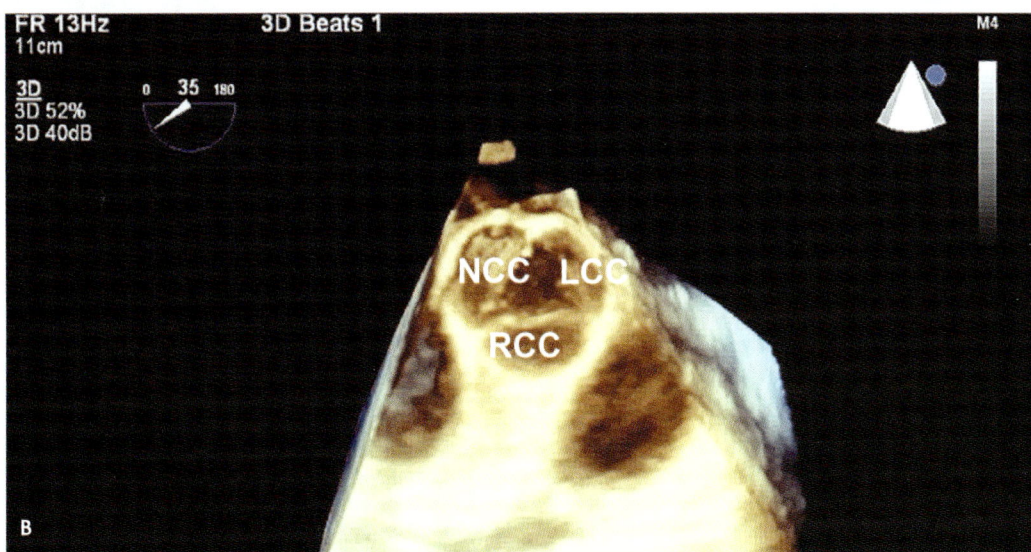

Fig. 14.3: Three-dimensional midesophageal aortic valve short-axis view showing a normal aortic valve: in closed position (A) and open position (B). All the 3 cusps are visible. (NCC: non-coronary cusp, LCC: left coronary cusp, RCC: right coronary cusp).

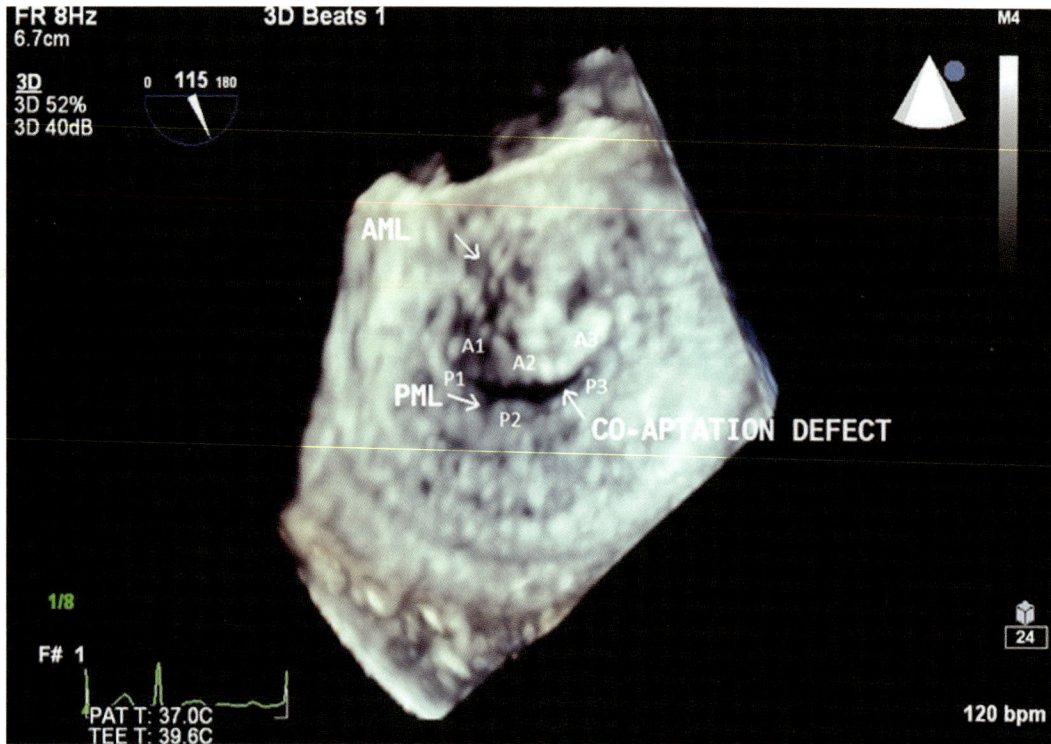

Fig. 14.4: Three-dimensional atrial view of the mitral valve in end-systole showing a co-aptation defect in a patient with severe mitral regurgitation. The three segments of the anterior mitral leaflet (AML) (A1, A2, A3) and the corresponding scallops of the posterior mitral leaflet (PML) (P1, P2, P3) can be identified.

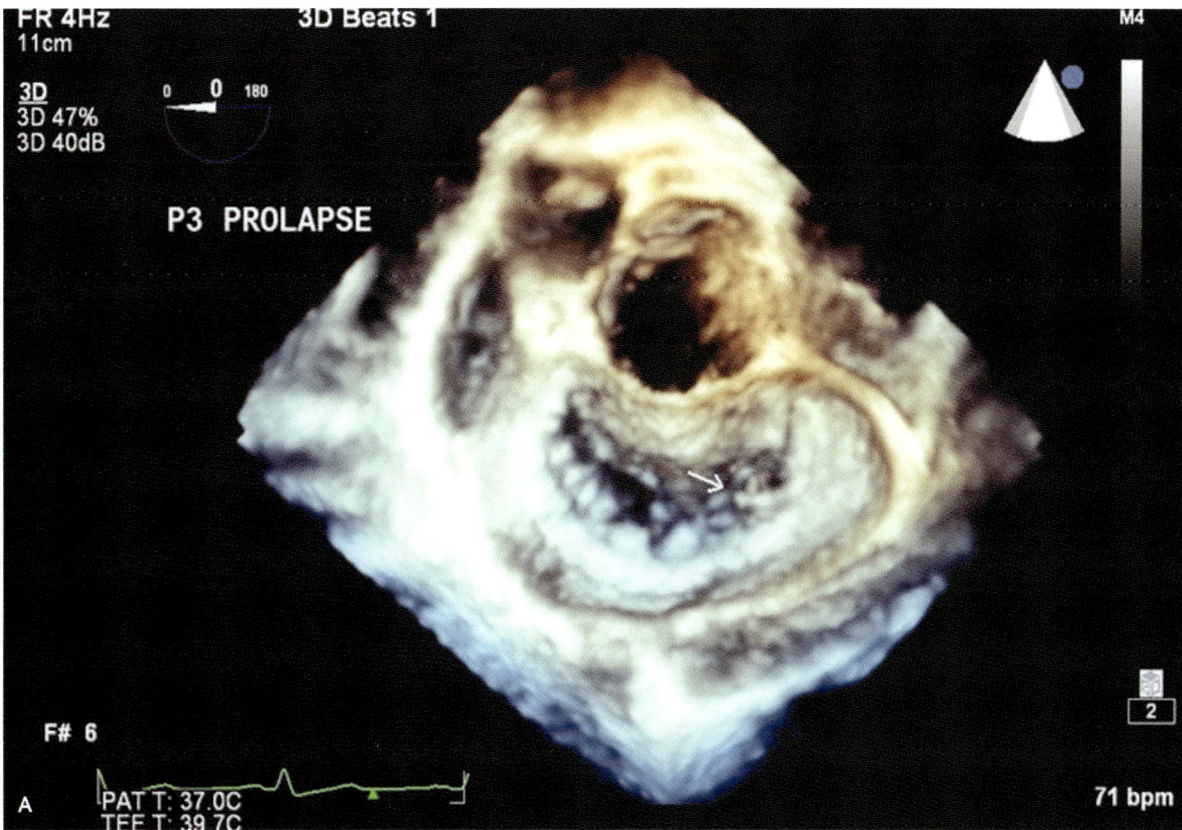

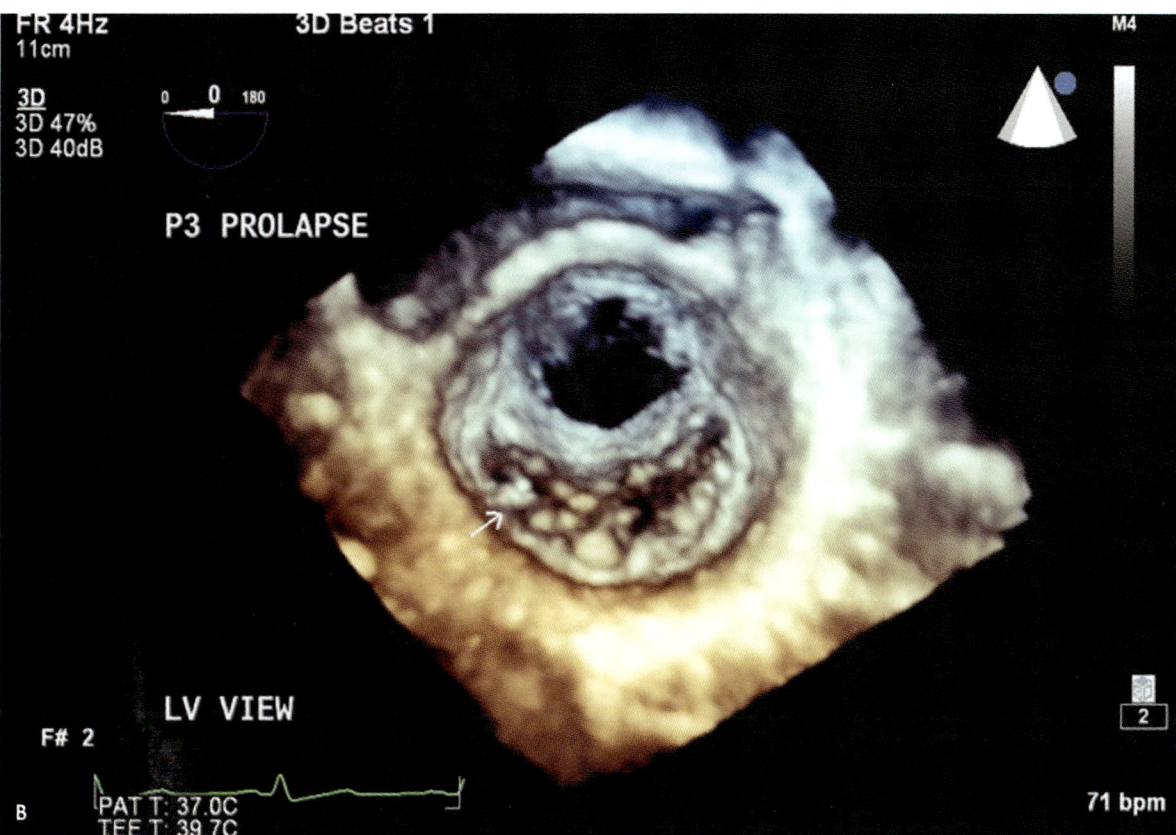

Fig. 14.5: Three-dimensional en-face view of the mitral valve from the atrial (A) and ventricular side (B) in a patient with mitral regurgitation showing P3 prolapse (arrow).

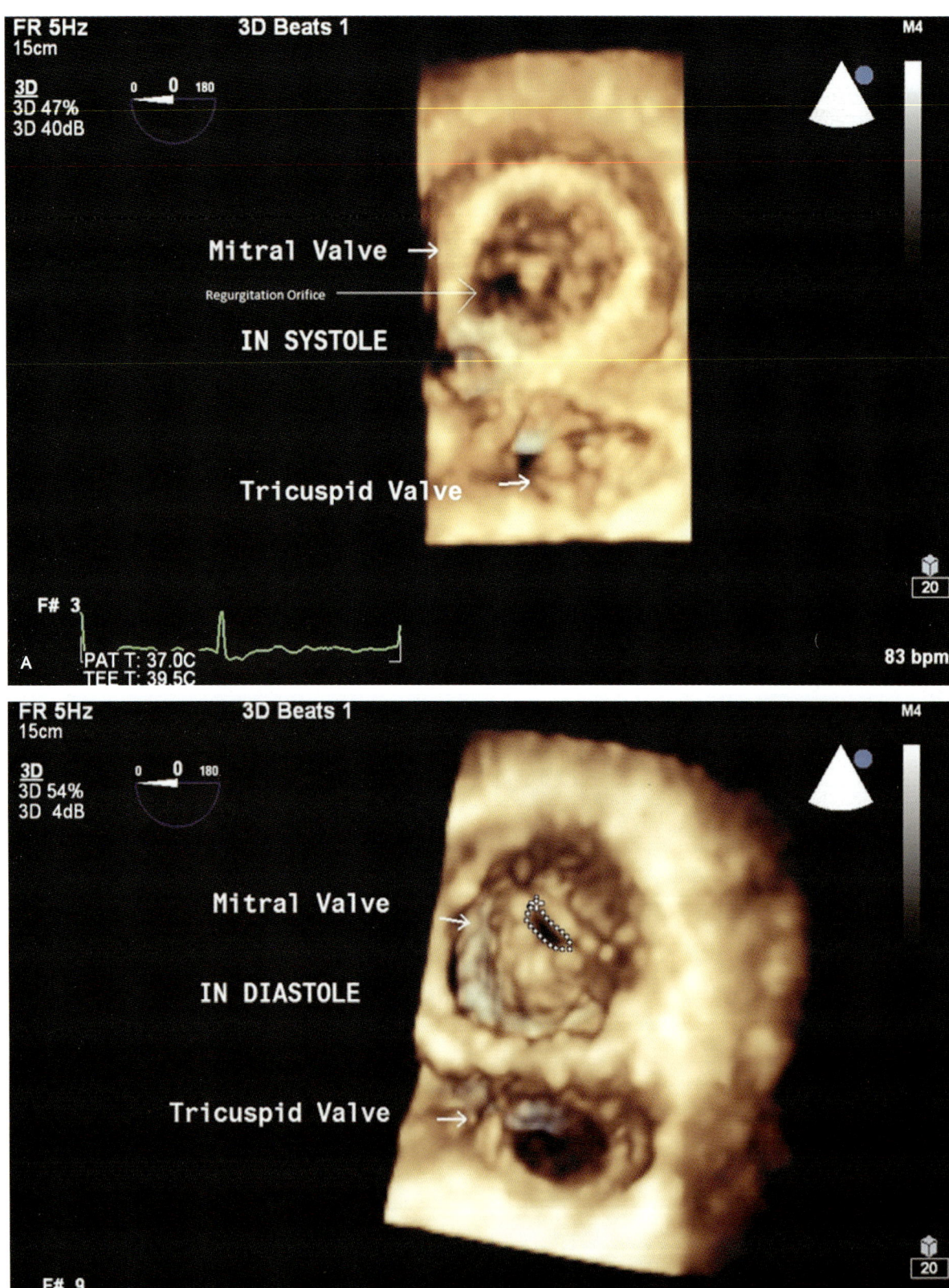

Fig. 14.6: Three-dimensional atrial view of the mitral and tricuspid valves in a patient with rheumatic mitral valve disease showing a regurgitation orifice in mitral valve in systole (A) and a stenosed orifice (mitral valve area by planimetry: 0.35 cm²) in diastole (B).

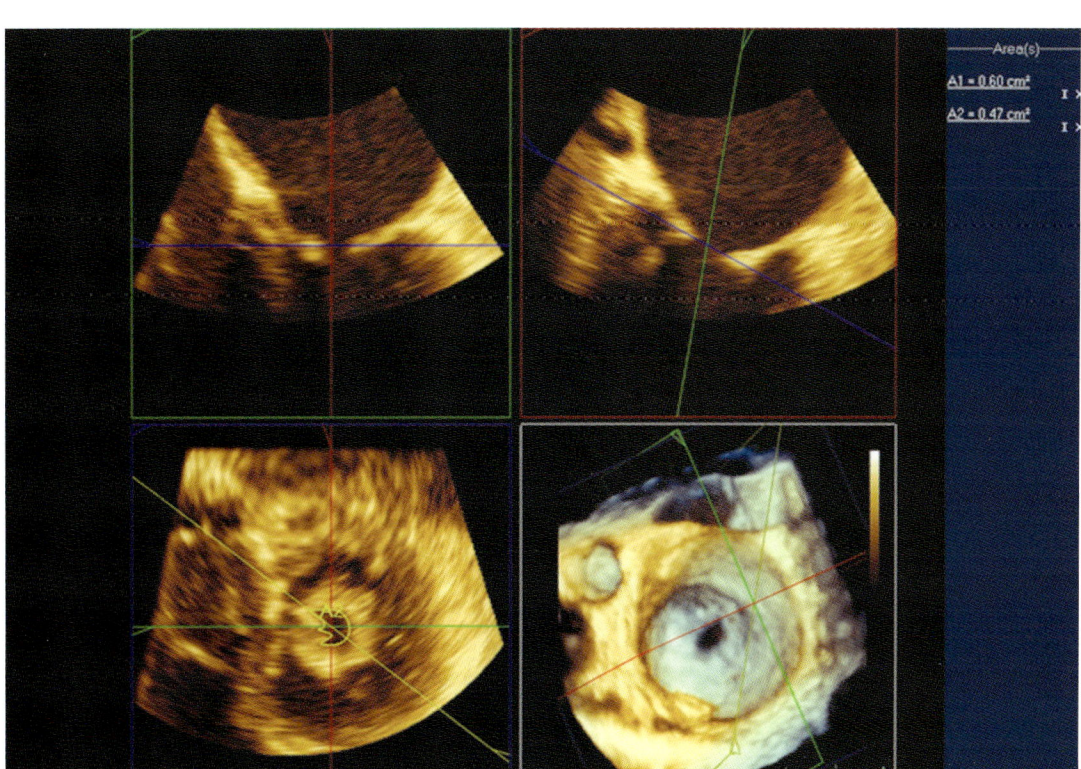

Fig. 14.7: Three dimensional measurement of mitral valve area. A full-volume image of the mitral valve was acquired in a patient with mitral stenosis. The mitral valve area was calculated by aligning three orthogonal planes (x, y and z shown in *red, green* and *blue*) at the minimal orifice area in diastole. The resulting image was traced to determine the mitral valve area (lower left).

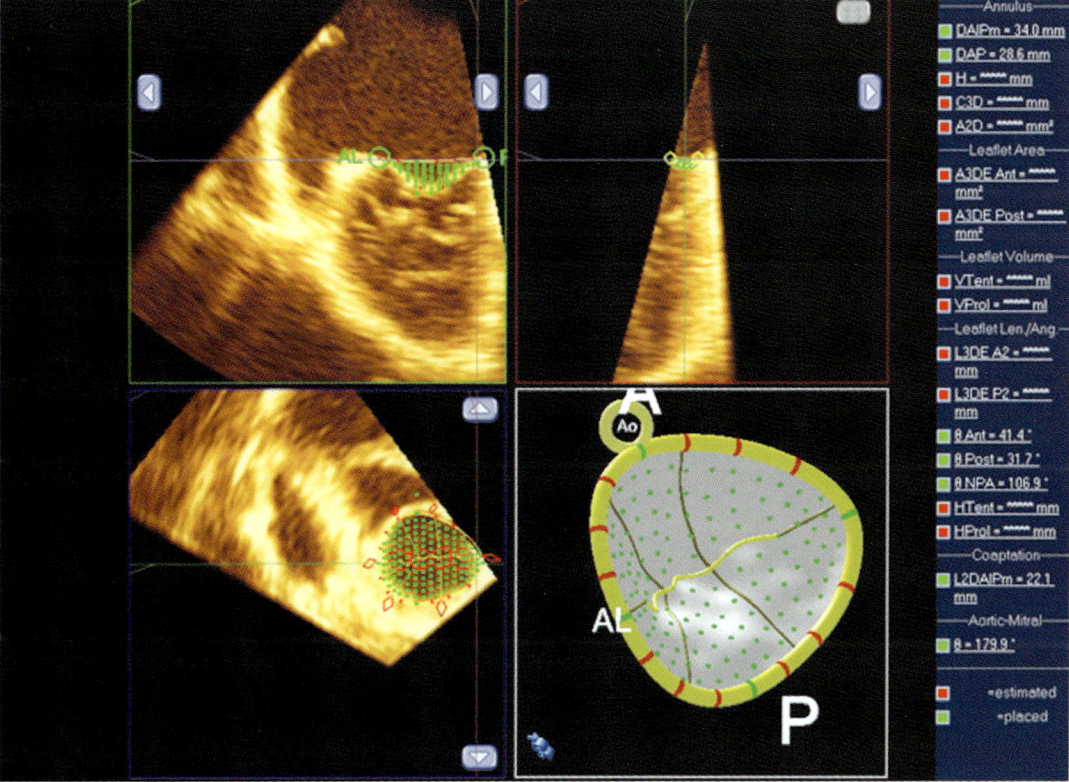

Fig. 14.8: Mitral valve quantification (MVQ) of a normal mitral valve showing the three-dimensional model of the leaflet surface along with coaptation line. (A: anterior, P: posterior, AL: anterolateral, Ao: aorta).

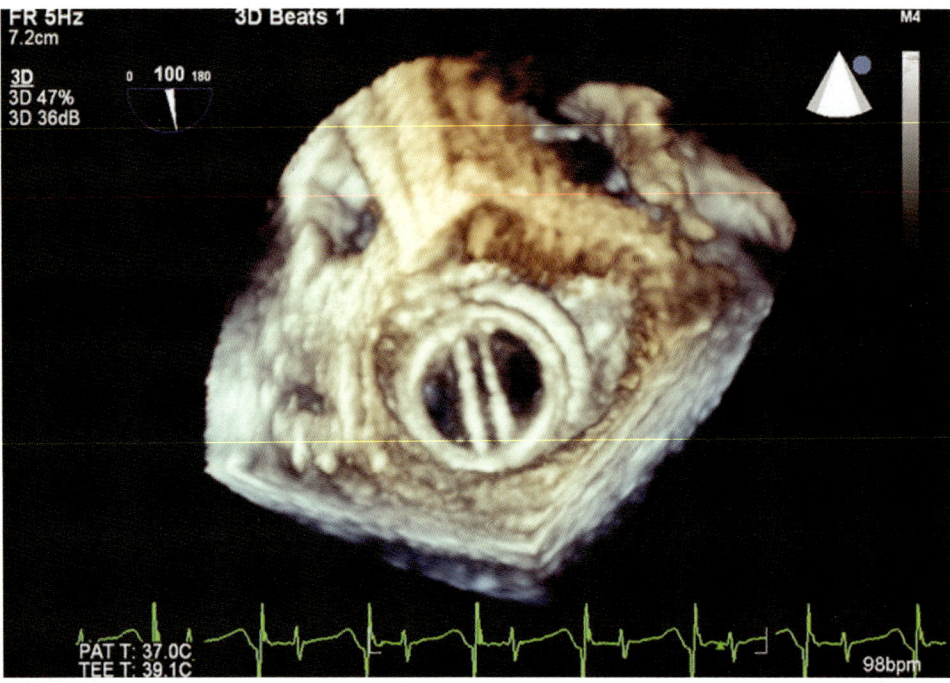

Fig. 14.9: Three-dimensional atrial view of a bileaflet prosthetic mitral valve in the open position at end-diastole.

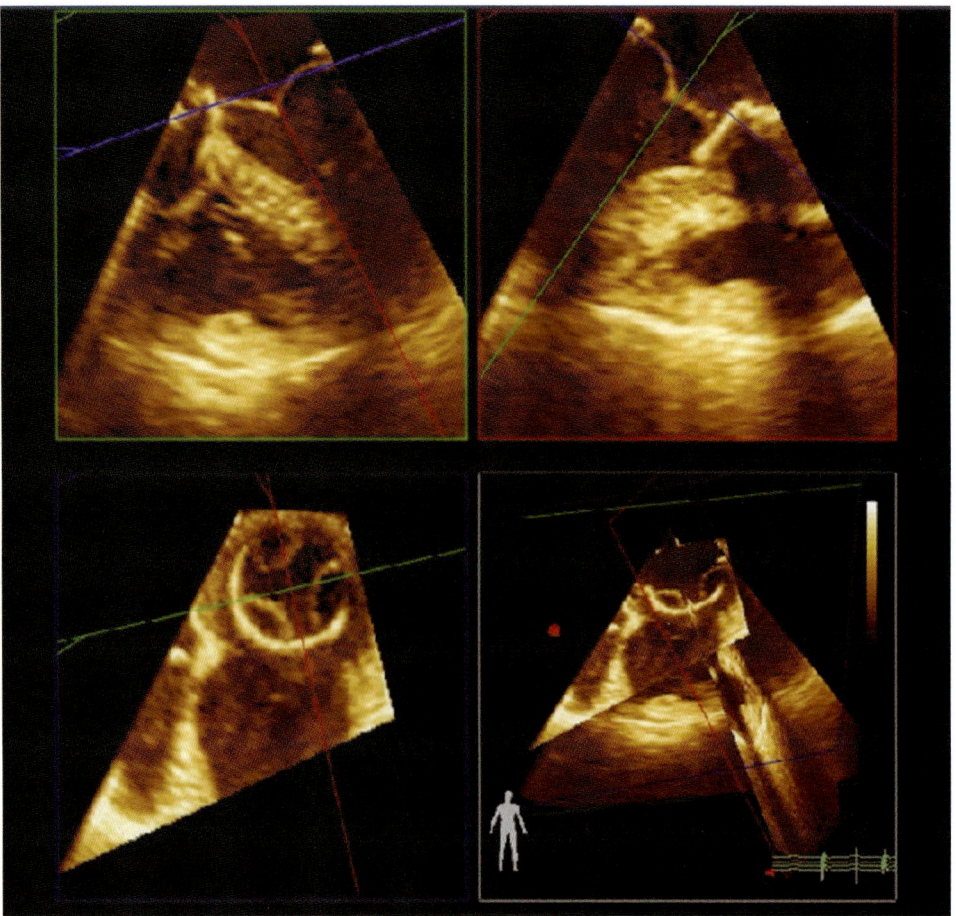

Fig. 14.10: Three-dimensional reconstructed view post-mitral valve replacement showing the three leaflets of the bioprosthesis.

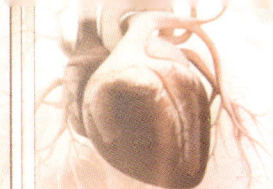

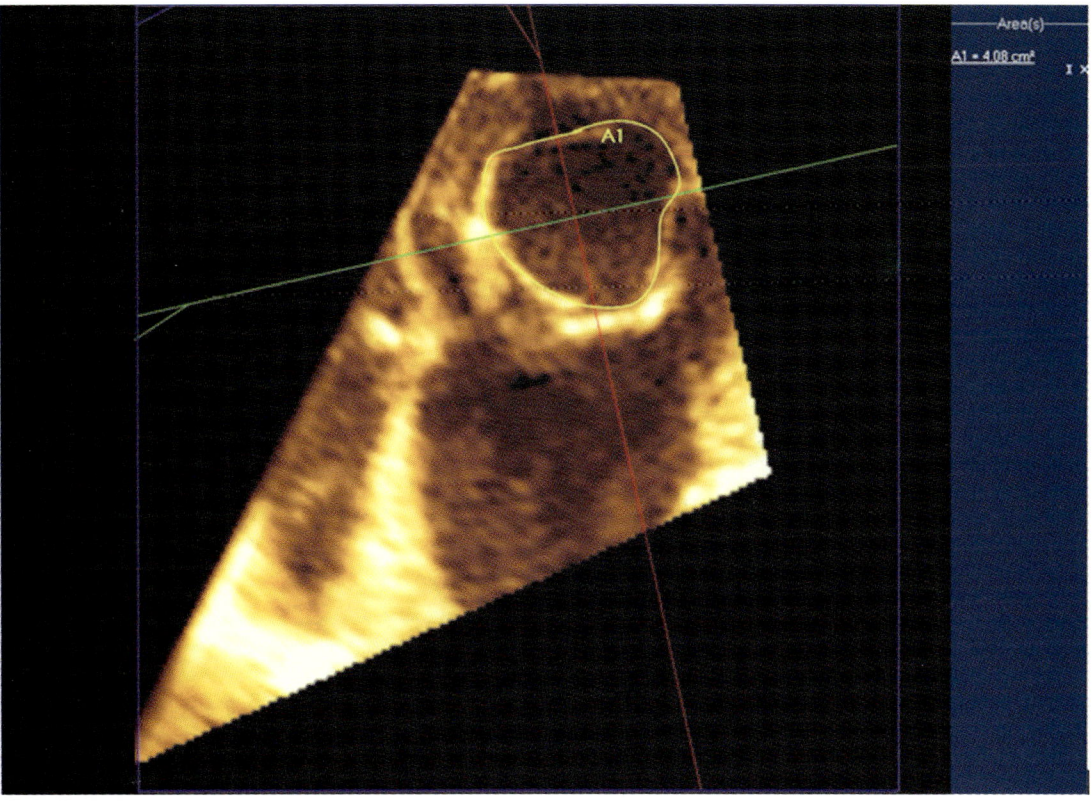

Fig. 14.11: Three-dimensional reconstructed view of the mitral bioprosthesis in short-axis (blue transverse plane) in the same patient showing the calculation of area by planimetry.

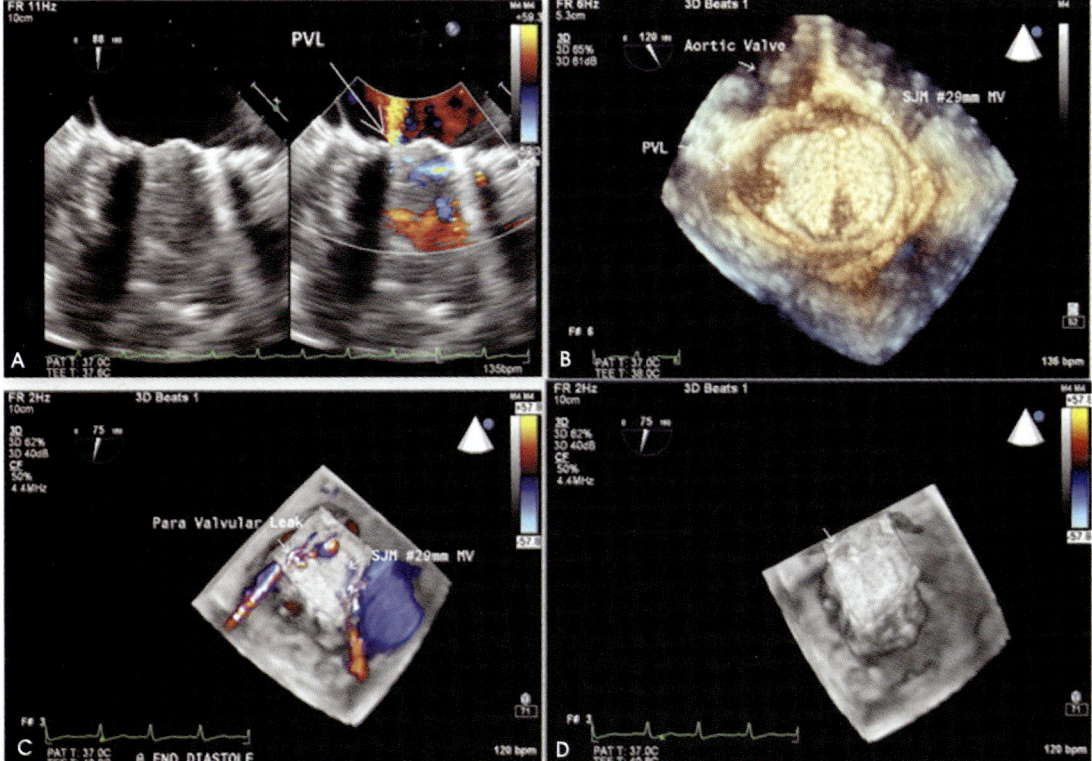

Fig. 14.12: Two-dimensional (A), corresponding three-dimensional (3-D) en-face (B), color Doppler (C), and color suppressed (D) views of a prosthetic mitral valve showing paravalvular leak (PVL).

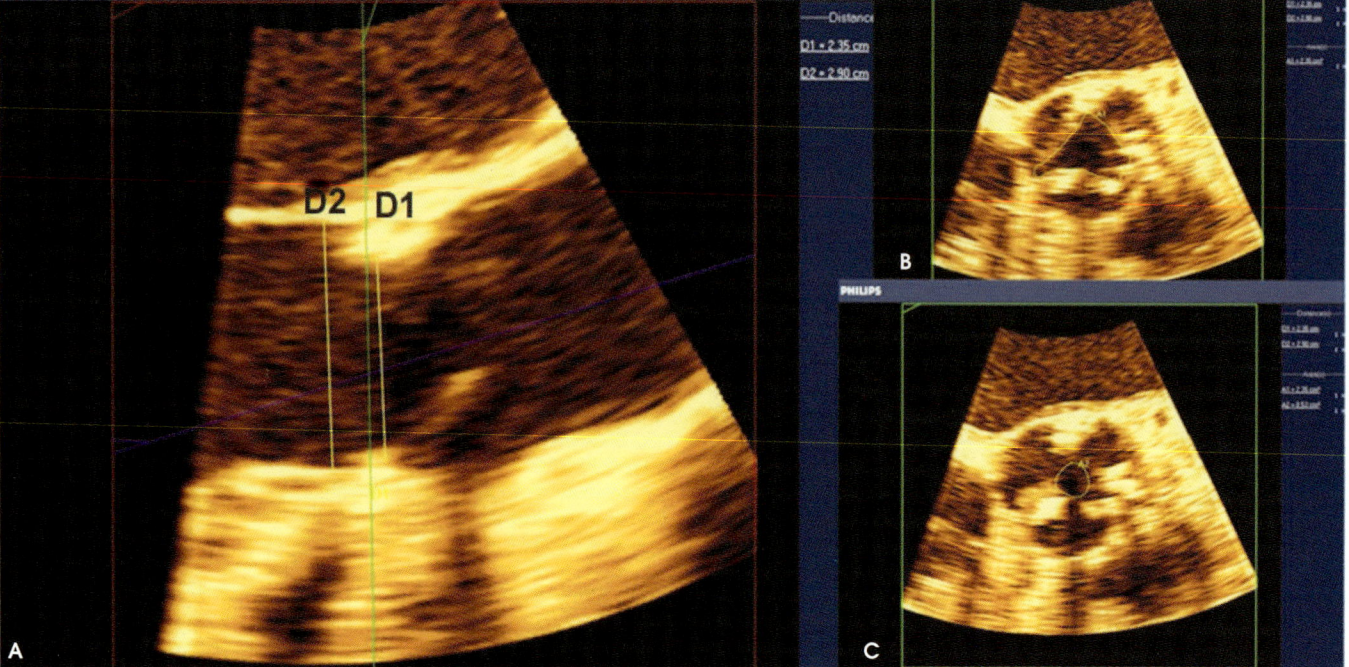

Fig. 14.13: Three-dimensional reconstructed view of the aortic valve in a patient with aortic regurgitation showing calculation of aortic root diameter (D1) and LVOT diameter (D2) in long-axis (A), and aortic valve area at end-systole (B) and effective regurgitant orifice area at end-diastole (C) in short-axis.

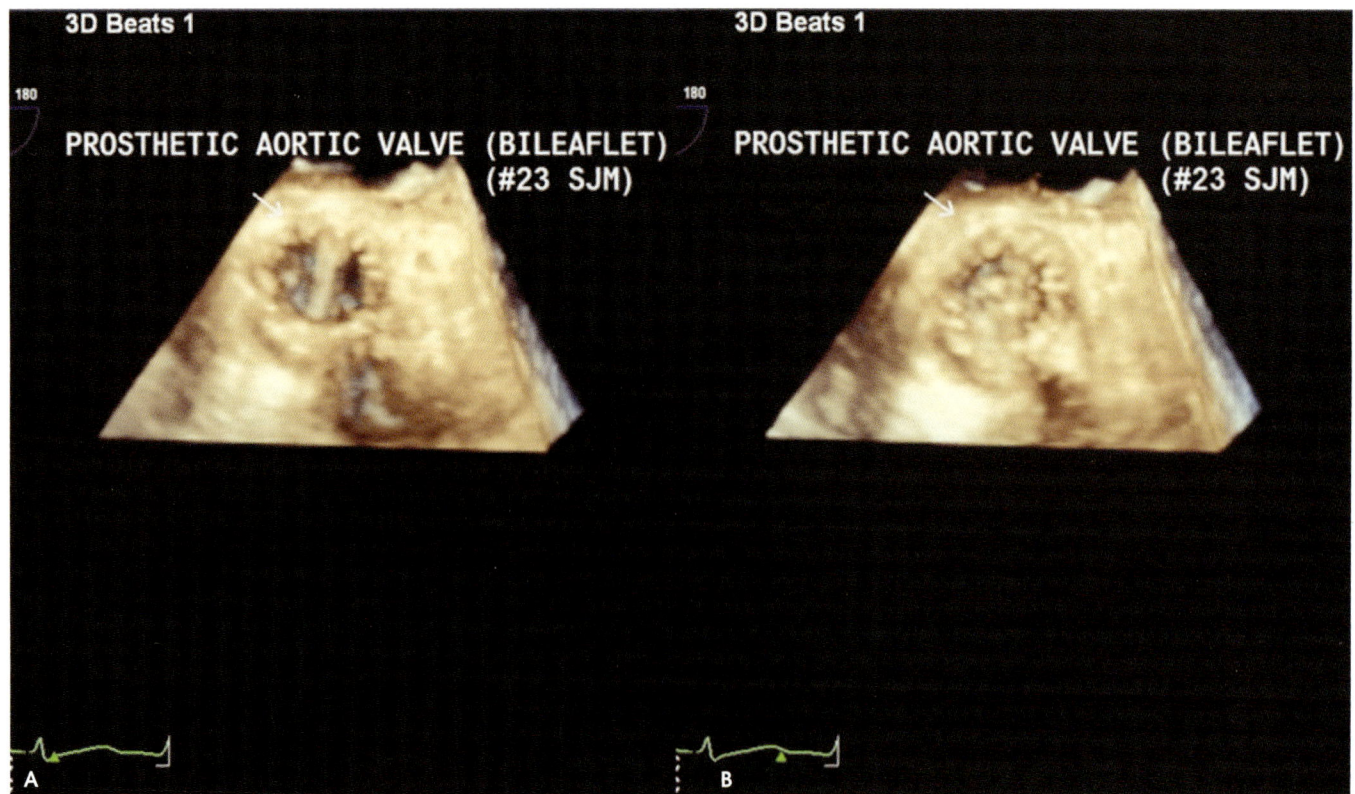

Fig. 14.14: Three-dimensioanl view of a prosthetic aortic valve in short-axis at end-systole (A) and end-diastole (B).

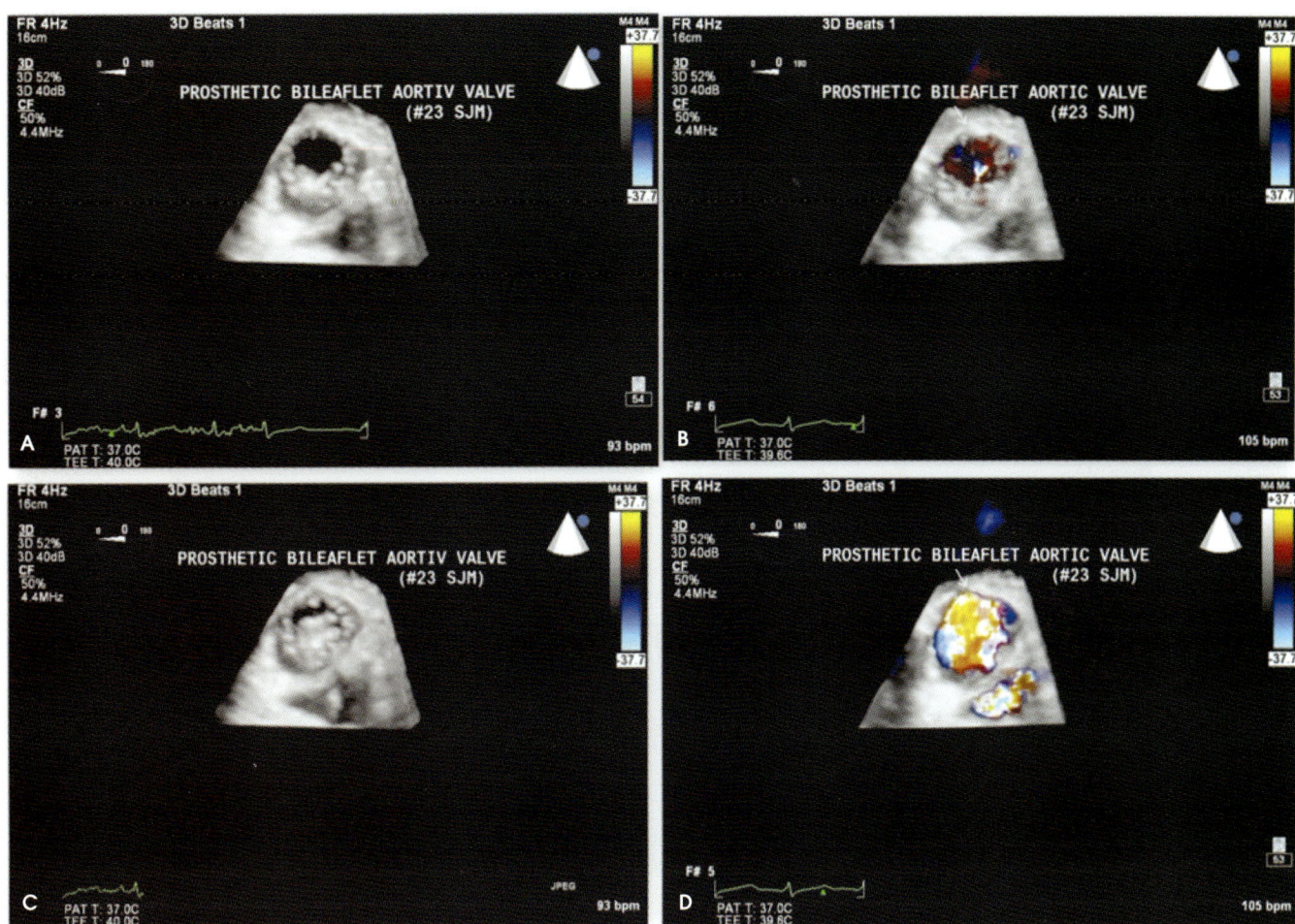

Fig. 14.15: Three-dimensional color Doppler view (along with corresponding color suppressed view) of a prosthetic aortic valve in short-axis at end-systole (A, B) and end-diastole (C, D). Turbulence caused by regurgitant washing jets can be appreciated in D.

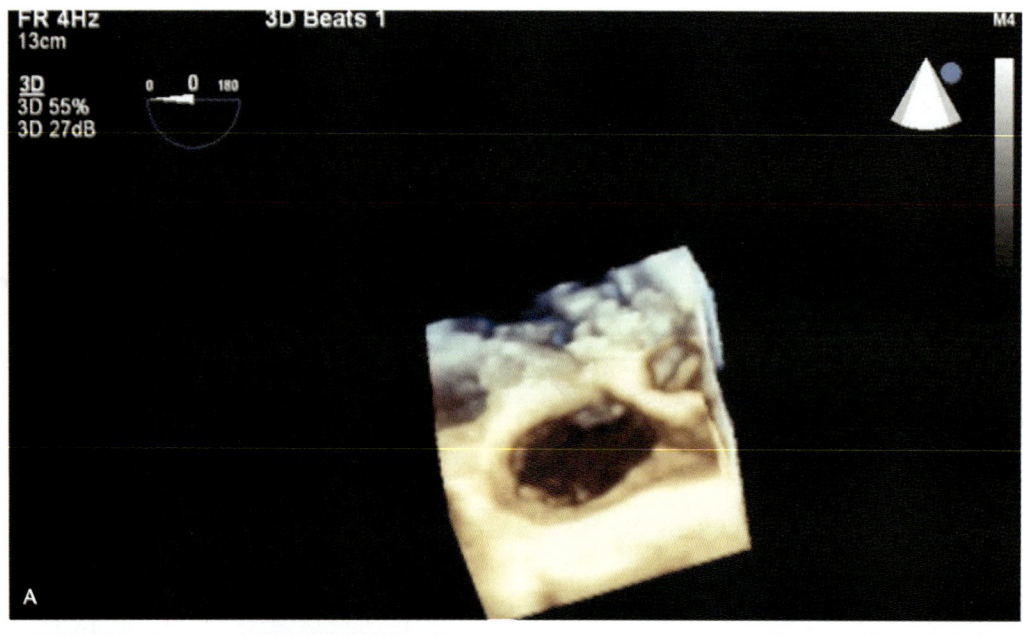

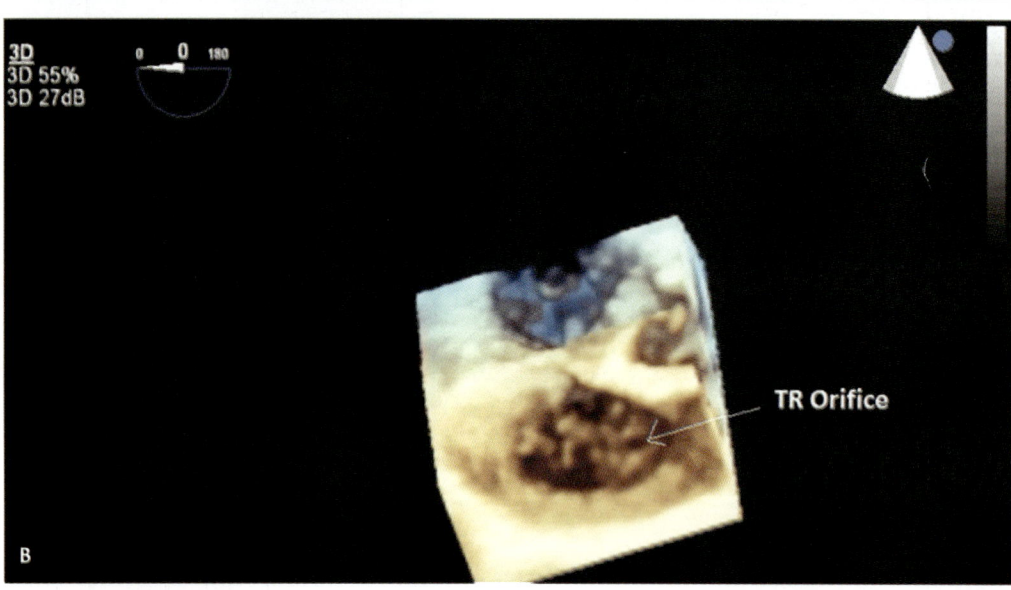

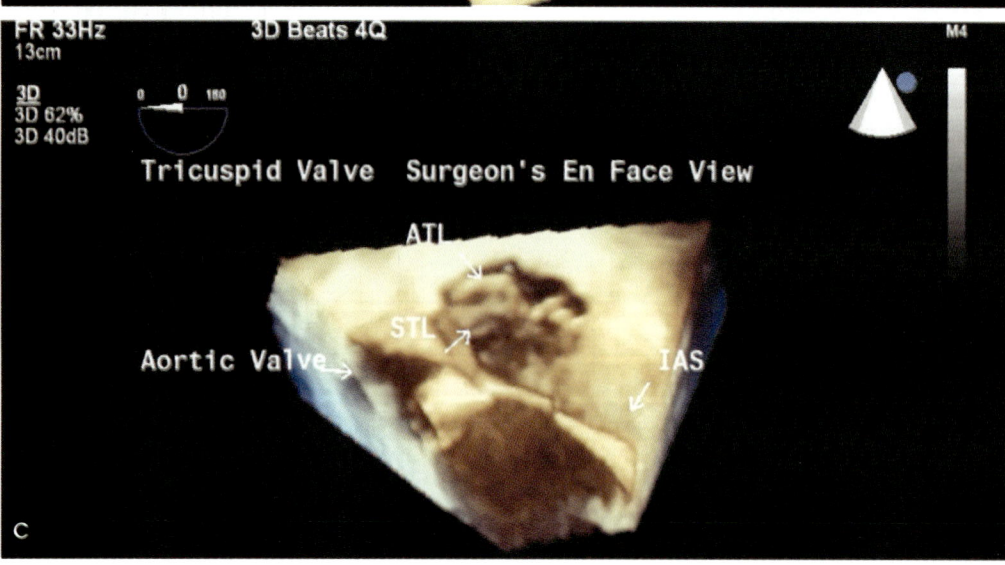

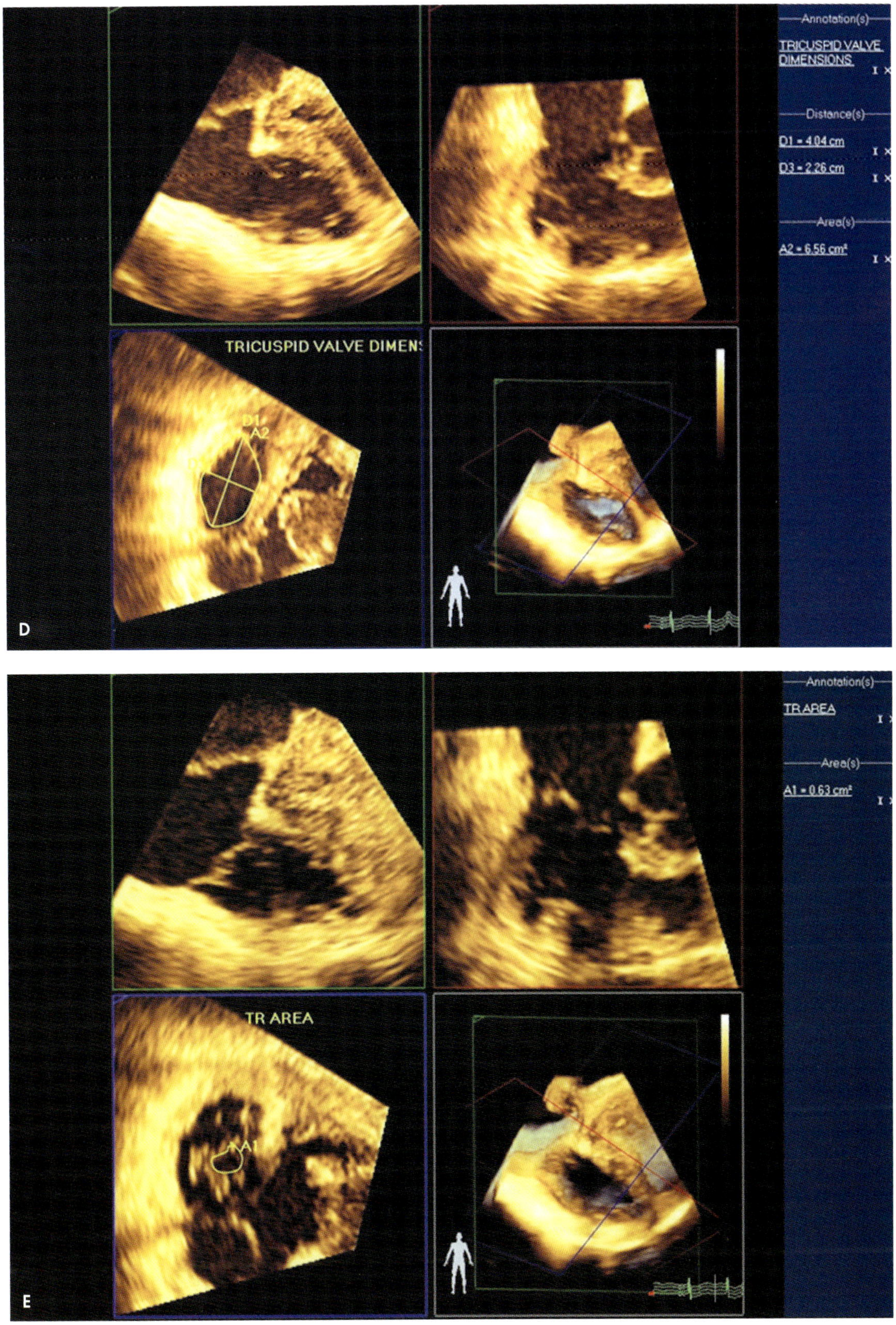

Fig. 14.16A to E: Three-dimensional (3-D) view of the tricuspid valve in open (A) and closed position (B) in a patient with severe mitral stenosis and tricuspid regurgitation (TR). The regurgitant orifice is visible with the tricuspid valve in closed position (B). (C) 3-D tricuspid valve en-face view. (D and E) 3-D reconstructed view of the tricuspid valve showing the annular dimension (D), and TR effective orifice area (E). (ATL: anterior tricuspid leaflet, STL: septal tricuspid leaflet, IAS: interatrial septum).

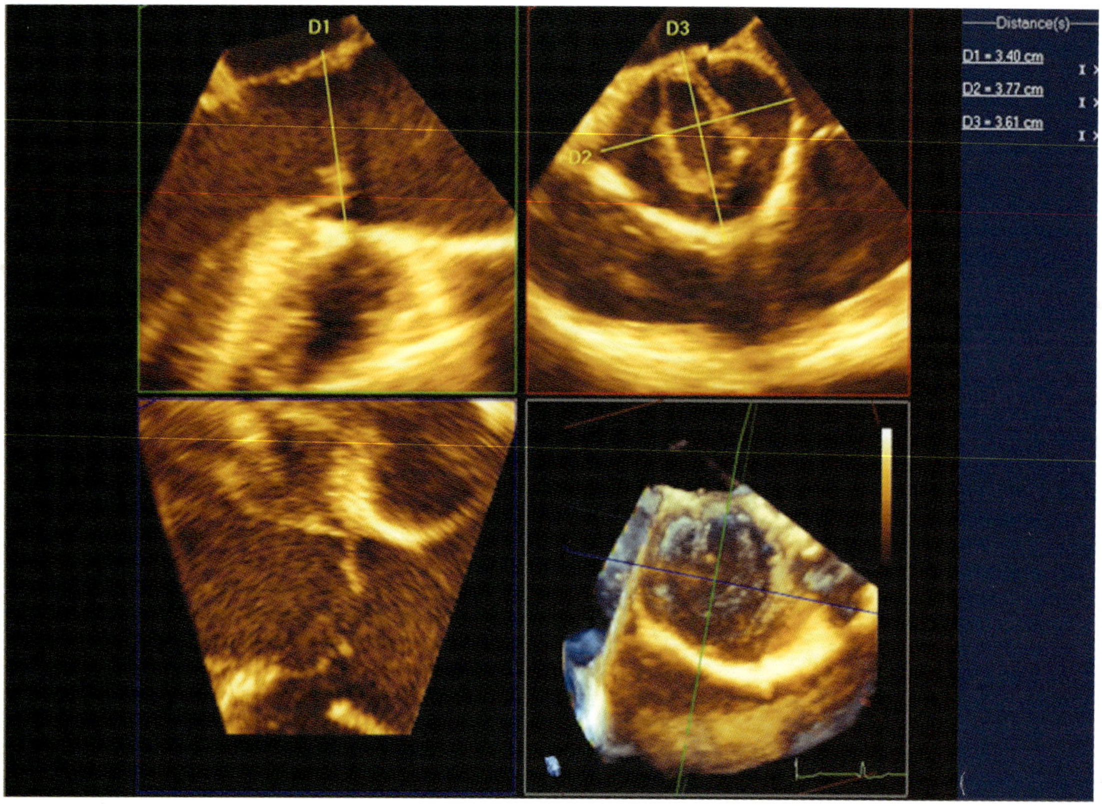

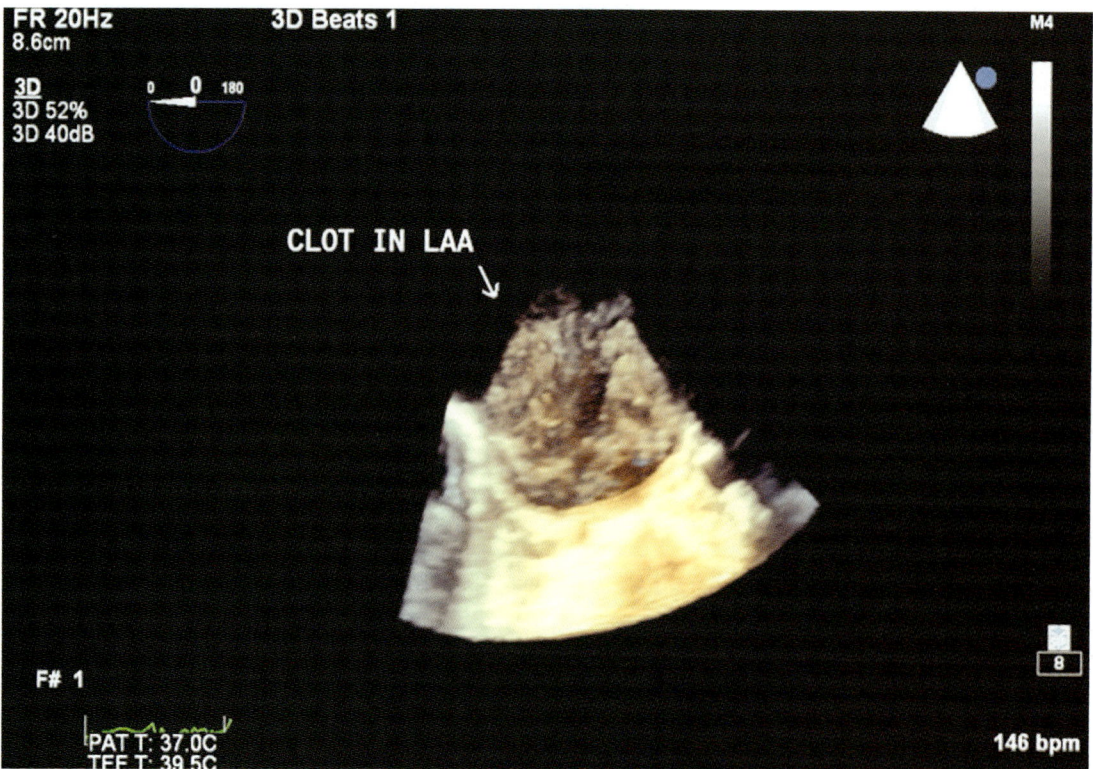

Fig. 14.17: Three-dimensional reconstructed view of the aortic valve at end-systole in a patient with an ascending aortic aneurysm. The aortic annulus measured 3.7 cm (D2) × 3.6 cm (D3).

Fig. 14.18: Three-dimensional view of an organized clot in the left atrial appendage (LAA) in a patient with severe mitral stenosis.

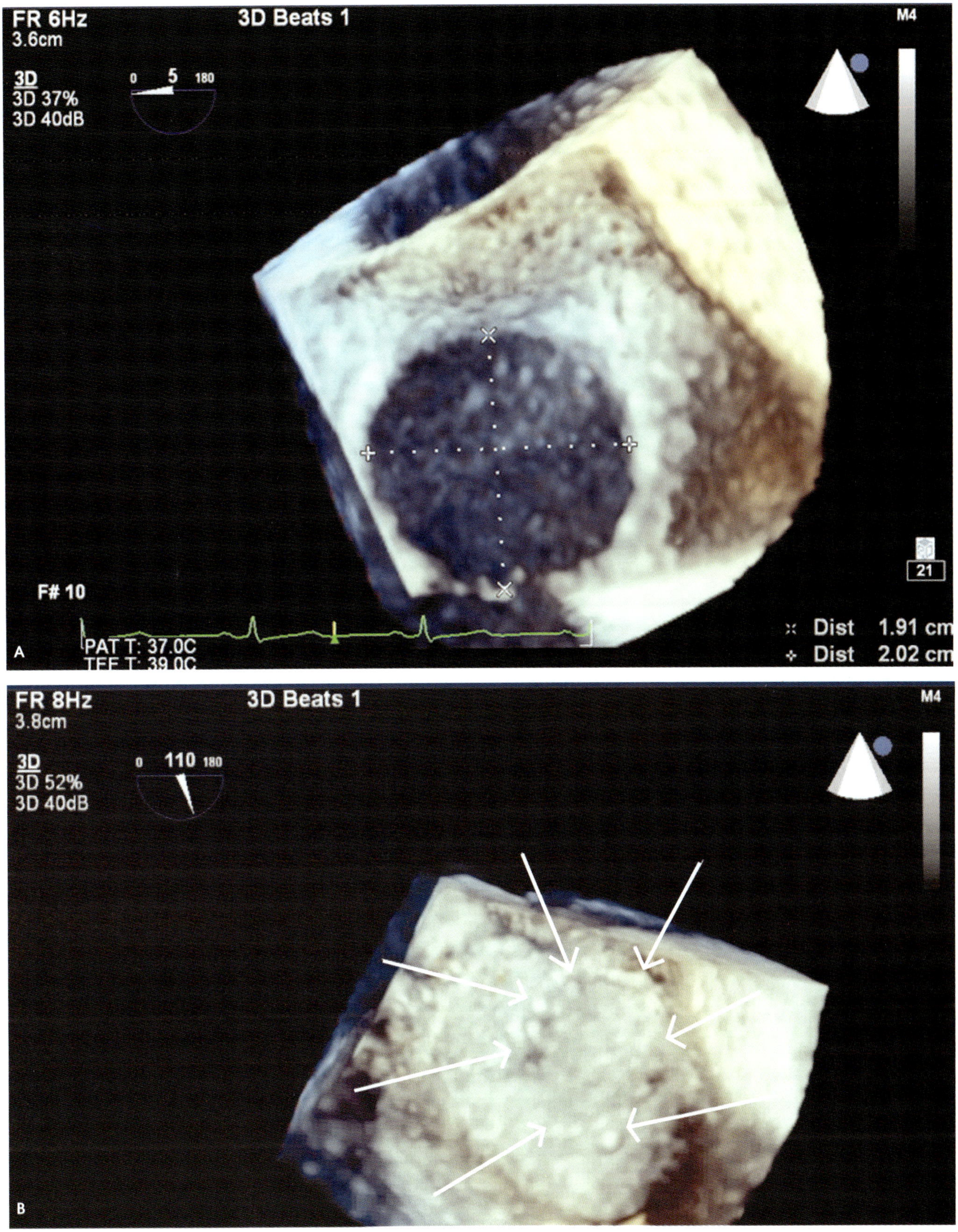

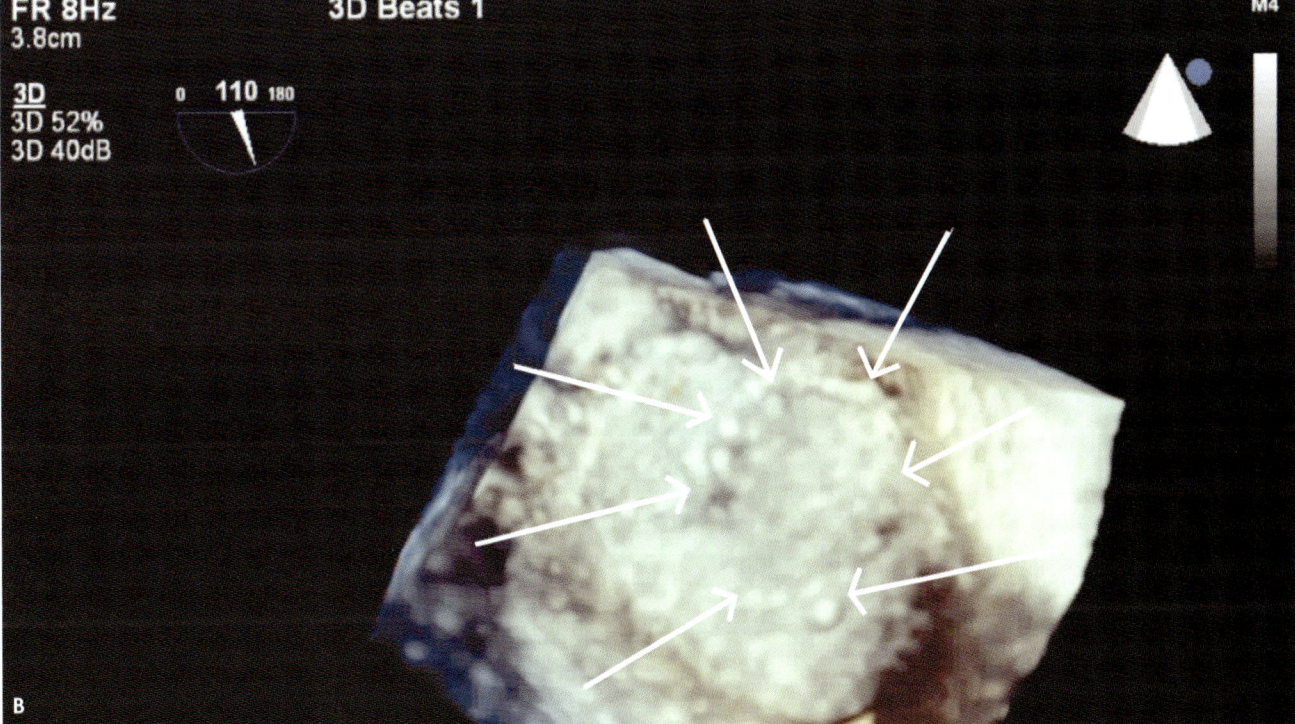

Fig. 14.19: Three-dimensional atrial view of a secundum atrial septal defect before (A) and after patch closure (B) with arrows showing the sutures of patch repair.

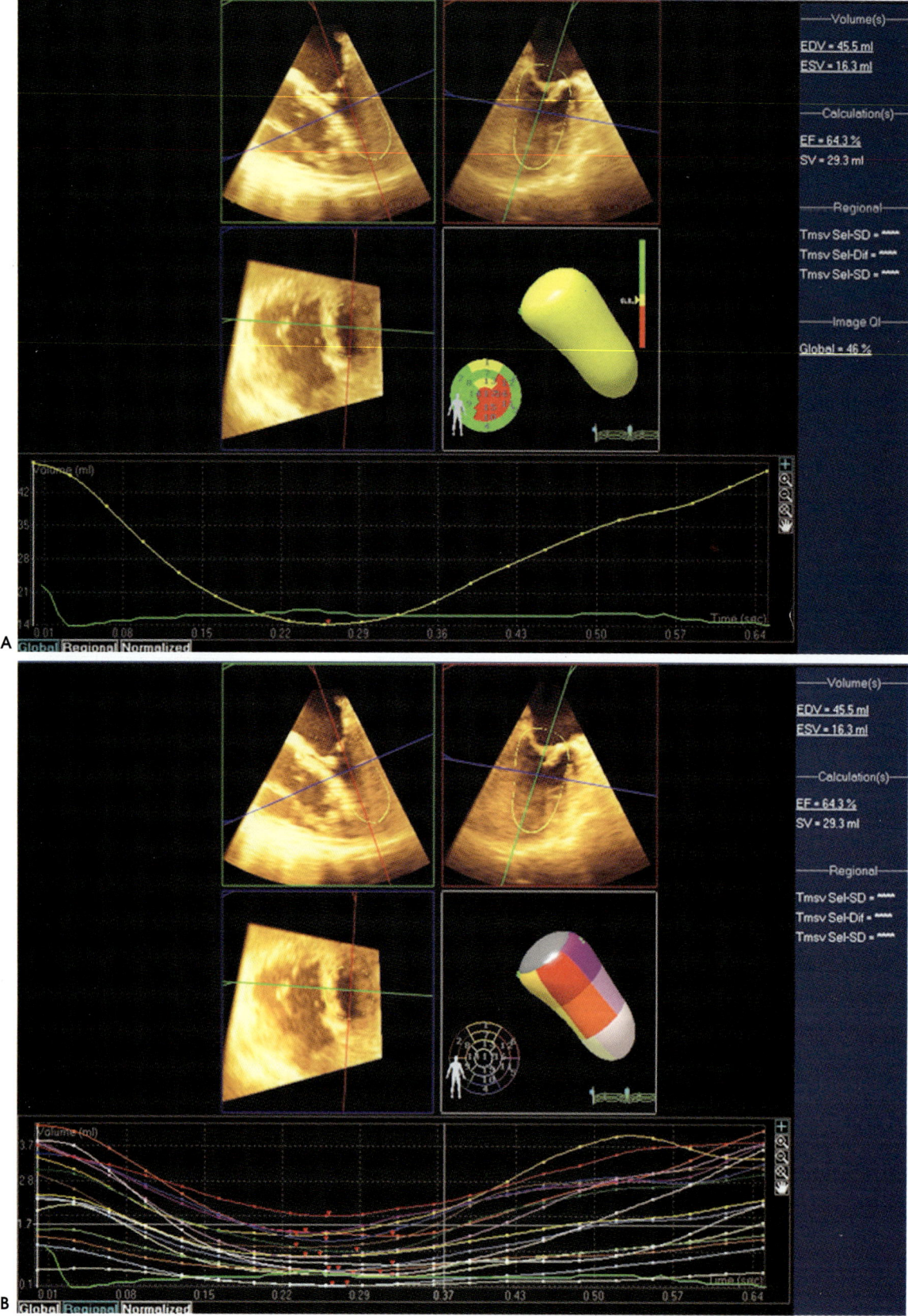

Fig. 14.20A and B: Three-dimensional global (A) and regional (B) volumetric measurement of the left ventricle constructed from images in different orthogonal planes (*x, y, z* shown in *red, green, blue*). The end-diastolic volume is 45.5 ml, end-systolic volume is 16.3 ml, stroke volume is 29.3 ml, and ejection fraction is 64.3%.

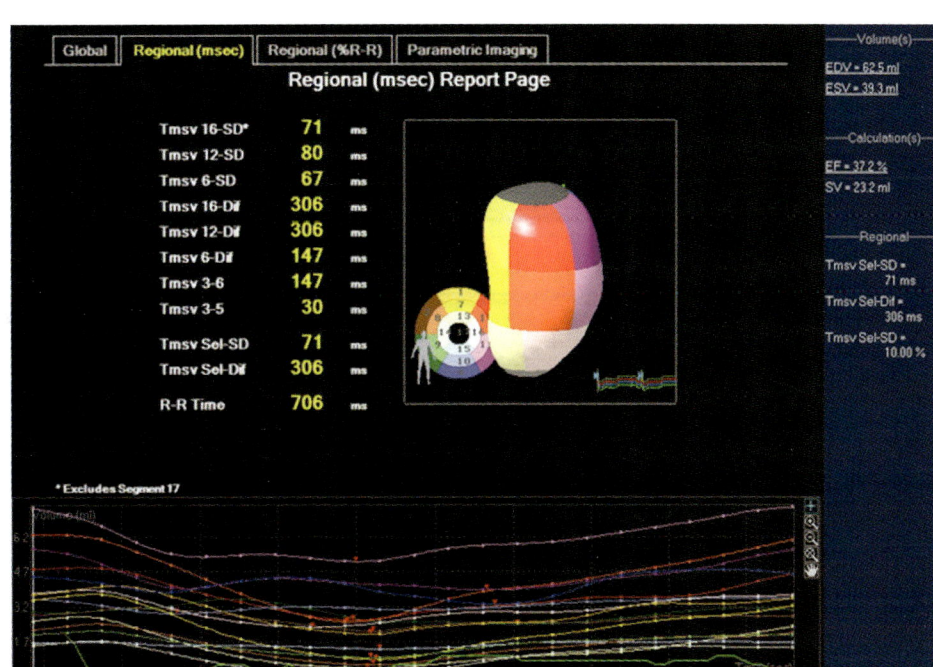

Fig. 14.21: Three-dimensional (3-D) echocardiographic analysis of left ventricular dyssynchrony in a patient with coronary artery disease. The 3-D model in the white box shows the color coded 16-segment analysis of left ventricle according to the American Heart Association/ American Society of Echocardiography 17-segment volumetric model. The blue panel on the right side gives the values of end-diastolic volume (EDV), end-systolic volume (ESV), stroke volume (SV) and ejection fraction (EF = 37.2%). Tmsv i.e., time to reach minimum systolic volume for different segments is calculated and displayed. The color-coded volume-time curves display the contribution of individual segments to the global left ventricular volume throughout the cardiac cycle. This patient had dyssynchrony of basal inferior, basal inferolateral and mid-papillary inferolateral segments (nos. 4, 5 and 11) relative to the rest of the myocardium as reflected by the delayed time to achieve minimum left ventricular systolic volume.

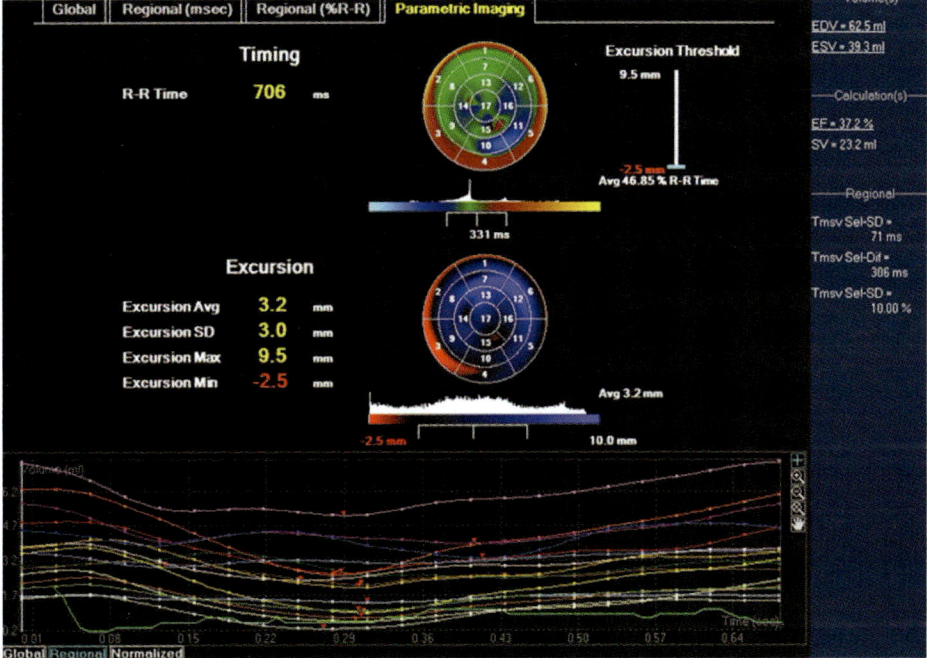

Fig. 14.22: Three-dimensional parametric imaging of left ventricle. The upper panel shows the timing of onset of contraction in individual segments (normal denoted as green, premature contraction denoted as blue, and delayed contraction as red). The middle panel shows excursion of individual segments towards the centre of the left ventricle (normal excursion displayed as blue, akinesis as black and dyskinesis as red). This patient had delayed onset of contraction and dyskinesis of the basal inferoseptal and inferior segments (nos. 3 & 4). Color brightness denotes the extent of the movement. The color-coded volume-time curves (already explained in the previous image) help corroborate the above findings.

Index

Acoustic shadows 205
Air bubble 165, 195
Aliasing 21
Aneurysm of the interatrial septum 157
Aorta 197
Aortic dissection 200
Aortic homograft 224
Aortic regurgitation 88, 90, 91, 94, 95, 174, 225, 281
Aortic root abscess 204
Aortic stenosis 80, 84, 87
  continuity equation 80
  jet velocity 80
  planimetry 80
  pressure gradient 80
  proximal isovelocity surface area (PISA) 80
Aortic valve 74
  anatomy 74
  sinuses of valsalva 74
Aortic valve area 78
  planimetry 78, 80
Aortic valve long-axis view 247
Aortic valve prosthesis 220, 226
Artifacts 17
  acoustic shadowing 147
  aliasing 152
  comet tail 149
  dissection flap 150, 151
  ghosting 153
  Nyquist limit 152
  reverberation artifact 149
  shadowing 153
  side-lobe artifact 150
Ascending aorta 197
Atheromas 197
Atheromatous plaque 148, 202
Atrial septal defect 233, 235, 239, 240
Atrio-ventricular septal defect 252

Basal transgastric view 34
Bernoulli equation 48
Biatrial myxoma 187
Bicaval view 29, 33
Bicuspid aortic valve 83, 172
Bifid papillary muscle 162
Bileaflet mitral valve prosthesis 207

Bileaflet prosthesis 214
Bioprosthetic valve 210
Bjork-Shiley tilting disc valve 208, 213, 220

Calcification 205
Cardiac output 128
Catheters and wires 158
Chiari network 155, 270
Color flow doppler 6
Color M-mode 144
Comprehensive transesophageal echocardiography 22, 23
Concentric left ventricular hypertrophy 84
Congenital heart disease 230
Congenitally corrected transposition of great arteries 263
Continuity equation 53, 80 (also see aortic stenosis)
Continuous wave Doppler 5, 21, 62, 72, 87, 88
Coronary artery disease 122
Coronary sinus 157
Coumadin ridge 161
Crista terminalis 154

Deceleration time 53
Deep transgastiric view 99
Deep transgastric long-axis view 36, 79, 88, 95
Deep transgastric RV apical view 101
Deep transgastric view 20, 128
Diastolic dysfunction 139–142
Diastolic function 137
Dilated right ventricle 121
Doppler echocardiography 3
  continuous wave Doppler 4
  Doppler equation 3
  Doppler shift 3
  pulsed wave Doppler 4
Double chamber right ventricle 269
dP/dt 129

Ebstein's anomaly 265–267
Eccentric jet 71
Echocardiography
  far zone 17
  frame rate 8
  principles 1

Ejection fraction 122, 127
End-diastolic area 125
End-systolic area 125
Enlarged coronary sinus 157
Eustachian valve 154
Evaluation of the aortic valve 74
Evaluation of the mitral valve 47

Four-chamber view 209
Fractional area change 122, 125
Fractional shortening 122, 124

Gerbode defect 238
Global RV function 101

Hepatic vein view 45
Hepatic venous flow 107, 108
Holodiastolic flow reversal 95

Image optimization 7
  color gain 8
  color scale 8
  depth 8, 14
  focus 8
  gain 8, 11, 12
  lateral gain control 8
  time gain compensation 8
Infective endocarditis 166
Inlet ventricular septal defect 245
Inoue balloon 66
Intracardiac masses 175
Inverted left atrial appendage 160
Isovolumetric relaxation time (IVRT) 143, 145
Isovolumic contraction time 145

Lambl's excrescences 162
Lateral gain control 17
Lateral mitral annulus 145
Left atrial appendage thrombus 190
Left atrial membrane 161
Left atrial thrombus 56, 58, 59, 188–189
Left atrial myxoma 177–185
Left to right shunt 239
Left ventricle 134, 286, 287
  anterior and inferior walls 134
  antero-septal and infero-lateral walls 135
  infero-septal wall 134

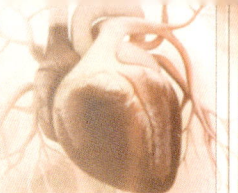

Left ventricular end-diastolic volume 126, 127
Left ventricular function 122
Left ventricular outflow tract 128
Left ventricular segments 133
  apical segments 136
  basal segments 135
  mid segments 136
  transgastric midpapillary short-axis view 136
Left ventricular thrombus 176
Left-to-right shunt 235, 237
Left-ventricular internal diameter 124
Lipomatous hypertrophy of the interatrial septum 156
Lower esophageal coronary sinus view 46

M mode 130
Mal-alignment of the aorta 256
Manipulation of the probe 23
Marfan's syndrome 91
Matrix array transducer 271
Midesophageal descending aortic long-axis view 39
Midesophageal 2-chamber view 23, 27, 28, 50, 70, 127, 134, 153, 157, 159, 160, 180
Midesophageal 4-chamber view 9, 23, 26, 54, 55, 64, 84, 96, 97, 102, 126, 134, 147, 153, 155–156, 160, 161, 187, 206, 207–209–212, 216, 235–238, 243–245, 247, 251, 253, 266, 267
Midesophageal 5-chamber view 40, 75, 173
Midesophageal aortic valve long-axis view 29, 32, 78, 85, 148, 150, 162, 167, 168, 174, 185, 209, 223, 227, 228, 242, 248, 254–256
Midesophageal aortic valve short-axis view 12, 29, 30, 76, 78, 82, 87, 92, 204, 220, 222, 224, 226, 227
Midesophageal ascending aorta long-axis view 197, 201
Midesophageal ascending aorta short axis view 37, 38, 111, 164, 198, 259
Midesophageal bicaval view 57, 155, 239–241
Midesophageal commissural view 23, 49
Midesophageal descending aorta long-axis view 199
Midesophageal descending aorta short-axis view 38, 148, 150, 198, 202
  aliasing 152
  comet tail 149
  dissection flap 150, 151
  ghosting 153
  midesophageal aortic valve long-axis view 150

midesophageal descending aorta short-axis view 150
  nyquist limit 152
  reverberation artifact 149
  shadowing 153
  side-lobe artifact 150
Midesophageal left atrial appendage view 45
Midesophageal long-axis view 23, 28, 50, 63, 100, 135, 158, 203, 250, 268
Midesophageal mitral commissural view 27
Midesophageal modified bicaval view 41
Midesophageal right ventricular inflow-outflow view 29, 31, 97, 115, 158, 163
Mid-papilary short-axis view 34
Mitral annular plane systolic excursion (MAPSE) 130
Mitral annular systolic velocity 132
Mitral regurgitation 68–72, 215
Mitral stenosis 57, 59, 189–190
Mitral subvalvular apparatus 52
Mitral valve 47
  anatomy 47
  carpentier nomenclature 47
  midesophageal commissural view 47
  midesophageal four-chamber view 47
  midesophageal long-axis view 47
  midesophageal two-chamber view 47
  transgastric basal short-axis view 47
  transgastric two-chamber view 47
Mitral valve prosthesis 206
Mitral valve quantification 277
M-mode 3, 124
Mobile vegetations 219
Moderator band 96, 161
Modified bicaval view 109, 112
Mullin's sheath 64, 66
Muscular ventricular septal defect 243, 248, 249
Mycotic aneurysm 88
Myocardial performance index 130, 131

Nyquist limit 4
  color Doppler 4
  spectral Doppler 4

Oblique sinus 164
Ostium primum atrial septal defect 238, 253
Ostium secundum atrial septal defect 230–234, 236, 237
Outlet ventricular septal defect 250
Over-riding aorta 255

Pannus 205, 211
Paravalvular defect 226
Paravalvular leak 224, 227, 229, 279

Patent foramen ovale 241
Pectinate muscle 159
Percutaneous balloon mitral valvuloplasty 64
Perimembranous ventricular septal defect 242–244, 247
Persistent left superior vena cava 164
Pitfalls 154
  chiari network 155
  coumadin ridge 161
  crista terminalis 154
  eustachian valve 154
  inverted left atrial appendage 160
  left atrial membrane 161
  lipomatous hypertrophy of the interatrial septum 156
  midesophageal four-chamber view 160
  midesophageal two-chamber view 159, 160
  moderator band 161
  pectinate muscle 159
  thebesian valve 156
  warfarin (Coumadin) ridge 159
Planimetry 48, 87
Pressure half time 48, 61
Probe insertion 22
Propagation velocity 144
Prosthesis-patient mismatch 205
Prosthetic aortic valve 222
Prosthetic mitral valve 278, 279
Prosthetic valve dysfunction 213
Prosthetic valve function 205
  degeneration 205
  dehiscence 205
Prosthetic valve stenosis 212
Prosthetic valve thrombosis 215
Proximal isovelocity surface area (PISA) 53, 63, 64, 70, 85 (*see* also aortic stenosis)
Pulmonary artery catheter 196
Pulmonary stenosis 259
Pulmonary thrombus 176
Pulmonary valve 96, 120
Pulmonary valve stenosis 120, 260
Pulmonary venous flow velocity 73
Pulmonary venous waveform 141
Pulse repetition frequency 8
Pulsed wave Doppler 5, 6, 79

Rate of rise of intraventricular pressure (dP/dt) 72, 129
Regional wall motion abnormality 133
Regurgitant jet 92
Regurgitant orifice 89
Right atrial myxoma 185–186
Right atrial thrombus 191

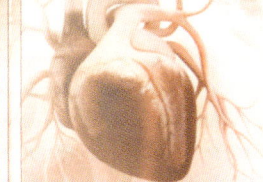

Right coronary cusp 93
Right pulmonary vein view 42
Right ventricle 96, 97
  crista supraventricularis 96
  diastolic function 105
    hepatic venous flow pattern 105
    RA pressure 105
  dilatation 101
  hypertrophy 101
  moderator band 96
  systolic function 104
    automated border detection 104
    fractional area change 104
    myocardial performance index 104
    RV dP/dt 104
    TEI index 104
    tissue Doppler 104
    tricuspid annular plane systolic
      excursion 104
Right ventricular inflow-outflow view 103,
  247
Right ventricular outflow tract 100, 119
Right ventricular systolic pressure 105
Ruptured sinus of Valsalva 261

Sector width 8
Secundum atrial septal defect 285
Severe mitral regurgitation 68
Severe mitral stenosis 58, 60–63
Simpson's rule 126, 127
Sinus venosus 239, 240
Spontaneous echo contrast 57, 113, 189,
  214
Spontaneous left atrial contrast 56
St. Jude bileaflet prosthesis 221
St. Jude prosthesis 209
St. Jude valve 212
Standard views 25
  deep TG LAX view (t) 25
  descending aorta LAX view (t) 25
  descending aorta SAX view (t) 25
  lower esophageal coronary sinus view
    (t) 25
  lower esophageal hepatic view (t) 25
  midesophageal 5-chamber view (t) 25
  midesophageal ascending aorta LAX
    view (t) 25
  midesophageal ascending aorta SAX
    view (t) 25
  midesophageal AV LAX view (t) 25
  midesophageal AV SAX view (t) 25
  midesophageal bicaval view (t) 25
  midesophageal four-chamber view (t) 25
  midesophageal left atrial appendage
    view (t) 25

  midesophageal LV LAX view (t) 25
  midesophageal mitral commissural view
    (t) 25
  midesophageal modified bicaval view (t)
    25
  midesophageal right pulmonary vein
    view (t) 25
  midesophageal RV inflow-outflow view
    (t) 25
  midesophageal two-chamber view (t) 25
  transgastric apical SAX view (t) 25
  transgastric basal SAX view (t) 25
  transgastric LAX view (t) 25
  transgastric midpapillary SAX view (t) 25
  transgastric RV basal view (t) 25
  transgastric RV inflow view (t) 25
  transgastric RV inflow-outflow view (t) 25
  transgastric two-chamber view (t) 25
  upper esophageal aortic arch LAX view
    (t) 25
  upper esophageal aortic arch SAX view
    (t) 25
  upper esophageal right and left
    pulmonary vein view (t) 25
Starr Edward prosthesis 218
Stenosed aortic valve 81
Stroke volume 122, 128
Stuck mitral valve prosthesis 213
Subaortic membrane 85, 268
Subaortic ventricular septal defect 254, 255
Sub-pulmonary membrane 118
Systolic function 122

Technique of TEE examination 22
TEI index 104
Temporal resolution 3
Tetralogy of Fallot 254, 256, 257, 259
Thebesian valve 156
Thickened aortic leaflets 82
Three-dimensional view of a prosthetic
  aortic valve 280
Three-dimensional atrial view 274, 278,
  285
Three-dimensional atrial view of the mitral
  valve 276
Three-dimensional atrial view of tricuspid
  valve 276
Three-dimensional color Doppler view 281
Three-dimensional echocardiography 271
Three-dimensional en-face view of the
  mitral valve 275
Three-dimensional midesophageal aortic
  valve short-axis view 272
Three-dimensional midesophageal right
  ventricular inflow-outflow view 272
Three-dimensional reconstructed view
  278, 279

Three-dimensional reconstructed view of
  the aortic valve 280, 284
Three-dimensional view of an organized
  clot 284
Three-dimensional view of the tricuspid
  valve 283
Three-dimensional volumetric
  measurement 286
Thrombosis 205
Thrombus 175, 213, 214
Tilting disc prosthesis 217
Tilting disc valve 208
Time gain compensation 15, 16
Tissue Doppler 104, 132, 145
Tissue Doppler imaging 144
Tissue valve 216
Transducer frequency 7
Transgastric apical short-axis view 45
Transgastric basal short-axis view 34, 51,
  135
Transgastric long-axis view 34, 79, 80, 143
Transgastric mid-papillary short axis view
  16, 34, 98, 123, 125, 137, 162
Transgastric right ventricular basal view 44
Transgastric right ventricular inflow view
  36, 99
Transgastric right ventricular inflow-outflow
  view 44
Transgastric RV inflow-outflow view 101
Transgastric RV-inflow view 36, 37
Transgastric short-axis view 84, 175
Transgastric two-chamber view 34, 52
Transgastric view 34, 121
Transmitral flow 53
Transmitral pulsed wave Doppler 138, 142
Transposition of great arteries 262
Transverse sinus 163
Tricuspid inflow pattern 107
Tricuspid regurgitation 109, 112–115, 117
Tricuspid valve 116–117
Triuspid annular plane systolic
  excursion 106
Truncus arteriosus 264
Tumour 175
Two-dimensional imaging 3
  B-mode 3

Ultrasound
  acoustic impedance 1
  contrast resolution 3
  physical properties 1
  spatial resolution 3
  temporal resolution 3
Unicuspid aortic valve 86
Upper esophageal aortic arch long-axis
  view 39

Upper esophageal aortic arch short-axis view 40, 192

Upper esophageal left pulmonary vein view 43

Upper esophageal right pulmonary vein view 43

Valve endocarditis 166

Velocity time integral 123

Vegetation 93, 166–170, 174, 205, 217, 218, 223

Venous cannula 193–194

Ventricular dysfunction 122

Ventricular dyssynchrony 287

Ventricular septal defect 246, 254, 256

VSD patch 251

Warfarin (Coumadin) ridge 159